Raman Spectroscopy
in Human Health and Biomedicine

Other Titles by Jürgen Popp

Handbook of Biophotonics (in 3 volumes)

Optical Nano- and Microsystems for Bioanalytics

Challenges in Molecular Structure Determination

Ex-vivo and In-vivo Optical Molecular Pathology

Modern Techniques for Pathogen Detection

Molecular Spectroscopy: A Quantum Chemistry Approach

Micro-Raman Spectroscopy: Theory and Application

Multimodal Optical Diagnostics of Cancer

Other Titles by Bayden R Wood

Vibrational Spectroscopy in Protein Research: From Purified Proteins to Aggregates and Assemblies

Other Titles by Yukihiro Ozaki

Raman, Infrared, and Near-Infrared Chemical Imaging

Frontiers of Surface-Enhanced Raman Scattering: Single Nanoparticles and Single Cells

Far- and Deep-Ultraviolet Spectroscopy

Molecular and Laser Spectroscopy: Advances and Applications (Volume 2)

Frontiers of Quantum Chemistry

Recent Developments in Plasmon-Supported Raman Spectroscopy: 45 Years of Enhanced Raman Signals

Molecular Spectroscopy: A Quantum Chemistry Approach

Vibrational Spectroscopy in Protein Research: From Purified Proteins to Aggregates and Assemblies

Near-Infrared Spectroscopy: Theory, Spectral Analysis, Instrumentation, and Applications

Spectroscopic Techniques for Polymer Characterization: Methods, Instrumentation, Applications

Spectroscopy and Computation of Hydrogen-Bonded Systems

Raman Spectroscopy
in Human Health and Biomedicine

Edited by

Hidetoshi Sato
Kwansei Gakuin University, Japan

Jürgen Popp
Friedrich-Schiller University Jena, Germany

Bayden R Wood
Monash University, Australia

Yukihiro Ozaki
Kwansei Gakuin University, Japan

World Scientific

NEW JERSEY • LONDON • SINGAPORE • BEIJING • SHANGHAI • HONG KONG • TAIPEI • CHENNAI • TOKYO

Published by

World Scientific Publishing Co. Pte. Ltd.
5 Toh Tuck Link, Singapore 596224
USA office: 27 Warren Street, Suite 401-402, Hackensack, NJ 07601
UK office: 57 Shelton Street, Covent Garden, London WC2H 9HE

Library of Congress Cataloging-in-Publication Data
Names: Sato, Hidetoshi, editor. | Popp, Jürgen, editor. | Wood, Bayden R., editor. | Ozaki, Y. (Yukihiro), editor.
Title: Raman spectroscopy in human health and biomedicine / edited by Hidetoshi Sato, Jürgen Popp, Bayden R Wood, Yukihiro Ozaki.
Description: New Jersey : World Scientific, [2024] | Includes bibliographical references and index.
Identifiers: LCCN 2023013424 | ISBN 9789811264603 (hardcover) | ISBN 9789811264610 (ebook for institutions) | ISBN 9789811264627 (ebook for individuals)
Subjects: MESH: Spectrum Analysis, Raman | Chemistry Techniques, Analytical
Classification: LCC RC270.3.D53 | NLM QY 90 | DDC 616.07/57--dc23/eng/20230720
LC record available at https://lccn.loc.gov/2023013424

British Library Cataloguing-in-Publication Data
A catalogue record for this book is available from the British Library.

For any available supplementary material, please visit
https://www.worldscientific.com/worldscibooks/10.1142/13094#t=suppl

Desk Editor: Shaun Tan Yi Jie

Typeset by Stallion Press
Email: enquiries@stallionpress.com

https://doi.org/10.1142/9789811264610_fmatter

Preface

About 50 years have passed since medical applications of Raman spectroscopy were born. In the first 20 years or so the development of Raman application to medical science was rather slow mainly due to the problems of fluorescence. Recently, applications of Raman spectroscopy to health and biomedical sciences have demonstrated remarkable progress in many aspects due to the rapid development of new Raman techniques, instruments, and spectral analysis methods. Many Raman spectroscopy methods such as SERS, TERS, and CARS, including their imaging equivalents, have all made significant advances. You can find the evolution of these spectroscopies and spectral analysis methods in detail in this book. This book has two unique attributes: one is that it treats applications to health science, lipid research in connection to human health, food science and cosmetic science, and another is that it put some emphasis on Raman data analysis.

Currently, we cannot find a contemporary book on medical applications of Raman spectroscopy. For the application of Raman spectroscopy to health science it is almost impossible to find a book at all. This book consists of 17 chapters, starting from the review of the history of medical applications of Raman spectroscopy, followed by a few chapters on the data analysis of Raman spectra. Then, chapters that are concerned with applications to health science are provided. In the later half one can find Raman and CARS imaging chapters as well as chapters on biomedical applications, from infection diagnosis to cancer diagnostics.

We succeeded in inviting active frontrunners in applications of Raman spectroscopy to health and biomedical sciences from many countries. This book is useful for scientists, engineers, and graduate students in numerous areas of science and engineering. One can use this book as a text, for example, at a graduate school seminar. We hope that many readers can learn much about applications of Raman spectroscopy to health and biomedical sciences from this book, and that this book can inspire readers to utilize various kinds of Raman spectroscopies and spectral analysis methods for a variety of novel investigations.

Last but not least, we would like to thank Mr. Shaun Tan Yi Jie of World Scientific for his continuous efforts in publishing this exciting book.

Hidetoshi Sato,
Jürgen Popp,
Bayden R. Wood,
Yukihiro Ozaki

April 2023

https://doi.org/10.1142/9789811264610_fmatter

About the Editors

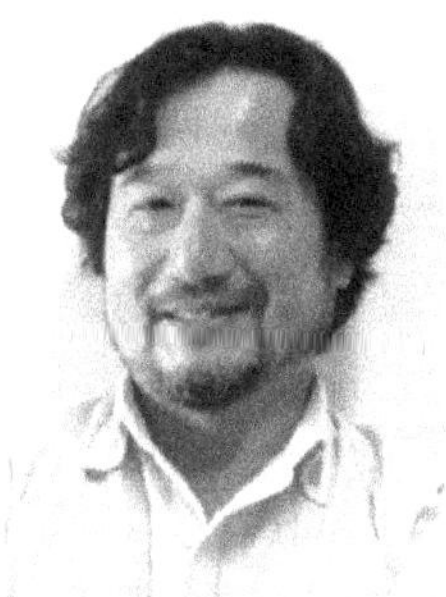

Professor Hidetoshi Sato is Professor at Kwansei Gakuin University, Japan. He was previously Research Unit Leader at RIKEN, Japan. His research focuses on the development of new instruments and analytical techniques of optical spectroscopy to explore mechanisms, dynamism and metabolism of live cells and tissues. He is a council member of The International Society for Clinical Spectroscopy (CLIRSPEC) and a member of the editorial committee of The Laser Society of Japan. He has published more than 60 peer-reviewed papers and 2 book chapters.

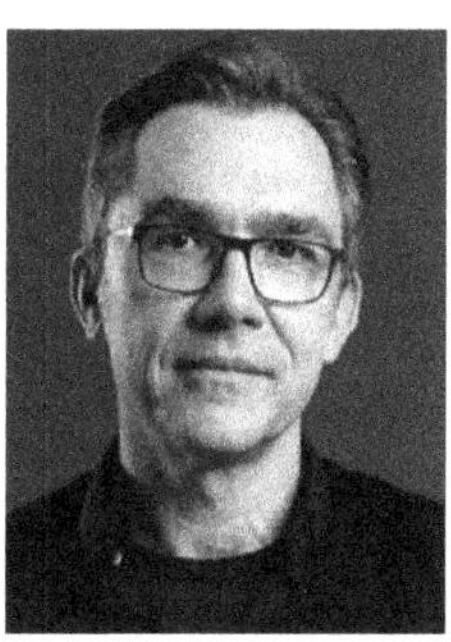

Professor Jürgen Popp FRSC is Chair Professor of Physical Chemistry at Friedrich-Schiller University Jena, Germany. He is also the Scientific Director of the Leibniz Institute of Photonic Technology, Germany. He is an Elected Fellow of the Royal Society of Chemistry, UK, and the American Institute for Medical and Biological Engineering, USA. He is Editor-in-Chief of the *Journal of Biophotonics*. Professor Popp is a world-leading expert in biophotonics/optical health technology covering the complete range from photonic basic research to translation into clinically applicable methods. He has published more than 960 journal papers, named as an inventor on 12 patents and given more than 200 invited talks on national and international conferences (among them more than 50 keynote/plenary lectures). He has received many prestigious accolades, including an honorary doctoral degree from Babeş-Bolyai University in 2012, the 2013 Robert Kellner Lecture Award, the 2016 Pittsburgh Spectroscopy Award, the 2018 Ioannes Marcus Marci Medal of the Czechoslovak Spectroscopy Society, the 2018 Kaiser Friedrich Research Prize, and the 2019 Ralf Dahrendorf Prize.

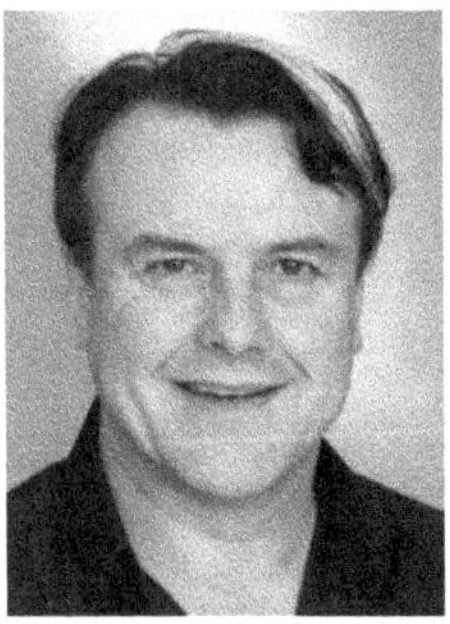

Professor Bayden R. Wood FRSC is Professor at Monash University, Australia, where he is also the Director for the Centre of Biospectroscopy. He is an Elected Fellow of the Royal Society of Chemistry, UK, and the Royal Australian Institute of Chemistry (RACI), Australia. He is Founder and Director of the International Society for Clinical Spectroscopy, and recipient of the 2014 RACI Doreen Clark Medal for Analytical and Environmental Chemistry. His research is focused on translating vibrational spectroscopic techniques to solve a range of biomedical and clinical research problems particularly associated with disease diagnosis. He has published over 180 papers, 11 book chapters and co-edited 1 book, with a h-index of 52.

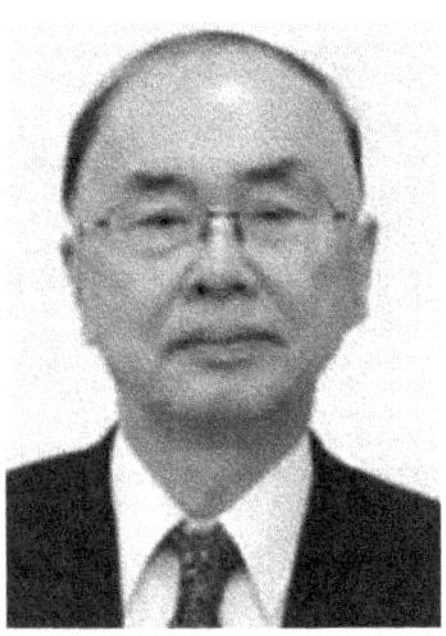

Professor Yukihiro Ozaki FRSC is Professor Emeritus at Kwansei Gakuin University, Japan, where he was previously Vice-President of the University. He is also Guest Professor at Kobe University, Japan; and Guest Scientist at RIKEN, Japan and Toyota Physical and Chemical Research Institute, Japan. He is an Elected Fellow of the Royal Society of Chemistry, UK, Society for Applied Spectroscopy, USA, Chemical Society of Japan, and International Council of Near-Infrared Spectroscopy.

Professor Ozaki has received many prestigious awards over the years, of which the most illustrious is the Medal of Honor bestowed by the Emperor of Japan in 2018. Others include the 2014 Bomem-Michelson Award, the 2017 Chemical Society of Japan Award, the 2019 Pittsburgh Spectroscopy Award, the 2020 Charles Mann Award of Applied Raman Spectroscopy, the 2021 Karl Norris Award, and the 2022 Ioannes Marcus Marci Medal. He has authored/edited 16 books and published more than 1,000 peer-reviewed papers, with a h-index of 84.

https://doi.org/10.1142/9789811264610_fmatter

About the Contributors

Chapter 2

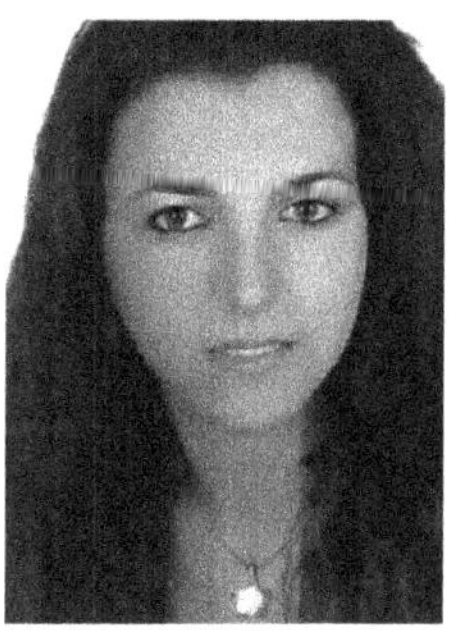

Dr. Rola Houhou is Post-Doctoral Researcher at the Photonic Data Science Department, Leibniz Institute of Photonic Technology, Germany. The principal focus of her research lies in the field of artificial intelligence (AI). More specifically, she is involved in investigating AI-driven solutions that have the potential to tackle some of the most complex problems in spectroscopy, including inverse and forward problems.

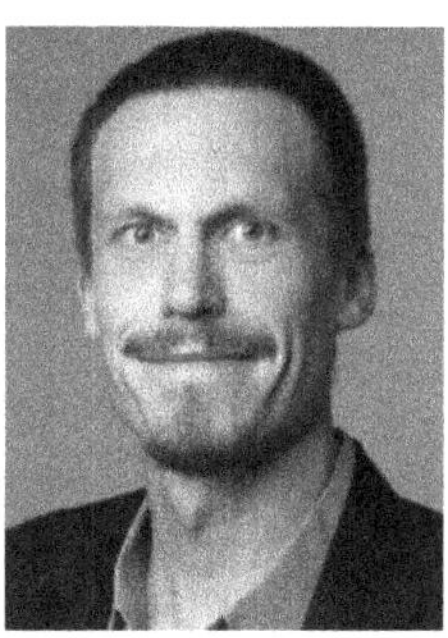

Professor Thomas Bocklitz is head of the UBT research group 'Artificial Intelligence in Spectroscopy and Microscopy' at the University of Bayreuth, and head of the IPHT 'Photonic Data Science' Department at the Leibniz Institute of Photonic Technology, Germany. His research is dedicated to exploring the entire life cycle of photonic data, including data generation, AI-based modeling and FAIR photonic data.

Chapter 3

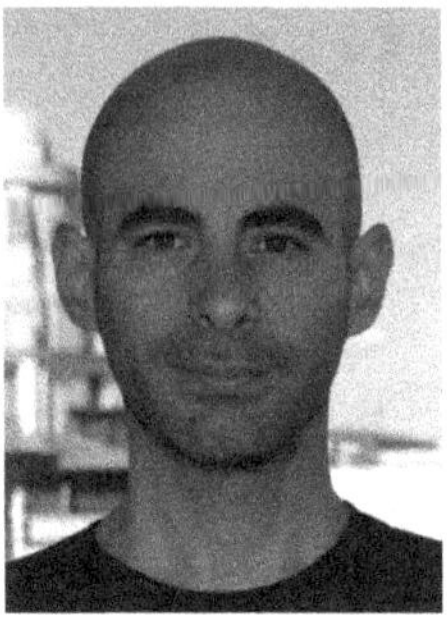

Dr. Ángel Sánchez-Illana is Post-Doctoral Researcher at the Department of Analytical Chemistry, University of Valencia, Spain. His current lines of research are using vibrational spectroscopy techniques and chemometric tools for the analysis of potentially bioactive lipids in novel oxidation and synthesis models, and development of point-of-care methods for the analysis of minimally invasive clinical samples.

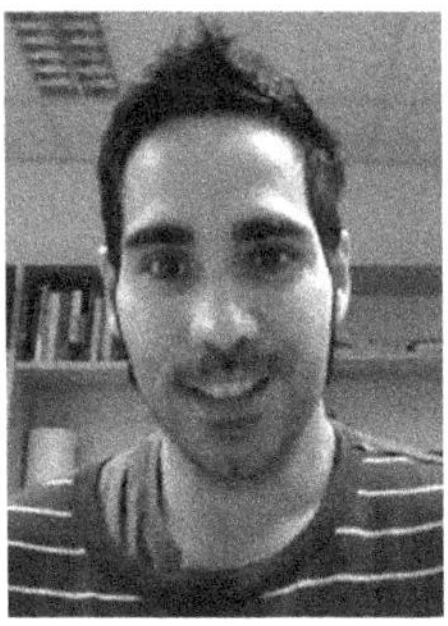

Dr. David Pérez-Guaita is a Ramon y Cajal researcher at the Department of Analytical Chemistry, University of Valencia, Spain. His research has focused on developing vibrational spectroscopic techniques to address a wide range of bioanalytical problems spanning the clinical and biological fields.

Chapter 4

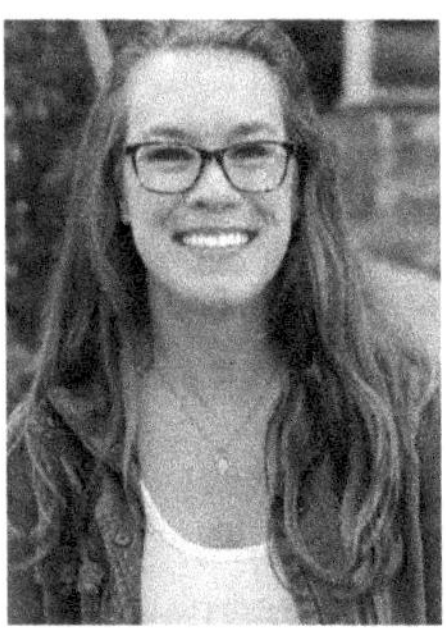

Dr. Nicole M. Ralbovsky is Senior Scientist at Merck, USA. She received two prestigious awards, the 2020 NY/NJ Society for Applied Spectroscopy's Graduate Student Award and the Eastern Analytical Symposium Graduate Student Research Award, for her PhD project which focuses on using surface-enhanced Raman spectroscopy for achieving single-molecule detection of DNA and RNA.

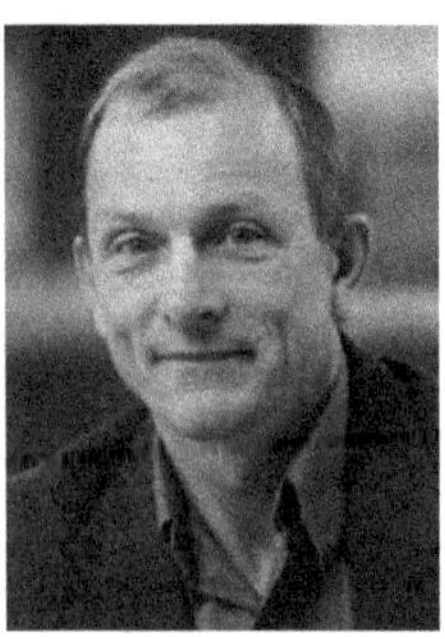

Professor Igor K. Lednev is Distinguished Professor at the Department of Chemistry, University at Albany, State University of New York, USA. He is a Fellow of the Royal Society of Chemistry and the Society for Applied Spectroscopy. His research is focused on the development of novel laser spectroscopy for medical diagnostics, forensic purposes and fundamental biophysics of protein folding and aggregation. He has authored over

260 publications in peer-reviewed journals, with an h-index of 71. He has received several prestigious awards including the Gold Medal Award from the NY/NJ Section of the Society for Applied Spectroscopy, and the Charles Mann Award from the Federation of Analytical Chemistry and Spectroscopy Societies. He served as an advisory member on the White House Subcommittee for Forensic Science, and Congressman Tonko acknowledged his research at the U.S. House of Representatives Hearing on the advancements in forensic science in September 2019. His work has been featured in the media over 100 times including TV and radio interviews, publications in the *Wall Street Journal, Chemical & Engineering News,* etc.

Chapter 5

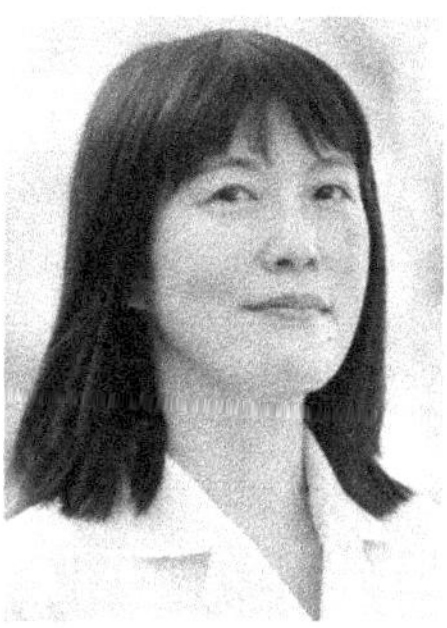

Dr. Mariko Egawa is an Executive Specialist at MIRAI Technology Institute, Shiseido Co., Ltd., Japan. To date, she has focused her research on the application of optics and spectroscopy techniques, including near-infrared spectroscopy, spontaneous Raman scattering microscopy, and coherent Raman scattering microscopy, for the evaluation of skin function. At present, she is also collaborating with occupational physicians on mental stress evaluation using facial image evaluation technology. She serves as a Editorial committee member for the Optical Society of Japan and as a Council member for The Japanese Society of Research Dermatology. She also contributes to the Laser Society of Japan, the Japan Association of Medical Spectroscopy, and the Spectroscopic Innovation Research Society as committee member and organizer. Her work has been recognized by several awards, including the NIR Advance Award in 2006, the best paper award of the 22nd International Federation of Societies of Cosmetic Chemists (IFSCC) International Conference in 2013, and the prestigious 2022 Award for Science and Technology from the Ministry of Education, Culture, Sports, Science and Technology (MEXT).

Chapter 7

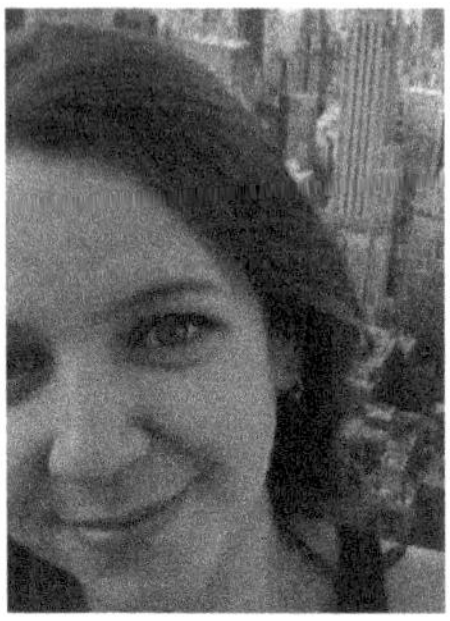

Dr. Sian Sloan-Dennison was awarded her MChem in Forensic and Analytical Chemistry at the University of Strathclyde, UK in 2013. During her final year she undertook a project with Professor Karen Faulds which led to a PhD focusing on the novel detection of biomolecules using SERS. She then spent two years as a research associate at the Ohio State University working with Professor Zac Schultz investigating protein receptor signaling with label-free SERS, before returning to the University of Strathclyde as a research associate with Professor Duncan Graham developing point-of-care biomarker assays coupled with handheld SERS detection.

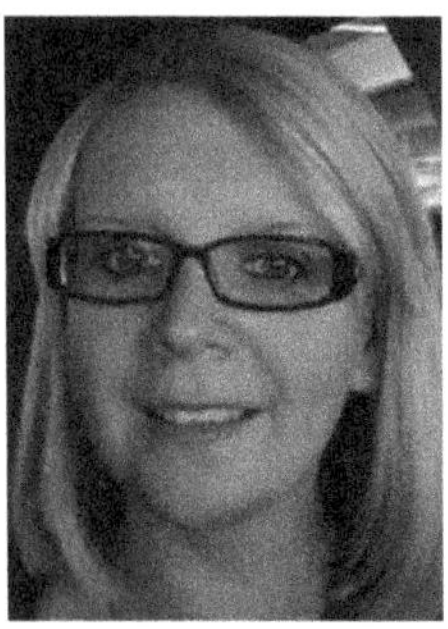

Dr. Hayleigh Kearns is a Postdoctoral Research Associate at the Department of Pure and Applied Chemistry, University of Strathclyde, UK. Her research is focused on the sensitive, selective and multiplexed detection of foodborne bacterial pathogens using SERS nanosensors. She holds a MSc in Forensic and Analytical Chemistry and a PhD in Pure and Applied Chemistry from the University of Strathclyde, UK.

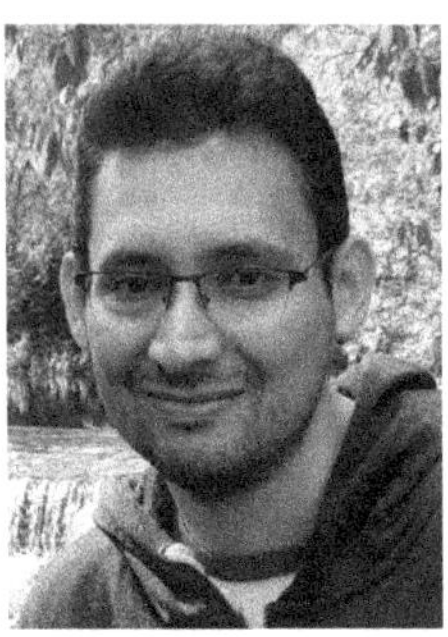

Dr. Waleed Hassanain is Postdoctoral Research Associate at the Centre of Molecular Nanometrology, University of Strathclyde, UK, where he is working on a project to create a sensitive, rapid and point-of-care assay for the assessment of antimicrobial resistance via monitoring specific bacterial DNA signatures using SERS technique.

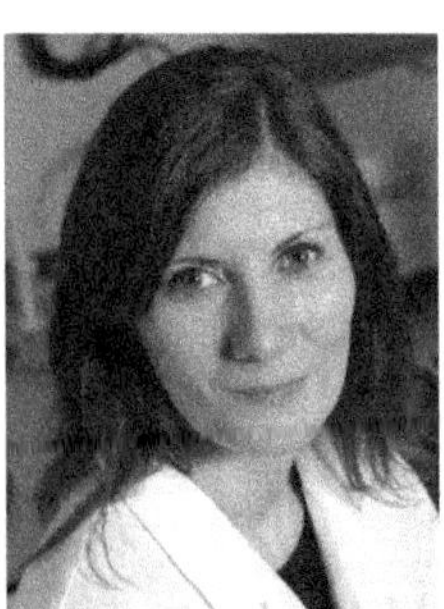

Professor Karen Faulds FRSC FRSE is Distinguished Professor at the Department of Pure and Applied Chemistry, University of Strathclyde, UK, where she is also the Strathclyde Director of the EPSRC and MRC Centre for Doctoral Training in Optical Medical Imaging. She is an elected Fellow of the Royal Society of Chemistry, Royal Society of Edinburgh, and Society for Applied Spectroscopy. She has received several prestigious awards including the Joseph Black Award and the Analytical Division Mid-Career Award from the Royal Society of Chemistry, the Charles Mann Award from the Federation of Analytical Chemistry and Spectroscopy Socicties, the Craver Award from the Coblentz Society, and the Robert Kellner Lecture Award from the Division of Analytical Chemistry of the European Chemical Societies. She has been named as one of the Top 50 Women in Analytical Science (2016), Top 10 Spectroscopists (2017) and Top 100 Influential Analytical Scientists (2019) by *The Analytical Scientist.*

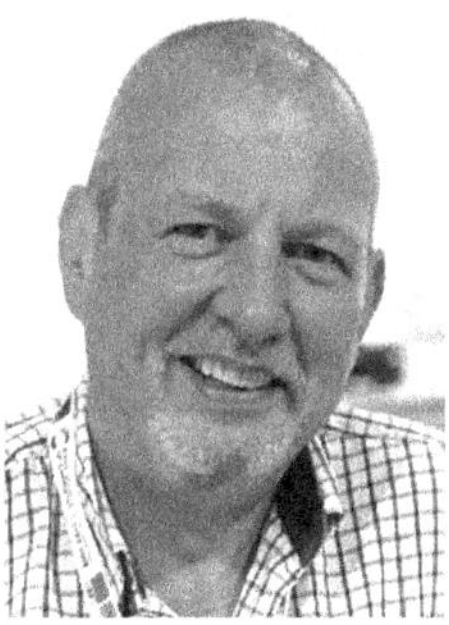

Professor Duncan Graham FRSC FRSE is Distinguished Professor and Research Chair of the Department of Pure and Applied Chemistry, University of Strathclyde, UK, where he is also Associate Principal & Executive Dean of the Faculty of Science. He is an elected Fellow of the Royal Society of Chemistry, Royal Society of Edinburgh, and Society for Applied Spectroscopy. He serves as Chair of the Publishing Board for the Royal Society of Chemistry, and is a trustee for the Royal Society of Chemistry and the Association of British Spectroscopists Trust fund. He has received several prestigious awards including the Theophilus Redwood Award and the Corday Morgan Prize from the Royal Society of Chemistry, the Charles Mann Award from the Federation of Analytical Chemistry and Spectroscopy Societies, the Craver Award from the Coblentz Society, and the Wolfson Research Merit Award from the Royal Society.

Chapter 8

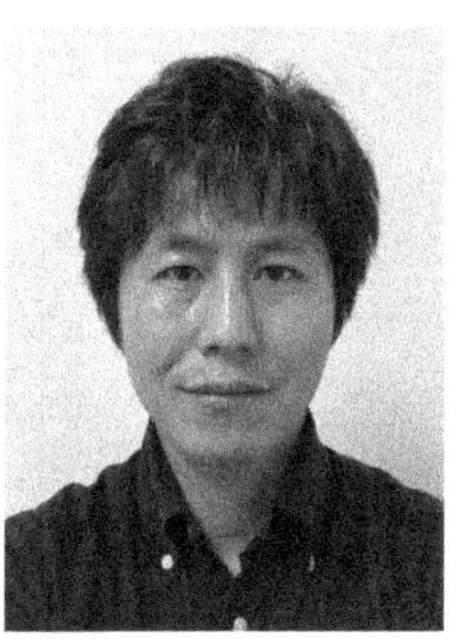

Professor Hiroyuki Yamakoshi is Assistant Professor at the Graduate School of Pharmaceutical Sciences, Tohoku University, Japan. He obtained his PhD degree from Tohoku University in 2010 working on the chemical biology research of bioactive natural products under the supervision of Professor Yoshiharu Iwabuchi. His research interests include chemical biology, medicinal chemistry, and total synthesis of biologically active natural products.

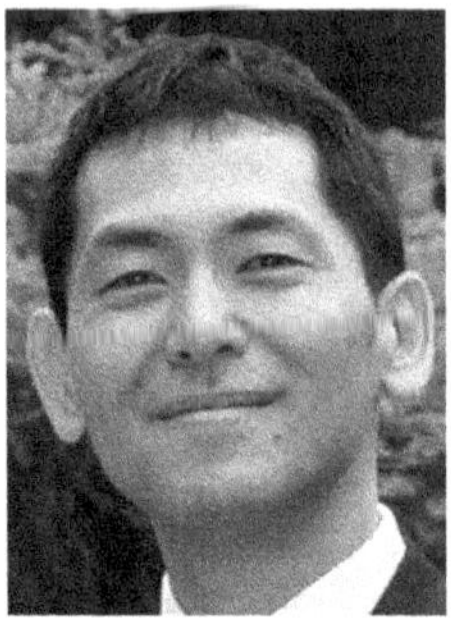

Dr. Jun Ando is a Research Scientist at the Molecular Physiology Laboratory, RIKEN, Japan. He received his PhD in Applied Physics from Osaka University in 2010. He was a JSPS research fellow, a post doctoral researcher at ERATO Sodeoka Live Cell Chemistry Project and Graduate School of Engineering, Osaka University, and an Assistant Professor at the Institute for Molecular Science. He has received the Spectroscopical Society of Japan Award for Young Scientists, and the Optics Award for Excellent Papers of the Optical Society of Japan. His research interests include biophotonics, vibrational spectroscopy, optical microscopy, biophysics, and plasmonics.

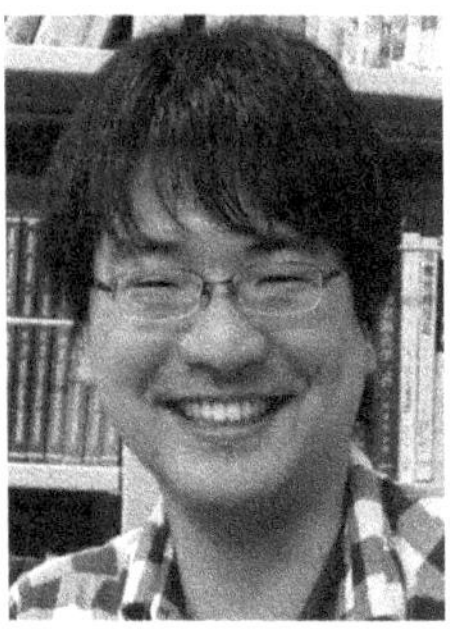

Dr. Syusuke Egoshi is Research Scientist at the Synthetic Organic Chemistry Laboratory and Catalysis and Integrated Research Group, RIKEN, Japan. His research interests are the development of unique chemical imaging technologies including Raman tags/probes and their application for elucidating the mode of action of small bioactive molecules.

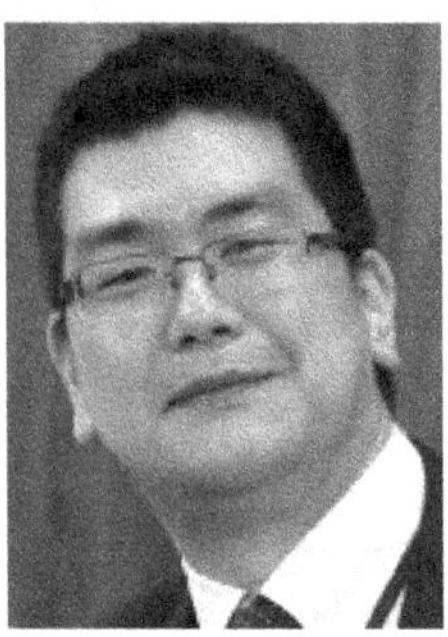

Dr. Kosuke Dodo is Senior Research Scientist at the Synthetic Organic Chemistry Laboratory and Catalysis and Integrated Research Group, RIKEN, Japan. His research interests span the development of unique chemical probes/technologies including Raman probes and their application for biological research related to cell death signaling.

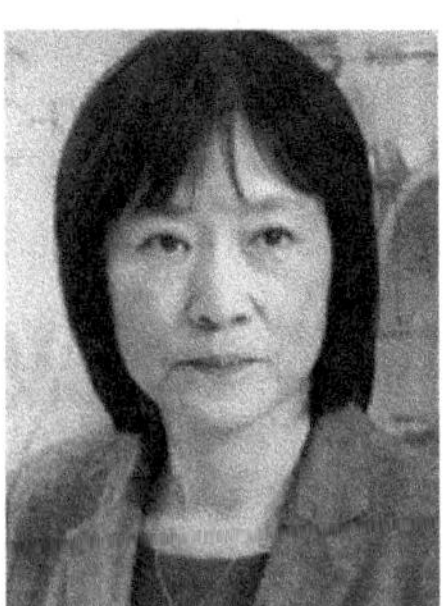

Professor Mikiko Sodeoka is Chief Scientist at RIKEN, Japan, where she is also Deputy Director of the RIKEN Center for Sustainable Resource Science. She is Visiting Professor at Saitama University and Tokyo Medical and Dental University, Japan. She is an Elected Fellow of the American Association for the Advancement of Science. She has received several prestigious awards including the Arthur C. Cope Scholar Award from the American

Chemical Society, ChemComm 40th Anniversary Lecture Award from the Royal Society of Chemistry, and the Pharmaceutical Society of Japan Award.

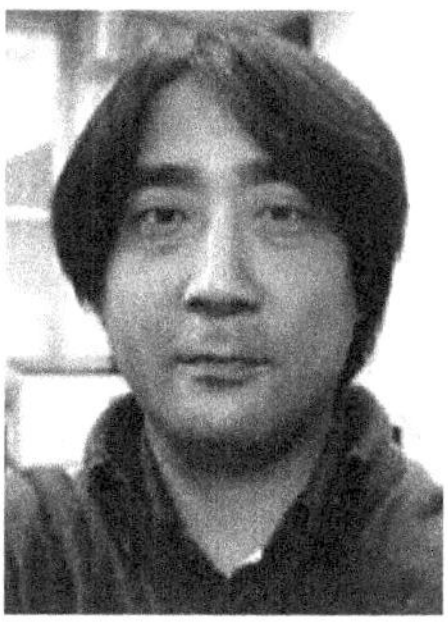

Professor Katsumasa Fujita is Professor at the Department of Applied Physics, Osaka University, Japan. His research interests are the development of optical techniques for bioimaging based on non-linear optics and vibrational spectroscopy. His current work is focused on improvement of the sensitivity and temporal resolution of Raman microscopy for molecular imaging of living cells and tissues.

Chapter 9

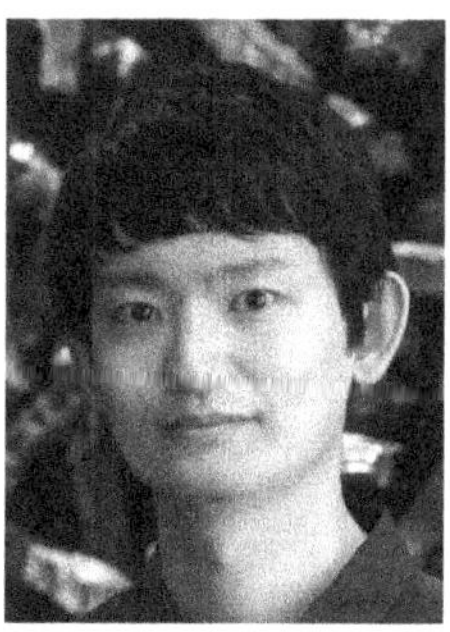

Professor Shinichi Miyazaki is Assistant Professor at the Department of Biological Sciences, University of Tokyo, Japan. He obtained his MD and PhD from the University of Tsukuba. In 2022, he received the Dean's Award from the School of Integrative and Global Majors in the University of Tsukuba. His current research interests include sleep medicine and nonlinear optical imaging.

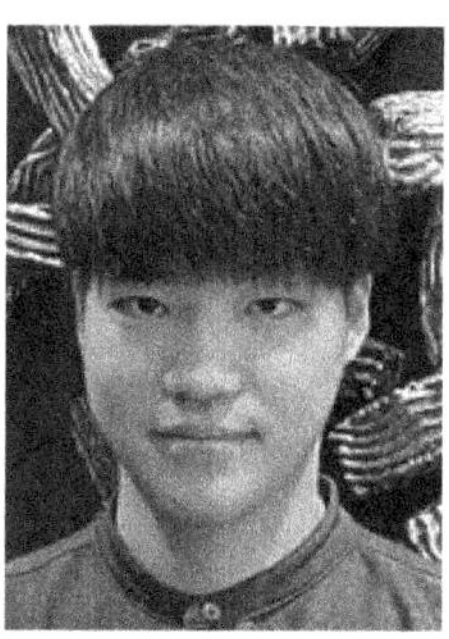

Mr. Yusuke Murakami is a PhD student in the PhD program in Humanics, University of Tsukuba, Japan. His major fields are physical engineering and neuroscience. His primary research interest lies in nonlinear optical imaging of the mouse brain.

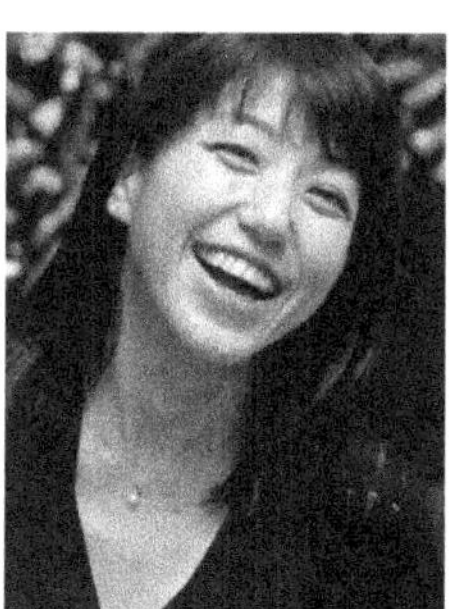

Professor Sakiko Honjoh is Assistant Professor at the International Institute for Integrative Sleep Medicine, University of Tsukuba, Japan. She has received the Young Scientists' Prize from the Ministry of Education, Culture, Sports, Science and Technology and the 1st Tachibana Award for the Most Outstanding Female Researcher from Kyoto University, amongst others. Her current focus is on homeostatic sleep/wake regulation in behavioral vigilance states and in cortical neural activity.

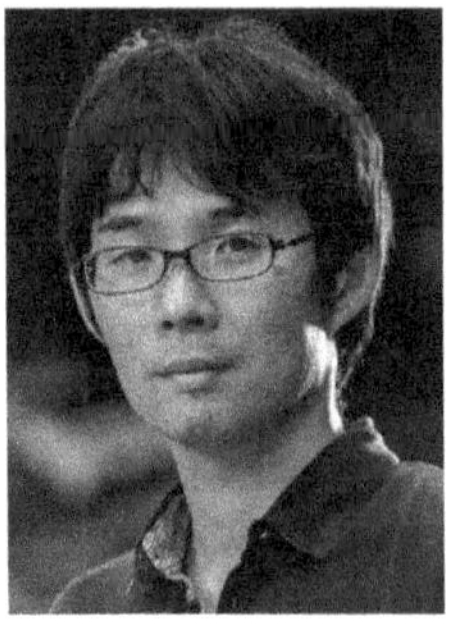

Professor Yu Hayashi is Professor at the Department of Biological Sciences, University of Tokyo, Japan, Specific Professor at the Department of Human Health Sciences, Kyoto University, Japan, and Visiting Professor at the International Institute for Integrative Sleep Medicine, University of Tsukuba, Japan. He has received the U.S. National Academy of Medicine Catalyst Award and the Young Scientists' Prize from the Ministry of Education, Culture, Sports, Science and Technology, amongst others. His current focus is on the function and evolution of sleep.

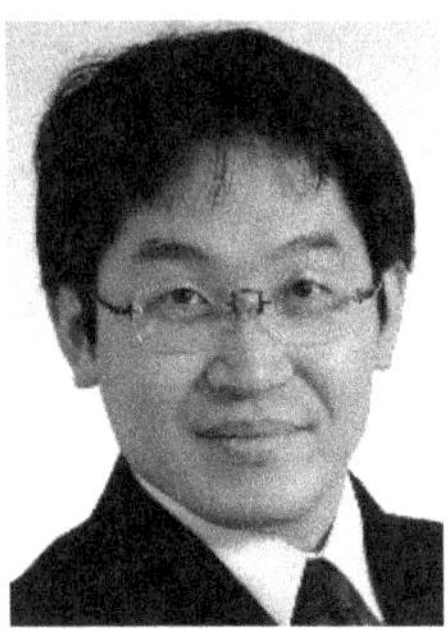

Professor Hideaki Kano is Professor at the Department of Chemistry, Kyushu University, Japan and Visiting Professor at the Department of Applied Physics, University of Tsukuba, Japan. He has received the Spectroscopical Society of Japan Award for Young Scientists and the Chemical Society of Japan Award for Young Chemists. He uses coherent Raman spectroscopy to create functional images of living cells and tissue. His research interests include nonlinear optical spectroscopy and imaging in biomedical studies.

Chapter 10

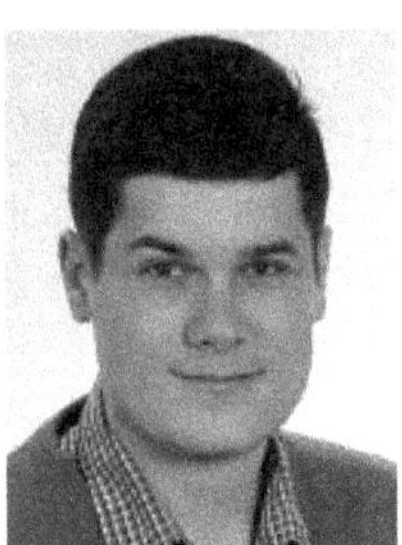

Mr. Markus Salbreiter is a PhD student at Friederich Schiller University Jena, Germany, where he previously studied Biology BSc and Microbiology MSc. His study focuses on the use of Raman spectroscopy to analyze clinically relevant aerobic and anaerobic microorganisms from the genera *Bacillus* and *Clostridium*.

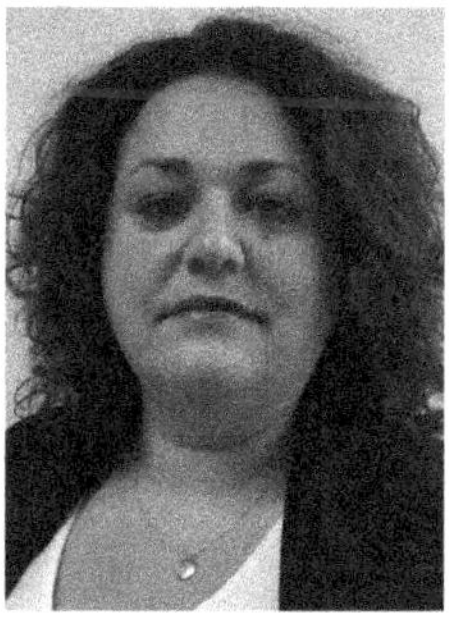

Dr. Aikaterini Pistiki is a researcher at Leibniz Institute of Photonic Technologies in Jena, Germany. She has been working for several years in the field of infectious diseases focusing in particular on microbiological documentation, antimicrobial resistance and host-pathogen interaction.

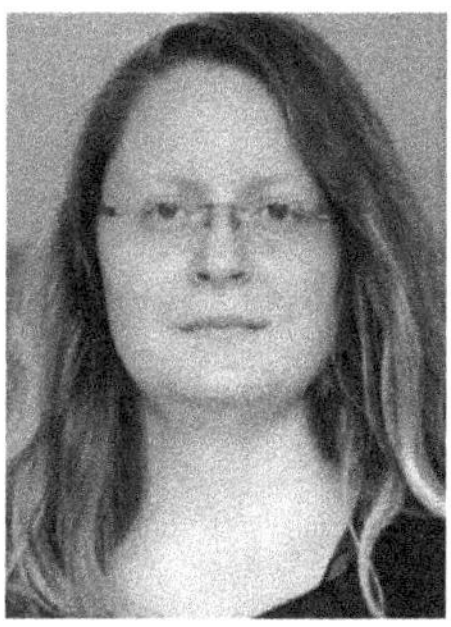

Dr. Dana Cialla-May is Group Leader at the Department of Spectroscopy and Imaging, Leibniz Institute of Photonic Technology, Germany. The research topics of her group include the development of powerful SERS substrates and their application towards clinical, food and environmental analytical tasks.

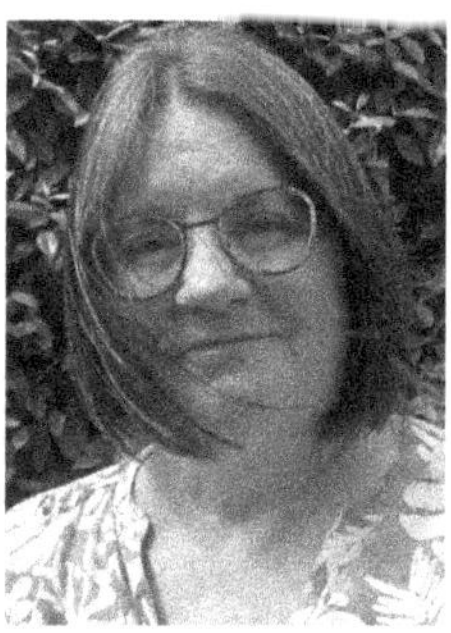

Dr. Petra Rösch is Principal Investigator at the Institute for Physical Chemistry, Friederich Schiller University Jena, Germany. Her main focus is on the cultivation-free characterization and identification of microorganisms with Raman.

Chapter 11

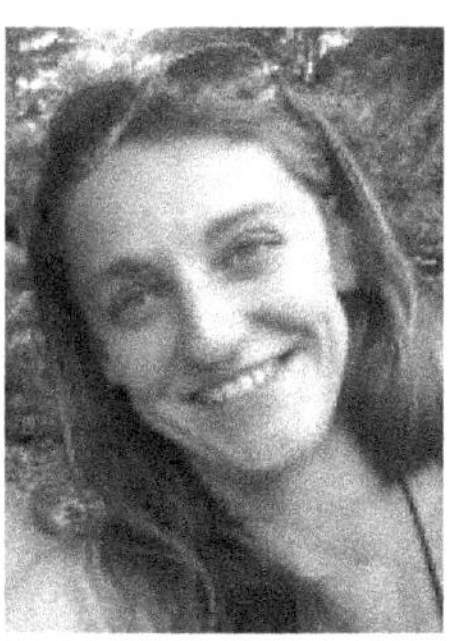

Dr. Kamila Kochan is Research Fellow at the Centre for Biospectroscopy, Monash University, Australia. She is named in *The Australian's Research* 2023 magazine as the research field leader in spectroscopy and molecular physics. Her research focuses on application of vibrational spectroscopy to biological materials, including micro- and nano-scale imaging as well as clinical diagnostic solutions.

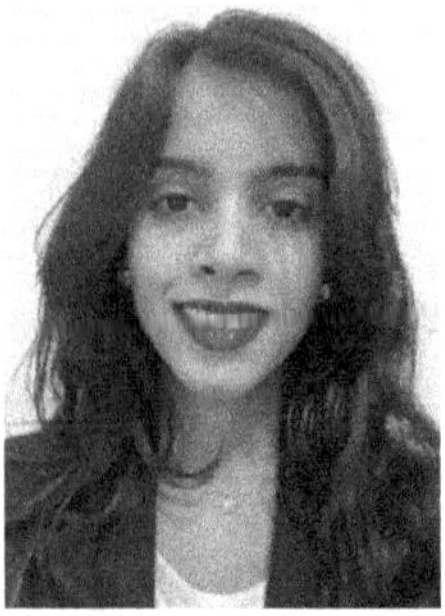

Ms. Savithri Pebotuwa is now pursuing her PhD at the Department of Microbiology and School of Chemistry in Monash University, Australia under the guidance of Prof. Anton Peleg and Prof. Bayden Wood. She completed her BSc (Hons.) at Monash University in 2018. Her PhD is an interdisciplinary project combining vibrational spectroscopy for the investigation of fungi with machine learning techniques.

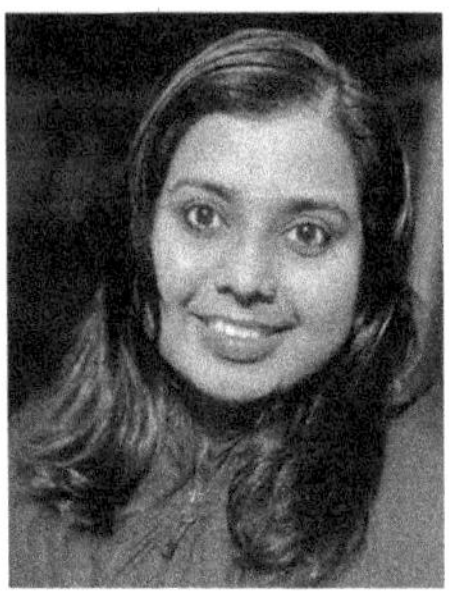

Ms. Thulya Chakkumpulakkal is pursuing a joint PhD degree in analytical chemistry from Monash University, Australia, and the University of Bath, UK, under the guidance of Prof. Bayden R. Wood (Monash University), Dr. Paul De Bank (University of Bath), Dr. Keith Bambery (Australian Synchrotron), and Prof. Karen J. Edler (Lund University, Sweden). In 2012, Thulya obtained her BSc in Physics with minors in Chemistry and Mathematics from the University of Calicut, India. Following that, she earned her MTech degree in Materials Science from the University of Mysore, India. In her PhD, Thulya has been working on a highly multidisciplinary project combining microfluidics, spectroscopy and machine modeling to develop new diagnostic tests for blood- and water-borne pathogens, particularly focusing on malaria parasites, leishmania parasites and bacteria. She has been awarded the following accolades: The Association of British Spectroscopists Trust (ABS Trust) Student Bursary Award for 2023, a Research Development Grant from the Royal Society of Chemistry, study away travel grant from Monash University, Doctoral Recognition Award for 2023 from the University of Bath, and the Coblentz Society Student Award 2023.

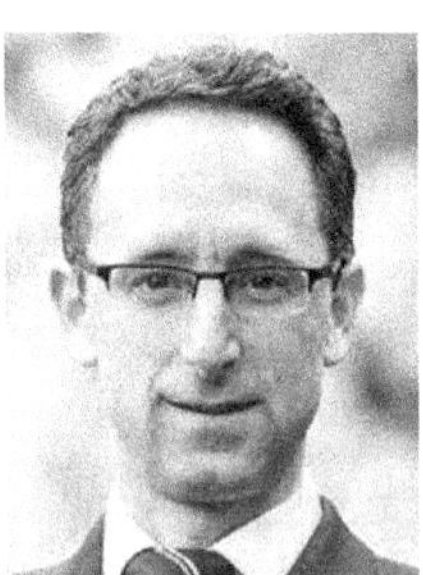

Professor Anton Y. Peleg is Professor of Infectious Diseases and Microbiology as well as Director of the Department of Infectious Diseases at the Alfred Hospital, Monash University, Australia, where he is also a research group leader in the Department of Microbiology. He is recognized as an expert on the clinical impact, epidemiology, and management of infections due to multidrug-resistant Gram-negative bacteria, specifically *Acinetobacter*. He provided the first description of carbapenemase genes in Australia and designed phenotypic methods for their detection in Gram-negative organisms. He also provided the first reports of tigecycline resistance in *Acinetobacter* and identified the mechanism of resistance as over-expression of a multi-drug efflux pump.

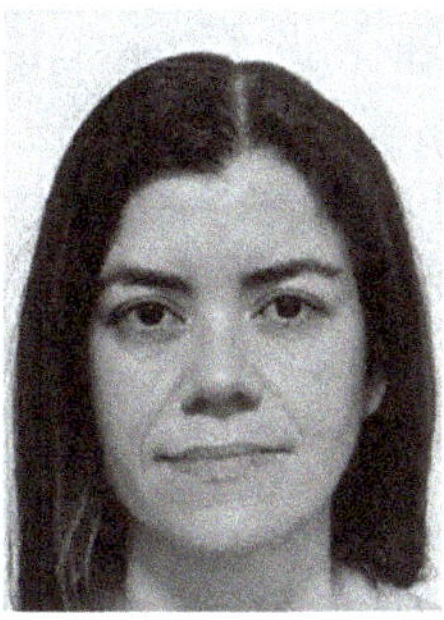

Dr. Xenia Kostoulias is a Research Assistant with the Department of Microbiology and the Department of Infectious Diseases, Monash University, Australia. She is interested in virulence and mechanisms of antimicrobial resistance in hospital-acquired organisms, with a special interest in the contribution of biofilms to this process. She uses a range of methods including molecular microbiology and *in vivo* infection models as well as static and dynamic biofilm models to conduct her investigations.

Chapter 12

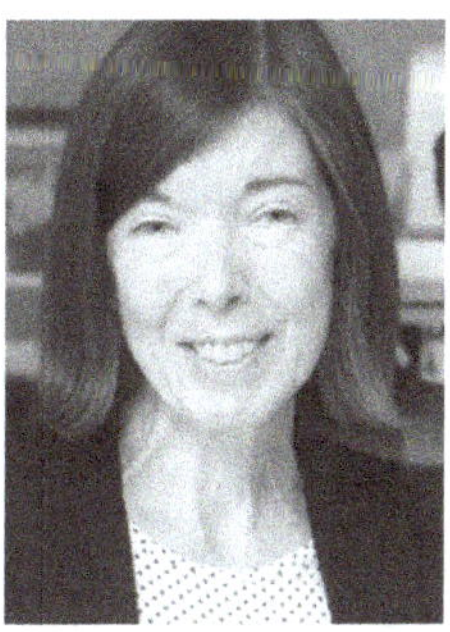

Professor Fiona M. Lyng is Manager of the Radiation and Environmental Science Centre in Technological University Dublin, Republic of Ireland. Her research is focused on non-targeted effects of ionizing and non-ionizing radiation, and the use of vibrational spectroscopy for disease diagnosis. She has published >200 peer-reviewed journal papers with a h-index of 51. She holds a BSc from University of Dublin (Trinity College) and a PhD from University College Dublin.

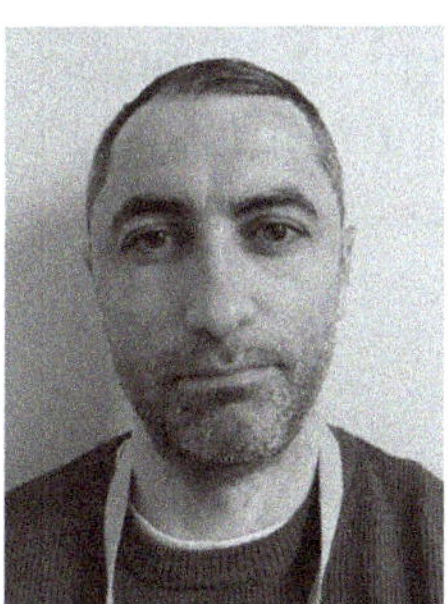

Dr. Damien Traynor is Project Lead for the organization of European Cancer Institute's accreditation program for the Mater Misericordiae University Hospital, Republic of Ireland. He has worked on the CERVIVA CARG program, specifically on the clinical evaluation of Raman spectroscopy for use in the diagnosis of cervical pre-cancer and cancer. He has a BA in Medical and Molecular Biology from Technological University Dublin and undertook his PhD in the FOCAS Research Institute, Technological University Dublin. He is a member of the Academy of Medical Laboratory Scientists in Cytology.

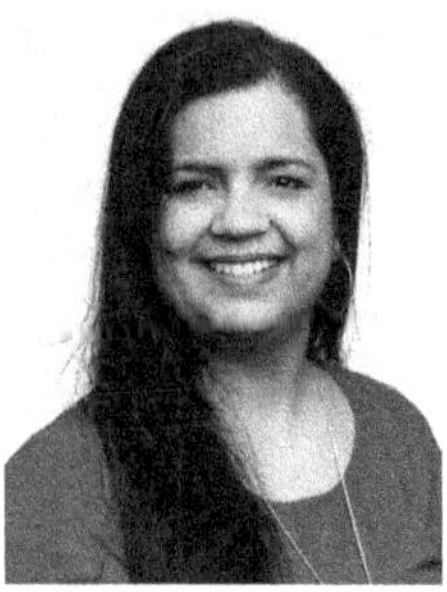

Dr. Isha Behl is a Research Fellow at University of Dublin (Trinity College), Republic of Ireland. After completing her MTech in Biotechnology, she was awarded the prestigious Women Scientist Fellowship by the Department of Science and Technology, Government of India. She was among only 10 women scientists honored with the fellowship until 2010. She completed her PhD in the biomedical application of vibrational spectroscopy for the early detection of oral cancer at Technological University Dublin. In 2022, she was awarded a Government of Ireland Postdoctoral Fellowship by the Irish Research Council to continue her research in oral cancer.

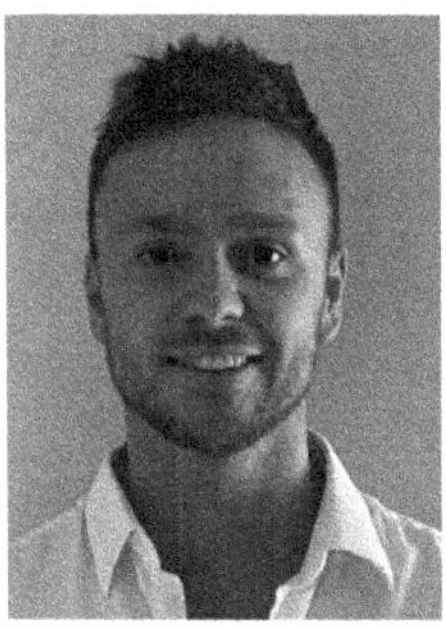

Dr. Declan O'Dea is currently a pharmaceutical project manager in Eli Lilly and Company. He received his BSc in Molecular Biology from Technological University Dublin, and his PhD, completed at the FOCAS Research Institute in Technological University Dublin, explored the use of Raman spectroscopy for the discrimination of thyroid and lung cancer subtypes for application in clinical cytopathology.

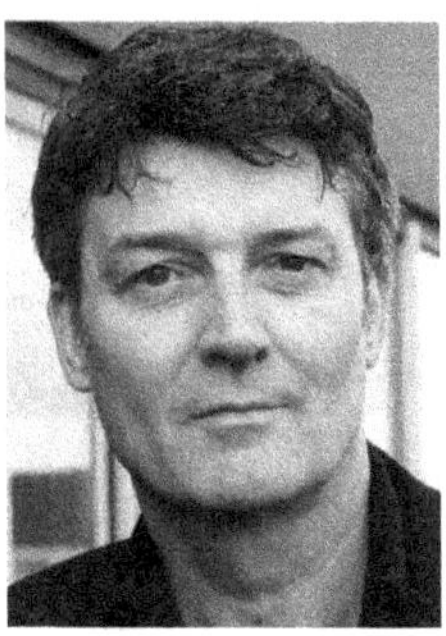

Professor Hugh J. Byrne is Head of the FOCAS Research Institute in Technological University Dublin, Republic of Ireland. He holds a BA (mod.) and PhD from University of Dublin (Trinity College). His principal research interests are in the applications of spectroscopy and the study of molecular and nanomaterials, most recently in biospectroscopy for diagnostics, cytological analysis and nano-bio interactions. He is a founding Director of the International Society for Clinical Spectroscopy (CLIRSPEC).

Chapter 13

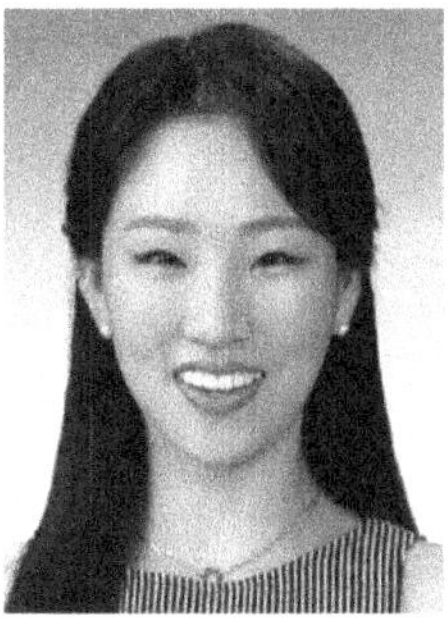

Ms. Jeong Hee Kim is a PhD candidate at Johns Hopkins University, USA. She holds a BSc from the Georgia Institute of Technology, USA and a MSc from Seoul National University, Republic of Korea.

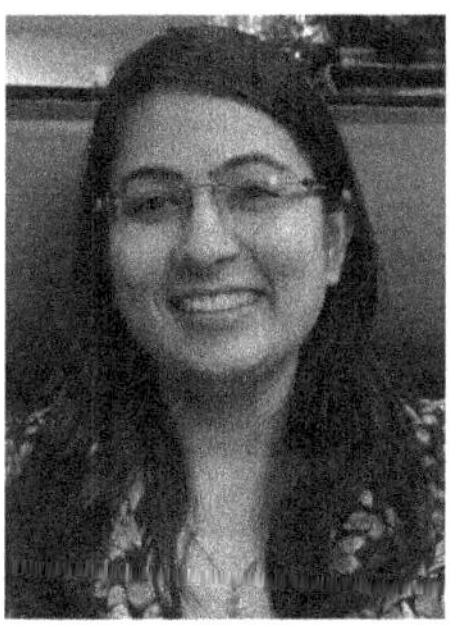

Dr. Swati Tanwar is a Postdoctoral Researcher at Johns Hopkins University, USA. She holds a BSc and MSc from Delhi University, India and a PhD from the Institute of Nano Science and Technology, India.

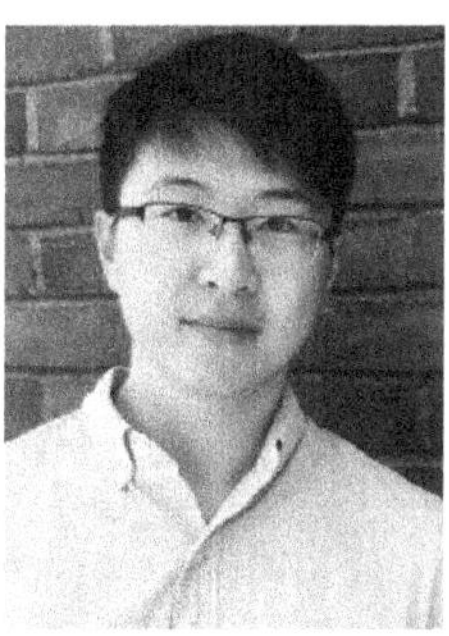

Mr. Zhenhui Liu is a PhD candidate in Mechanical Engineering at Johns Hopkins University, USA. He holds a BSc in Mechanical Engineering and a BA in Economics from Tsinghua University, China.

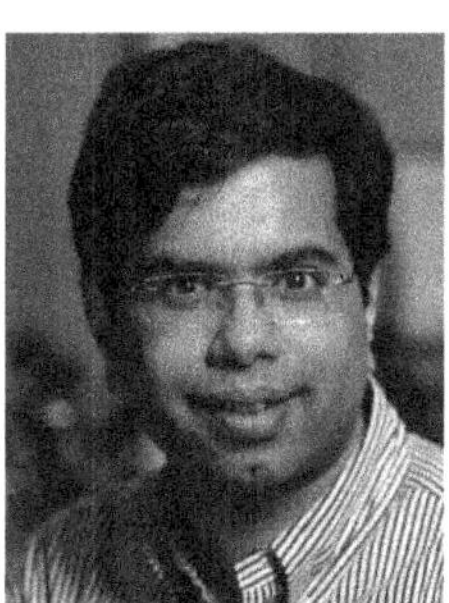

Professor Ishan Barman is Associate Professor at the Department of Mechanical Engineering, Johns Hopkins Whiting School of Engineering, USA, with a joint appointment in the Johns Hopkins Sidney Kimmel Comprehensive Cancer Center. He seeks to advance photonics methods for applications in clinical diagnosis, on the comprehensive characterization of biomolecules, the investigation of pharmaceutical drugs and their interaction with biological systems, and on rapid measurements in microfluidic platforms. He holds a BTech from the Indian Institute of Technology, India and a MSc and PhD from the Massachusetts Institute of Technology, USA.

Chapter 14

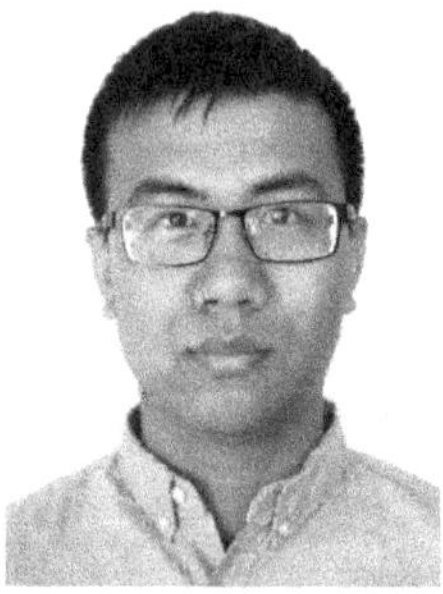

Dr. Chi Shu is a Research Fellow at the Department of Biomedical Engineering, National University of Singapore, Singapore. His research interest is in developing optical imaging and spectroscopy systems, especially Raman spectroscopy systems for biological tissue characterization and *in vivo* clinical disease detection.

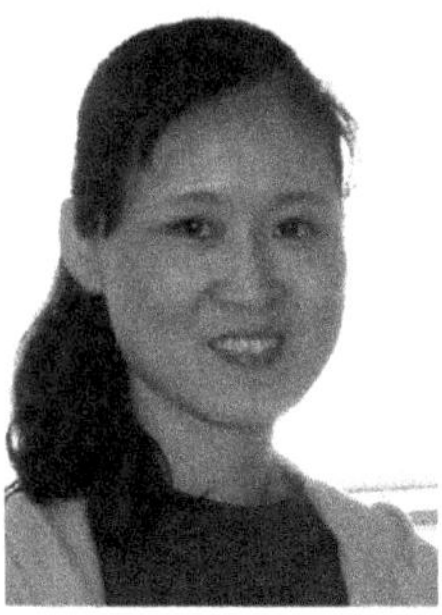

Dr. Wei Zheng is a Research Fellow at the Department of Biomedical Engineering, National University of Singapore, Singapore. Her research interests are focused on biomedical optics, biophotonics and optical bioimaging. She is particularly dedicated to the development of fiber-optic Raman and fluorescence spectroscopy, endoscope imaging, and full-field OCT imaging techniques, and their translations for biomedical applications.

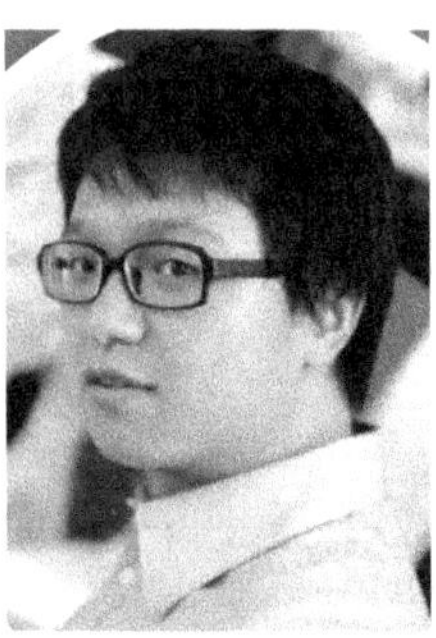

Dr. Kan Lin is a Research Fellow at the Department of Biomedical Engineering, National University of Singapore. His research interest is in biomedical and optical spectroscopy, imaging systems, and data analytics, as well as their applications for early cancer and pre-cancer diagnosis and detection in clinical settings.

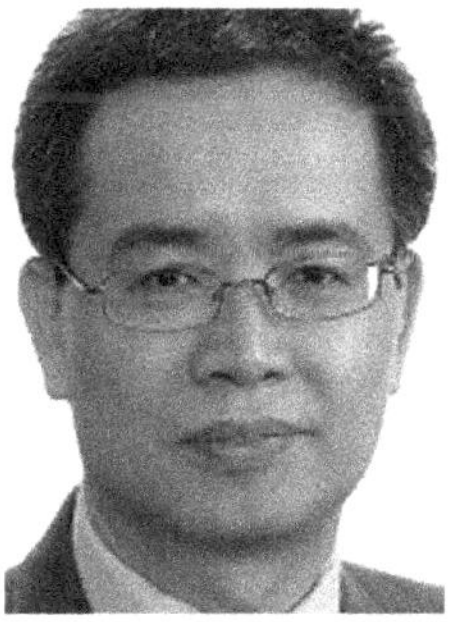

Professor Zhiwei Huang is Associate Professor at the Department of Biomedical Engineering, National University of Singapore, Singapore. His research interests include optical spectroscopy and imaging in medical diagnostics and treatment, modeling of light propagation in turbid media, nonlinear microscopy, optical coherence microscopy, and single-molecule imaging.

Chapter 15

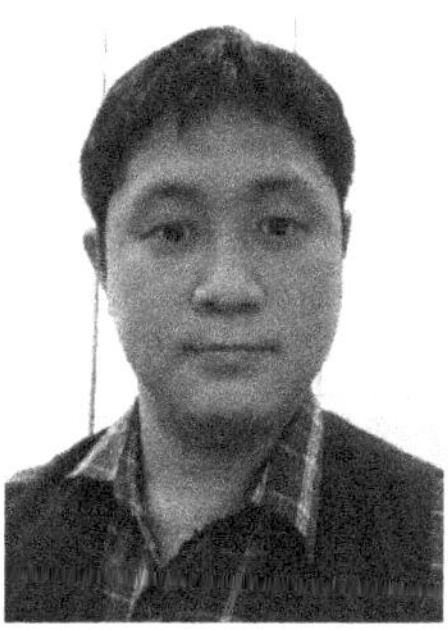

Dr. Akinori Taketani is Specially Appointed Assistant Professor at Research Center for Pre-Disease Science, University of Toyama, Japan. He holds a PhD in Science from Kwansei Gakuin University, Japan. His research focuses on the identification of pre-disease state using Raman spectroscopy and mathematical analysis.

Chapter 16

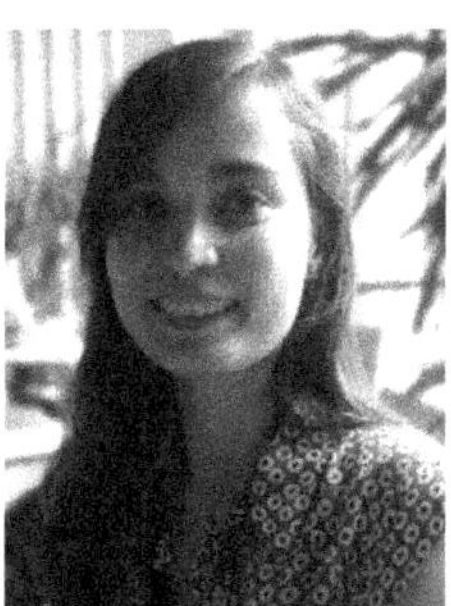

Dr. Katherine Ember is a Postdoctoral Fellow at Polytechnique Montréal, Canada. She holds a PhD in Optical Medical Imaging from the University of Edinburgh, UK and an MSc in Biochemistry and Molecular Biology from the University of Oxford, UK.

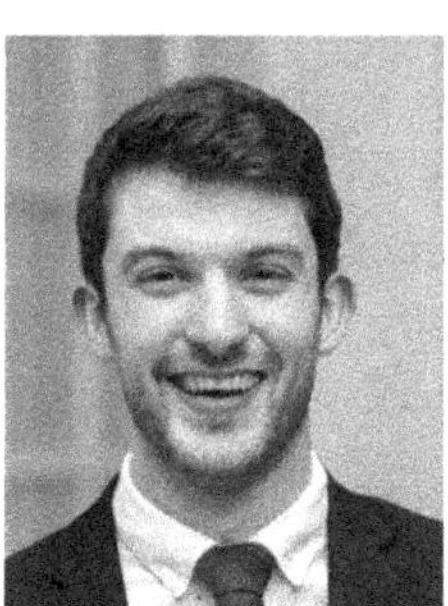

Dr. Jean-Philippe Dulude is a senior General Surgery resident at the Université de Montréal, Canada. He is also completing a Master's degree in biomedical engineering in the LUMED Lab at Polytechnique Montréal. His work focuses on the *in vivo* use of Raman spectroscopy in soft tissue sarcoma resection surgery.

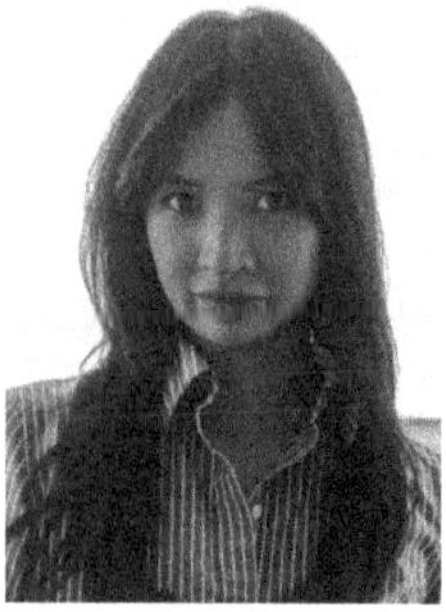

Dr. Trang Tran is a research scientist at the CRCHUM medical research center and has honed her expertise in neurosciences and biomedical research, with a particular focus on clinical applications. She currently oversees several clinical research projects in the LUMED Lab. Her interests lie at the intersection of molecular biology and neurosurgery. Her ultimate goal is to contribute to the development of novel therapeutic approaches that can improve the lives of patients affected by neurological disorders.

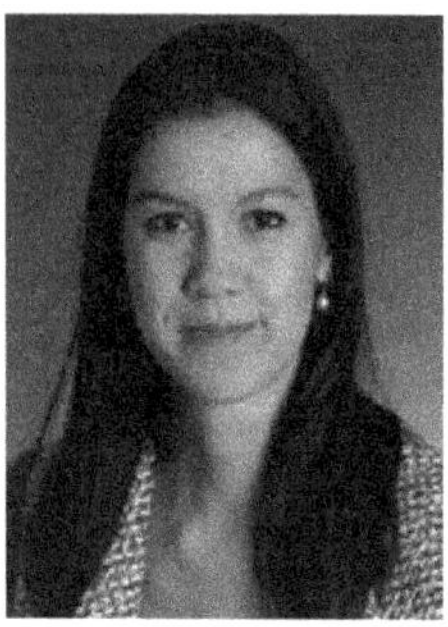

Professor Mai-Kim Gervais is Professor in the Department of Surgery at the Université de Montréal, Canada and Surgical Oncologist at Maisonneuve-Rosemont Hospital, Canada. She chairs a subcommittee in the establishment of guidelines for the management of retroperitoneal sarcomas under the Quebec Cancer Program of the Quebec Ministry of Health. Her areas of expertise include retroperitoneal sarcoma, melanoma, gastric cancer and breast cancer.

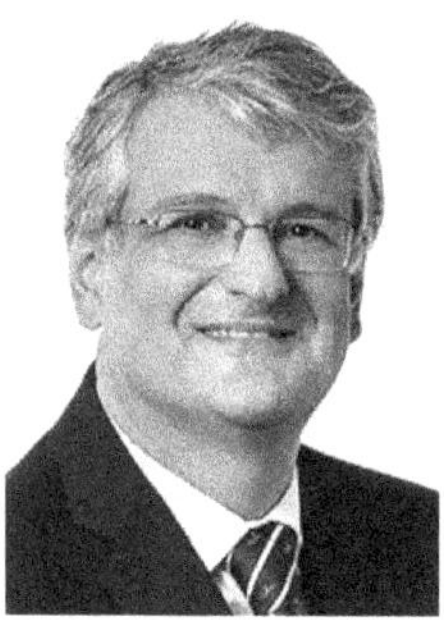

Professor Sarkis Meterissian is Professor in the Department of Surgery at McGill University, Canada and Director of the Breast Cancer Clinic of McGill University Health Centre. His research focuses on the diagnosis, pathogenesis and prognosis of breast cancer.

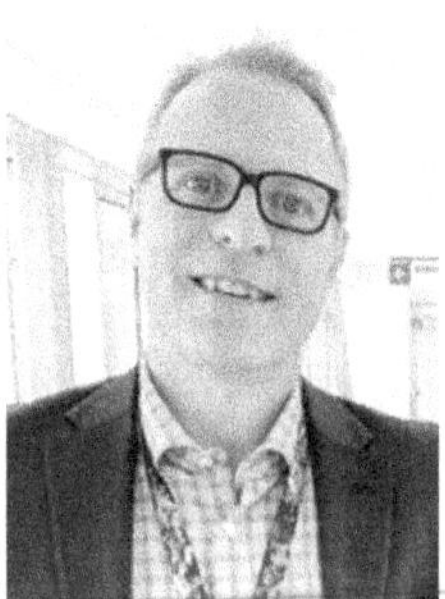

Dr. Roy Dudley is a pediatric neurosurgeon and epilepsy surgeon at the Montreal Children's Hospital and the Montreal Neurological Institute of McGill University, Montreal, Canada. His research focuses on multimodal pre-surgical investigations for focal epilepsy including seizure semiology analysis, novel neuroimaging and electrophysiology techniques, advanced magnetoencephalography methods, stereo-electroencephalography, as well as intra-operative surgical adjuncts such as intra-operative magnetic resonance imaging and Raman spectroscopy.

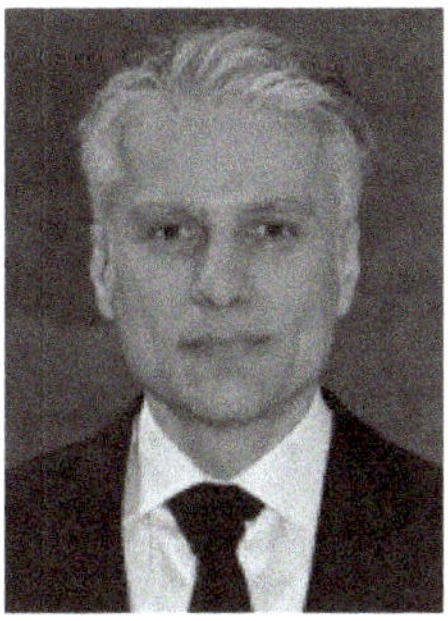

Professor Kevin Petrecca is Associate Professor and William Feindel Chair in Neuro-Oncology in the Department of Neurology and Neurosurgery at McGill University, Canada and Chief of the Department of Neurosurgery at McGill University Health Centre. He is an Elected Fellow of the American Association of Neurological Surgeons and the Royal College of Physicians and Surgeons of Canada. He is dedicated to treating brain cancer patients and his research program focuses on studying the origin, development, and properties of brain cancer stem cells and developing new tools for brain cancer surgery.

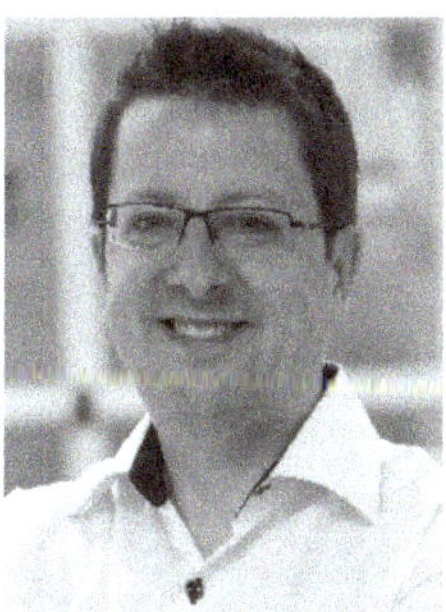

Professor Frédéric Leblond is head of the LUMED Lab and Professor in the Department of Engineering Physics at Polytechnique Montréal, Canada. He is also a researcher at the CRCHUM medical research center and is co-Founder of the companies Reveal Surgical Inc and Exclaro-Tridan Inc. Reveal Surgical is tasked with commercialization of his Raman spectroscopy-based cancer cell detection device, while Exclaro-Tridan focuses on the development of biofluid-based spectroscopic diagnostic testing. The emphasis of his research is the development of molecular optical imaging techniques applied to the detection and characterization of cancer and infectious diseases for clinical applications.

Chapter 17

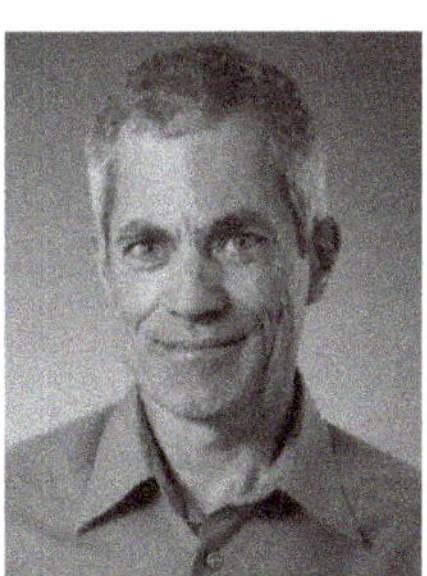

Dr. Christoph Krafft is Research Group Leader at the Leibniz Institute of Photonic Technology, Germany. He is working on optical cell and tissue identification, in particular using Raman imaging, FTIR imaging and nonlinear microscopy.

https://doi.org/10.1142/9789811264610_fmatter

Contents

https://doi.org/10.1142/9789811264610_0001

Chapter 1

History of Challenges of Raman Spectroscopy to Medical Science — From 1970s to 2000

Yukihiro Ozaki[1,2]

[1]School of Biological and Environmental Sciences,
Kwansei Gakuin University,
Sanda, Hyogo 669-1330, Japan
[2]Toyota Physical and Chemical Research Institute,
Nagakute, Aichi 480-1192, Japan
ozaki@kwansei.ac.jp

1.1 Introduction

The purpose of this chapter is to describe the history of challenges of Raman spectroscopy to medical science from the 1970s to 2000. Since laser was introduced to Raman spectroscopy in 1968 in Brazil, Raman spectroscopy has faced various exciting challenges, such as challenges to ultra-high speed, ultra-small amount, ultra-trace amount, ultra-high spatial resolution, ultra-thin, and ultra-high pressure, as well as challenges to a wide range of the excitation from deep ultraviolet to near-infrared (NIR) [1–3]. Challenges to various materials including nanomaterials and those to biomedical sciences have received keen interest. Medical application is one of the most difficult challenges of Raman spectroscopy in terms of interferences from strong fluorescence, sample decomposition, small amounts of samples, and complexity of samples [4–13]. Nowadays, Raman spectroscopy has become a potentially important clinical tool for real-time diagnosis of disease and *in situ* evaluation of living tissue. Raman spectroscopy can provide detailed information about the chemical compositions of the tissue under study. As the first chapter of this book, this chapter has tried to find a guide into tomorrow by taking lessons from the past. I put emphasis on the studies from the 1970s to around 2000 because the investigations carried out after 2000 are reviewed in other chapters in this book.

The 1970s were the age when light shined on Raman spectroscopy thanks to the developments of lasers, gratings, and detectors. Moreover, it was the 1970s that the application of Raman spectroscopy to biological molecules and materials started [1–3, 13–16]. However, for medical application it was still the dark age because of strong fluorescence from disease tissues and damage by strong laser light. Even so several scientists tried to open a new age of medical applications [4]. For example, Larsson and Hellgren [17] measured Raman spectra of blood plasma with homologous serum hepatitis. Yu *et al.* [18, 19] measured Raman spectra of eye lenses, and Thomas *et al.* [20, 21] obtained Raman spectra of several kinds of viruses non-destructively. The latter two studies were not true medical applications but they demonstrated the potential of Raman spectroscopy in medical science. In the 1980s Ozaki *et al.* [4, 22–24] reported Raman studies of cataract formation. This may be the first example that Raman spectroscopy has ever been applied to the study of the mechanism of disease. Ishida *et al.* [25] revealed the usefulness of micro-Raman spectroscopy for gallstone research in 1987. However, the 1970s and 1980s were still a dark age of Raman spectroscopy for medical applications because of two difficulties. One was strong fluorescence from disease tissues and organs, and another was decomposition and denaturation of samples by laser irradiation. Therefore, it was difficult to find true medical applications of Raman spectroscopy except for a few exceptions.

It was the 1990s that the medical application of Raman spectroscopy made truly important progress [5, 7–12]. NIR-excited Raman spectroscopy emerged from the end of the 1980s [5, 7, 11, 26–34]. The development of NIR-excited Raman spectroscopy overcame considerably the problem of fluorescence. In the 1990s diode lasers, charge-coupled device (CCD) detectors, optical filters, optical fibers, and gratings showed remarkable advances, and chemometrics was introduced to Raman spectroscopy [5]. After 2000 the developments in medical applications were expanded to many different fields, and so many innovations in techniques appeared [12]. Therefore, it is not easy to describe the history after 2000. In this chapter the evolutions in the medical application of Raman spectroscopy until around 2000 are described, and for those after 2000 one can find them in other chapters in this book. In this chapter the history of the development of various Raman spectroscopies such as resonance Raman spectroscopy and micro-Raman spectroscopy, and the history of the instrumentations, techniques, and spectral analysis methods are also described.

1.2 Dawn of Medical Application of Raman Spectroscopy — 1970s

1.2.1 *Development of New Raman Spectroscopies and Instrumentation in the 1970s*

Since laser was introduced to Raman spectroscopy in 1968, great innovations of Raman spectroscopy began [1–3]. The 1970s are called the "renaissance" of Raman spectroscopy. During the 1970s not only lasers, but also photomultipliers and gratings made remarkable progress. Note that in the 1970s we had already pulsed lasers, dye lasers, and UV lasers. A number of new Raman methods such as resonance Raman scattering, surface-enhanced Raman scattering (SERS), micro-Raman spectroscopy, Raman optical activity, and time-resolved Raman spectroscopy were initiated in the 1970s (note that it was the 1960s when nonlinear Raman spectroscopy started). It was also the 1970s when the applications of Raman spectroscopy to biochemistry and biology became active [13–16]. One of the most shocking events in the early 1970s was the observation of resonance Raman effect using cytochrome *c* and hemoglobin by Spiro and Strekas [35]. This lighted investigations of resonance Raman spectroscopy both in theoretical studies and applications [13–15]. Raman spectroscopy was used actively to the study of almost all kinds of biological molecules. For examples, structure, functions, and intermolecular interactions of proteins, enzymes, nucleic acids, carbohydrates, and lipids were explored extensively. Applications to medical science followed those to biochemistry and biology [4]. Among the above new spectroscopies, resonance Raman spectroscopy and micro-Raman spectroscopy were important for medical applications in the 1970s and 1980s.

Raman microprobes or micro-Raman systems were established in 1973–1975 by three groups: Black Engineering Inc. and NBS in the U.S. and CNRS at Lille, France [13–16]. Even in the 1970s the spatial resolution of micro-Raman systems reached 1μm. There was an important progress of micro-Raman systems around 1980: a multichannel optical detector was attached, shortening measurement time and avoiding excess heat absorption by samples.

1.2.2 *Some Trials of Clinical Application of Raman Spectroscopy in the 1970s*

In the 1970s application of Raman spectroscopy to clinical problems was still in its infant stage [4, 5]. However, one can find several innovative trials in them. For example, Larsson and Hellgren [17] attempted to use Raman spectroscopy to investigate normal human blood plasma and that with homologous serum hepatitis as described later. Webb *et al.* [36] reported low-frequency Raman spectra (200–50 cm^{-1}) of human mammary carcinoma. According to them, the spectra were significantly different from those of normal human mammary tissues in band shifts and band widths. There were some studies concerning the application of Raman spectroscopy to clinical analysis. Morris [37] reported resonance Raman spectra of some biochemically important catecholamines. In his study catecholamines were first oxidized to the corresponding aminochromes by ferricyanamide. A band due to the $C=N^+$ stretching mode of aminochromes was strongly enhanced by the resonance Raman effect. Aminochromes were determined at 1480 cm^{-1} for adrenaline, 1425 cm^{-1} for noradrenaline, and 1415 cm^{-1} for dopamine.

Larsson and Hellgren [17] applied Raman spectroscopy to disease samples in 1974. This may be the first trial that Raman spectroscopy was applied to disease samples. Figure 1.1(a) shows a Raman spectrum of blood plasma from a 23-year-old healthy woman. Fluorescence is not so serious in this spectrum, and one can observe a band due to water in the region of 3800–2800 cm^{-1} and two sharp bands in the 1600–1000 cm^{-1} region due to carotenoid. Thus, this is a resonance Raman spectrum of carotenoid; nothing else is observed. Figure 1.1 (b) and (b') depict Raman spectra of blood plasma from a 20-year-old woman with homologous serum hepatitis. They were measured during the icteric period (b) and taken 20 days later (b') when the patient was clinically recovered. The spectrum (b) is practically a fluorescence spectrum of blood plasma but the spectrum (b') is similar to that of the healthy woman. Raman spectra (c) and (d) were obtained from a 62-year-old woman with infiltrating mammary carcinoma and from a 64-year-old woman with pseudomucinous papillary cyatadeno carcinoma, respectively. These spectra were also practically fluorescence spectra. Larsson and Hellgren could not measure Raman spectra from the blood plasma of patients but they could use resonance Raman spectra of carotenoid nicely for the marker of healthy samples.

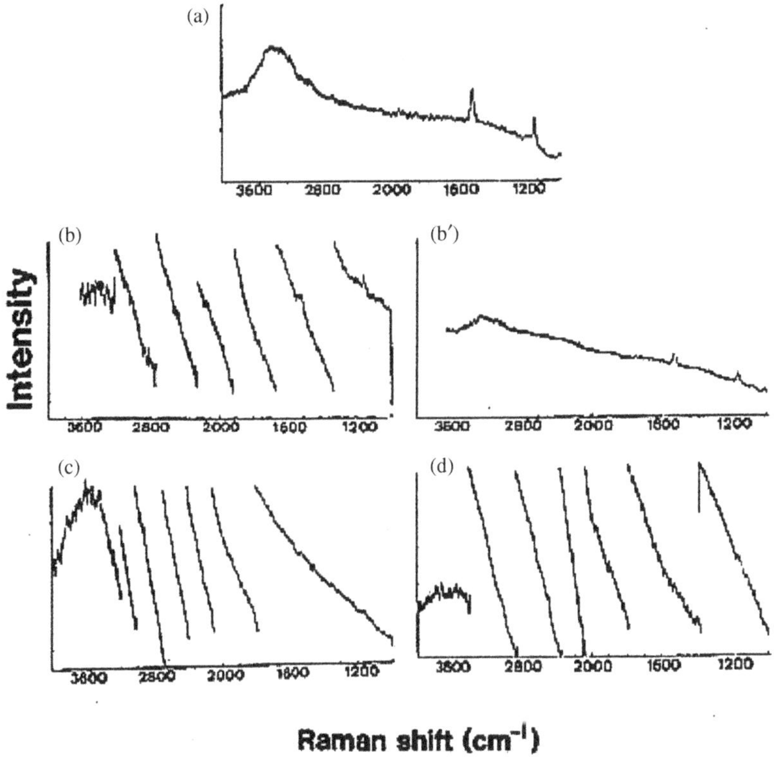

Figure 1.1. (a) A Raman spectrum of blood plasma from a 23-year-old healthy woman. (b) and (b') Raman spectra of blood plasma from a 20-year-old woman with homologous serum hepatitis measured during the icteric period (b) and taken 20 days later (b') when the patient was clinically recovered. (c) and (d) Raman spectra obtained from a 62-year-old woman with infiltrating mammary carcinoma and from a 64-year-old woman with pseudomucinous papillary cyatadeno carcinoma, respectively. Reproduced from Ref. [17] with permission.

1.2.3 *Non-destructive Raman Studies of Eye Lenses and Viruses*

Two great investigations on non-destructive analysis of biological materials were reported by Yu *et al.* [18, 19, 38] (eye lenses) and Thomas *et al.* [20, 21] (viruses) in the 1970s. These studies are really pioneering works in biomedical applications of Raman spectroscopy. Fortunately, young animal lenses and viruses did not show severe fluorescence.

1.2.3.1 *Eye Lens Research*

The main dry components of lens fiber are three lens proteins named α-, β-, and γ-crystallin. Their combined weight accounts for about 33% of the total weight of the lens. Yu *et al.* [18, 19, 38] investigated Raman spectra of whole lenses *in vivo* and also three kinds of crystallines *in vitro*. They showed that using Raman spectroscopy it is possible to monitor *in vivo* or *in vitro* the secondary structure of lens proteins and microenvironments of protein side chains such as tyrosine, tryptophan, and sulfhydryl. They investigated, for example, position-dependent changes in the Raman spectra of whole eye lenses. Figure 1.2 shows variations of SH group content (monitored by SH stretching band at 2582 cm^{-1}) along the visual axis of a six-month-old mouse lens [38]. (For Raman spectra in the whole region of eye lenses, see Figure 1.5). The intensity at 2731 cm^{-1} was used as an indicator of protein concentration. It was revealed from Figure 1.2 that the protein concentration is high at the lens nucleus while the SH content has two maxima in the cortex. The SH groups come from both the proteins and glutathione. The SH content decreases with aging, suggesting that SH to S–S conversion occurs, but the decrease in the SH content is not always equivalent to the increase of the S–S content. This

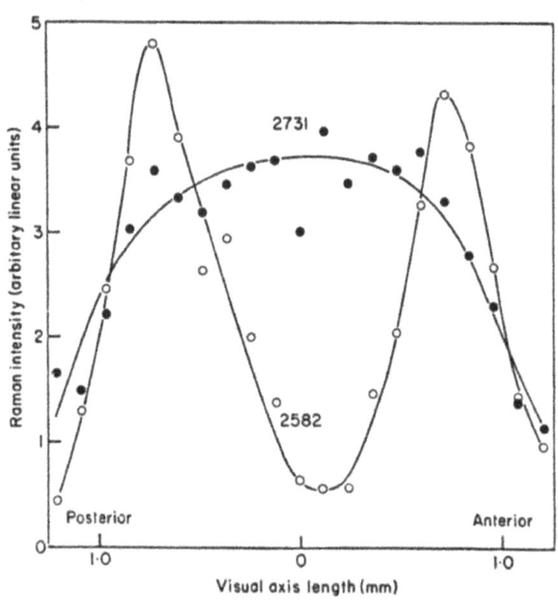

Figure 1.2. Variations of SH group content monitored by the SH stretching band at 2582 cm^{-1} along the visual axis of a six-month-old mouse lens. Reproduced from Ref. [38] with permission.

indicates that α- and β-crystallins, which are low in –SH, have faster synthesis rates of S–S bonds than γ-crystallin, which is high in –SH.

Yu *et al.* [39] also carried out a preliminary experiment for clinical application of Raman spectroscopy for eye lenses. Mathies and Yu were able to measure the Raman spectra of a bovine lens with only 1 mW of laser power, which is below the threshold for retinal damage, using sensitive multichannel detectors.

1.2.3.2 *Virus Research*

Figure 1.3 shows Raman spectra of the native MS2 virus in (a) H_2O and (b) D_2O solutions with band assignments [20]. The virus concentration was ~38 mg/mL. Since the middle of the 1970s Thomas and his coworkers [20, 21] were very active in virus research by Raman spectroscopy. This may be the first example of non-destructive analysis of biological materials. Viruses are relatively simple entities consisting of well-defined proteins and nucleic acid components, and their Raman spectra contain the contributions from both components [20, 21]. MS2 consists of 180 identical coat-protein molecules

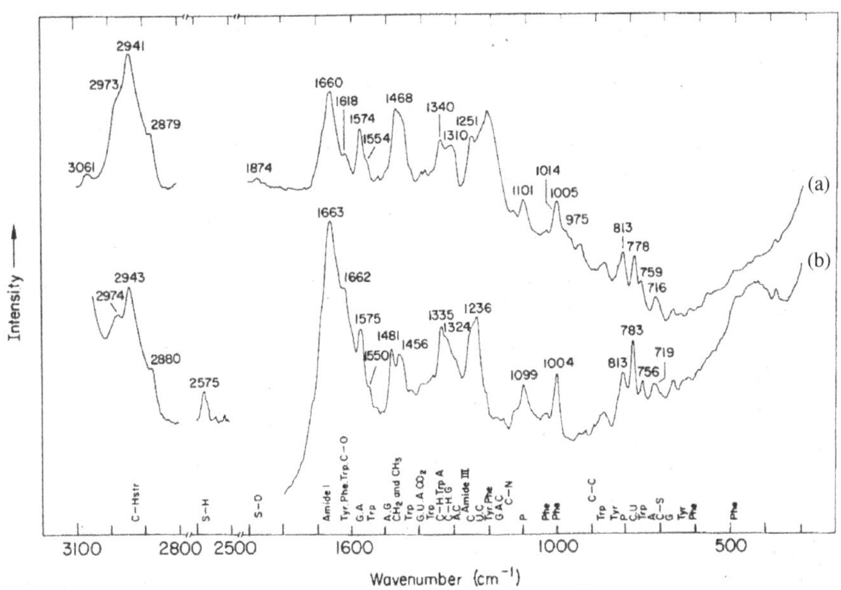

Figure 1.3. Raman spectra of the native MS2 virus in (a) H_2O and (b) D_2O solutions with band assignments. Reproduced from Ref. [20] with permission.

each of molecular weight (MW) 13,750 which make up the capsid or "coat" of the virus, one additional protein molecule of MW 38,000, and one RNA strand of MW 1.1×10^6. When the virus infects its bacterial host, a single protein is thought to enter the host with the RNA, leaving the capsid protein outside.

Thomas *et al.* [20] also measured Raman spectra of the capsid protein with the RNA removed and of the RNA in the absence of capsid. They found that the Raman spectrum of intact MS2 was almost the same as the sum of the spectra of capsid protein and free RNA, indicating that both the protein and RNA did not experience major conformational changes upon separation of these components. From the amide I band at 1660 cm^{-1} and the amide III band at 1236 cm^{-1} (Figure 1.3), Thomas *et al.* concluded that the protein had β structure and random coil structure. A band due to S–S stretching was not observed clearly but a band ascribed to the S–H stretching mode was clearly detected at 2575 cm^{-1}. Thus, it is very likely that most of the cysteine residues assume the reduced S–H forms. As for the RNA moiety, the intensity of the 813 cm^{-1} band in the spectra of intact phase (Figure 1.3) and RNA alone indicates that in both forms more than 85% of the RNA nucleotide residues participate in base-paring and/or base-staking interactions.

In the 1970s *in vivo* Raman spectra of cornea, teeth, dentine, bovine Achilles and muscle including whole muscle, which exhibited relatively little fluorescence background, were also reported [4, 5, 13, 14].

1.2.4 *Studies of Abnormal Hemoglobins by Resonance Raman Spectroscopy*

Resonance Raman spectroscopy played an important role in exploring the structure and function of abnormal hemoglobins (Hb) even in the 1970s. Brunner *et al.* [40] reported resonance Raman spectra of Hb M Iwate ($\alpha^{87\text{His}\rightarrow\text{Tyr}}\beta$) and Hb Zurich ($\alpha\beta^{63\text{His}\rightarrow\text{Arg}}$). The resonance Raman studies, particularly the studies of oxidation state marker bands of hemes in the 1375–1350 cm^{-1} region, revealed that despite the marked differences in O_2 affinity, cooperativity, and preferred quaternary structure among Hb A (normal hemoglobin), Hb M Iwate, and Hb Zurich, the position of the iron atom relative to the heme plane is independent of the quaternary state of these different hemoglobins in either the non-liganded or met forms. In 1980 Nagai and Kitagawa [41] investigated differences in Fe(II)-N_ε(His-F8) stretching frequencies between deoxyhemoglobins in the two alternative quaternary structures using not only normal hemoglobin but also abnormal hemoglobins (Hb M Boston and Hb M Milwakee). These were pioneering studies of molecular medicine.

1.2.5 *Raman Spectroscopy Studies of Biological Molecules and Materials Related to Medical Applications*

The 1970s was the age when Raman studies of biological molecules and materials showed marked progress. Raman spectra of proteins, nucleic acids, lipids, carbohydrates, various chromophores such as carotenoids and chlorophyll, and so on were investigated in detail [13–16]. Those of biomembranes, protein-nucleic acid complexes, visual pigments and photosynthetic pigments were also explored [13–16]. These provided a strong base for medical applications.

Tu *et al.* [42] investigated Raman spectra of snake toxin. This study is a typical Raman study of a protein and is a somewhat related medical application. Figure 1.4 shows Raman spectra of native and heat-denatured *Pelamis platurus*

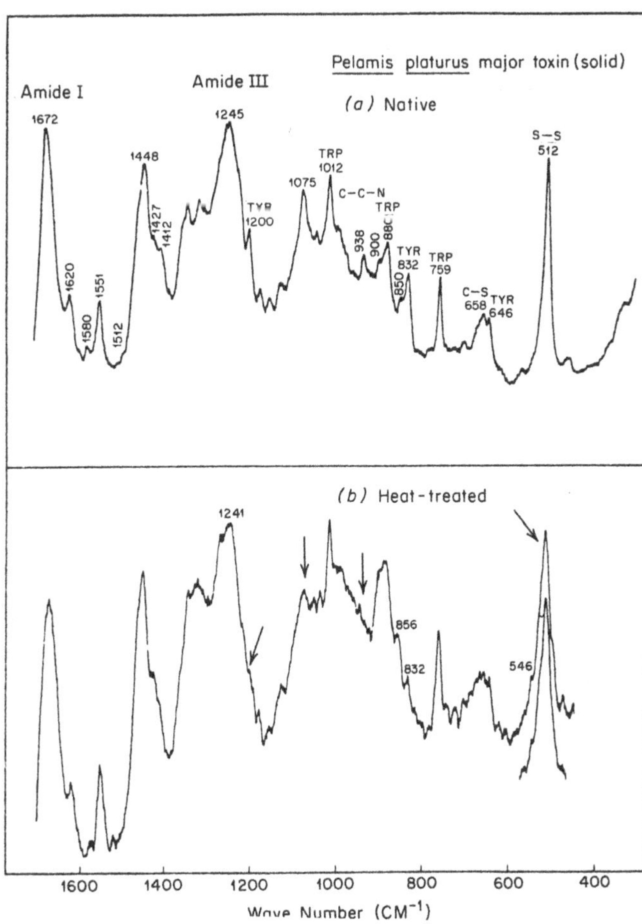

Figure 1.4. Raman spectra of native and heat-denatured *Pelamis platurus* neurotoxin. Reproduced from Ref. [42] with permission.

neurotoxin. The detailed band assignments are given in the figure. It is noted that upon denaturation there are little changes in the frequencies and relative intensities of Amide I and Amide III bands, suggesting that the secondary structure of the protein changes little. A significant change is observed in the relative intensity of the tyrosine doublet at 853 and 832 cm^{-1}. This indicates that tyrosine side chains become exposed upon the heat denaturation. Moreover, in the S–S stretching band region a new band appears at 546 cm^{-1}; note that the S–S stretching band becomes broader upon denaturation. Thus, it is very likely that a small fraction of disulfides, C–C–S–S–C–C, changes to the *trans-gauche-trans* conformation.

In the 1970s low-frequency Raman spectroscopy was already applied to long-chain fatty acids such as lauric acid and stearic acid. Lippert and Peticolas [43] measured Raman spectra in the region of 700–100 cm^{-1} of lauric acid at −12 and 57°C and those of stearic acid at 27 and 77°C. They observed bands due to the accordion vibrations and investigated temperature-dependent structural variations of alkyl chains of these fatty acids.

1.3 Progress in Medical Application of Raman Spectroscopy in the 1980s

In 1982 two great books on biochemical and biological applications of Raman spectroscopy were published [13, 14]. These were milestones in the history of applications of Raman spectroscopy in the life sciences. One could find many applications of Raman spectroscopy to medicine-related fields. In 1988 Ozaki [4] published the first review on application of Raman spectroscopy to medicine. Applications of Raman spectroscopy for cellular analysis were reviewed in 1986 [6].

However, even in the 1980s progress in medical application of Raman spectroscopy was rather slow. Raman spectroscopists battled the fluorescence issue, but the fight was not successful. Resonance Raman spectroscopy was actively used for biochemical and biological applications but not for medical applications. In the 1980s micro-Raman spectroscopy showed significant progress and was used for some medical applications as described later.

1.3.1 *Raman Studies of Lens Aging and Cataractogenesis*

Ozaki *et al.* [4, 22–24] explored the mechanism of cataract formation at the molecular level non-destructively using Raman spectroscopy in 1980s. Their

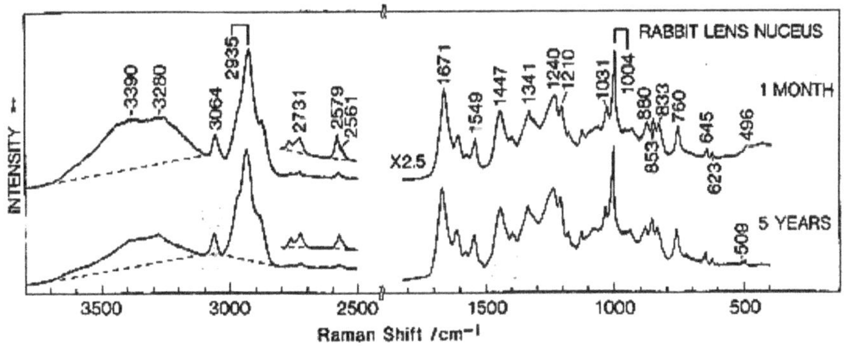

Figure 1.5. Raman spectra of rabbit lenses (nucleus center, one month and five years old). Reproduced from Ref. [22] with permission.

studies demonstrated for the first time the potential of Raman spectroscopy in investigations of disease mechanisms.

Figure 1.5 shows Raman spectra of rabbit lenses (nucleus center, one month and five years old) [22]. The spectra have broad bands in the 3800–3100 cm^{-1} region due to OH stretching modes of water in the lenses, bands in the 3100–2800 cm^{-1} region are assigned to CH stretching modes of lens proteins, and bands at 2579 and 2561 cm^{-1} are ascribed to SH stretching modes of cysteine residues of the proteins. The existence of the two bands at 2579 and 2561 cm^{-1} indicate that there are two kinds of cysteine residues having hydrogen bonds with different strength.

It is noted that the intensities of bands due to water become weak significantly with lens aging. These results suggest that the water content in the eye lenses decreases with lens aging. It was found that one can monitor water content *in situ* by Raman spectroscopy. The intensity decreases in the SH stretching bands, and concomitant intensity increase at 509 cm^{-1} due to the S–S stretching mode of disulfide bonds show the formation of S–S bridges in the lens proteins.

Raman spectral features in the 1800–400 cm^{-1} region are typical protein spectra, consisting of many bands due to Amide I, Amide III, and amino acid residues such as tyrosine, tryptophane and phenylalanine. Amide I and Amide III are observed at 1671 and 1240 cm^{-1}, respectively. Thus, it is very likely that the lens proteins take largely β structure. The Amide I and Amide III bands change little with aging, suggesting that the protein secondary structure varies little with aging.

Figure 1.6(a) and (b) depict age-dependent Raman spectral variations in the 3800–2800 and 2800–2500 cm^{-1} regions of SD-strain rat lens nuclei,

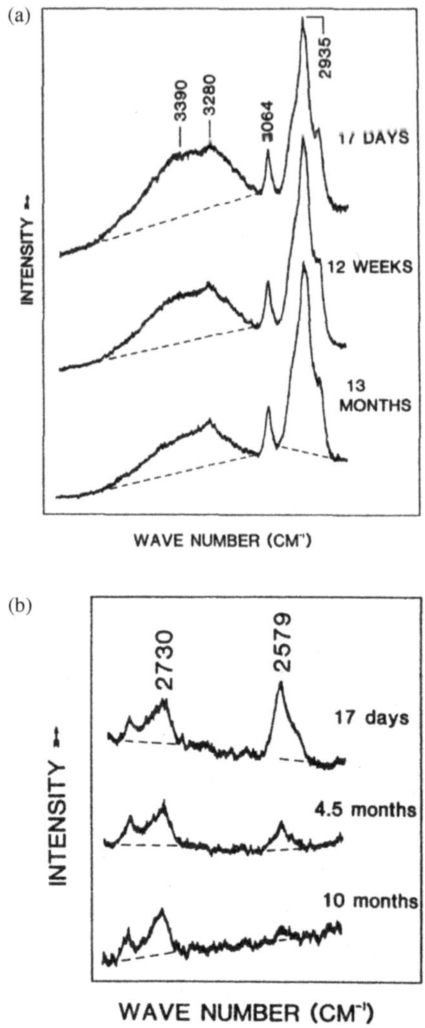

Figure 1.6. Age-dependent Raman spectral variations in the (a) 3800–2800 and (b) 2800–2500 cm^{-1} regions of SD-strain rat lens nuclei. Reproduced from Ref. [23] with permission.

respectively [23]. Figure 1.7(a) and (b) plot the intensity ratio of the two bands at 2579 and 2731 cm^{-1} and that of the two bands at 3390 and 2935 cm^{-1}, respectively. It is noted that both intensity ratios decrease almost in parallel to each other, showing that the formation of S–S stretching bonds proceed with the decrease of water content.

Ozaki *et al.* [24(a)–(b)] explored cataractogenesis *in vivo* using Raman spectroscopy. The causes and processes of lens opacification had been investigated by biochemical and morphological standpoints [24(a)–(b)].

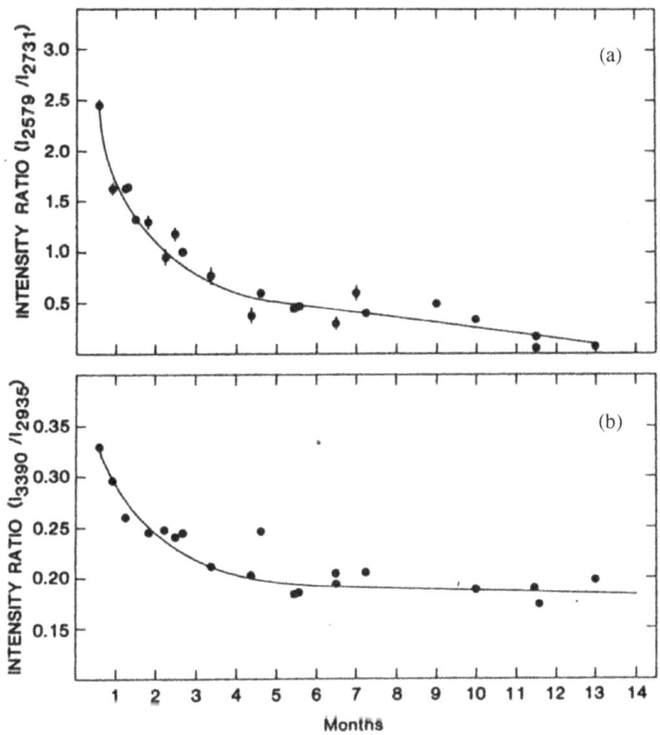

Figure 1.7. (a) The intensity ratio of the two bands at 2579 and 2731 cm^{-1} and (b) that of the two bands at 3390 and 2935 cm^{-1}. Reproduced from Ref. [23] with permission.

The most prominent physicochemical event bringing about lens opacification is the formation of protein aggregates. Figure 1.8 shows Raman spectra of lens nuclei of the cac-strain mice (2.5, 5, and 9 weeks old) [24a]. The cac-strain mice possesses a hereditary defect in the lens; in the mice a cataract appears in the nuclear portion of the lens approximately three weeks after birth, and nuclear opacity is completed within a few weeks. It can be seen from Figure 1.8 that although Amide I and Amide III do not show significant change, the relative intensity of the two bands due to tyrosine residues at 856 and 830 cm^{-1} and that of the two bands ascribed to tryptophan residues at 880 and 760 cm^{-1} vary clearly with the cataract formation. Figure 1.9(a) and (b) plot changes in the relative intensity of the two bands at 880 and 760 cm^{-1} (I_{880}/I_{760}) and that of the two bands at 832 and 855 cm^{-1} (I_{832}/I_{855}) versus age, respectively. It is well known that the relative intensity of the tyrosine doublet is very sensitive to the microenvironment of a tyrosine residue [13, 14]. That of the two tryptophan bands may also reflect the environment of tryptophan residues. Therefore, these results suggest that some buried

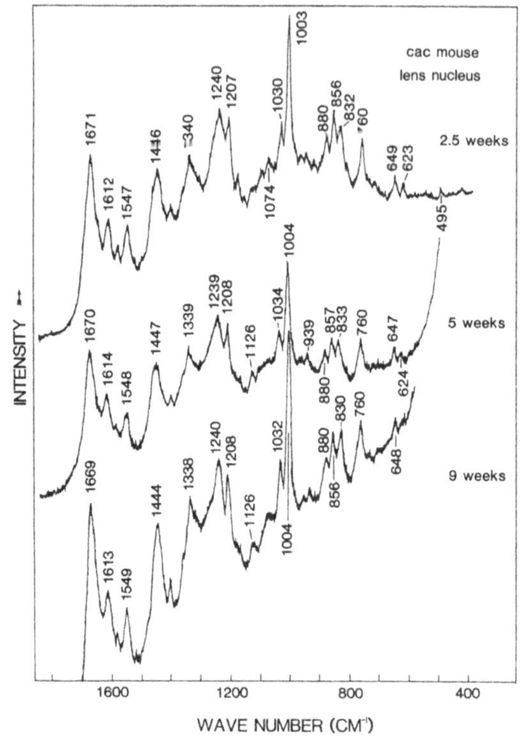

Figure 1.8. Raman spectra of lens nuclei of the cac-strain mice (2.5, 5, and 9 weeks old). Reproduced from Ref. [24a] with permission.

tyrosine and tryptophan residues become exposed with protein aggregation during the formation of cataract [24a].

Emory mouse cataract is a late appearing hereditary cataract. Figure 1.10 presents Raman spectra in the 3800–2800 cm^{-1} region of Emory mice lens nuclei (41 days, 6 and 8 months) [24b]. The lens nuclei for 41 days, 6 and 8 months were clear, hazy, and lightly opaque, respectively. It is interesting to note that the intensity of water band decreases upon going from the 41 days to the 6 months, and then increases upon going from the 6 months to the 8 months. The first decrease indicates that the water content decreases with aging as in the case of ICR-strain mice lens nuclei, while the subsequent increase suggests that the water content increases with the development of cataract. The water content in a lens sensitively reflects the physiological conditions of the lens. For many kinds of cataracts, it is known that the break of the balance of water efflux and influx through the lens membrane initiates a series of physicochemical events that ultimately lead to lens opacification [24b].

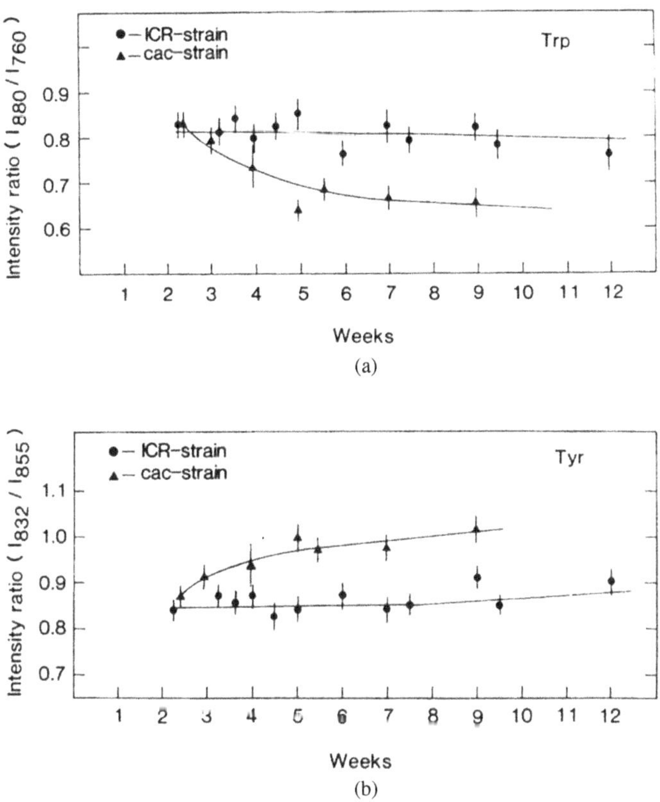

Figure 1.9. (a) Changes in the relative intensity of the two bands at 880 and 760 cm^{-1} (I_{880}/I_{760}) and (b) that of the two bands at 832 and 855 cm^{-1} (I_{832}/I_{855}) versus age. Reproduced from Ref. [24a] with permission.

The idea of using the intensity ratio of OH and CH stretching bands for estimating water content was employed after 2000. For example, Figure 1.11 displays a series of Raman spectra in the CH and OH stretching band region of (a) normal cornea and (b) drug-treated cornea obtained as a function of probing depth into the cornea [44]. The spectra were obtained along the axis of the cornea by a confocal Raman spectrometer. It can be seen from Figure 1.11(b) that hydration in the cornea changes with depth and the drug affects it significantly. Sato *et al.* [45] investigated water content and water structure in brain tissue using the OH stretching bands. Figure 1.12 shows Raman spectra of mice brain in the 3800–2600 cm^{-1} region measured under (a) anesthesia, (b) inhalation of diethyl ether, and (c) within one minute after euthanasia. Of note is that the relative intensity of two water bands at 3397 and 3297 cm^{-1} in the spectrum in Figure 1.12(c) changes significantly. The result

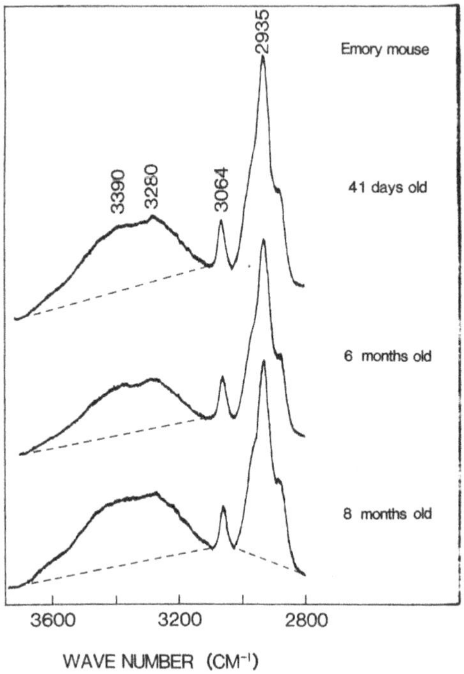

Figure 1.10. Raman spectra in the 3800–2800 cm^{-1} region of Emory mice lens nuclei (41 days, 6 and 8 months). Reproduced from Ref. [24b] with permission.

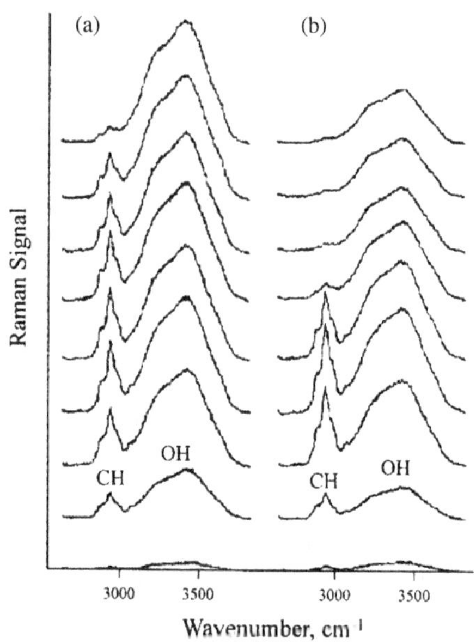

Figure 1.11. A series of Raman spectra in the CH and OH stretching band region of (a) normal cornea and (b) drug-treated cornea obtained as a function of probing depth into the cornea. Reproduced from Ref. [44] with permission.

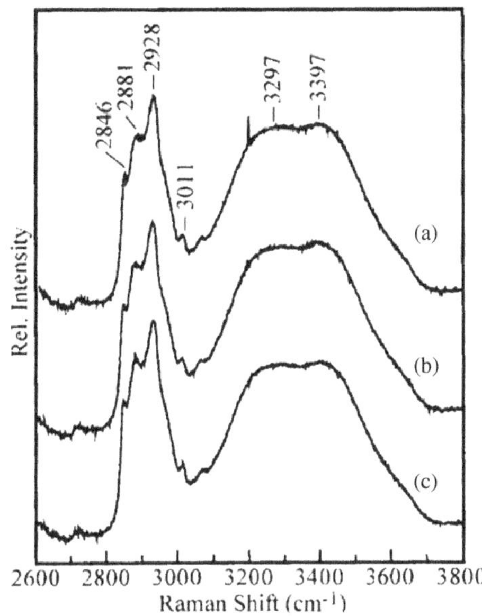

Figure 1.12. Raman spectra of mice brain in the 3800–2600 cm^{-1} region measured under (a) anesthesia, (b) inhalation of diethyl ether, and (c) within one minute after euthanasia. Reproduced from Ref. [15] with permission.

indicates that cluster structure of water changed a little within one minute after euthanasia.

In Chapter 5 Egawa describes her investigation about water content in skin which was based on the 3800–2800 cm^{-1} region of Raman spectra of skin.

1.3.2 *Clinical Applications of Micro-Raman Spectroscopy in the 1980s*

In the 1980s micro-Raman spectroscopy was employed for various applications to biology. Just before the 1980s, in 1979 micro-Raman spectroscopy was used to detect foreign material within a lymph node from a patient with silicon elastomer finger-joint prosthesis [46]. It was found that the Raman spectra of the foreign inclusions in the lymph node and those of prosthesis were identical.

In 1987 Ishida *et al.* [25] reported micro-Raman studies of a cholesterol-type gallstone and a bilirubin-type gallstone using visible excitation. They succeeded in obtaining high-quality Raman spectra because the Raman scattering cross-sections of inorganic and organic substances in the stones were relatively large, and their fluorescence was relatively weak. Moreover, they made combined use of electron probe X-ray microanalysis, Raman microprobe, and IR spectroscopy for the study of the microstructure of gallstones. The microstructure of the cholesterol-type gallstone with a layered structure was studied with particular emphasis. By Raman microprobe it was found that small white particles contained in both cholesterol-type and bilirubin-type gallstones consist of calcium salt of a fatty acid, probably calcium palmitate. Figure 1.13(a) shows Raman spectra of white microcrystalline parts in the bilirubin and cholesterol gallstones, dipalmitoyl phosphating choline (DPPC),

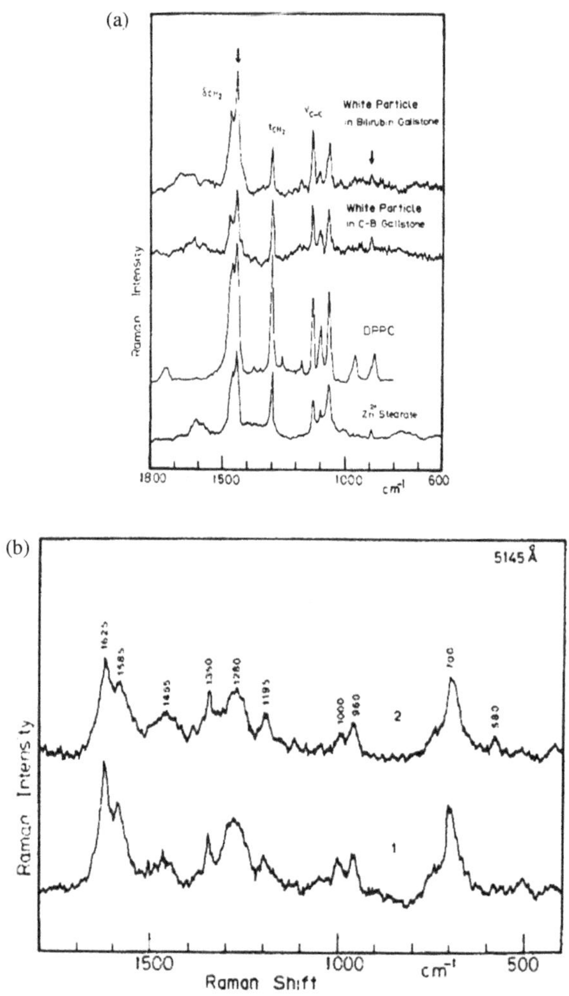

Figure 1.13. (a) Raman spectra of white microcrystalline parts (white particles) in the bilirubin gallstone, those in the cholesterol gallstone, dipalmitoyl phosphating choline (DPPC), and zinc stearate, from top to bottom. (b) Raman spectra of (1) reddish-brown and (2) blackish-brown crystalline parts of the bilirubin-type gallstone. Reproduced from Ref. [25] with permission.

and zinc stearate. It is noted that the spectra of white microcrystalline parts in the two gallstones are similar to each other. They are also similar to that of DPPC, but the formers do not have characteristic bands due to ester and phosphoester groups. In the spectra of white microcrystalline parts in the two gallstones the relative intensity of a band at 1450 cm^{-1} due to the CH_2 bending mode is very intense, and thus Ishida *et al.* concluded that the white microcrystalline parts are long-chain fatty acid salts. The combined use of Raman microprobe, electron probe X-ray microanalysis, and IR suggested that the crystalline parts are palmitic calcium. Figure 1.13(b) depict Raman spectra of (1) reddish-brown and (2) blackish-brown crystalline parts of the bilirubin-type gallstone, respectively. Both spectra are a spectrum of bilirubin, so it was confirmed that the bilirubin gallstone consisted mainly of bilirubin. Electron probe X-ray microanalysis indicated the existence of calcium. Therefore, it was very likely that the stone contained insoluble bilirubin as a calcium salt. These results obtained were very useful for understanding the mechanism of the gallstone formation process.

In 1987 and 1988 Clarke *et al.* [47, 48] carried out the first Raman studies of cardiovascular tissues using 514.5 nm excitation. They could subtract a broad, featureless fluorescence background from the Raman spectra. They ascribed observed Raman bands of calcified tissue and fatty plaques to hydroxyapatites and carotenoids, respectively.

1.4 Innovations in Medical Application of Raman Spectroscopy in the 1990s

In the 1990s there were several innovative advances in the medical application of Raman spectroscopy [5–11]. One was the development of NIR-excited Raman spectroscopy, and another was the development of instruments and devices such as lasers, CCDs, gratings, optical filters and optical fibers. Yet another was to introduce multivariate analysis (at the end of the 1990s) [5, 12]. The advances in confocal micro-Raman spectroscopy are also noted.

1.4.1 *NIR-excited Raman Spectroscopy*

NIR excitation reduces tissue background fluorescence markedly [5–11]. Another advantage is that NIR light can penetrate deeply (of the order of millimeters) into the tissues. This advantage produces a "diagnostic window" into tissues due to its minimal absorption. NIR-excited Raman spectroscopy was initiated with Fourier Transform (FT) Raman spectroscopy in the latter half of the 1980s [26]. Medical application of FT-Raman spectroscopy started with the investigations of artery, aorta, ocular lenses and tissues [5–11, 27–29, 33, 34, 49–51]. Using FT-Raman spectroscopy, Yu *et al.* [49] were able to measure fluorescence-free Raman spectra from pigmented animal and human lenses. They investigated pathological processes such as senile cataract formation, lipid peroxidation, and protein glycation. Feld *et al.* [5, 27, 28] applied FT-Raman spectroscopy to aortic tissues and later an *in situ* quantitative biochemical analysis of normal and diseased tissues for diagnosing atherosclerosis. Various tumor tissues were also investigated by FT-Raman spectroscopy [34, 50, 51]. Here, I introduce our studies of FT-Raman spectra of cancer tissues in some detail as a good example of a medical application of FT-Raman spectroscopy.

Mizuno *et al.* [34] reported non-destructive examination of several kinds of human brain tumors using 1064 nm excited FT-Raman spectroscopy in 1994. Figure 1.14(A) depicts Raman spectra of human glioma (a) grade II and (b) grade III. Of note is that using 1064 nm excitation Mizuno *et al.* could obtain high-quality Raman spectra even from the disease issues. Histological examination of the glioma grade III tissue revealed extracellular PAS-positive materials. There are clear differences between the two spectra in Figure 1.14(A). The spectrum of grade III (Figure 1.14(A)(b)) yields several bands in the 1150–800 cm^{-1} region. These bands may be due to polysaccharides, indicating that the polysaccharides are accumulated in the grade III tissue. Other significant differences between the Raman spectra of the grade II and grade III tissues are a change in the intensity ratio of the two bands at 1664 (Amide I) and 1446 cm^{-1} (CH_2 bending) and an appearance of a sharp band at 1006 cm^{-1} (phenylalanine). These results indicate that the relative content of proteins increases and that of lipids decreases with the procession of the cancer [34].

Raman spectra of human acoustic neurinoma from a 36-year-old female and 43-year-old female patients are shown in Figure 1.14(B)(a) and (b), respectively. The two spectra are relatively similar to each other except for two intense bands at 1527 and 1157 cm^{-1}. These two bands originate from carotenoid, and thus it was concluded that acoustic neurinoma from the 43-year-old female patient contained a small amount of carotenoid.

Figure 1.14(C) presents a Raman spectrum of human central neurocytoma. In this spectrum a band due to hydroxyapatite is observed at 960 cm^{-1}, indicating that calcification occurred in the cancer tissue.

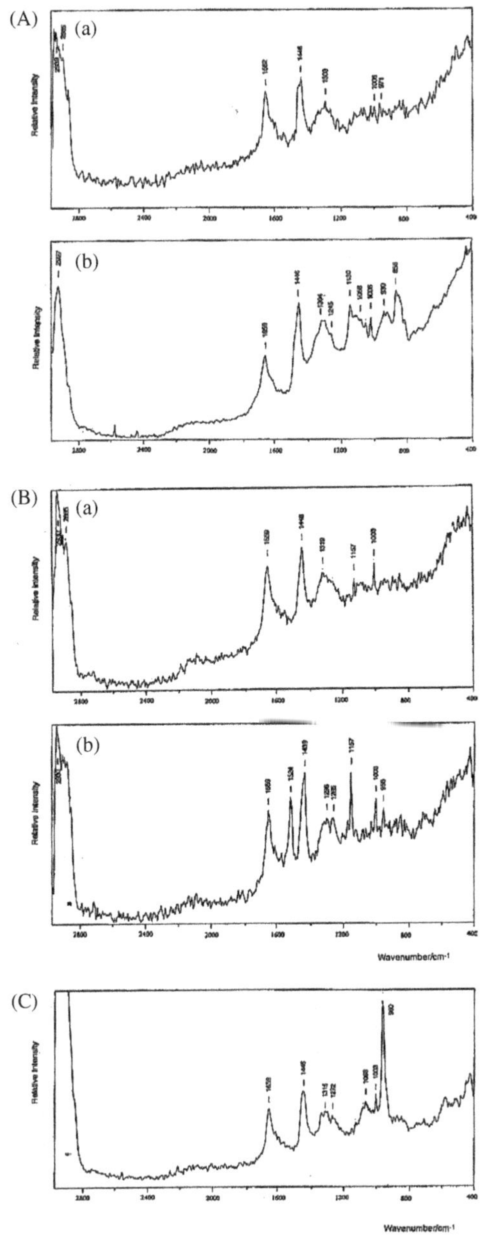

Figure 1.14. (A) Raman spectra of human glioma (a) grade II and (b) grade III. (B) Raman spectra of human acoustic neurinoma from (a) 36-year-old female and (b) 43-year-old female patients. (C) A Raman spectrum of human central neurocytoma. Reproduced from Ref. [34] with permission.

FT-Raman spectroscopy played important roles in medical application of Raman spectroscopy in the first half of the 1990s. However, it has a few disadvantages [5]. First of all, it takes a long time to get a Raman spectrum because InGaAs detectors exhibit substantial noise, requiring long data collection times, usually 30 minutes or so. Another issue for FT-Raman spectroscopy is that it requires high laser power, 200–500 mW. Moreover, one must be careful about the temperature increase of water included in a sample by the 1064 nm excitation.

NIR-excited CCD-based dispersive Raman spectroscopy gradually took over FT-Raman spectroscopy in the middle of the 1990s [5, 30–32], with the developments of compact solid state semiconductor lasers, optical filters, and CCD detectors. Already in the early 1990s Feld *et al.* showed that excitation wavelengths in the 800 nm range were optimal to minimize tissue fluorescence while best taking advantage of cooled CCD detectors [5]. There were many examples of NIR-excited CCD-based dispersive Raman studies of biological tissues. For example, in 1992 *in vitro* laboratory analysis of aorta tissues was carried out using 810 nm excitation [5]. The 830 nm excitation was also tried, which reduced fluorescence interference further, and in 1997 Brennan *et al.* described a NIR Raman *in vitro* laboratory system and a prototype *in vitro* clinical system for tissue analysis [52]. They have also demonstrated the usefulness of NIR Raman spectroscopy with CCD detection for exploring cancerous changes in the colon, urinary bladder, breast and soft tissue sacromas [5]. Puppels and co-workers [53, 54] used NIR Raman spectroscopy to characterize esophageal cancer and various skin lesions using a fiber-optic Raman instrument. Richards-Kortum's group [7, 11, 55] investigated NIR Raman spectroscopy to differentiate cervical pre-cancers from non-malignant variations.

Fiber-optic Raman probes for biomedical applications started to develop from the mid-1990s [56–61]. For example, Feld *et al.* [57], Wach and Marple [58], Puppeles *et al.* [59] and Sim *et al.* [60] developed a fiber-optic Raman probe for medical applications. In 1998 Richards-Kortum's group proposed a fiber-optic Raman probe for *in vivo* studies of cervical pre-cancers and collected initial spectra during colposcopy [61]. Sato *et al.* developed a thinner Raman microprobe with a diameter of only 0.6 mm in 2005 [56(a)–(b)] (for more details, see Chapter 16).

1.4.2 *UV resonance Raman Spectroscopy*

UV resonance Raman spectroscopy is another useful method to overcome the fluorescence issue. Since the middle of the 1970s, it was used extensively to study biological molecules such as proteins and nucleic acids and later to investigate even bacteria cells [62–64]. Using UV resonance Raman spectroscopy, one can expect a remarkable increase in Raman intensity partly due to the resonance Raman effect and partly due to the fourth-power frequency dependence of Raman scattering intensity. On the other hand, UV resonance Raman has two major disadvantages: one is that the tissue penetration depth is of the order of microns, so this technique is only suitable for probing superficial abnormalities. Another disadvantage is that UV light may induce mutagenesis. In comparison with NIR excitation, the applications of UV resonance Raman are limited. However, one can find some interesting results. Nelson's group [63(a)] was the first who investigated the applications of UV resonance Raman spectroscopy for quantitative *in situ* assay of chemical markers such as quinones, lipids, nucleic acids and proteins in microorganisms and for potential detection and identification of bacterial cells. Turpin *et al.* [63(b)] succeeded in exciting selectively nucleic acids from a single T84 cancer cell using 257 nm excitation. Richards-Kortum's group [64] reported the 257 nm excited resonance Raman spectra of normal and malignant breast and cervical cell cultures.

1.4.3 *Developments of Raman Instruments and Devices in the 1990s*

FT-Raman spectroscopy played a significant role in the biomedical application of Raman spectroscopy in the former half of the 1990s, but dispersive NIR Raman spectroscopy took over in the middle of the decade. CCDs showed remarkable progress during the 1990s [5]. Different types of CCDs such as front-illuminated, thinned back-illuminated and front- or back-illuminated deep depletion types were developed for different purposes. For NIR excitation, deep-depletion CCDs were most suitable. It was widely recognized that liquid nitrogen-cooled, silicon-based CCD detectors are efficient up to wavelengths of about 1100 nm, and have extremely low dark noise [5].

Clinical applications of Raman spectroscopy require rapid acquisition of high-quality spectral data using low-power laser excitation. The development of CCD induced the advances in spectrographs. Both the high-throughput and flat image field at the detector plane with high spectra resolution were obtained by fiber optic f-number matched holographic spectrographs. We should not forget the marked progress of holographic gratings in the 1990s.

The appearance of holographic notch filters enabled one to eliminate the need for low-throughput, multistage scanning spectrometers, and it was critical for rapid spectral data acquisition. For clinical applications, all components of the optical fibers must have suitable size for incorporation into needles, endoscopes, angioscopes and other clinical devices. One of the most serious problems of optical fiber probes is spectral interferences from the optical fibers themselves. The problems of fiber fluorescence and absorption can be minimized by selecting readily available, high-purity, low-hydroxyl fibers, but generation of Raman-scattered light in the optical fibers was more serious. It interfaces with Raman signals from the tissue investigated. Raman scattering was generated both in the excitation and collection fibers. Nowadays, these problems have almost been solved by attaching a filter at the top of each fiber.

1.4.4 *Application of Confocal Raman Microscopy to Medical Samples in the 1990s*

Confocal Raman microscopy was already used extensively in the 1990s. In confocal Raman microscopy, only a small, well-defined volume of tissue is sampled, thus giving rise to increased spatial resolution and rejection of background light (see, for example, [65(a)–(b)]). Using confocal Raman microscopy, Greve *et al.* investigated DNA in chromosomes [66(a)–(b)] and pigments in granulocytes and lymphocytes with very high spatial resolution [67]. Confocal Raman microscopy was also applied to the analysis of changes in cholesterol, phospholipid and protein in cataract lens [68]. Morris *et al.* [69] started Raman studies of bone and cartilage at the end of the 1990s and extended them in the 2000s using Raman microscopy.

1.4.5 *Developments of Clinical Raman Systems in the 1990s*

In the latter half of the 1990s several research groups developed clinical Raman systems using different configurations to obtain *in vivo* Raman spectra [61, 70–75]. Puppels *et al.* [72, 73] measured *in vivo* Raman spectra of the esophagus using an optical fiber probe. Feld and his coworkers [5, 74, 75] developed a portable Raman system, which is simple to operate and fully functional in a hospital catheterization laboratory or operating room. Figure 1.15 illustrates a clinical Raman system designed for rapid data acquisition, portability, and safety in a hospital environment [5]. In the system a single-mode diode laser operating at 830 nm coupled to an optical fiber probe was used. The probe was directly coupled to a high-throughput *f*-number matched holographic imaging spectrograph, giving 10 cm^{-1} resolution. A liquid nitrogen-cooled,

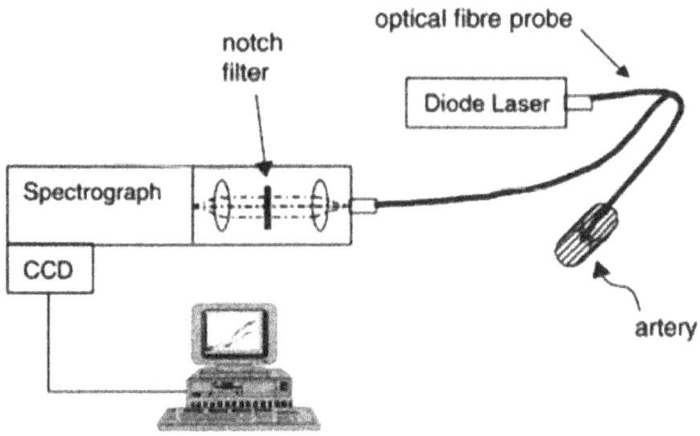

Figure 1.15. A clinical Raman system designed for rapid data acquisition, portability, and safety in a hospital environment. Reproduced from Ref. [5] with permission.

back-thinned, deep-depletion CCD with 1024 × 256 pixels was used, and they could measure *in vivo* Raman spectra of peripheral arteries in only a few seconds.

1.4.6 *Developments of Spectral Analysis Methods in the 1990s*

Raman spectral analysis methods have long been investigated. In the 1970s one can say conventional Raman spectral analysis was already established. They were advanced further in the 1990s thanks to the developments of Raman instruments, computers, and software. The conventional spectral analysis methods used in the 1990s are summarized as follows:

(1) Spectral analysis based on group frequencies

(2) Calculation of derivative spectra

(3) Calculation of difference spectra

Calculations of derivative spectra and difference spectra became much easier from the 1990s.

(4) Spectra-structure correlations

(5) Spectral analysis based on perturbation

(6) Spectral interpretation by polarization measurement

(7) Isotope exchange experiments

A new spectral analysis method used in medical application of Raman spectroscopy in the 1990s was chemometrics [76,77]. Chemometrics was born around 1960s–70s. It developed markedly in the 1980s. Application of chemometrics to medical applications of Raman spectra started at the end of the 1990s [5]. Principal component analysis and partial least squares regression were used for classification and quantitative analysis of Raman data. Quantum chemical calculations were introduced to Raman spectroscopy in the second half of the 1980s, and in the 1990s they were used for Raman spectra analysis of rather simple biological molecules.

In the 1990s development of spectral pre-treatment methods was also noted. Four kinds of data pre-treatment methods — noise reduction methods, baseline correction methods, resolution enhancement methods, and centering and normalization methods — were investigated and used.

1.4.7 *The use of CARS and SERS in Medical Applications in the 1990s*

Coherent Anti-Stokes Raman Spectroscopy (CARS) was first reported in 1964 and 1965 by Yajima and Takasuji [78] and by Maker and Terhune [79], respectively. In the 1970s it was used as a useful Raman technique to avoid fluorescence [80, 81]. One can find some examples in biochemical applications such as those to flavin adenine dinucleotide and bacteriorhodopsin. It was in 1982 that Duncan *et al.* [82] first demonstrated CARS microscopy using non-collinear pump, Stokes visible dye laser beams and two-dimensional detector to collect anti-Stokes beam in the phase-matching direction. In 1999 Zumbusch *et al.* [83] revived CARS microscopy using tightly focused, collinearly propagating pump and Stokes NIR laser beams for CARS detection in the forward direction. Hashimoto *et al.* [84] also developed a new type of CARS microscope. Application of CARS microscopy to biomedical problems has become popular after 2000. Kano *et al.* describes the principles and applications of CARS in Chapter 9.

SERS made remarkable progress in the 1990s, particularly after the observations of single-molecule SERS by Kneipp *et al.* [85] and Nie *et al.* [86]. Application of SERS to biomedical applications thus became active in the 1990s. Vo-Dinh *et al.* [87] developed SERS gene probe in 1994 for HIV detection [88]. Several interesting SERS immunoassay studies were carried out in the 1990s [89, 90]. For example, our group reported enzyme immunoassay utilizing SERS of the enzyme reaction product [90]. In this study we proposed the "indirect SERS" method. We also carried out SERS-based quantitative analysis of double-stranded DNA amplified by polymerase chain reaction [91]. At that time, it was not easy to measure SERS of DNA. SERS was also applied to the study of bacteria in the 1990s [92]. In 1998 nanoparticles were prepared *in situ* in bacteria suspension for SERS [92].

Acknowledgement

I would like to thank Prof. Hidetoshi Sato of Kwansei Gakuin University, Japan, for fruitful discussion during the preparation of this review.

References

1. Long, D. A. (2002) *The Raman Effect*, John Wiley & Sons.
2. Vandenabeele, P. (2013) *Practical Raman Spectroscopy: An Introduction*, John Wiley & Sons.
3. Smith, E. and Dent, G. (2019) *Modern Raman Spectroscopy: A Practical Approach*, John Wiley & Sons.
4. Ozaki, Y. (1988) Medical application of Raman spectroscopy. Appl. Spectrosc. Rev. **24**, 259–312.
5. Hanlon, E. B., Manoharan, R., Koo, T.-W., Schafer, K. E., Motz, J. T., Fitzmaurice, M., Kramer, J. R., Itzkan, I., Dasari, R. R. and Feld, M. S. (2000) Prospects for *in vivo* Raman spectroscopy. Phys. Med. Biol. **45**, 1–59.
6. Butterfield, D. A. (1986) Spectroscopic methods in degenerative neurological diseases. CRC Crit. Rev. Clin. Neurobiol. **2**, 169–240.
7. Mahadevan-Jensen, A. and Richards-Kortum, R. (1996) Raman spectroscopy for the detection of cancers and precancers. J. Biomed. Opt. **1**, 31–70.
8. Schrader, B., Dippel, B., Fendel, S., Keller, S., Lochte, T., Riedl, M., Schulte, R. and Tatsch, E. (1997) NIR FT Raman spectroscopy — a new tool in medical diagnostics. J. Mol. Struct. **408**, 23–31.
9. Lawson, E. E., Barry, B. W., Williams, A. C. and Edwards, H. G. (1997) Biomedical applications of Raman spectroscopy. J. Raman Spectrosc. **28**, 111–117.
10. Manoharan, R., Wang, Y., Dasari, R. R., Singer, S., Rava, R. P. and Feld, M. S. (1995) UV resonance Raman spectroscopy for detection of colon cancer. Lasers Life Sci. **6**, 217–227.
11. Richards-Kortum, R. and Sevick-Muraca, E. (1996) Quantitative optical spectroscopy for tissue diagnosis. Ann. Rev. Phys. Chem. **47**, 455–606.
12. Matousek, P. and Morris, M. D. (2010) *Emerging Raman Applications and Techniques in Biomedical and Pharmaceutical Fields*, Springer.
13. Tu, A. T. (1982) *Raman Spectroscopy in Biology: Principles and Applications*, John Wiley & Sons.
14. Carry, P. R. (1982) *Biochemical Applications of Raman and Resonance Raman Spectroscopies*, Academic Press.

15. Spiro, T. G. (Ed.) (1988) *Biological Applications of Raman Spectroscopy*, John Wiley & Sons.
16. Diem, M. (1993) *Modern Vibrational Spectroscopy*, John Wiley & Sons.
17. Larsson, K. and Hellgren, L. (1974) A study of the combined Raman and fluorescence scattering from human blood plasma. Experientia **30**, 481–483.
18. Yu, N. T. and East, E. J. (1975) Laser Raman spectroscopic studies of ocular lens and its isolated protein fractions. J. Biol. Chem. **250**, 9126.
19. Yu, N. T., DeNagel, D. C. and Kuck, J. F. R. (1987) Ocular Lenses. In *Biological Applications of Raman Spectroscopy* (Spiro, T. G., ed.), pp. 47–80, John Wiley & Sons.
20. Thomas, Jr. G. J., Prescott, B., Macdonald-Ordzie, P. E. and Harman, K. A. (1976) Studies of virus structure by laser Raman spectroscopy II. MS2 phase, MS2 capsid, and MS2 RNA in aqueous solutions. J. Mol. Biol. **102**, 103.
21. Thomas, Jr. G. J. and Murphy, P. (1975) Structures of coat proteins in Pfl fd virions by laser Raman spectroscopy. Science **188**, 1205.
22. Ozaki, Y., Mizuno, A., Kamada, Y., Itoh, K. and Iriyama, K. (1982) Laser Raman spectroscopic study of a diabetic cataract. Chem. Lett. **1982**, 887–890.
23. Ozaki, Y., Mizuno, A., Itoh, K., Yoshiura, M., Iwamoto, T. and Iriyama, K. (1983) Raman spectroscopic study of age-related structural changes in the lens proteins of an intact lens. Biochemistry **22**, 6254–6259.
24. (a) Itoh, K., Ozaki, Y., Mizuno, A. and Iriyama, K. (1983) Structural changes in lens proteins of hereditary cataract monitored by Raman spectroscopy. Biochemistry **22**, 1773–1778. (b) Ozaki, Y., Mizuno, A., Itoh, K., Matsushima, S. and Iriyama, K. (1982) Raman spectroscopic study of cataract formation: Emory mouse cataract. Appl. Spectrosc. **41**, 597–605.
25. Ishida, H., Kamoto, R., Uchida, S., Ishitani, A., Ozaki, Y., Iriyama, K., Tsukie, T., Shibata, K., Ishihara, F. and Kameda, H. (1987) Raman microprobe and Fourier transform-infrared microsampling studies of the microstructure of gallstones. Appl. Spectrosc. **41**, 407–412.
26. Hirschfeld, T. and Chase, B. (1986) FT-Raman spectroscopy — development and justification. Appl. Spectrosc. **40**, 133–137.
27. Rava, R. P., Baraga, J. J. and Feld, M. S. (1991) Near-infrared Fourier-transform Raman-spectroscopy of human artery. Spectrochim. Acta A **47**, 509–512.
28. Manoharan, R., Baraga, J. J., Feld, M. S. and Rava, R. P. (1992) Quantitative histochemical analysis of human artery using Raman spectroscopy. J. Photochem. Photobiol. B **16**, 211–233.
29. Liu, C. H., Glassman, W. L. S., Zhu, H. R., Akins, D. L., Deckelbaum, L. I., Stetz, M. L., O'Brien, K., Scott, J. and Alfano, R. R. (1992) Near-IR Fourier transform Raman spectroscopy of normal and atherosclerotic human aorta. Lasers Life Sci. **4**, 257–264.
30. Wang, Y. and McCreery, R. L. (1989) Evaluation of a diode-laser charge coupled device spectrometer for near-infrared Raman-spectroscopy. Anal. Chem. **61**, 2647–2651.

31. Williamson, J. M., Bowling, R. J. and McCreery, R. L. (1989) Near-infrared Raman-spectroscopy with a 783-nm diode-laser and CCD array detector. Appl. Spectrosc. **43**, 372–375.
32. McCreery, R. L. (1995) *Raman Spectroscopy for Chemical Analysis*, John Wiley & Sons.
33. Mizuno, A., Hayashi, T., Tashibu, K., Maraishi, S., Kawauchi, K. and Ozaki, Y. (1992) Near-infrared FT-Raman spectra of the rat-brain tissues. Neurosci. Lett. **141**, 47–52.
34. Mizuno, A., Kitajima, H., Kawauchi, K., Muraishi, S. and Ozaki, Y. (1994) Near infrared Fourier transform Raman spectroscopic study of human brain tissues and tumours. J. Raman Spectrosc. **25**, 265–269.
35. Spiro, T. G. and Strekas, T. C. (1972) Resonance Raman spectra of hemoglobin and cytochrome *c*: Inverse polarization and vibronic scattering. Proc. Natl Acad. Sci. **69**, 2622.
36. Webb, S. J., Lee, R. A. and Stoneham, M. E. (1977) Possible viral involvement in human mammary carcinoma: A microwave and laser Raman study. Int. J. Quant. Chem. **4**, 277.
37. Morris, M. D. (1975) Resonance Raman spectra of the aminochromes some biochemically important catecholamines. Anal. Chem. **47**, 2457.
38. Askren, C. C., Yu, N. T. and Kuck, Jr. J. F. R. (1979) Variation of concentration sulfhydryl along the visual axis of aging lenses by laser Raman optical dissection technique. Exp. Eye Res. **29**, 647.
39. Mathies, R. and Yu, N. T. (1978) Raman spectroscopy with intensified vidicon detections: A study of intact bovine lens proteins. J. Raman Spectrosc. **7**, 349.
40. Brunner, H., Mayer, A. and Gersonde, K. (1974) A Resonance Raman study of Hb M Iwate ($\alpha^{87His \rightarrow Tyr}\beta$) and Hb Zurich ($\alpha\beta^{63His \rightarrow Arg}$). FEBS Lett. **48**, 141–144.
41. Nagai, K. and Kitagawa, T. (1980) Differences in Fe(II)-N_ε(His-F8) stretching frequencies between deoxyhemoglobins in the two alternative quaternary structures. Proc. Natl. Acad. Sci. **77**, 2033–2037.
42. Tu, A. T., Jo, B. H. and Yu, N. T. (1976) Laser Raman spectroscopy of snake venom neurotoxin: Conformation. Int. J. Pept. Prot. Res. **8**, 337.
43. Lippert, J. L. and Peticolas, W. L. (1972) Raman active vibrations in long-chain fatty acid and phospholipid sonicates. Biochim. Biophys. Acta **282**, 8.
44. Erekens, R. G., Jongsma, F. H. M., Wicksted, J. P., Hendrikse, F. and Motamedi, M. (2001) Drug-induced corneal hydration changes monitored in vivo by non-invasive confocal Raman spectroscopy. J. Raman Spectrosc. **32**, 733–737.
45. Sato, H., Yamamoto, S. Y., Maruyama, A., Katagiri, T., Matsuura, Y. and Ozaki, Y. (2009) Raman study of brain functions in live mice and rats: A pilot study. Vib. Spectrosc. **50**, 125–130.
46. Abraham, J. L. and Etz, E. S. (1979) Molecular microanalysis of pathological specimens in situ with a laser Raman microprobe. Science **206**, 716–718.
47. Clarke, R. H., Hanlon, E. B., Isner, J. M. and Brody, H. (1987) Laser Raman spectroscopy of calcified atherosclerotic lesions in cardiovascular tissue. Appl. Opt. **26**, 3175–3177.

48. Clarke, R. H., Wang, Q. and Isner, J. M. (1988) Laser Raman spectroscopy of atherosclerotic lesions in human coronary artery segments. Appl. Opt. **27**, 4799–4800.
49. Nie, S. M., Bergbauer, K. L., Kuck, J. F. R. and Yu, N. T. (1990) Near-infrared Fourier-transform Raman-spectroscopy in human lens research. Exp. Eye Res. **51**, 619–623.
50. Alfano, R. R., Liu, C. H., Sha, W. L., Zhu, H. R., Akins, D. L., Cleary, J., Prudente, R. and Clemer, E. (1991) Human breast tissues studied by IR Fourier transform Raman spectroscopy. Lasers Life Sci. **4**, 23–28.
51. Keller, S., Schrader, B., Hoffman, A., Schrader, W., Metz, K., Rehlaender, A., Pahnke, J., Ruwe, M. and Budach, W. (1994) Application of near-infrared Fourier-transform Raman spectroscopy in medical research. J. Raman Spectrosc. **25**, 663–671.
52. Brennan, J. F., Wang, Y., Dasari, R. R. and Feld, M. S. (1997) Near-infrared Raman spectrometer systems for human tissue studies. Appl. Spectrosc. **51**, 201–208.
53. Puppels, G. J. (1997) Development of in vivo diagnostic tools based on Raman spectroscopy. *24th Annual Conference of the Federation of Analytical Chemistry and Spectroscopy Societies (FACSS)*. Santa Fe, NM.
54. Caspers, P. J., Lucassen, G. W., Wolthuis, R., Bruining, H. A. and Puppels, G. J. (1998) *In vitro* and *in vivo* Raman spectroscopy of human skin. Biospectroscopy **4**, S31–S39.
55. Mahadevan-Jensen, A., Mitchell, M. F., Ramanujam, N., Malpica, A., Thompsen, S., Utzinger, U. and Richards-Kortum, R. (1998) NIR Raman spectroscopy for *in vitro* detection of cervical precancers. Photochem. Photobiol. **68**, 123–132.
56. (a) Sato, H., Shinzawa, H. and Komachi, Y. (2010) Fiber-optic Raman Probes for Biomedical and Pharmaceutical Applications. In *Emerging Raman Applications and Techniques in Biomedical and Pharmaceutical Fields* (Matousek, P. and Morris, M. D., Eds.), pp. 25–46, Springer. (b) Komachi, H., Sato, H., Matsuura Y., Miyagi, M. and Tashiro, H. (2005) Raman probe using a single hollow waveguide. Opt. Lett. **30**, 2942–2944.
57. Kittrell, C., Cothren, R. M. Jr. and Feld, M. S. (1994) U. S. Patent 5304173.
58. Wach, M. L. and Marple, E. T. (1997) Patent application WO 97/34175.
59. Buschman, H. P., Marple, E. T., Wach, M. L., Benett, B., Bakker Schut, T. C., Bruining, H. A., Bruschke, A. V., van der Laarse, A. and Puppels, G. J. (2000) In vivo determination of the molecular composition of artery wall by intravascular Raman spectroscopy. Anal. Chem. **72**, 3771–3775.
60. Shim, M. G., Wilson, B. C., Marple, E. and Wach, M. (1999) Study of fiber-optic probes in vivo medical Raman spectroscopy. Appl. Spectrosc. **53**, 619–627.
61. Mahadevan-Jensen, A., Mitchell, M. F., Ramanujam, N., Utzinger, U. and Richards-Kortum, R. (1998) Development of a fiber optic probe to measure NIR Raman spectra of cervical tissue in vivo. Photochem. Photobiol. **68**, 427–431.

62. (a) Asher, S. A. and Johnson, C. R. (1984) Raman-spectroscopy of a coal liquid shows that fluorescence interference is minimized with ultraviolet excitation. Science **225**, 311–313. (b) Fodor, S. P. A., Rava, R. P., Copel, R. A. and Spiro, T. G. (1986) H-2Raman-shifted YAG laser ultraviolet Raman spectrometer operating at wavelengths down to 184 nm. J. Raman Spectrosc. **17**, 471–475. (c) Asher, S. A. (1988) UV resonance Raman studies of molecular-structure and dynamics — applications in physical and biophysical chemistry. Ann. Rev. Phys. Chem. **39**, 537–558.
63. (a) Nelson, W. H., Manoharan, R. and Sperry, J. F. (1992) UV resonance Raman studies of bacteria. Appl. Spectrosc. Rev. **27**, 67–124. (b) Sureau, F., Chinsky, L., Amirand, C., Ballini, J. P., Duquesne, M., Laigle, A., Turpin, P. Y. and Vigny, P. (1990) An ultraviolet micro Raman spectrometer — resonance Raman spectroscopy within single living cells. Appl. Spectrosc. **44**, 1047–1051.
64. Yazdi, Y., Ramanujam, N., Lotan, R., Mitchell, M. F., Hittelman, W. and Richards-Kortum, R. (1999) Resonance Raman spectroscopy at 257 nm excitation of normal and malignant cultured breast and cervical cells. Appl. Spectrosc. **53**, 82–85.
65. (a) Turrell, G. and Corset, J. (Eds.) (1996) *Raman Microscopy*, John Wiley & Sons. (b) Puppels, G. J., Demul, F. F. M., Otto, C., Greve, J., Robertnicoud, M., Arndtjovin, D. J. and Jovin, T. M. (1990) Studying single living cells and chromosomes by confocal Raman microspectroscopy. Nature **347**, 301–303.
66. Puppels, G. J., Otto, C., Greve, J., Robert-Nicoud, M., Arndt-Jvin, D. J. and Jovin, T. M. (1994) Raman microspectroscopic study of low pH induced changes in DNA structure of polytene chromosomes Biochemistry **33**, 3386–3395. (b) Puppels, G. J., Garristen, H. S. P., Kummer, J. A. and Greve, J. (1993) Carotenoids located in human lymphocyte subpopulations and natural killer cells by Raman microspectroscopy. Cytometry **14**, 251–256.
67. Bakker Schut, T. C., Puppels, G. J., Kraan, Y. M., Greve, J., van der Maas, L. L. and Figdor, C. G. (1997) Intracellular carotenoid levels measured by Raman microspectrocopy: comparison of lymphocytes from lung cancer patients and healthy individuals. Int. J. Cancer **74**, 20–25.
68. Duindam, J. J., Vrensen, G. F., Otto, C. and Greve, J. (1998) Cholesterol, phospholipids, and protein changes in focal opacities in the human eye lens. Invest. Ophthalmol. Vis. Sci. **39**, 94–103.
69. Morris, M. D. (2010) Raman Spectroscopy of Bone and Cartilage. In *Emerging Raman Applications and Techniques in Biomedical and Pharmaceutical Fields* (Matousek, P. and Morros, M. D., Eds.), pp. 347–364, Springer.
70. Shim, M. G. and Wilson, B. C. (1997) Development of an in vivo Raman spectroscopic system for diagnostic applications. J. Raman Spectrosc. **28**, 131–142.
71. Mahadevan-Jensen, A., Mitchell, M. F., Ramanujam, N., Malpica, A., Thompsen, S., Utzinger, U. and Richards-Kortum, R. (1998) NIR Raman spectroscopy for in vivo detection. Photochem. Photobiol. **68**, 123–132.

72. Puppels, G. J., Otto, C., Greve, J., Robert-Nicoud, M., Arndt-Jovin, J. and Jovin, T. M. (1994) Raman microspectroscopic study of low-pH-induced changes in DNA structure of polytene chromosomes. Biochemistry **33**(11), 3386–3395.
73. Puppels, G. J., van Aken, T., Wolthuis, R., Caspers, P. J., Bakker Schut, T. C., Bruining, H. A., Romer, T. J., Buschman, H. P. J., Wach, M. L. and Robinson, J. S. J. (1998) *In vivo* tissue characterization by Raman spectroscopy. Proc. BIOS/SPIE **3257**, 78–83.
74. Brennan, J. F., Wang, Y., Dasari, R. R. and Feld, M. S. (1997) Near-infrared Raman spectrometer systems for human tissue studies. Appl. Spectrosc. **51**, 201–208.
75. Salenius, J. P., Brennan, J. F., Miller, A., Wang, Y., Aretz, T., Sacks, B., Dasari, R. R. and Feld, M. S. (1998) Biochemical composition of human peripheral arteries using near infrared Raman spectroscopy. J. Vasc. Surg. **27**, 710–719.
76. Martens, H. and Martens, M. (2000) *Multivariate Analysis of Quality — An Introduction*, John Wiley & Sons.
77. Brereton, R. G. (2018) *Chemometrics: Data Driven Extraction for Science* 2nd ed., John Wiley & Sons.
78. Yajima, T. and Takatsuji, M. (1964) Higher order optical mixing of raman laser light in nonlinear dielectric media. J. Phys. Soc. Japan. **19**, 2343–4344.
79. Marker, P. D. and Terhune, R. W. (1965) Study of optical effects due to an induced polarization third order in the electric field strength. Phys. Rev. **137**, A801.
80. (a) Dutta, P. K., Nestor, J. R. and Spiro, T. G. (1977) Resonance coherent anti-Stokes scattering spectra of fluorescent biological chromophores: vibrational evidence for hydrogen bonding of flavin to glucose oxidase and for rapid solvent exchange. Proc. Natl. Acad. Sci. **74**, pp. 4146. (b) Dutta, P. K., Nestor, J. R. and Spiro, T. G. (1978) Resonance coherent anti-Stokes scattering (CARS) spectra of flavin adenine dinucleotide, riboflavin binding protein and glucose oxidase. Biochem. Biophys. Res. Comm. **83**, 209.
81. Carreira, L. A., Maguire, C. and Malloy, Jr. T. B. (1977) Excitation profile of the coherent anti-Stokes Raman spectrum of β carotene. J. Chem. Phys. **66**, 2621–2626.
82. Duncan, M. D., Reintjes, J. and Manuccia, T. J. (1982) Scanning coherent anti-Stokes Raman microscope. Opt. Lett. **7**, 350–352.
83. Zumbusch, A., Holtom, G. R. and Xie, X. S. (1999) Three-dimensional vibrational imaging by coherent anti-Stokes Raman scattering. Phys. Rev. Lett. **82**, 4142.
84. Hashimoto, M., Araki, T. and Kawata, S. (2000) Molecular vibration imaging in the fingerprint region by use of coherent anti-Stokes Raman scattering microscopy with a collinear configuration. Opt. Lett. **25**, 1768–1770.
85. Kneipp, K., Wang, Y., Kneipp, H., Perelman, L. T., Itzkan, I., Dasari R. R. and Feld M. S. (1997) Single molecule detection by surface-enhanced Raman scattering (SERS). Phys. Rev. Lett. **78**, 1667.
86. Nie, S. R. (1997) Probing single molecule and single nanoparticles by surface-enhanced Raman scattering. Science **275**, 1102–1106.

87. Vo-Dinh, T., Houck, K. and Stokes, D. L. (1994) Surface-enhanced Raman gene probes. Anal. Chem. **66**, 3379–3383.
88. Isola, N. R., Stokes, D. L. and Vo-Dinh, T. (1998) Surface-enhanced Raman gene probe for HIV detection. Anal. Chem. **70**, 1352–1356.
89. Cotton, T. M., Kim, J.-H. and Chumanov, G. D. (1991) Application of surface-enhanced Raman spectroscopy to biological systems. J. Raman Spectrosc. **22**, 729–742.
90. Dou, X., Takama, T., Yamaguchi, Y., Yamamoto, H. and Ozaki, Y. (1997) Enzyme immunoassay utilizing surface-enhanced Raman scattering of the enzyme reaction product. Anal. Chem. **69**, 1492–1495.
91. Dou, X., Takama, T., Yamaguchi, Y., Hirai, K., Yamamoto, H., Doi, S. and Ozaki, Y. (1998) Quantitative analysis of double-stranded DNA amplified by polymerase chain reaction employing surface-enhanced Raman spectroscopy. Appl. Opt. **37**, 759–763.
92. Efrima, S. and Bronk, B. V. (1998) Silver colloid impregnating or coating bacteria. J. Phys. Chem. B **102**, 5947–5950.

https://doi.org/10.1142/9789811264610_0002

Chapter 2
Photonic Data Science for Raman Data Analysis

Rola Houhou,[1,2] Thomas Bocklitz[1-3,*]

[1]*Leibniz Institute of Photonic Technology, Member of Leibniz Health Technologies, Member of the Leibniz Centre for Photonics in Infection Research (LPI), Albert-Einstein-Strasse 9, 07745 Jena, Germany*
[2]*Institute of Physical Chemistry (IPC) and Abbe Center of Photonics (ACP), Friedrich Schiller University Jena, Member of the Leibniz Centre for Photonics in Infection Research (LPI), Helmholtzweg 4, 07743 Jena, Germany*
[3]*Institute of Computer Science, Faculty of Mathematics, Physics & Computer Science, University Bayreuth Universitaetsstraße 30, 95447 Bayreuth, Germany*
**Corresponding author: thomas.bocklitz@uni-jena.de*

2.1 Introduction

The field of Raman spectroscopy continues to grow due to its wide range of applications covering pharmaceuticals and cosmetics, geology and mineralogy, carbon materials, semiconductors, and life science. Its non-destructive nature is considered one of the most crucial characteristics where numerous information about materials is revealed, including but not limited to their chemical structure, identity, contamination, and purity. Raman spectroscopy probes matter at the molecular level for a wide range of sampling media and environments. In particular, its low dependency to water is an advantage over other techniques, for instance, infrared spectroscopy, and makes it suitable for various examinations such as *in vivo* analysis. Throughout the years, Raman spectroscopy not only expanded into other areas but the method itself was improved. This involved advancements in the design and control of lasers, improvement of Raman instrumentation, and progress in the creation of nanomaterials and nanoparticles. These developments resulted in a variety of Raman techniques which can be grouped into linear and nonlinear Raman spectroscopy based on their dependency on the excitation intensity. In linear Raman spectroscopy, molecular polarizability P is linearly related to the electric field E of the incident light which implies that the signal intensity and the irradiating light intensity are linearly dependent. Within the scope of the linear Raman methods, several techniques were developed such as spontaneous Raman spectroscopy and resonance Raman spectroscopy. Other methods like surface-enhanced Raman scattering (SERS) are hard to assign to either of the categories. On th other hand, in nonlinear Raman spectroscopy, the electric field of high intensity contributes nonlinear effects to molecular polarizability which can be expressed by a power series as follows:

$$\mathrm{P}/\varepsilon_0 = \chi^{(1)}E^1 + \chi^{(2)}E^{(2)} + \chi^{(3)}E^3 + \cdots, \tag{2.1}$$

where $\chi^{(i)}$ represents the ith electric susceptibility tensor. Further innovations are also well noticed for the nonlinear Raman processes which overcome the limitations in the linear processes, and include coherent anti-Stokes Raman scattering (CARS) and stimulated Raman scattering (SRS). These linear and nonlinear Raman methods have been widely implemented and assist in the understanding of complex architecture and chemical information of samples. Accordingly, the complexity of the generated data from these linear and nonlinear Raman processes is enormous and often the data cannot be easily understood. Therefore, these data need specific treatments to extract the underlying information from a sample. To do so, photonic data science is utilized. The cycle of photonic data science is illustrated in Figure 2.1, and it starts with the experimental design where a protocol is created, under which the associated experiments are performed. Afterward, linear and/or nonlinear Raman techniques can be applied to the sample in the measurement step. Subsequently, the corresponding data are collected from the setups used for measurement, and finally, useful information is extracted in the photonic data science step.

Typically, photonic data science includes the development of mathematical and statistical methods that could extract meaningful information from the measured data. Therefore, the importance of photonic data science increases with the increasing size of the measured data. Since the measured data are not directly expressive and pose significant challenges for complex systems, a diversity of methods including machine learning and deep learning are

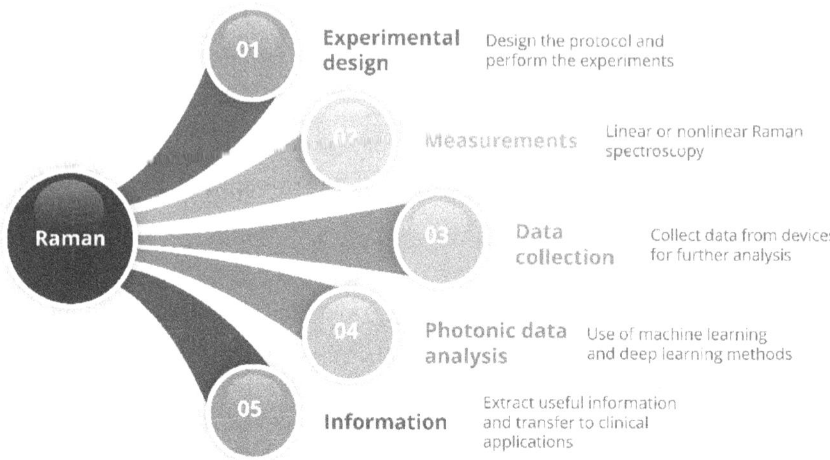

Figure 2.1. Photonic data science: from experimental design to artificial intelligence. A typical study is started by design of the experiment. Then, Raman spectroscopy is implemented, and data is collected. Afterward, artificial intelligence methods including machine learning and deep learning are applied to the measured data to extract relevant information. This aims to produce automated systems and help in rapid decision making based on the data.

developed. These methods are task- and data-dependent. Consequently, photonic data science methods can be grouped into three categories: inverse modeling, preprocessing, and data modeling. First, the inverse modeling category includes methods that aim to recover the parameters of a physical system from the measured data of that system. Since linear and nonlinear Raman measurements depend on detectors, laser power, environment, or sample, the measured data are disrupted by side contributions, artifacts, and noises derived from various sources. Therefore, the preprocessing category consists of constructing an improved version of the data where unwanted variations are removed. The last category is data modeling in which supervised and unsupervised methods can be implemented depending on the task to be solved. As previously stated, photonic data science methods are data-dependent which implies that a specific type of data requires specific treatment which can be combined at the end in a data pipeline. In this chapter, the focus is on data acquired in the form of images or spectra. Therefore, we organized two separate sections entitled image analysis pipeline and spectral analysis pipeline. We structured the image pipeline into preprocessing and data modeling methods. In the spectral pipeline, we divided it into inverse modeling, preprocessing, and data modeling as well. Afterward, a model evaluation section is presented which concentrates on the cross-validation approach and popular metrics for model evaluation.

2.2 Image Analysis Pipeline

Often Raman imaging data, whether acquired based on linear or nonlinear methods, are not directly understandable and require treatment using mathematical and statistical functions. However, these treatments are task-dependent; for instance, if the task is to detect the level of disorders or classify diseases, different approaches should be considered. In the image analysis pipeline, several methods exist which can be grouped into two main categories: image preprocessing and data modeling, and these are summarized in Figure 2.2.

In this section, we define an image as a two-dimensional function denoted $X(i,j)$ where i and j are indices representing spatial coordinates, and the intensity at any pair of coordinates (i,j) is given by X, which is also known

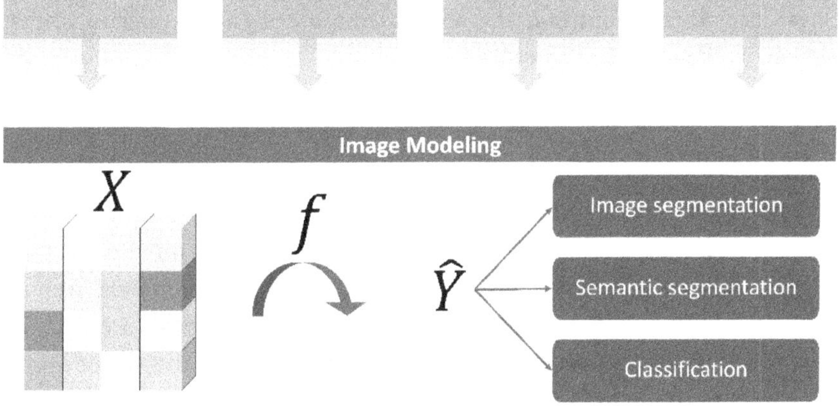

Figure 2.2. Image Raman analysis pipeline from data preprocessing to data modeling. Data preprocessing approaches include denoising, registration, normalization, and object detection. One or a combination of these techniques can be utilized, which is crucial for further analysis. The next step is to implement data modeling techniques, and this is task-dependent and involves the application of either image segmentation, semantic segmentation, or classification methods.

as a pixel value. For simplicity, we refer to the image as X. The mathematical notations Y and $\widehat{Y}$ refer to the true class (or label) and the estimated one, respectively. In addition, x represents the features extracted from the data used in the form of vectors.

In the following sections, details of the methods characterizing each category are discussed.

2.2.1 *Preprocessing*

The linear and nonlinear Raman images are usually affected by noise and artifacts coming from various sources such as sample environments and CCD detectors. These noises and artifacts compromise the quality of the Raman images, which makes Raman image preprocessing one of the most important prerequisites needed for further analysis. In general, image preprocessing consists of reconstructing an improved version of the original disrupted image which can be more easily interpreted afterward. It highlights features in the images which result in the efficient extraction of information from the data. Hence, the application of suitable methods for enhancing images became a must and has been one of the major interests in image processing. For instance, in medical applications, image preprocessing is very crucial since images affected by noise, blurriness, poor contrast and sharpness may result in false diagnoses. Therefore, various processes in image preprocessing are tackled below where in each of them, the most used methods are explained, and an overview is sketched in Figure 2.3.

2.2.1.1 *Denoising*

The loss of information is very common during the acquisition of linear and nonlinear Raman images, and this is due to the contamination of these images with noise originating from the process itself and influence from the environment. Therefore, image denoising takes a leading role in enhancing Raman data, which is needed for further Raman image analysis. The idea of image denoising consists of restoring an original image by removing noise from the disrupted image while minimizing the loss of the original features. This denoising problem can be translated mathematically as

$$\widetilde{X} = X + \eta, \tag{2.2}$$

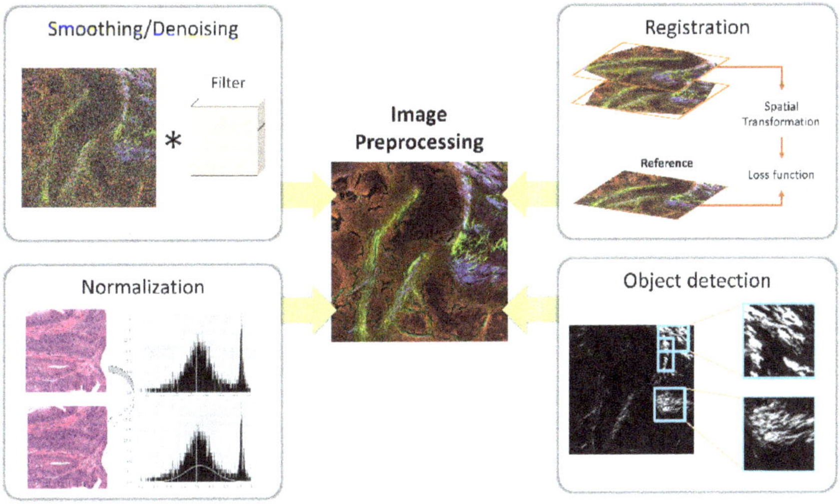

Figure 2.3. An overview of the preprocessing methods of Raman images. The smoothing or denoising methods remove unwanted variations from images. On the other hand, the registration techniques aim to align the images to a reference, which makes further analysis more efficient. In addition, the normalization methods are techniques that are crucial for further analysis. Finally, object detection aims to detect abnormalities in an image. (H&E images were reproduced from https://portal.gdc.cancer.gov with permission).

where $\widetilde{X}$ is the noisy image, X is the unknown clean image, and η represents an additive noise term often assumed to be white noise. Although image denoising is quite popular and used in multiple disciplines, it is still a challenging task since it falls under the inverse problem umbrella where the result of the reconstruction of a clean image is not unique. The reconstruction of clean images should smooth flat areas, preserve edges from blurring, preserve the textures in the image, and prevent the occurrence of new artifacts [1]. Hence, a variety of methods exists, and we can group them into three main categories: classical methods, transform-based methods, and deep learning-based methods. Classical methods include spatial domain filtering-based methods and variational denoising methods. The former consists of constructing pixels by applying directly either linear or nonlinear filters to the observed noisy image, and many can be utilized such as mean filtering, Wiener filtering, median filtering, and bilateral filtering. An alternative to the use of filters is the implementation of variational denoising methods which consist of constructing an energy function E and finding a suitable image prior, where a denoised image $\widehat{X}$ is calculated through a mapping procedure as follows:

$$\widehat{X} = \underset{\widetilde{X}}{\operatorname{argmin}}\, E(\widetilde{X}). \tag{2.3}$$

Popular variational denoising methods were developed such as total variation regularization, sparse representation, and nonlocal regularization. On the other hand, transform-based methods consist of transforming the noisy image to another domain and then applying a denoising procedure to the converted image. One crucial insight about the transform-based denoising technique is that in the transform domain, the characteristics of the image differ from those of the noise. These methods were widely developed, and they depend on the choice of basis transform functions which include cosine transform, wavelet domain methods, independent component analysis (ICA), and principal component analysis (PCA) [2]. Apart from the aforementioned methods, deep learning (DL) approaches and in particular convolutional neural network (CNN)-based methods have been widely utilized as a denoising method. This CNN approach consists of learning a mapping from the noisy images to the clean image by optimizing a loss function. This optimization is done using a training dataset that consists of several noisy $\widetilde{X}$ and clean X. The loss function can be formulated as follows:

$$\min_{\theta} \mathcal{L}\left(\widetilde{X}, X\right), \tag{2.4}$$

where $\mathcal{L}$ is the loss function and θ represents the model parameters. Although the time complexity for the learning process in DL is quite high, the CNN-trained networks are getting more popular for their effectiveness and enhancement of the extracted detailed features in the denoised images.

2.2.1.2 *Registration*

One of the common problems that arise in image analysis is that images are sometimes measured at different times, from different viewpoints, and with different devices where their alignment is needed to detect differences and compare different images. To solve this issue, image registration methods can be implemented. Image registration is the process of aligning two or more images with a reference one. It consists of a mapping between two images spatially and intensity-wise. This mapping procedure can be translated mathematically as

$$X_1(i,j) = g(X_2(p(i,j))), \tag{2.5}$$

where X_1, X_2 are the intensity of two images, p is the spatial coordinate transformation, and g represents the intensity transformation [3, 4]. The procedure of image registration starts with feature detection where common features must be extracted from the reference and the non-aligned images. The next step involves matching the extracted features from the reference image on one hand and the non-aligned image on the other hand, which is also known as the feature matching step. Afterward, the matched features are used to estimate the parameters of the transformation function that aligns between the reference image and the non-aligned image. And finally, the aligned image is obtained by using the optimized transformation. Since image registration implies multiple choices from the feature to the similarity metric, various methods from standard to advanced are developed such as correlation-based methods, point mapping methods, wavelet-based methods, and artificial neural networks.

2.2.1.3 *Normalization*

Intensity normalization is also considered a preprocessing step which is important for later analysis such as pattern recognition, segmentation, and classification. There exist two classes of normalization methods: intensity and geometric normalization. First, intensity normalization is used to reduce the changes between a set of measured images, which might be introduced by the optical setup itself, by different noise contributions, etc., which might affect even the color of the images. Therefore, the intensity normalization transforms the intensity values in the observed image into a standardized intensity range. In this context, various methods can be used such as min-max, z-score, z-score standard deviation, and decimal scaling normalization [5–7]. For instance, the z-score normalization on an image X is calculated as

$$X_{SNV} = \frac{X - \overline{X}}{\sigma_X} \tag{2.6}$$

where X_{SNV} is the normalized image, $\overline{X}$ is the mean of the image, and σ_X represents the standard deviation in the image. On the other hand, geometric normalization consists of geometrically transforming an image into a normalized form that is invariant to geometric distortions such as rotation, scaling, and translation. Moment-based, feature extraction-based, and affine transformation-based methods are some of the various techniques that can be implemented in this context which are useful, for instance, in the pattern recognition task.

2.2.1.4 *Object detection*

One of the challenging tasks in Raman image analysis is to detect and evaluate objects existing in the studied sample, for instance, in cells. Although object detection has become one of the growing research fields in computer vision, it is also beneficial for Raman image analysis. Object detection involves both object localization and object classification [8]. In object localization, the position of the target object is determined, and then object classification is used to discriminate between the target object classes based on their size, shape, and other characteristics. Again, these methods depend on the studied task. The complex structure in linear and nonlinear Raman images leads to more difficulty in object detection, where standard methods became less effective. Therefore, CNN-based DL networks have gained a lot of popularity for the object detection task and were able to successfully improve the performance in comparison with traditional object detection techniques. In combination with transfer learning, the CNNs could be used for Raman images [9]. In this regard, several CNN networks were developed and became dominant in object detection tasks such as Region-based Convolutional Neural Network (R-CNN), Single Shot Detector (SSD), and Fast R-CNN.

2.2.2 *Data modeling*

After the application of various data preprocessing techniques on linear and nonlinear Raman images, the improved Raman images are used at this stage for data modeling. Data modeling is the approach of learning from images, and it consists of building a model that best represents the Raman images and can extract relationships or discriminate between these images. In data modeling, the choice of methods is again task-dependent, and it involves the application of one or more of the following tasks: object detection, semantic segmentation, segmentation, and classification.

2.2.2.1 *Semantic Segmentation*

The application of semantic segmentation in linear and nonlinear Raman images is promising and challenging at the same time. It is based on clustering sections from the images which belong to the same class. Therefore, semantic segmentation intends to classify each pixel of an image to its appropriate class, and this is achieved by creating masks of the image, which segment the classes

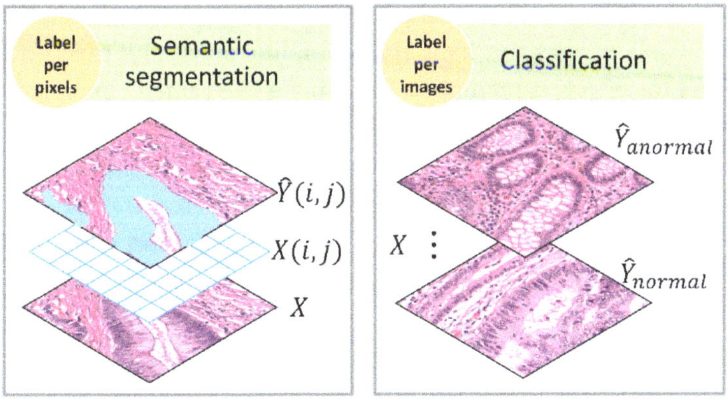

Figure 2.4. Semantic segmentation and classification for image analysis. In semantic segmentation, each pixel of the image is predicted where a region of interest is the focus of the study. In the classification case, the aim is to label the whole image. Both methods could use supervised or unsupervised methods. (H&E images were reproduced from https://portal.gdc.cancer.gov with permission).

from each other. However, these maps of masks should segment a region accurately and assign it to its proper class. Figure 2.4 summarizes the main difference between semantic segmentation and classification methods. For an image X, the problem in semantic segmentation is to learn the function that accurately maps the image to its corresponding mask of classes, and it can be formulated mathematically as

$$f(X(i,j)) = M(i,j), \tag{2.7}$$

where M represents the map of classes and f represents the mapping function to be learned. Classical techniques were used to solve this problem such as graph-based segmentation algorithms, gradient ascent-based algorithms, and the simple linear iterative clustering (SLIC) segmentation algorithm [10, 11]. For instance, graph-based segmentation algorithms consist of constructing a graph where each pixel is used as a node and the edge weight between two nodes is calculated as proportional to the similarity between the pixels. Additionally, superpixel segments are obtained by minimizing a cost function defined on this graph. However, in the SLIC segmentation algorithm, the superpixel segments are generated by clustering pixels based on their color similarity and proximity in the image. On the other hand, DL and in particular CNN-based networks have outperformed the classical methods and become a very famous tool for solving semantic segmentation problems. In studies,

CNN-based networks were used either by training a specific architecture on the available images and their corresponding labels and then tuning the parameters for effective prediction, or using a pretrained CNN network as a transfer learning technique [12–14]. All these methods require *a priori* knowledge of the set of classes in the image, which categorizes these methods as supervised semantic segmentation.Another form of semantic segmentation exists which is called unsupervised semantic segmentation, and it aims to localize semantically meaningful classes within the image without any form of annotation.

2.2.2.2 *Segmentation*

Image segmentation is an important technique which can highlight the region of interest and abnormalities in the image. It consists of partitioning an image into homogenous segments that incorporate similar features or attributes. To choose the appropriate technique for image segmentation, there is no unique approach, and several methods can be implemented in this regard. All these techniques can be grouped into threshold-based, edge-based, region-based, clustering-based, watershed-based, partial differential equation (PDE)-based, and DL-based methods [15–19]. Briefly, threshold-based methods consist of finding threshold values based on the histogram of the image. These methods do not require previous information and are considered the simplest methods for image segmentation. However, they depend highly on the shape of the histogram, and the spatial information is not considered. Edge-based methods perform well when images contain better contrast between objects. In edge-based methods, all edges are detected first, and the object boundaries are formed by bonding the edges together. These methods are based on discontinuity detection and are not suitable for too many edges. On the other hand, region-based methods consist of dividing an image into homogenous regions that incorporate similar characteristics. These methods are almost immune to noise, but they are time- and memory-consuming. Another group that can be applied for image segmentation is the clustering method. It consists of partitioning an image into homogeneous clusters. In this group, hard and soft clustering can be implemented where hard clustering divides an image into clusters such that each pixel belongs to one cluster, and soft clustering partitions pixels into a cluster based on partial membership. For instance, k-means and fuzz c-means clustering are types of hard and soft clustering, respectively (more details about clustering methods can be found in the spectral analysis pipeline section). Watershed- and PDE-based methods use topological interpretation and partial differential equations, respectively. These two groups require more complex calculations and computation. Finally, DL-based methods are also very famous for image segmentation and consist of estimating a function that maps between pairs of input and output, for instance between an image and its background, by training a specific network architecture.

2.2.2.3 *Classification*

Image classification is one of the most important tasks in linear and nonlinear Raman image analysis. It consists of classifying the acquired images into their corresponding predefined classes. However, the classification step directly applied to images leads to poor performance if features were not extracted beforehand. Therefore, feature extraction or feature selection is critical for the classification procedure. This step aims to acquire relevant attributes that assist in distinguishing between classes and are independent of unrelated variations in the data. Methods that are used for selecting or extracting important features for further use in classification tasks are aplenty and here we mentioned some; more details are presented in the section on spectral analysis pipeline. For instance, statistical measures such as chi-squared, F-test, and analysis of variance (ANOVA) are implemented to select the relevant features that influenced the discrimination procedure. Other methods such as forward and backward selection can also be utilized. These methods consist of searching for a set of features that improve the performance of the desired classifier. Other than feature selection methods, feature extraction techniques consist of transforming the data into a new subspace by reducing the dimensionality of the data and preserving important information. In this context, one of the popular methods to use is PCA, which transforms data into subspace in a linear and orthogonal manner by generating features that consist of a linear combination of the data. However, it is important to mention that the selection of these relevant features is not often straightforward and the choice of the best methods is not simple. Afterward, image classification is implemented, which can be understood as the process of finding a mapping function that connects these image features or images to their classes. To find the mapping function, various machine learning methods were developed, and we present here the most commonly used [20].

Support vector machine (SVM) is well-known for Raman image classification, and it consists of finding the optimal hyperplane that best separates images into their classes. In SVM, the mapping function is specified by a subset of the training images which are called support vectors. The support vectors are critical elements in the optimization, and the hyperplane depends only on these support vectors where the margin from these supports to the hyperplane should be maximized. In most cases, we need to find a nonlinear hyperplane h that separates the data; therefore, we define a feature space ϕ that transforms the data into a new space where it is linearly separable. The general optimization problem can be formulated as

$$\begin{cases} \max\left[\sum \alpha_i - \frac{1}{2}\sum\sum \alpha_i \alpha_k Y_i Y_k \langle \varphi(x_i) | \varphi(x_k) \rangle\right], \\ 0 < \alpha_i < C; \sum \alpha_i Y_i = 0 \end{cases} \quad (2.8)$$

where α_i, Y_i, C represent the weights, classes, and margin, respectively. The solution for this problem is the equation of the hyperplane and it can be written as

$$h(x) = \sum_{i=1}^{n} \alpha_i Y_i \langle \varphi(x_i) | \varphi(x) \rangle + b. \quad (2.9)$$

However, the solution can be also formulated without the feature space as

$$h(x) = \sum_{i=1}^{n} \alpha_i Y_i K(x_i, x) + b, \quad (2.10)$$

where K represents the kernel function that we can choose from polynomial, radial basis, and sigmoid functions. The most used kernel is the radial basis or the Gaussian kernel which is given by the following equation:

$$K(x_i, x) = \exp\left(-\frac{\|x_i - x\|^2}{\sigma^2}\right). \quad (2.11)$$

In SVM, various choices should be made such as the choice of the kernel, the penalty term, and the multi-class training method.

On the other hand, k-nearest neighbor classification is a supervised method that is considered one of the simplest classification techniques among various machine learning methods. It is based on calculating the Euclidean distance between training images:

$$d(x_i, x_k) = \sqrt{\Sigma_{j=1}^{p} \left(x_{ij} - x_{kj}\right)^2}, \quad (2.12)$$

where x_i, x_k represent two sample images and p is the number of features. In this regard, the classification rule consists of assigning the testing image to the class from the majority of votes given by its k neighbors. There are several other classification algorithms available such as decision trees, random forests, and hidden Markov models. Nowadays, DL methods are booming and particularly for classification and pattern recognition tasks. Similar to machine learning, DL consists of learning from data and involves nonlinear connections between multiple layers. It reveals effective representations of data through multiple levels of nonlinear transformations. Additionally, DL methods are characterized by their implicit feature extraction, which is part of the learning procedure that consists of extracting important features from data while training the network. The most common architecture used for classification tasks involves CNN that intends to capture the spatial and temporal attributes in an image by applying certain filters. A basic CNN includes a convolutional layer, pooling layer, and fully connected layer. The convolutional layer converts the input into a representation of the data, and this is achieved by performing a convolution operation between the input and a learned kernel. On the other hand, the dimension of the input is reduced through the pooling layer where a specific method is selected, and it aims to conserve as much information as possible. Finally, the fully connected layer is often added between the output layer and the previous to model nonlinear connections of the input features. However, the use of such a layer is being questioned since it may lead to overfitting, and researchers are considering removing the fully connected layer from the CNN architecture. Nevertheless, when using DL, different approaches can be considered to train these methods. In the case of a large dataset, the training of the models can be performed from scratch using certain neural network architectures. Or, in the case of smaller datasets, the transfer learning concept can be implemented. Transfer learning consists of using pretrained networks and transferring them to the small dataset of interest. This transfer can be done by using directly the pretrained weights from a specific DL network, or by freezing some layers and training on the remaining with the studied data.

2.3 Spectral Analysis Pipeline

The generated data from linear and nonlinear Raman optical measurements can be also acquired in the form of spectral data. These spectral data are also not directly utilized and need specific treatments to extract the underlying information, which follow a specific data analysis pipeline. Again, the whole

Raman spectral analysis pipeline depends on the data and the task, and all steps within the pipeline belong to one of the three main categories of analysis: inverse modeling, preprocessing, and data modeling. Methods belonging to the three categories use mathematical and statistical functions and details of each of the categories are presented below. In the following, one spectrum is denoted by S, while the set of Raman spectra is stored in a matrix $X = \{X_1, \cdots, X_p\} \in \mathbb{R}^{n \times p}$ where p is the number of variables and n is the sample size.

2.3.1 *Inverse Modeling*

Inverse modeling consists of using the Raman spectral data and estimating the parameters of the physical system. For instance, in CARS, we often encounter the problem of finding an accurate estimation of the phase, which is challenging and sometimes impossible [21–25]. Since the phase often contains a lot of information and only the square modulus of a signal is measured, phase retrieval methods can be implemented to recover the phase from the given magnitude and subsequently reconstruct the full signal. Generally, sophisticated measurement setups, e.g., holography, directly measure the phase by requiring interference with another known field. Since these methods are expensive and time-consuming, algorithmic methods can be used as an alternative to recover the phase from the measured magnitude. An overview of the phase extraction methods for CARS data is visualized in Figure 2.5.

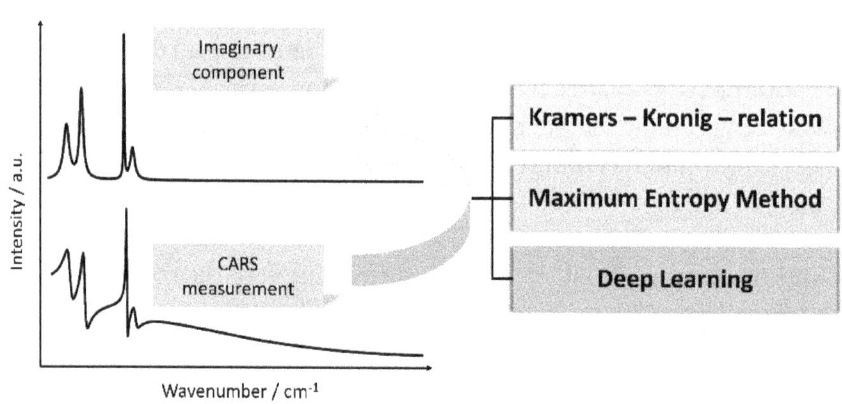

Figure 2.5. Phase retrieval methods of CARS measurements. To extract the Raman-like spectrum from the CARS measurement, the Kramers-Kronig relation (KK), the maximum entropy method (MEM), and deep learning or CNN-based methods can be implemented. KK and MEM are standard techniques that are popular but suffer from the persistence of the non-resonant background while DL shows more promises concerning the efficiency of the reconstruction of the Raman-like spectra.

The maximum entropy method (MEM) and the Kramers–Kronig relation (KK) are standard methods that are used to extract the phase from the CARS spectral data. First, MEM is a probability-based method which considers that any inference made from incomplete information should be based on the probability distribution, with the maximum entropy permitted by the available data. In CARS only the intensity spectrum $S = I_{CARS}$ is measured, which is given by the following equation:

$$I_{CARS} \propto |\chi^{(3)}|^2 \, I_{pu}{}^2 I_S, \tag{2.13}$$

where $\chi^{(3)}$, I_{pu}, I_s represent the nonlinear third-order susceptibility, and the pump and Stokes intensity, respectively. The calculation in MEM starts by approximating the power spectrum $S(v)$ on a defined normalized frequency range v

$$S(v) \approx \frac{b_0}{\left|1 + \sum_{k=1}^{M} b_k \exp(-i2\pi v)\right|^2}, \tag{2.14}$$

where b_0, b_k for $1 \le k \le M$ and M represent the coefficients and the number of poles of the approximation, respectively. The right side of the approximation can be written in terms of the autocorrelation function R_l:

$$\frac{b_0}{\left|1 + \sum_{k=1}^{M} b_k \exp(-i2\pi v)\right|^2} \approx \sum_{l=-M}^{M} R_l \exp(-i2\pi v l), \tag{2.15}$$

where $R_l = \int S(v) \exp(i2\pi v l) dv$ since the power spectrum is equal to the Fourier transform of the autocorrelation function R_l. Afterward, the coefficients b_0 and b_k are estimated by solving the following Toeplitz matrix:

$$\begin{pmatrix} R_0 & R_{-1} & \cdots & R_{-M} \\ R_1 & R_0 & & R_{-M} \\ \vdots & & \ddots & \vdots \\ R_M & R_{M-1} & \cdots & R_0 \end{pmatrix} \begin{pmatrix} 1 \\ b_1 \\ \vdots \\ b_M \end{pmatrix} = \begin{pmatrix} b_0 \\ 0 \\ \vdots \\ 0 \end{pmatrix} \tag{2.16}$$

Finally, the phase $\phi(v)$ is retrieved by imposing a physical constraint at a specific frequency position, such as if v_0 is far from any resonances or the imaginary part has a local maximum at a resonance v_r. Consequently, the real and imaginary components of $\chi^{(3)}$ are calculated. On the other hand, KK is implemented differently since it consists of a mathematical relationship between the real and the imaginary components of any analytical function like $\chi^{(3)}$ that was developed according to the Cauchy residue theorem. If the real component is available, the imaginary component can be calculated by the KK relation and vice versa:

$$\begin{aligned} \mathrm{Re}\left(\chi^{(3)}(i\nu)\right) &= -\frac{1}{\pi}\wp\int\frac{\mathrm{Im}\left(\chi^{(3)}(ix)\right)}{x-\nu}dx \\ \mathrm{Im}\left(\chi^{(3)}(i\nu)\right) &= \frac{1}{\pi}\wp\int\frac{\mathrm{Re}\left(\chi^{(3)}(ix)\right)}{x-\nu}dx \end{aligned}, \tag{2.17}$$

where $\wp$ represents the Cauchy principal value. However, in CARS spectral data, only the intensity is measured, therefore the KK relation can be modified to connect the intensity to the phase:

$$\phi(\nu) = -\frac{1}{\pi}\wp\int\frac{\ln\left(\sqrt{S(\nu')}\right)}{\nu'-\nu}d\nu'. \tag{2.18}$$

The phase can be extracted by applying the discrete Hilbert transform on $\ln\left(\sqrt{S(\nu)}\right)$, and subsequently the real and imaginary components can be estimated. In addition, DL-based methods are becoming popular for retrieving the phase from CARS spectral data. For instance, the long short-term memory (LSTM) method, which is a type of recurrent neural network, was utilized for phase retrieval. Its parameters were optimized on pairs of artificial CARS spectra and their corresponding imaginary components. The method showed great performance in extracting the Raman-like spectra directly from the CARS spectra [26]. Another DL technique, a CNN-based network, showed promising results to generate the imaginary components from the squared modulus of $\chi^{(3)}$ [27–29].

2.3.2 *Preprocessing*

Similar to images, linear and nonlinear Raman spectral data are contaminated by artifacts and unwanted variations which make the extraction of useful information difficult. The origin of these artifacts and noises is either from the experimental setup or the sample environment and the measurements themselves. Therefore, it is crucial to remove all artifacts and unwanted

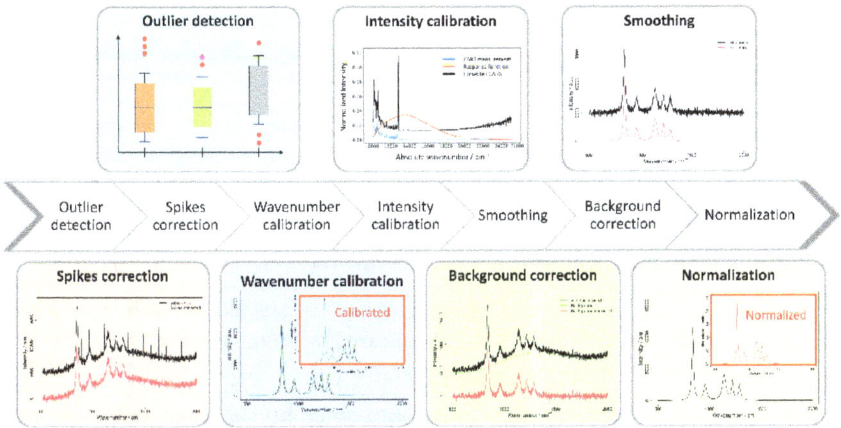

Figure 2.6. An overview of spectral Raman pipeline analysis. The analysis starts by improving the Raman spectra and several steps are implemented from spike removal, wavenumber and intensity calibration, background correction, to normalization.

variations for better analysis and understanding of the data. In the following, common preprocessing techniques for linear and nonlinear Raman spectral analysis are presented. These methods were chosen based on the work published by Guo *et al.* [30], which describes a protocol for the analysis of spontaneous Raman measurements. A summary of the preprocessing methods is presented in Figure 2.6.

2.3.2.1 *Outlier Detection*

An outlier is a measurement that is characterized by its non-conformity in comparison to the rest of the data. These outliers should be detected and removed from the datasets since their presence will compromise further analysis such as feature selection and classification. In the case of spectral Raman data, burning and contamination of the samples can result in such an outlier. For instance, biological samples can be contaminated by small undesired particles and due to their different chemical composition, they will result in additional peaks in the spectra. This fact will affect the classifier and may result in a false prediction. On the other hand, due to the contamination, another problem may occur which is the burning of the samples. Therefore, these signals should be excluded from the analysis and various methods can be used in this regard, for instance, Z-scores or the modified Z-score, and the area under the curve for a set of peaks.

2.3.2.2 *Spike removal*

The acquired Raman spectra are often affected by cosmic rays which originate from the high-energy photons hitting the detector, e.g., CCD array. The interaction between these photons and the CCD array results in high-intensity, positive, and narrow bandwidth peaks, known as cosmic spikes. However, these cosmic spikes are typically more intense than the Raman spectrum, and depending on the integration time, one or more cosmic spikes occur randomly within the Raman spectral range. Due to the random nature of their occurrence and their independence from the sample or the measurement system, it is impossible to directly detect their spectral positions. Since these cosmic spikes are often more intense, the signal level becomes higher than the measured spectra which compromises the data analysis steps such as normalization. Therefore, the removal of these spikes is necessary and considered one of the initial techniques in the pipeline. Apart from using a special instrument that aims to avoid the occurrence of these spikes, various algorithmic methods are considered to remove these cosmic spikes. Straightforward methods can be implemented in the case of multiple recorded spectra and consist of comparing sequentially a spectrum with either each measured spectrum or with a reference, e.g., the mean or a smoothed spectrum. More sophisticated techniques, e.g., polynomial filters, smoothing methods, and wavelet transform [31–35] can be implemented. After the detection and removal of the cosmic spikes, the region around the detected spikes requires interpolation to restore the original intensity value altered by the spike or by smoothing using a wide window.

2.3.2.3 *Baseline Correction*

One of the challenges in Raman data analysis is the presence of a fluorescence background in the Raman spectra. Theoretically, Raman and fluorescence spectroscopy follow a scattering and absorption process, respectively. While the Raman bands in the wavenumber domain do not depend on laser excitation, the fluorescence is affected by the laser frequency. In this way, a suitable excitation frequency can be chosen to minimize the fluorescence background. Even after optimizing the excitation frequency, a fluorescence background could still exist, which distorts the spectra. This fluorescence background can be several orders of magnitude more intense than the Raman peaks, which results in a broad background that hides Raman features. Therefore, it is necessary to separate the Raman spectrum from the background [36]. A simple technique that can be applied to avoid fluorescence background contribution is by using near-infrared wavelength light as the excitation source, in which case the excitation energy is generally insufficient to induce strong fluorescence. Additionally, computational methods could be used to perform background removal, e.g., first and second derivatives, wavelet transformation, and polynomial filtering. The polynomial fitting method consists of fitting the Raman spectrum with a low-order polynomial and then subtracting it from the Raman spectrum, which is reasonable since the Raman spectrum is a series of Lorentzian peaks and most computational methods are based on the fact that the Raman peaks vary faster in the wavenumber domain than the background does. This method preserves the original shapes of Raman peaks after the suppression of the background. However, the optimal choice of order for polynomial fitting varies and depends on the user experience. On the other hand, the wavelet transform is based on the fact that the fluorescence background is mainly composed of slowly changing and low-frequency components compared to the Raman signal. The measured spectrum can be decomposed into different frequency components first and then those low-frequency components corresponding to the fluorescence background can be removed. Unfortunately, many parameters need to be optimized, which is often difficult and time-consuming. The method of derivatives is based on the fact that a small number of derivatives removes the fluorescence background which is only composed of slowly varying components compared to those of Raman peaks. Therefore applying this method will eliminate the background components and enhance the sharp Raman signals, but at the same time, the high-frequency noises are often amplified as well. Additionally, the spectrum can be distorted because of the derivative process. Other prominent methods can be implemented, e.g., the sensitive nonlinear iterative peak (SNIP) [37] clipping algorithm, asymmetric least squares smoothing (ALS) [38], and extended multiplicative signal correction (EMSC) [39, 40]. To select the baseline parameters leading to an optimal analysis model, an optimization of the parameters with respect to the model performance is carried out. This optimization can only be performed if the available amount of data and the computational power is sufficient and a supervised analysis task with known response values of the training data is studied.

2.3.2.4 *Calibration*

Spectrometer calibration in Raman spectroscopy is needed due to the instrumental bias on the Raman spectra which will result in a shift in the wavenumber position and changes in the intensity. Therefore, it is important to standardize the Raman spectra with higher wavenumber and intensity precision. This can be achieved via accurate calibration of spectrometers that estimate the relationship between observed wavenumber positions and Raman intensities to their theoretical values. Below the details on the intensity calibration and wavenumber calibration in Raman spectroscopy are presented [41–43].

2.3.2.5 *Intensity calibration*

Significant variations in the measured Raman intensities can be observed when acquired by different instruments. These variations can be large when different laser excitations are used but also can occur when the same laser excitation is used. However, the Raman spectra collected on the same sample under the same conditions should be identical. An intensity calibration tries to accomplish long-term stability and provide reliable relative intensities. These intensities are utilized for spectral library searches and quantitative analysis. To perform the intensity calibration, a standard material with known emission intensity over the wavenumber range is employed. First, a measured dark spectrum $D(v)$ is subtracted from the observed Raman intensities $S(v)$, and afterward, it is divided by the intensity response function $R(v)$ as shown in the following equation:

$$S_I^c(v) = \frac{S(v) - D(v)}{R(v)}, \tag{2.19}$$

where S_I^c is the corrected Raman spectrum after intensity calibration and the intensity response function $R(v)$ is calculated as follows:

$$R(v) = \frac{S_{sd}(v) - D(v)}{S_{sd}^{th}(v)}, \tag{2.20}$$

where S_{sd} is the observed emission intensity of the standard material and S_{sd}^{th} represents its theoretical intensity. Usually, the intensity calibration step is ignored due to the assumption that all measurements acquired from the same device will not show changes in intensity over time. However, this fact is not accurate, particularly for clinical applications where the intensity response function might change with time due to long measurement campaigns. Thus, it is proposed to perform intensity calibration since it assists with the removal of unwanted spectral variations, which leads to better Raman data quality and subsequently good model performance.

2.3.2.6 *Wavenumber calibration*

Wavenumber calibration consists of using a measured standard material with the same device that acquired the studied Raman data. Since spectra from highly related samples show small Raman shifts which are susceptible to calibration errors, wavenumber calibration is regarded as an important step for further analysis. It consists of using the measured standard material and fitting a mathematical function to the deviations between the observed and theoretical Raman band positions of the standard material and afterward using this estimated function to correct the wavenumber axis. In the end, this new wavenumber axis is utilized for all Raman spectra acquired on the same device and at the same time. For fitting the calibration function, a polynomial function with degree p can be employed as follows:

$$P(\Delta v) = a_0 + a_1 \Delta v + a_2 \Delta v^2 + \cdots + a_p \Delta v^p, \tag{2.21}$$

where Δv represents the Raman shift position and p can be chosen between 3 and 5; in addition, the peak positions are determined by a Gaussian or Lorentzian profile which is used to fit all the Raman bands of the standard materials. The performance of the wavenumber calibration is dependent on the standard material used, the quality of the peak search, the peak fit, and the fit of the calibration function.

2.3.2.7 *Smoothing*

Spectral Raman data often includes a contribution from several types of noise that corrupt the spectra. This contribution needs to be reduced so that the Raman features are well preserved for further analysis. Although changes in the experimental conditions might reduce the level of noise, using algorithmic methods can be beneficial as well. Generally, filtering methods are implemented to reduce the noise from spectra such as mean, median, and Gaussian filters. These filtering methods remove high-frequency variations associated with noise contributions. However, careful use of these methods is required since a change in the peak shape and amplitude might be introduced.

On the other hand, Savitzky-Golay filtering [44] can be used as an alternative due to its maintenance of the Raman features. The idea in the Savitzky-Golay smoothing technique is based on least squares polynomial approximation First, a polynomial of degree p is defined as

$$P(t)=\sum_{m=0}^{p} a_m t^m, \tag{2.22}$$

and the sum of the squared residuals ξ is minimized in a given window,

$$\xi=\sum_{i=1}^{n}\left(S_i-P(\Delta v_i)\right)^2=\sum_{i=1}^{n}\left(S_i-\Sigma_{m=0}^{p} a_m \Delta v_i^{\,m}\right)^2. \tag{2.23}$$

There is no suggested polynomial degree to use, and it is data-dependent and should be chosen cautiously so that the smoothed spectra do not lose important Raman features.

2.3.2.8 *Normalization*

Normalization is the last step in preparing the data for further analysis. This step is crucial since it intends to eliminate variations resulting from differences in sample thickness, laser focus, and optical path length. A variety of normalization techniques exist that were mentioned in the Raman image analysis section. Briefly, spectral Raman data can be normalized by applying one of the following: division by norm (Eq. (2.24)), min-max normalization (Eq. (2.25)), and SNV (Eq. (2.26)).

$$S_{norm}=\frac{S}{\|S\|^p} \tag{2.24}$$

$$S_{min-max}=\frac{S-\min(S)}{\max(S)-\min(S)} \tag{2.25}$$

$$S_{SNV}=\frac{S-\bar{S}}{\sigma_S} \tag{2.26}$$

where $\bar{S}$ and σ represent the mean and standard deviation of the spectrum S. On the other hand, EMSC can also be used to normalize the Raman spectra. The basic EMSC model is written as

$$S(v) = a + S_{ref}(v).b + \Sigma_{i=1}^{q} d_i v^i + e(v), \tag{2.27}$$

where $e(v)$ is residual in the model, S_{ref} is a reference spectrum, v is the wavenumber position, q indicates the polynomial degree of the baseline, and a, b, d_i are unknown additive and multiplicative terms. The parameters a, b and d_i are estimated by ordinary or weighted least squares regression and finally, the spectra are corrected according to:

$$S_{corr}(v) = \frac{S(v) - a}{b}. \tag{2.28}$$

The normalization step should be performed after the removal of the background since the strength of the fluorescence background will influence the normalization coefficient.

2.3.2.9 *Feature extraction*

Spectral Raman data is a high-dimensional data type that is complex to understand and difficult to directly analyze. Therefore, feature extraction techniques can be implemented, which involve methods that reduce the dimensionality of the Raman data while preserving important information [45]. Generally, in feature extraction methods, the Raman spectral data are transformed into a new subspace of variables of lower dimension that are easier to deal with. A variety of techniques are used to do such a transformation and we can group them into two groups: linear and nonlinear methods [46]. For instance, one of the most popular linear feature extraction methods is PCA. PCA is a dimension reduction technique that transforms data into a subspace in a linear and orthogonal manner. It generates new variables called principal components as a linear combination of the original variables which show the largest variation in the dataset. The methods start by calculating the covariance matrix $\Sigma \in \mathbb{R}^{p \times p}$ which is given by the following equation:

$$\hat{\Sigma} = \frac{1}{n-1} X^t X. \tag{2.29}$$

Then the eigenvalues and the eigenvectors of the covariance matrix are computed as follows:

$$\hat{\Sigma} = U \Lambda U^t, \tag{2.30}$$

where $\Lambda = \text{diag}(\lambda_1, \cdots, \lambda_m)$ is the diagonal matrix of the ordered m eigenvalues λ_i, and U is a $p \times m$ orthogonal matrix containing the eigenvectors. Finally, the principal components which represent a set of uncorrelated features of the original variables are then computed by the following:

$$Z = XU. \tag{2.31}$$

Another example of a feature extraction method is ICA [47], which consists of finding an unmixing matrix and then projecting the data onto that matrix for extracting independent components. The unmixing matrix is estimated either by a maximum likelihood estimation or by maximizing measures for the non-Gaussianity, such as Kurtosis and negative entropy. Other standard methods for extracting features from Raman spectra such as factor analysis (FA), nonlinear PCA, simultaneous component analysis, and non-negative matrix factorization [46] can be implemented as well. Additionally, DL techniques, in particular CNN-based architectures, are attracting more attention for extracting meaningful Raman features and promising results can be noticed in this respect.

2.3.2.10 *Feature selection*

Feature selection is similar to feature extraction in terms of their aim, as both aim to reduce dimensionality. However, in feature selection, no transformation to a new space is required. In feature selection, a set of features within the Raman dataset are chosen which are needed for building models for classification, regression, or clustering analysis. Feature selection methods are divided into three main groups: filter, wrapper, and embedded methods [48, 49]. First, the filter-based methods select the most relevant features based on certain characteristics of the data. These methods are known for their speed and scalability, and they consist of implementing either statistical tests that determine the relationship between the variables and the response, or selecting features based on their importance. In this regard, Pearson correlation [50], Spearman correlation [51], and ANOVA [52] can be utilized. For instance, Pearson correlation is implemented to check the extent of the linear correlation between the variables X_i and the dependent variable Y and it is defined by the following coefficient:

$$r_{X_i,Y} = \frac{cov(X_i, Y)}{\sigma_{X_i}\sigma_Y}, \tag{2.32}$$

where $cov(X_i, Y)$ represents the covariance between X_i and Y, σ_{Xi} is the standard deviation of X_i, and σ_Y represents the standard deviation of Y. The closer $r_{Xi,Y}$ is to 1 and −1, the more X_i is positively and negatively correlated with Y, respectively. On the other hand, the Spearman correlation measures the relationship between X_i and Y using a monotonic function. Therefore, the difference between Pearson and Spearman is that Pearson evaluates for a linear relationship between dependent and independent variables while Spearman assesses whether a relationship is linear. The Spearman correlation coefficient is defined as the Pearson correlation between the rank variables as follows:

$$\rho_{R_{X_i}, R_Y} = \frac{cov\left(R_{X_i}, R_Y\right)}{\sigma_{R_{X_i}} \sigma_{R_Y}}, \tag{2.33}$$

where R_{Xi} is the rank of the variable X_i and R_Y is the rank of the variable Y. Additionally, ANOVA is quite popular in feature selection which consists of finding whether there are statistically significant differences between more than two variables. There are different types of ANOVA such as one-way and two-way ANOVA. Briefly, one-way ANOVA is given by the following coefficient:

$$F = \frac{\frac{1}{K-1}\sum_{i=1}^{K} n_i \left(\overline{X}_i - \overline{\overline{X}}\right)^2}{\frac{1}{n-K}\sum_{i=1}^{K} \left(n_i - 1\right) s_i^2}, \tag{2.34}$$

where s_i is the ith sample variance, K is the number of groups, and n is the total sample size which is equal to $n = n_1 + \cdots + n_K$. ANOVA is derived from a t-test and similarly, it consists of calculating a p-value that will indicate which variables have a statistically significant influence on the dependent variable. In contrast, the wrapper-based method consists of searching for the optimal subset of features by evaluating them with a machine learning method. Hence, the wrapper method involves training multiple models with all possible combinations of features against an evaluation criterion. The most used techniques under wrapper methods are forward selection, backward elimination, and stepwise selection. These types of selection iteratively fit a model with a combination of features and evaluate its performance. So, for instance, in the forward selection, the model starts to fit each feature at a time and selects the feature with the minimal p-value. While in the backward selection, all features are used first, and then features with the highest p-value are removed and this is repeated until all features are significant. On the other hand, the stepwise selection is similar to the forward selection, but it also verifies the significance of selected features from the previous iteration and removes them through backward selection if insignificant. Although these wrapper methods can construct an optimal set of features in comparison with the filter-based methods, they require a high computation time and need careful attention for the overfitting problem.

The last group of feature selection is the embedded methods, which are also iterative methods that look at each iteration of the model training process and extract features that contribute the most to the training for a particular iteration. Compared with the filter- and wrapper-based methods, this group performs better and reduces the computation cost. Various techniques can be implemented in this regard such as LASSO regularization [53] and Random Forest importance. In addition to the standard methods previously introduced, DL techniques are attracting more attention for selecting the significant features in spectral Raman data.

2.3.3 *Data modeling*

Data modeling is the last step in the analysis of spectral Raman data, which consists of extracting valuable information from the data, e.g., relevant information for diagnosing diseases. Previously, the important features from the Raman spectra were either extracted by dimension reduction techniques or selected using one of the feature selection tools. Afterward, these features or the original data need further analysis which is achieved by either unsupervised or supervised methods. The unsupervised methods consist of using an unlabeled dataset that aims to unravel hidden patterns in the data with minimal external intervention, while the supervised methods use labeled datasets that train models either to classify or predict parameters of the data. These standard techniques involve clustering, regression, and classification. An overview of the data modeling methods and the dimension reduction techniques used beforehand is shown in Figure 2.7.

2.3.3.1 *Clustering*

Clustering is an unsupervised learning technique that is based on similarities and constructs groups of data known as clusters. It is widely used for spectral Raman data that can find similar patterns within the data without the need for labels or classes. Generally, various types of clustering methods exist but

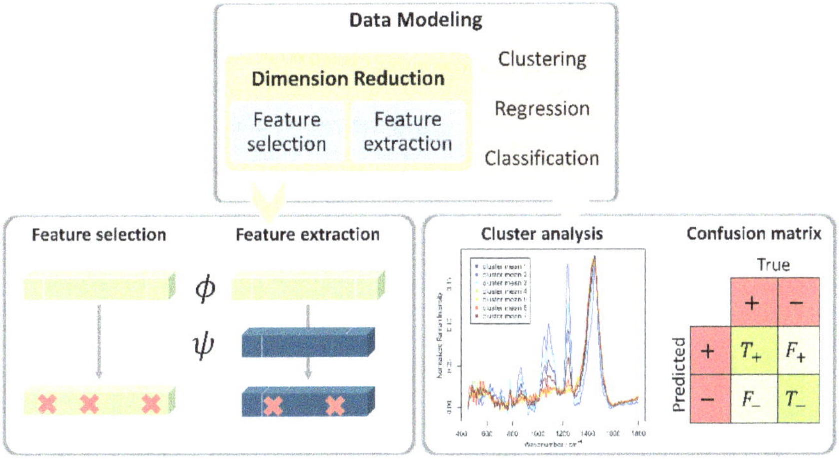

Figure 2.7. Overview of data modeling techniques for spectral Raman data. Depending on the task, either clustering, regression, or classification can be implemented. However, due to the high dimensionality of the spectral data, it is always recommended to use either feature extraction or feature selection techniques beforehand. In the feature selection methods, a set of features are selected based on their importance to the dependent variable, while in the feature extraction techniques the Raman data is transformed to a new subspace, and then features are selected.

here only hierarchical clustering, partition clustering, and fuzzy clustering are discussed. First, hierarchical cluster analysis (HCA) is one of the popular and easy-to-understand methods that consider each data to be related to its neighbors based on certain distances and criteria. In HCA, two approaches can be implemented: the agglomerative and divisive approaches. In the agglomerative approach, the distance matrix is computed, and each data point is considered at the beginning as a separate cluster. Then K clusters are formed by iteratively merging similar points. Therefore, two spectral data points belong to the same cluster if the distance between them is minimal while they belong to different clusters if the distance is maximal. On the contrary, in the division approach, all data are considered as a single cluster and then at each iteration, the data are separated forming dissimilar clusters. As previously stated, two measures should be computed: the distance matrix and the similarity criterion. The choice of the distance between two data points $d(X_1, X_2)$ used in HCA varies and includes, but is not limited to, Euclidean, maximum, and Mahalanobis distances. For the similarity criterion, various choices also exist including maximum linkage, minimum linkage, and Ward's methods. The second approach that can be applied is the partition-based method where the most famous technique is K-means clustering. K-means clustering is also one of the very simple and frequently used techniques. It consists of defining *a priori* K clusters and iteratively assigning each data point to one of these clusters and updating the centroid of each cluster c_K. Initially, the clusters c_K are randomly assigned and the centroid is calculated. Then the distance between each data point (spectrum) and the centroids $d(X_i, c_K)$ are computed and the data is re-sorted by the minimal distance. Similar to the HCA method, the choice of distance varies and includes Euclidean, Manhattan, and cosine similarity. Afterward, we use the following equation to assign each data to the closet centroid:

$$\underset{c_K \in C}{\operatorname{argmin}}\, d^2(X_i, c_K), \tag{2.35}$$

where C is a set of the K centroids. Consequently, new centroids are computed by updating the old one as an average of the data that exist in each cluster. These steps are repeated until the centroids are not changed. The drawback of K-means is that it requires setting *a priori* the number of clusters and it is sensitive to small variations in the data. Another approach for clustering is fuzzy c-means clustering (FCM) [54], which is a generalization of the partition-based clustering method. The principle of the fuzzy approach is that each data point can belong to more than one cluster. In FCM, a cluster membership to all clusters is introduced which takes a value between 0 and 1 and the following function should be minimized:

$$J_m = \sum_{i=1}^{n} \sum_{j=1}^{C} u_{i,j}^{m} d^2\left(X_i, c_j\right), \tag{2.36}$$

where m is any real number greater than 1, $u_{i,j}$ is the degree of membership of X_i to the cluster j, c_j is the centroid of the cluster j, and d represents the distance between the variables and the centroid. FCM also iteratively optimizes the function defined previously and updates both the membership term and the centroids of the clusters.

2.3.3.2 *Classification*

Mainly, the classification task consists of training a model that best approximates a mapping function, which maps between the input data, e.g., the spectral Raman data, and its corresponding label or classes. This trained model is used afterward to classify a new input to the appropriate label. However, there are several types of classification algorithms where their use is data-dependent. For instance, the most intuitive method is the linear discriminant analysis (LDA) [55] which is used quite frequently in Raman spectral data analysis. LDA is a robust supervised classification method that consists of finding a direction that best discriminates between the classes. Therefore, LDA transforms the data by linearly projecting it into a lower-dimensional subspace where the labels L are distinct. These projections are completed by defining $L - 1$ discriminant functions ζ_l as a linear combination of the original variables:

$$\zeta_l = \omega_l^t . X + \beta_{l_0}, \tag{2.37}$$

where ω_l represents the weight vector for the lth discriminant function and β_{l_0} is the lth bias. These functions are estimated to maximize the between-group variance S_b and minimize the within-group variance S_w and this can be combined to find the solution for the following optimization problem:

$$\max_{V:\|V\|=1} \frac{V^t S_b V}{V^t S_w V}; \tag{2.38}$$

$$S_b = \sum_{l=1}^{L} n_l \left(\overline{X}_l - \overline{X}_g\right)\left(\overline{X}_l - \overline{X}_g\right)^t \tag{2.39}$$

$$S_w = \sum_{l=1}^{L} \sum_{i=1}^{n_l} \left(X_i^l - \overline{X}_l\right)\left(X_i^l - \overline{X}_l\right)^t \tag{2.40}$$

where $\overline{X}_l$ is the mean spectra per class, $\overline{X}_g$ is the mean of the whole data, n_l represents the number of spectra in each class, and X_i^l is the ith spectra in class l. The solution for this problem is given by the largest eigenvector of $S_w^{-1} S_b$, i.e.,

$$S_w^{-1} S_b V_1 = \lambda_1 V_1, \tag{2.41}$$

where λ_l is the eigenvalue that indicates the directions in which the groups should be separated. Similar to the Raman image analysis, SVM is also used frequently for spectral Raman data which consists of finding a hyperplane that features the largest margin between the classes and hence best separates the classes (details of the methods are presented in the image analysis pipeline section). Another machine learning method used for classification is the random forest (RF) [56]. RF is a supervised learning technique known for its simplicity and good performance. It consists of building several decision trees using bootstrap samples where the prediction from each is stored and the majority votes of prediction represent the final class. If $\widehat{C}_b$ represents the class prediction of the bth RF tree, then the final prediction of the RF model is given by the following:

$$\widehat{C}_{RF}^{B} = majority\,vote\left\{\widehat{C}_1,\cdots,\widehat{C}_B\right\}. \tag{2.42}$$

One of the growing fields for the classification task is DL, which is defined as a learning process between a network of functions to understand the connection between the input and output data. DL attempts to learn a mapping function between the input and output through a combination of data, weights, and bias. These elements interact to accurately classify input data. It consists of multiple layers of interconnected nodes that iteratively try to improve the learning procedure. Although DL overcomes standard machine learning methods, they are still very complex and computationally exhaustive [12, 57, 58].

2.3.3.3 *Regression*

In the previous section, the classification task was introduced for spectral Raman data analysis; however, quantitative data analysis is also well-known where a quantity or proportion of a substance or concentration, for instance, is predicted. In this regard, several regression techniques can be implemented which are supervised learning methods that explore the relationship between the Raman data X and a certain dependent variable Y. Frequently, partial least squares (PLS) regression [59, 60] is applied to spectral Raman data since Raman data involves a high number of components. PLS is an efficient and optimal regression technique that works by combining two techniques: PCA and multiple regression. Therefore, PLS aims to find a set of components that performs a simultaneous decomposition of X and Y where these components should explain as much as possible the covariance between X and Y. Hence, the first step is to decompose X and Y by using a set of orthogonal factors and loadings as follows:

$$\begin{array}{c} X = TP^t;\; T^tT = I \\ \widehat{Y} = TBC^t \end{array}, \tag{2.43}$$

where T is called the score matrix. In T the columns are the latent vectors, I is the identity matrix, P is the loading matrix, and B is a diagonal matrix with the weights as diagonal elements. Afterward, a regression step is performed where the decomposition of X is used to predict Y. The first set of PLS components and loadings $t = Xw$ and $u = Yc$ are calculated such that $w^t w = 1$, $t^t t = 1$, and $t^t u$ are maximal. Then, this first latent vector t is subtracted from both X and Y, and the procedure is repeated until X becomes a null matrix. Another popular method is principal component regression (PCR) [61] which is similar to PLS since both utilize a dimension reduction technique before applying the regression method; however, the main difference is that the PLS transformation is supervised, i.e., the components are obtained so that they explain as much as possible Y. Theoretically, the regression model can be written as

$$Y = XB + \xi, \tag{2.44}$$

where B contains the estimated regression coefficients and ξ represents the residuals. The coefficients are estimated by applying ordinary least squares which are formulated as

$$\hat{B} = \left(X^t X\right)^{-1} X^t Y. \tag{2.45}$$

However, in PCR the independent variables are transformed into the principal component space as

$$X^t X = PDP^t = Z^t Z, \tag{2.46}$$

where D is a diagonal matrix of eigenvalues of $X^t X$, P is the eigenvector matrix of $X^t X$, and Z contains the principal components. Afterward, a regression model is fitted to Y using Z, where the regression coefficient Q is estimated by applying the least squares method. Then the original coefficients are computed via $B = PQ$. Moreover, the RF method can be also applied for regression tasks and this by following the same steps explained in the RF classification task, but the final prediction is given by

$$\hat{f}_{RF}^{B} = \frac{1}{B}\sum_{b=1}^{B} T_b, \tag{2.47}$$

where $\{T_1, \cdots, T_B\}$ is the ensemble of trees.

2.4 Model evaluation

All methods mentioned earlier are used to either reconstruct real Raman data from observation or generate models that extract features from data, classify, and predict certain classes and components. However, the aim is to achieve results that are as close as possible to the real measurements and to generate models that demonstrate high predictive performance. Therefore, it is important to check how close the reconstruction is to the real data and to determine how general and robust the trained models are. For these reasons, two subsections are described below that include the most common evaluation techniques used in Raman data analysis.

2.4.1 *Cross-validation*

Once a learning function is trained on initial data a prediction model is obtained; however, information on its quality is missing. Before relying on its prediction, it is essential to assess its performance. Additionally, each method described above depends on one or more (hyper-)parameters and their choice has a strong impact on the final performance. That leads to the problem of selecting a model and its hyper-parameter. Evaluation methods provide an answer to these problems [62, 63]. All are resampling techniques that consist of splitting the original data into subsamples where a model is trained on a subset and then the model is evaluated by measuring the error made when predicting the remaining data. However, several approaches exist to implement these evaluation methods, which are dependent on the way the dataset is split. In this regard, holdout validation, *k*-fold cross-validation (CV), leave-*p*-out CV, and Monte Carlo CV are common methods used for evaluating the trained models. First, holdout validation is the simplest version of CV where the data is shuffled first and then divided once into two sets of training and testing, where usually the training size is twice the testing size. Afterward, the model is trained using the training set and the trained model is used to predict the testing set. Although this approach is straightforward to implement, in reality the testing set might contain important features of the whole data that were excluded. Another type of CV is *k*-fold CV, which is one of the most popular approaches that is used in various fields. *k*-fold CV consists of randomly dividing the data into *k* folds or subsets where iteratively each fold is considered a testing set and left aside for prediction while the model is trained on the remaining folds, and this is repeated for the *k* folds. On the other hand, in leave-*p*-out CV, randomly selected data that constitute the testing set are maintained for the prediction purpose while the remaining $N - p$ data are used to train the model. All possible combinations of *p* samples are checked and aggregated to evaluate the model. Finally, the Monte Carlo CV randomly selects a subset to train the model and the remaining data are used for prediction. This procedure is repeated several times to ensure high accuracy and unbiased validation. To choose an evaluation approach, its algorithmic complexity should be considered when the computation time is limited. In addition, some problems arise when the assumptions made by the CV concept are violated. For instance, when the data is dependent, the training and the testing datasets are no longer independent which can induce a strong bias in the prediction of the performance of the trained model.

2.4.2 *Metrics*

Plenty of evaluation metrics are available that are data- and task-dependent. For instance, classification or clustering models can be evaluated using a confusion matrix, which is a representation of the prediction output and the true values of the testing set. From the confusion matrix, various metrics can be derived which indicate how well the model performed such as sensitivity, specificity, accuracy, precision, and F1 score:

$$sensitivity = \frac{T_+}{T_+ + F_-} \tag{2.48}$$

$$specificity = \frac{T_-}{T_- + F_+} \tag{2.49}$$

$$accuracy = \frac{T_+ + T_-}{T_+ + T_- + F_+ + F_-} \tag{2.50}$$

$$Precision = \frac{T_+}{T_+ + F_+} \tag{2.51}$$

$$F_1 score = \frac{2T_+}{2T_+ + F_+ + F_-} \tag{2.52}$$

where T_+, T_-, F_+ and F_- represent the number of true positive, true negative, false positive, and false negative predictions, respectively. Moreover, the receiver operating characteristic curve can also be useful since it shows the performance of a classification model at different thresholds where it visualizes the 1-specificity against the sensitivity. On the other hand, for regression models, metrics that calculate the distance between the predicted and the true data can be implemented such as mean absolute error, mean-squared error, root-mean-squared error (RMSE), and R-squared (R^2). For instance, RMSE and R^2 are given by the following equations, respectively:

$$RMSE\left(Y,\hat{Y}\right)=\sqrt{\frac{1}{n}\sum_{i=1}^{n}\left(Y_i-\hat{Y}_i\right)^2} \tag{2.53}$$

$$R^2=1-\frac{\sum_{i=1}^{n}\left(Y_i-\hat{Y}_i\right)^2}{\sum_{i=1}^{n}\left(Y_i-\overline{Y}\right)^2}, \tag{2.54}$$

where Y_i is the ith true value, $\hat{Y}_i$ is the predicted one, and $\overline{Y}$ is the mean value. These evaluation metrics can also be used for checking the quality of the reconstruction in inverse problems or preprocessing tasks. In image analysis, additional metrics are developed and some details about the commonly used ones are presented here. For instance, the structural similarity index (SSIM) [64] is used to quantify the similarity of a constructed image to its original. This metric highlights the difference between the two images in terms of luminence, contrast, and structure and it is given by

$$SSIM\left(Y,\hat{Y}\right)=\frac{\left(2\overline{Y}\overline{\hat{Y}}+C_1\right)\left(2\sigma_{Y\hat{Y}}+C_2\right)}{\left(\overline{Y}^2+\overline{\hat{Y}}^2+C_1\right)\left(\sigma_Y^2+\sigma_{\hat{Y}}^2+C_2\right)}, \tag{2.55}$$

where $\overline{Y}$ is the mean of the true image, $\hat{Y}$ is the mean of the reconstructed image, σ_Y is the standard deviation of the true image, $\sigma_{\hat{Y}}$ is the standard deviation of the reconstructed image, C_1 and C_2 are two constants, and $\sigma_{Y\hat{Y}}$ represents the covariance of the true image Y and the predicted one $\hat{Y}$. On the other hand, peak signal-to-noise ratio (PSNR) [65] is one of the popular metrics that is implemented to compare the effects of image preprocessing methods on the quality of the image, and it can be translated mathematically as follows:

$$PSNR\left(Y,\hat{Y}\right)=20\log_{10}\left(\frac{Max_Y}{\sqrt{\frac{1}{IJ}\sum_{i=0}^{I-1}\sum_{j=0}^{J-1}\left\|Y(i,j)-\hat{Y}(i,j)\right\|^2}}\right), \tag{2.56}$$

where I represents the number of rows of pixels of the image and J is the number of columns of pixels of the image. For the segmentation task, the quality of the segmented image can be measured by using various statistical parameters such as the rand index, global consistency error, and variations of information [66]. In conclusion, for each task different evaluation metrics are used and it is a common practice to combine several metrics which can provide a more reliable model evaluation.

2.5 Summary

Photonic data acquired from linear and nonlinear Raman devices are large and of different forms, e.g., images and spectra. They are complex and cannot be easily understandable and informative. Therefore, specific treatments of these data are needed which include the application of machine learning and DL methods. These methods are task- and data-dependent and consist of a variety of techniques. In this chapter, the most important techniques that are implemented for image and spectral Raman data analysis are presented. These two different forms of Raman data require distinct data pipelines, therefore separate pipelines were presented for each. Regardless of the form of the acquired Raman data, preprocessing steps should be implemented before further analysis such as feature extraction and classification. Due to the presence of artifacts and noise originating from the Raman setup and the sample environment, the acquired Raman data are often disrupted. Therefore, various methods that remove artifacts and improve the quality of the Raman data should be implemented which are dependent on the type of data.

For instance, in the case of Raman images, denoising techniques such as filter-based methods, variational denoising methods, and transform-based methods are implemented to remove unwanted variations from the images. Another important step in the analysis of Raman images is to detect differences between images and potential changes, therefore image registration methods can be implemented to solve this problem. Moreover, object detection consists of methods that are crucial in Raman data which can detect abnormalities in the sample, for instance, in the cells. Finally, the normalization step is crucial for further analysis such as classification and it is divided into intensity- and geometric-based methods.

On the other hand, for spectral data analysis, burned and contaminated Raman spectra should be removed since they will compromise further analysis, and this is achieved by applying outlier detection methods such as z-score or modified z-score. The next step consists of removing spikes from the data since these cosmic spikes are extremely large, and the signal level becomes many orders of magnitude larger than the measured spectra which compromises spectral data analysis steps such as normalization. One of the challenges in

Raman spectra is the presence of a fluorescence background which needs to be removed, and this can be achieved by implementing baseline correction techniques such as SNIP, ALS, and EMSC. Because of instrumental bias on the Raman spectra, a shift in the wavenumber position and changes in the intensity can be observed. Therefore, intensity and wavenumber calibration are also crucial steps. Intensity calibration removes unwanted spectral variations which leads to better Raman data quality and subsequently good model performance, and wavenumber calibration corrects the Raman spectra to the same wavenumber axis. Smoothing can also be implemented to remove noises from the Raman spectra, but the method should be chosen cautiously so that the smoothed spectra do not lose important Raman features. Finally, normalization methods are utilized since it is necessary to eliminate variations resulting from differences in sample thickness, laser focus, and optical path length. Since Raman data involves an enormous number of components where not all of them are playing a role in further analysis, feature extraction and feature selection methods are implemented to acquire important features in the Raman spectra. While feature extraction consists of reducing dimensionality in the data by applying a transformation to a new subspace, feature selection selects a set of features that best describe the Raman data. A lot of methods can be implemented in this regard: PCA, ICA, and FA are implemented to extract features by projecting the data to new subspaces, and ANOVA, Spearman, and Pearson coefficients are used to choose components that best describe the Raman data. An inverse problem step is needed when CARS spectra are acquired, which consists of extracting the Raman-like spectrum by applying phase retrieval methods such as MEM and KK.

The final step for image and spectral Raman data analysis is data modeling, which is task-dependent. For instance, in Raman images, semantic segmentation can be implemented which intends to classify each pixel of an image to its appropriate class. This is achieved by creating masks of the image segments that correspond to each class, and various methods are considered such as graph-based segmentation algorithms, gradient-based algorithms, and SLIC algorithms. Additionally, image segmentation methods such as clustering-based, threshold-based, and edge-based methods can be utilized, and they consist of analyzing Raman images which can highlight the region of interest and abnormalities in the image.

Image classification is an important task where acquired images are classified into their corresponding predefined classes. Methods such as SVM,

RF, and Hidden Markov models are implemented in this regard. For spectral Raman data, clustering techniques such as hierarchical, partition, and fuzzy clustering are implemented which consist of finding similar patterns within the data without the need for labels. Classification methods are similar to the case of Raman images which consists of training a model that best approximates the mapping function between the input data and its corresponding label. Additionally, quantitative data analysis via regression is much employed for spectral Raman data, which explore the relationship between the Raman data and a certain dependent variable such as concentration values. Most important is the rise of the DL networks in all these tasks where either a pretrained network is used as a transfer learning technique or a new architecture is developed according to the data in hand.

References

1. Alisha, P. B. and Sheela, K. G. (2016) Image denoising techniques-an overview. IOSR J. Electr. Commun. Eng. **11**, 78–84.
2. Fan, L., Zhang, F., Fan, H. and Zhang, C. (2019) Brief review of image denoising techniques. Vis. Comput. Ind. Biomed. Art **2**, 1–12.
3. Brown, L. G. (1992) A survey of image registration techniques. ACM Comput. Surv. **24**, 325–376.
4. Nag, S. (2017) Image registration techniques: a survey. arXiv preprint arXiv:1712.07540.
5. Patro, S. G. K. and Sahu, K. K. (2015) Normalization: a preprocessing stage. arXiv preprint arXiv:1503.06462.
6. Liao, C.-J. and Chen, S.-Y. (2002) Complementary retrieval for distorted images. Pattern Recognit. **35**, 1705–1722.
7. Shinohara, R. T., Sweeney, E. M., Goldsmith, J., Shiee, N., Mateen, F. J., Calabresi, P. A., Jarso, S., Pham, D. L., Reich, D. S. and Crainiceanu, C. M. (2014) Statistical normalization techniques for magnetic resonance imaging. NeuroImage Clin. **6**, 9–19.
8. Zhang, Q., Yun, K. K., Wang, H., Yoon, S. W., Lu, F. and Won, D. (2021) Automatic cell counting from stimulated Raman imaging using deep learning. PLOS One **16**, e0254586.
9. Zhiqiang, W. and Jun, L. (2017) A review of object detection based on convolutional neural network. In 2017 36th Chinese Control Conference (CCC), pp. 11104–11109.
10. Thoma, M. (2016) A survey of semantic segmentation. arXiv preprint arXiv:1602.06541.
11. Radhakrishna, A., Shaji, A., Smith, K., Lucchi, A., Fua, P. and Süsstrunk, S. (2010) SLIC Superpixels. EPFL Technical Report 149300.

12. Pradhan, P., Guo, S., Ryabchykov, O., Popp, J. and Bocklitz, T. W. (2020) Deep learning a boon for biophotonics? J. Biophotonics **13**, e201960186.
13. Hamilton, M., Zhang, Z., Hariharan, B., Snavely, N. and Freeman, W. T. (2022) Unsupervised semantic segmentation by distilling feature correspondences. arXiv preprint arXiv:2203.08414.
14. Pradhan, P., Meyer, T., Vieth, M., Stallmach, A., Waldner, M., Schmitt, M., Popp, J. and Bocklitz, T. (2019) Semantic segmentation of non-linear multimodal images for disease grading of inflammatory bowel disease: a segnet-based application. In ICPRAM, pp. 396–405.
15. Sathya, B. and Manavalan, R. (2011) Image segmentation by clustering methods: performance analysis. Int. J. Comput. Appl. **29**, 27–32.
16. Kaur, D. and Kaur, Y. (2014) Various image segmentation techniques: a review. Int. J. Comput. Sci. Mob. Comput. **3**, 809–814.
17. Pal, N. R. and Pal, S. K. (1993) A review on image segmentation techniques. Pattern Recognit. **26**, 1277–1294.
18. Haralick, R. M. and Shapiro, L. G. (1985) Image segmentation techniques. Comput. Vis. Graph. Image Process. **29**, 100–132.
19. Sharma, N. and Aggarwal, L. M. (2010) Automated medical image segmentation techniques. J. Med. Phys. **35**, 3.
20. Nath, S. S., Mishra, G., Kar, J., Chakraborty, S. and Dey, N. (2014) A survey of image classification methods and techniques. In 2014 International Conference on Control, Instrumentation, Communication and Computational Technologies (ICCICCT), pp. 554–557.
21. Camp Jr., C. H., Lee, Y. J. and Cicerone, M. T. (2016) Quantitative, comparable coherent anti-Stokes Raman scattering (CARS) spectroscopy: correcting errors in phase retrieval. J. Raman Spectrosc. **47**, 408–415.
22. Kuzmenko, A. B. (2005) Kramers–Kronig constrained variational analysis of optical spectra. Rev. Sci. Instrum. **76**, 083108.
23. Gornov, E., Vartiainen, E. M. and Peiponen, K.-E. (2006) Comparison of subtractive Kramers-Kronig analysis and maximum entropy model in resolving phase from finite spectral range reflectance data. Appl. Opt. **45**, 6519–6524.
24. Cicerone, M. T., Aamer, K. A., Lee, Y. J. and Vartiainen, E. (2012) Maximum entropy and time-domain Kramers–Kronig phase retrieval approaches are functionally equivalent for CARS microspectroscopy. J. Raman Spectrosc. **43**, 637–643.
25. Vartiainen, E. M. (1992) Phase retrieval approach for coherent anti-Stokes Raman scattering spectrum analysis. JOSA B **9**, 1209–1214.
26. Houhou, R., Barman, P., Schmitt, M., Meyer, T., Popp, J. and Bocklitz, T. (2020) Deep learning as phase retrieval tool for CARS spectra. Opt. Express **28**, 21002–21024.
27. Valensise, C. M., Giuseppi, A., Vernuccio, F., De la Cadena, A., Cerullo, G. and Polli, D. (2020) Removing non-resonant background from CARS spectra via deep learning. APL Photonics **5**, 061305.

28. Wang, Z., O' Dwyer, K., Muddiman, R., Ward, T., Camp Jr., C. H. and Hennelly, B. M. (2022) VECTOR: Very deep convolutional autoencoders for non-resonant background removal in broadband coherent anti-Stokes Raman scattering. J. Raman Spectrosc. **53**, 1081–1093.
29. Junjuri, R., Saghi, A., Lensu, L. and Vartiainen, E. M. (2022) Effect of non-resonant background on the extraction of Raman signals from CARS spectra using deep neural networks. RSC Adv. **12**, 28755–28766.
30. Guo, S., Popp, J. and Bocklitz, T. (2021) Chemometric analysis in Raman spectroscopy from experimental design to machine learning–based modeling. Nat. Protoc. **16**, 5426–5459.
31. Ehrentreich, F. and Sümmchen, L. (2001) Spike removal and denoising of Raman spectra by wavelet transform methods. Anal. Chem. **73**, 4364–4373.
32. Maury, A. and Revilla, R. I. (2015) Autocorrelation analysis combined with a wavelet transform method to detect and remove cosmic rays in a single Raman spectrum. Appl. Spectrosc. **69**, 984–992.
33. Tian, Y. and Burch, K. S. (2016) Automatic spike removal algorithm for Raman spectra. Appl. Spectrosc. **70**, 1861–1871.
34. Ryabchykov, O., Bocklitz, T., Ramoji, A., Neugebauer, U., Foerster, M., Kroegel, C., Bauer, M., Kiehntopf, M. and Popp, J. (2016) Automatization of spike correction in Raman spectra of biological samples. Chemom. Intell. Lab. Syst. **155**, 1–6.
35. Katsumoto, Y. and Ozaki, Y. (2003) Practical algorithm for reducing convex spike noises on a spectrum. Appl. Spectrosc. **57**, 317–322.
36. Wei, D., Chen, S. and Liu, Q. (2015) Review of fluorescence suppression techniques in Raman spectroscopy. Appl. Spectrosc. Rev. **50**, 387–406.
37. Ryan, C. G., Clayton, E., Griffin, W. L., Sie, S. H. and Cousens, D. R. (1988) SNIP, a statistics-sensitive background treatment for the quantitative analysis of PIXE spectra in geoscience applications. Nucl. Instrum. Methods Phys. Res. Sect. B **34**, 396–402.
38. Peng, J., Peng, S., Jiang, A., Wei, J., Li, C. and Tan, J. (2010) Asymmetric least squares for multiple spectra baseline correction. Anal. Chim. Acta **683**, 63–68.
39. Martens, H. and Stark, E. (1991) Extended multiplicative signal correction and spectral interference subtraction: New preprocessing methods for near infrared spectroscopy. J. Pharm. Biomed. Anal. **9**, 625–635.
40. Afseth, N. K. and Kohler, A. (2012) Extended multiplicative signal correction in vibrational spectroscopy, a tutorial. Chemom. Intell. Lab. Syst. **117**, 92–99.
41. Raj, A., Kato, C., Witek, H. A. and Hamaguchi, H. (2020) Toward standardization of Raman spectroscopy: Accurate wavenumber and intensity calibration using rotational Raman spectra of H2, HD, D2, and vibration–rotation spectrum of O2. J. Raman Spectrosc. **51**, 2066–2082.
42. Choquette, S. J., Etz, E. S., Hurst, W. S., Blackburn, D. H. and Leigh, S. D. (2007) Relative intensity correction of Raman spectrometers: NIST SRMs 2241 through 2243 for 785 nm, 532 nm, and 488 nm/514.5 nm excitation. Appl. Spectrosc. **61**, 117–129.

43. Hutsebaut, D., Vandenabeele, P. and Moens, L. (2005) Evaluation of an accurate calibration and spectral standardization procedure for Raman spectroscopy. Analyst **130**, 1204–1214.
44. Press, W. H. and Teukolsky, S. A. (1990) Savitzky-Golay smoothing filters. Comput. Phys. **4**, 669–672.
45. Zhao, X. Y., Liu, G. Y., Sui, Y. T., Xu, M. and Tong, L. (2021) Denoising method for Raman spectra with low signal-to-noise ratio based on feature extraction. Spectrochim. Acta. A **250**, 119374.
46. Fodor, I. K. (2002) A survey of dimension reduction techniques. https://doi.org/10.2172/15002155.
47. Stone, J. V. (2002) Independent component analysis: an introduction. Trends Cogn. Sci. **6**, 59–64.
48. Li, J., Cheng, K., Wang, S., Morstatter, F., Trevino, R. P., Tang, J. and Liu, H. (2017) Feature selection: A data perspective. ACM Comput. Surv. CSUR **50**, 1–45.
49. Guyon, I. and Elisseeff, A. (2003) An introduction to variable and feature selection. J. Mach. Learn. Res. **3**, 1157–1182.
50. Benesty, J., Chen, J., Huang, Y. and Cohen, I. (2009) Pearson Correlation Coefficient. In *Noise Reduction in Speech Processing* (Cohen, I., Huang, Y., Chen, J., and Benesty, J., Eds.), pp. 1–4, Springer.
51. Myers, L. and Sirois, M. J. (2006) Differences between Spearman Correlation Coefficients. In *Encyclopedia of Statistical Sciences*, John Wiley & Sons.
52. St, L. and Wold, S. (1989) Analysis of variance (ANOVA). Chemom. Intell. Lab. Syst. **6**, 259–272.
53. Zhang, H., Wang, J., Sun, Z., Zurada, J. M. and Pal, N. R. (2020) Feature selection for neural networks using group lasso regularization. IEEE Trans. Knowl. Data Eng. **32**, 659–673.
54. Karim, E., Madani, S. P. V. S. K. and Yun, F. (2010) *Fuzzy Clustering Analysis.* Master's Thesis, Blekinge Institute of Technology, Blekinge.
55. Balakrishnama, S. and Ganapathiraju, A. (1998) Linear discriminant analysis-a brief tutorial. Inst. Signal Inf. Process. **18**, 1–8.
56. Speiser, J. L., Miller, M. E., Tooze, J. and Ip, E. (2019) A comparison of random forest variable selection methods for classification prediction modeling. Expert Syst. Appl. **134**, 93–101.
57. Luo, R., Popp, J. and Bocklitz, T. (2022) Deep learning for Raman spectroscopy: a review. Analytica **3**, 287–301.
58. Lussier, F., Thibault, V., Charron, B., Wallace, G. Q. and Masson, J.-F. (2020) Deep learning and artificial intelligence methods for Raman and surface-enhanced Raman scattering. Trends Anal. Chem. **124**, 115796.
59. Ng, K. S. (2013) A simple explanation of partial least squares. https://users.cecs.anu.edu.au/~kee/pls.pdf.

60. Abdi, H. (2003) Partial Least Square Regression (PLS Regression). In *Encyclopedia of Social Sciences Research Methods* (Lews-Beck, M., Bryman, A. and Futing, T., Eds.), pp. 792–795, SAGE.
61. Ortabaş, N. (2001) *Principal Components in the Problem of Multicollinearity.* PhD Thesis, DEÜ Fen Bilimleri Enstitüsü.
62. Kohavi, R. (1995) A study of cross-validation and bootstrap for accuracy estimation and model selection. In IJCAI, pp. 1137–1145.
63. Xu, Q.-S., Liang, Y.-Z. and Du, Y.-P. (2004) Monte Carlo cross-validation for selecting a model and estimating the prediction error in multivariate calibration. J. Chemom. **18**, 112–120.
64. Zujovic, J., Pappas, T. N. and Neuhoff, D. L. (2013) Structural texture similarity metrics for image analysis and retrieval. IEEE Trans. Image Process. **22**, 2545–2558.
65. Korhonen, J. and You, J. (2012) Peak signal-to-noise ratio revisited: Is simple beautiful? In 2012 Fourth International Workshop on Quality of Multimedia Experience, pp. 37–38.
66. Küçükkülahli, E., Erdoğmuş, P. and Polat, K. (2016) Brain MRI segmentation based on different clustering algorithms. Int. J. Comput. Appl. **155**, 37–40.

https://doi.org/10.1142/9789811264610_0003

Chapter 3

Chemometric Treatment of Raman Spectra in Biomedicine and Food Science

Ángel Sánchez-Illana, David Pérez-Guaita*

Department of Analytical Chemistry, Chemistry Faculty, Universtitat de València, Doctor Moliner 50, 46100 Burjassot, Spain
**Corresponding author: david.perez-guaita@uv.es*

3.1 Introduction

Biomedicine and food science are active fields of research with deep economic and social implications. Both fields require analytical methodologies which provide quantitative and qualitative information about the chemical components of the samples and thus, new analytical improvements are continuously developed to drive innovative lines of research as well as to perform routine analysis.

In this context, Raman spectroscopy is a versatile technique that provides a wide range of tools to investigate the composition of biological samples, from high-throughput microscopes for the analysis of cells and bacteria to handheld portable instruments to investigate the composition of bulk samples *in situ*. Although clinical and food sciences are very distinct fields, both deal with complex biological samples containing several components such as water, carbohydrates, proteins, or lipids.

Raman spectroscopy has many advantages when it comes to the analysis of food and clinical samples. The characteristic Raman spectrum of a biological sample constituent, caused by the unique vibrational modes of each Raman active molecule, provides enough selectivity to identify biological molecules, pharmaceuticals, adulterants, and contaminants. Furthermore, since Raman intensities are proportional to the concentration of the molecules under study, quantification methodologies can be developed to predict the concentration of a nutrient or a clinical parameter. In addition, the weak Raman scattering of water facilitates direct measurement on aqueous samples.

However, biological samples are diverse matrices containing a wide range of components, and their Raman spectrum is normally composed by a set of overlapped bands. This hampers the proper assignment of bands to specific molecular vibrations. Consider as an example the Raman shifts depicted in Figure 3.1 for the different moieties of lipids, nucleic acids, and proteins. A combination of these signals would result in a spectrum rich in chemical information, but it would be virtually impossible to extract this information with the naked eye. In practice, the experimental Raman spectra of biological samples are even more complicated because other molecules are also present [1–3].

Moreover, Raman spectra are acquired employing a variety of techniques including classical non-resonant Raman, resonant Raman, surface-enhanced Raman scattering (SERS), surface-enhanced resonance Raman scattering, and Fourier transform Raman spectroscopy. In these techniques, different experimental parameters are adjusted to optimize the analytical features.

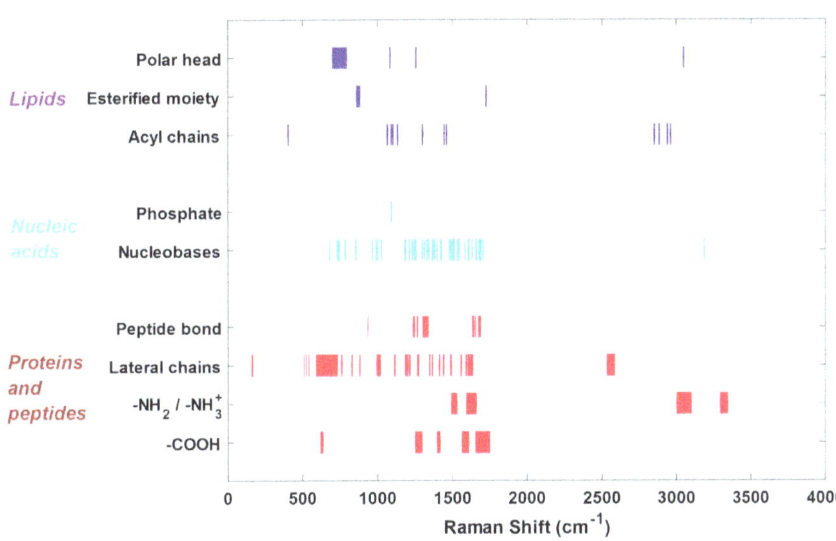

Figure 3.1. Raman shifts of different moieties of lipids, nucleic acids, and proteins. Data extracted from Niaura *et al.* [1].

These technical parameters include the laser (e.g., wavelength, continuous/pulsed, power) and the chemistry of SERS substrates (e.g., metal composition, nanoparticle type, colloidal/solid) and cause different enhancements for each vibrational mode, which adds variability to the spectra. In summary, the extraction of information from the Raman spectra of clinical samples and foodstuffs is challenged by the intrinsic complexity of the overlapped Raman bands and, in most of the cases, the univariate study of a single Raman variable is not enough. In this context, the use of chemometric approaches that can provide an integrated analysis of the whole spectra using multivariate approaches becomes indispensable.

A plethora of data analysis workflows employing multivariate statistics are currently being developed in the field of chemometrics, which has been influenced by the emergence of machine learning, deep learning, and data mining. These methods have been applied to the analysis of Raman spectra of biological samples and foodstuffs and used for the discrimination (i.e., classification) or the determination (i.e., quantification) of parameters. In this regard, comprehensive reviews and tutorials have been published in recent years, and the field aims to move towards the standardization of methodologies [4–7]. Here we provide a brief description of the modeling process for the reader, and we refer to dedicated chapters in this book for further information.

The first step is preprocessing, which is used to reduce the noise and technical variations and enhance the signals related to the analyte or class of interest. This can include basic operations (e.g., spectral range selection, scaling) or more sophisticated routines such as baseline correction, random noise reduction or spectral differentiation [4, 7]. Preprocessed spectra are then used in the model training, which is, in general, a function approximation [8]. Thus, any model considered is used to approximate a function that assigns one element of response space y from the spectra space x. Given a spectrum matrix $\boldsymbol{X} \in x$, and a model $f\colon x \rightarrow y$, the response matrix $\boldsymbol{Y} \in y$ is approximated by the prediction of $\widehat{\boldsymbol{Y}} \in y$ as:

$$\boldsymbol{Y} \approx \widehat{\boldsymbol{Y}} = f(\boldsymbol{X}) \tag{3.1}$$

In the spectrum matrix $\boldsymbol{X}$, each x is a spectrum vector. Likewise, $\hat{y}$ is a predicted vector in the matrix $\widehat{\boldsymbol{Y}}$ of predicted responses (i.e., class or concentrations).

Then, validation approaches are used for optimizing the model fitting (i.e., optimizing the parameters of the model) and for a first evaluation of the results and significance of the model. For the former, different types of cross-validation are the most common methods. For the latter, resampling approaches are the most popular (e.g., a single evaluation set, leave-one-out, leave-more-out, single and double cross-validation, bootstrapping and permutation tests). Finally, independent testing (i.e., test set validation) is used to assess the actual predictive performance on new samples and it is the penultimate step towards the final implementation of the method in routine analysis [4, 7, 9]. It should be noted that a proper test set validation, including samples as independent from the calibration sample set, is the only way to estimate error metrics [10].

In this chapter we wanted to provide an overview about one of the most popular applications of the chemometric analysis of Raman data: the elucidation of chemical information contained in Raman spectra from biological matrices. To that end, we discuss state-of-the art chemometric workflows for most common scenarios in the fields of biomedicine and food science, assessing specific challenges and pitfalls and providing an outline on recent and future trends. Section 3.2 describes the use of chemometrics in the Raman analysis of food contamination, authentication, and in the prediction of nutritional parameters, while Section 3.3 focuses on applications in diagnosis of diseases, prediction of clinical parameters, and analysis of clinical longitudinal studies as well as data fusion.

3.2 Analysis of Raman Datasets in Food Science

When the first Raman analysis of foodstuffs was published in the pre-chemometrics era (i.e., early 1970s), Raman bands were being integrated from paper records using a classical planimeter. In this context, the implementation of early computers such as the IBM1800 for spectra processing was a breakthrough [11] that enabled faster analysis and minimized human-related errors. Since then, the development of computing and chemometrics have allowed the study of an increasing number of food matrices qualitatively and quantitatively.

Different chemometric approaches have revealed the potential of Raman spectroscopy to the food and nutritional science community. However, these tools are still being used exclusively for research purposes and they are rarely employed in official food safety laboratories. A lack of method harmonization of chemometric methods applied to Raman, and the need of technicians trained on advanced multivariate analysis could explain the marginal use of these tools in official institutions. This section presents state-of-the-art chemometrics methodologies for food Raman datasets covering their use, validation, and transferability to official laboratories in three main fields: 1) Analysis of food contamination, 2) Analysis of food authentication, and 3) Nutritional quality assessment.

For further clarification on food terminology, analytical guidelines, and limits we refer the reader to the publications made by Codex Alimentarius (FAO/WHO): https://www.fao.org/fao-who-codexalimentarius.

3.2.1 *Analysis of Food Contamination*

Analysis of contaminants in foodstuffs allows the detection of harmful microbiological agents and the quantitative and qualitative evaluation of pesticide and pollutant residues. Due to the large variability among each class of contaminants and matrices, a wide range of methodologies based on the chemometric analysis of Raman data have been developed. Multivariate analysis of Raman bands can be used as a label-free approach which identifies spectral fingerprints of bacteria (i.e., composition of the outer surface of bacteria and the excretions of small molecules), fungi (i.e., excreted mycotoxins) or the contaminant itself (i.e., antibiotic, pesticide, or pollutant residues). Besides, multivariate analysis can also be used in labeled approaches for extracting the reporter signal within the matrix. Furthermore, more complex recognition methods have also been developed, combining the separation and enrichment of the analyte with label-free or label-based Raman approaches [12].

Table 3.1 exemplifies that standard Raman and other related techniques such as SERS, Raman imaging or single-cell Raman spectroscopy (SCRS) have been coupled with different chemometric workflows for the analysis of different types of contaminants and matrices. Among these chemometric approaches, classification models are the most common, but quantitative models have also been carried out. Preprocessing steps include baseline correction, Savitzky–Golay (SG) smoothing with or without derivatization, and standard normal variate (SNV) normalization. Regarding classification and regression, various methods have been proposed including principal component analysis (PCA), partial least squares (PLS), support vector machines (SVM) for both discriminant analysis (SVMDA) and regression (SVR), convolutional neural network (CNN), and recurrent neural network (RNN) among others.

Table 3.1. Examples of recent publications employing Raman and chemometrics for contamination assessment.

Contamination	Analyte(s)	Type of Sample	Raman Technique	Chemometric Technique(s)			Software	Ref.
				Preprocessing	*Training*	*Validation*		
Bacteria	Bacteria Species	Cultures	SCRS	SNV, SG	KPCA-DT and PCA-SVM	kf-CV	Scikit-Learn (Python)	[13]
	Cyanobacteria	Spirulina	RS	Norm, SG	PCA, SVMDA and SVR	Validation set	PLS toolbox (MATLAB)	[14]
Fungi	Aflatoxin B_1	Peanut oil	RS	ASN-SMOTE	CNN and RNN	Validation set	Tensorflow and Keras (Python)	[15]
	Zearalenone	Maize	RS	SG	PLS, siPLS, ACO-PLS, siPLS-ACO	Validation set	MATLAB	[16]
Antibiotic residue	Chloramphenicol	Pork meat	SERS	Raw, SNV, MSC	PLS, VCPA-PLS, ACO-PLS, UVE-PLS, CARS-PLS	Validation set	MATLAB	[17]
	Chlortetracycline and oxytetracycline	Spiked animal feed	SERS	Norm, SG	KNN, LDA, MLR, PLS	Validation set	SAS	[18]
Pesticide residue	Thiabendazole	Citrus	SERS	SNV, SG, MSC, MC, airPLS	PLS, GA-PLS, CARS-PLS, ACO-PLS	Validation set and reference method	MATLAB	[19]
Heavy metals	Mercury	Tea-spiked samples	SERS	SNV, SG	ACO-PLS	Validation set	MATLAB	[20]
Microplastics	Microplastics	Caryfish	RS	CR, Baseline corr., SG	PVR*	—	WIRE and ImageJ	[21]

Abbreviations: **SCRS**: Single-Cell Raman Spectroscopy; **SNV**: Standard Normal Variate; **SG**: Savitzky-Golay; **K-PCA**: Kernel Principal Component Analysis-Decision Tree; **PCA**: Principal Component Analysis; **SVM**: Support Vector Machines; **kf-CV**: Cross-Validation; **RS**: Raman Spectroscopy; **Norm**: Normalization; **SVR**: Support Vector Regression; **SMOTE**: Synthetic Minority Class Oversampling Technique; **CNN**: Convolutional Neural Network; **RNN**: Recurrent Neural Network; **PLS**: Partial Least Squares; **SiPLS**: Synergy Interval PLS; **ACO-PLS**: Ant Colony Optimization-PLS; **MSC**: Multiplicative Scattering Correction; **UVE-PLS**: Uninformative Variable Elimination-PLS; **LDA**: Linear Discriminant Analysis; **KNN**: k-Nearest Neighbors; **MLR**: Multiple Linear Regression; **MC**: Mean Center; **airPLS**: adaptive iteratively reweighted-PLS; **GA-PLS**: Genetic Algorithm-PLS; **SERS**: Surface-Enhanced Raman Spectroscopy; **PVR**: Pixel Value Ratio.

For bacterial contamination analysis, SCRS offers an interesting alternative to traditional microbiological cultures, especially in terms of analysis time. However, Raman signals of bacteria are complex due to the low scattering efficiency of single cells, the high number of bands in their spectra, and the heterogeneity of bacteria individuals within the same strain. In order to overcome these challenges, models based on kernel principal component analysis-decision tree (KPCA-DT) and PCA-SVM were implemented by Yan *et al.* to classify among different genera and strain of bacteria cultures [13]. The main advantage of the applied methodologies was that, while standard PCA extracted only linear information, PCA-SVM or KPCA-DT were able to exploit nonlinear features for the discrimination. Figure 3.2 shows the high discrimination performance of the KPCA-DT algorithm applied for the different bacteria strains.

Other methods based on machine learning for analyzing bacteria and mycotoxins include SVMDA, SVR, and deep learning neural networks such

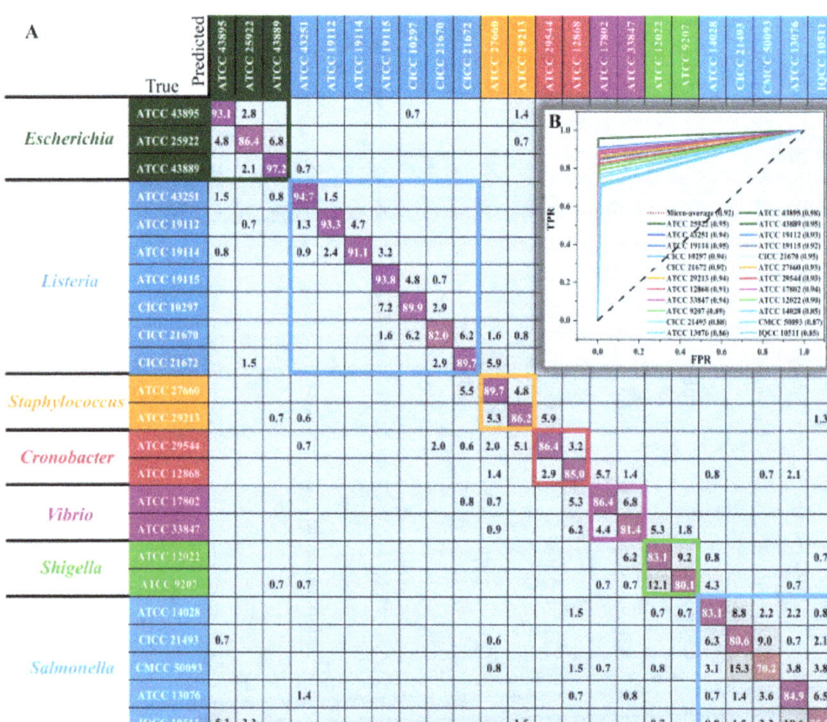

Figure 3.2. Discrimination performance of a KPCA-DT classification model for all bacterial strains analyzed with SCRS by Yan *et al.* Reproduced from Ref. [13] with permission.

as CNN and RNN for both classification and quantification. Adejimi *et al.* [14] used SVMDA in spirulina samples for the classification of several species of cyanobacteria at concentration levels of 10^4 cells/mL. Furthermore, SVR allowed the quantification of bacteria within the 10^4–10^8 range with acceptable root mean square error of prediction (RMSEP) values. For hazardous mycotoxin analysis, CNN and RNN models were proposed by Deng *et al.* in peanut oil samples [15]. It was observed that with CNN and RNN the complex spectra preprocessing steps were not necessary, but the dataset had to be balanced (i.e., same elements of each class) to obtain proper results. To that aim, a synthetic minority class oversampling technique (ASN-SMOTE) was implemented to generate new similar data of the minority class. The methodology reported a perfect classification and a quantification with ratio of performance to deviation values of 3.58 and 4.86 for CNN and RNN, respectively.

Variable selection strategies for PLS models have been applied to different contaminant analysis as shown in Table 3.1. For zearalenone mycotoxin detection, variable selection strategies were applied prior to PLS models (i.e., synergy interval-PLS [siPLS], ant colony optimization-PLS [ACO-PLS], and siPLS-ACO), and these models were compared to the PLS with the full spectral range [16]. The results suggested that siPLS-ACO model produced the best results among the four models with an R^2 of 0.9 and RMSEP of 87.9 μg/kg. However, the authors only proposed their method for screening approaches due to high limit of detection.

Application of variable selection approaches for PLS in SERS methods have also been published recently for antibiotic residues, pesticide residues, and heavy metals [17–20]. Moreover, Pan *et al.* also proposed the use of adaptive iteratively reweighted Penalized Least Squares (airPLS) for baseline correction [19]. Figure 3.3(a-d) exemplifies the application of airPLS for preprocessing of SERS spectra of citrus samples. Genetic algorithm-partial least squares (GA-PLS) prediction was then applied for the quantification of thiabendazole (Figure 3.3(a-b)). The method was validated by method comparison (i.e., comparison with HPLC reference method) using a t-test which showed no significant differences and the limit of detection obtained met the corresponding official standard.

3.2.2 *Analysis of Food Authentication*

International authorities commit significant resources to evaluate the inauthenticity of food [22] in order to prevent fraud and ensure food safety.

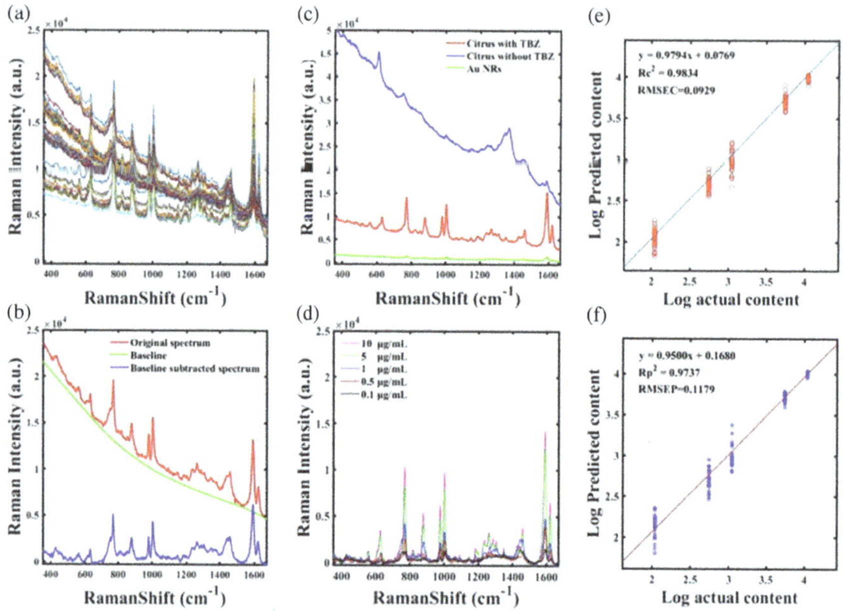

Figure 3.3. (a) Raman spectra of thiabendazole (TBZ) residues with different concentrations in citrus, (b) SERS spectra of gold nanorods (SERS substrate), citrus without TBZ and citrus with TBZ, (c) airPLS-fitted baseline and the baseline-subtracted spectra, and (d) the average spectra of TBZ residues with different concentrations after baseline correction. Scatter plots of predicted versus experimental values by the GA-PLS model for (e) the calibration and (f) prediction sets. Reproduced from Ref. [19] with permission.

Adulteration could compromise human health as manifested by well-known foodborne illnesses and mass food poisoning such as the aniline adulteration in the toxic oil syndrome in 1981 in Spain (more than 20,000 people affected and 2,500 deaths) [23] and the melamine scandal in 2008 in China (more than 300,000 people affected and six infant deaths) [24]. In this regard, Raman spectroscopy and chemometrics have emerged as valuable techniques providing several analytical methods, as was recently reviewed by Xu *et al.* [25] and Hu *et al.* [26].

Table 3.2 summarizes recent publications of methodologies based on Raman and chemometrics for food authentication with potential effects in human health. Classification methods such as linear discriminant analysis (LDA), PCA, soft independent modeling of class analogies (SIMCA), KNN or partial least squares-discriminant analysis (PLSDA) are the most popular. Besides, PLS models are generally used for the quantification of certain adulterants.

Table 3.2. Examples of recent publications employing Raman and chemometrics for food adulteration.

Adulteration Issue	Type of Sample(s)	Raman Technique	Chemometric Technique(s)			Software	Ref.
			Preprocessing	*Training*	*Validation*		
Grapefruit adulteration	Orange juice	RS	SNV	PCA, PC-DFA, PLSDA, PLS	CV	MATLAB	[27]
Egg falsification	Eggs	RS	MSC, airPLS	PCA, PLSDA	—	MATLAB	[28]
Sudan dye adulteration	Paprika powder	RS	IPF	PCA, PLS	Validation set	MATLAB and Unscrambler	[29]
Waste cooking oil	Edible oils spiked with waste oil	RS	Baseline corr., SG, SNV	iPLS, siPLS	Validation set	OptoTrace	[30]
Melamine adulteration	Powder milk	RS	SG, SNV	PCA, SIMCA	Validation set	SOLO	[31]

Abbreviations: **RS**: Raman Spectroscopy; **SNV**: Standard Normal Variate; **PCA**: Principal Component Analysis; **CV**: Cross-Validation; **PLS**: Partial Least Squares; **PLSDA**: PLS Discriminant Analysis; **MSC**: Multiplicative Scattering Correction; **IPF**: Polynomial Fitting; **Corr.**: Correction; **SG**: Savitzky-Golay; **iPLS**: Interval PLS; **SiPLS**: Synergy Interval PLS; **SIMCA**: Soft Independent Modeling by Class Analogy.

Grapefruit adulteration in juices is, surprisingly, a serious adulteration since this juice has dangerous interactions with some pharmaceuticals. Employing a portable handheld Raman spectrometer, Varnasseri *et al.* [27] developed different models based on PCA, principal component-discriminant function analysis (PC-DFA), PLSDA and PLS for the classification of adulterated juices and for the quantification of the adulterant. PCA and PC-DFA were used for exploratory analysis and for identifying sources of variation associated with the origin of the juice that could interfere with the quantitative model. This effect was mitigated via PLSDA/PLS hierarchical model to predict the juice origin followed by a regression to assess the adulteration degree.

Another important application recently developed is the detection of melamine adulteration in milk [31]. Figure 3.4 depicts the Raman spectra of melamine-adulterated milk powder samples, acquired with two different portable Raman spectrometers, before and after spectra preprocessing (see insets). As is shown, the derivatization of the spectra allowed the resolution of characteristic melamine bands (e.g., 676 cm^{-1}). Results also indicated that one of the portable devices (Figure 3.4(b)) was less sensitive due to their poor linear dependence with the melamine concentration. The chemometric approach proposed in this work was based on the SIMCA classification model, which allowed the classification of all control samples with no false negatives

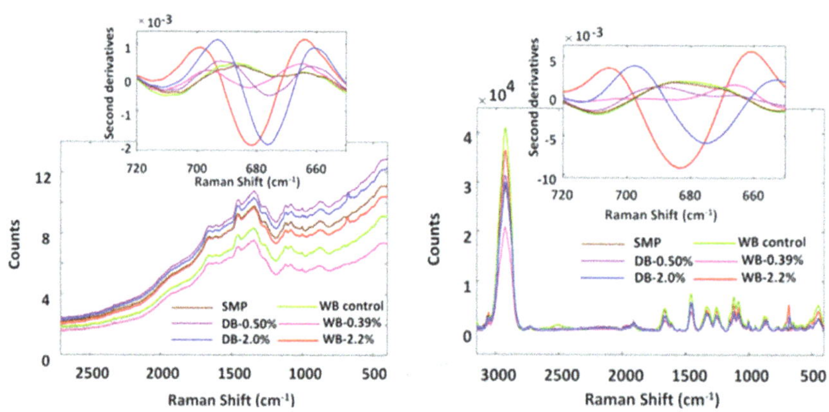

(a) (b)

Figure 3.4. Raman spectra for two representative milk powder (labeled standard milk powder (SMP) and wet blend (WB)) samples and four milk powder blends measured with the (a) TrueScan and (b) Bravo devices. WB and dry blend (DB) were measured with two different concentrations of melanine adulteration. Left inset are the second derivative spectra for the same samples. Right inset are the second derivative spectra for the corresponding samples. Reproduced from Ref. [31] with permission.

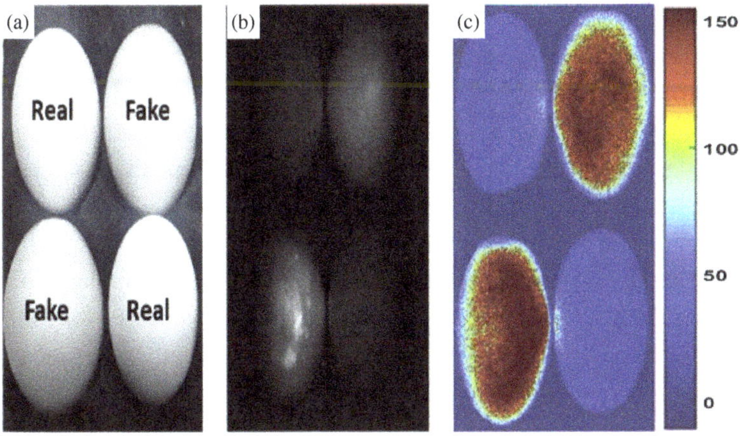

Figure 3.5. (a) Original, (b) selected waveband, and (c) fluorescence-corrected Raman image at 1295 cm^{-1} for real and fake egg samples. Reproduced from Ref. [28] with permission.

and the detection of adulterated milk samples (i.e., ≥ 1% of adulteration) with no false positives.

Furthermore, Raman imaging has also been used in adulteration studies. Joshi *et al.* [28] have developed an interesting method for the detection of fake eggs, which is a dangerous falsified food that contains substances with potentially harmful effects on human health. The authors demonstrate that PCA of hyperspectral images of real and fake eggs allowed the detection of fake eggshells, albumens and yolks. Additionally, they also employed airPLS and a fluorescence correction algorithm to monitor a characteristic Raman shift found for the fake eggshell, enabling the prompt detection of fake eggs (see Figure 3.5). Finally, other studies have focused on edible oil adulteration [26]. In this regard, Li *et al.* [30] developed a method for analyzing waste oil (i.e., used cooking oil) contamination employing interval PLS (iPLS) and siPLS models. Results showed that the use of siPLS enables the prediction of waste oil concentration with adequate RMSEP and a limit of detection of 0.5%.

3.2.3 *Assessment of Nutritional Parameters*

Vibrational spectroscopy has been widely applied for the fast evaluation of nutritional parameters of food. Chemometrics has played a key role in the development of these methodologies, allowing the multicomponent quantification of parameters on complex liquid and solid matrices. Recent examples include *in situ* Fourier transform infrared spectroscopy (FTIR) methods for quantitative profiling [32]. Some of them have been implemented into commercial analyzers such as the Miris HMA system for human milk (Miris Human Milk Analyzer, Miris AB, Uppsala, Sweden). In this context, Raman spectroscopy has also emerged as a fast technique for analyzing nutritional profiles [33]. Table 3.3 summarizes different methods recently published which involved the chemometric treatment of Raman spectra of food. Considering the need for fast and cost-effective approaches in the food industry, standard Raman spectroscopy has been the most popular approach. Regarding the multivariate methodologies, conventional PCA, PLS, and PLSDA models [34, 35] are normally applied, although other methods based on spectral deconvolution have also been proposed [36].

For example, nutritional studies feature the use of Raman spectroscopy for the nutritional evaluation of extremely complex samples such as bee pollen or infant formula. In these approaches, the corresponding reference methods were firstly used for the analysis of the parameters. These values were used for the calibrations of PLS models and then, models were validated with external validation sets or cross-validation. In pollen analysis, the relative errors of prediction reported for macronutrients quantification (i.e., total protein, red sugars, fats) were in the 1.9%–2.6% range, comparable with the prediction errors obtained with FTIR models of 1.7%–3.6% [34]. Similar results were obtained in the analysis of the nutritional profile of infant formula by Wang *et al.* [35], which employed the same approach for the prediction of preheat and storage temperatures, formula storage time, FAST index, soluble protein, fat content and surface free fat content. Similarly, Yazgan *et al.* [37] used PLSDA for the prediction of preheat treatment and animal origin of milk.

Spectral deconvolution algorithms have also demonstrated their applicability to nutritional quantitative profiling. Recently, Pezzotti *et al.* [36] proposed Voigtian deconvolution as a spectral processing step to obtain characteristic signals (i.e., deconvoluted bands) of nutritional parameters in rice samples. The authors carried out a detailed band assignment based on previous literature and density functional theory calculations (see Figure 3.5(a)). Then, the bands corresponding to each nutritional component were integrated and fitted via least squares to the "actual values" obtained by the reference method. Moreover, an algorithm was developed to plot each deconvoluted profile in a barcode-like plot as shown in Figure 3.5(b-c). These types of representations can provide an appealing approach for fast quality control assessment and product matching with quality control purposes.

Table 3.3. Examples of recent publications employing Raman and chemometrics for nutritional parameters assessment.

Parameters	Type of Sample(s)	Raman Technique	Chemometric Technique(s)			Software	Ref.
			Preprocessing	*Training*	*Validation*		
Amylose fraction, Phe fraction, Trp fraction, succ. substitution	Rice	RS	Voigtian deconvolution, FFT smoothing, SG	LS of integrated areas	Reference method correlation	LabSpec and Origin	[36]
Total protein, red sugars, fat, total polyphenols, antioxidant activity, color	Bee pollen	RS	MSC, MC	PCA, PLS	Validation set	PLS Toolbox (MATLAB) and TQ Analyst	[34]
Preheat treatment, storage temperature, storage time, FAST index, sol. protein, fat, SFF	Infant formula	RS	Raw, Baseline Correction, SNV	PCA, PLSDA, PLS	CV	OMNIC and Unscrambler	[35]
Preheat treatment and animal origin	Milk	RS	Baseline Correction, MC	PLSDA	Validation set	SOLO	[37]

Abbreviations: **succ.**: succinate; **FAST**: Fluorescence of Advanced Maillard products and Soluble Tryptophan; **sol.**: soluble; **SFF**: Surface Free Fat; **RS**: Raman Spectroscopy; **FFT**: Fast Fourier Transform; **SG**: Savitzky-Golay; **LS**: Least Squares; **MSC**: Multiplicative Scattering Correction; **MC**: Mean Center; **PCA**: Principal Component Analysis; **PLS**: Partial Least Squares; **CV**: Cross-Validation; **PLSDA**: PLS Discriminant Analysis.

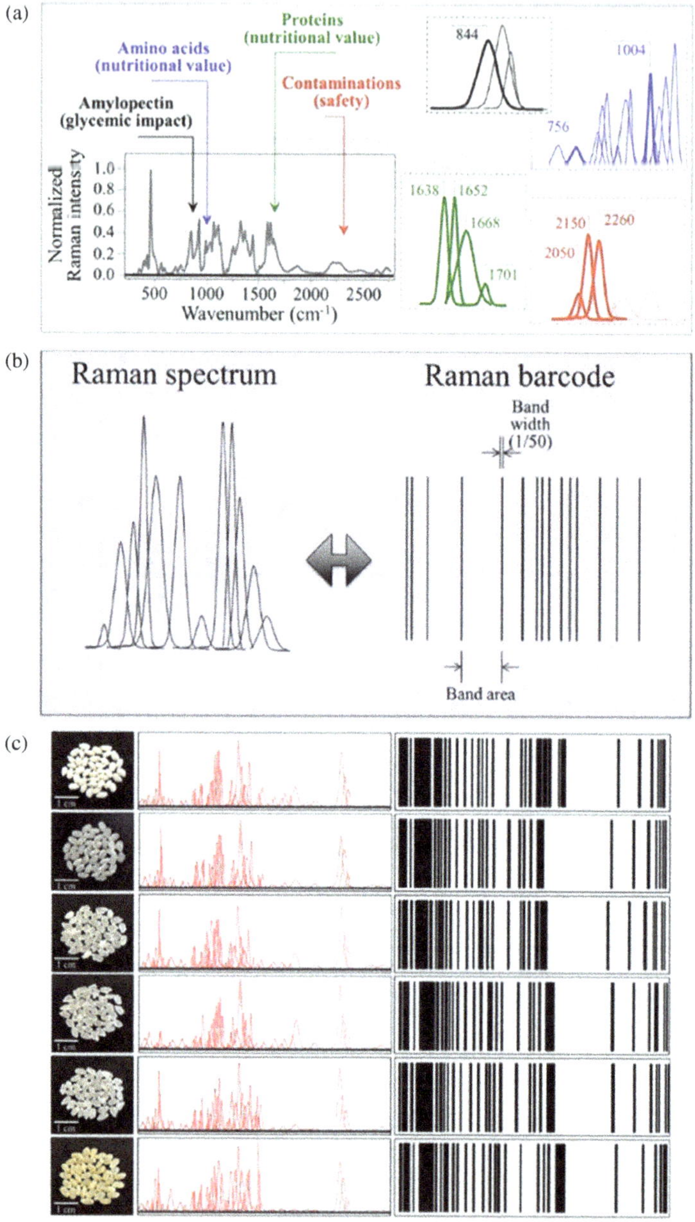

Figure 3.6. (a) Schematic drafts locating different zones of the Raman spectrum representing different nutritional and quality characteristics and their deconvoluted sub-band components. (b) A proposed algorithm to convert the sub-band sequence into a linear barcode. (c) Images of different rice cultivars and associated Raman barcodes. Adapted from Ref. [36], CC BY 4.0.

3.3 Analysis of Raman Datasets in Biomedicine and Health Science

3.3.1 *Use of Discriminant Analysis for Diagnosis*

Effective disease treatment depends on quick and correct diagnosis. If the illness causes detectable changes in the composition of a clinical sample, Raman bands can be used to determine if a disease is present. However, due to the complex nature of the Raman spectra of biological samples, the diagnosis is generally carried out by creating multivariate classification models using the Raman variables. To that end, LDA, PLSDA, or SVMDA are common chemometric discrimination methods which are used to classify the data into "positive" and "negative" categories [38].

According to our analysis in the Web of Science database (November 2022) using the queries "Raman or SERS", "Diagnostic or Diagnosis", and "Chemometrics or Machine Learning", more than 500 papers have been published since 2010 dealing with the use of chemometrics and machine learning methodologies for the development of diagnostic tools. Figure 3.7(a) depicts the evolution of the number of papers published per year during the last decade, evidencing an exponential increase of studies clearly driven by the irruption of machine learning. On the other hand, the term "chemometrics", while it was the preferred keyword in the first five-year period, has experienced a more modest increase followed by a plateau in the beginning of the new

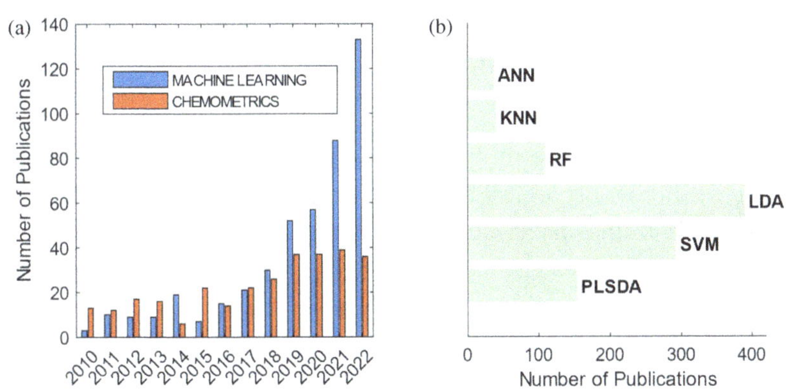

Figure 3.7. Results of a bibliographic analysis in the Web of Science database (November 2022) searching the topics "Raman or SERS", "Diagnostic or Diagnosis" and "Chemometrics or Machine Learning" since 2010. (a) Evolution of the use of "Machine Learning" and "Chemometrics". (b) Number of articles which included the terms "ANN", "KNN", "RF", "LDA", "SVM" and "PLSDA".

decade. Indeed, "machine learning" is considered a more appealing keyword and is used to attract interest from scientists in the clinical field (which are often not familiar with the term "chemometrics"). Furthermore, this change in nomenclature indicates that chemometricians are taking advantage of the artificial intelligence trend to adapt sophisticated machine learning algorithms to treat Raman spectroscopy signals [9]. The same analysis also showed that, among the different classification methodologies, LDA and SVM are the most popular techniques to create diagnostic models (see Figure 3.7(b)).

The creation of diagnostic methods requires the consideration of specific aspects related to the clinical implantation of the models. The most important, considering the strong impact of the treatment and decisions resulting from the analysis outcome, is the need for an accurate assessment of the true positive and true negative rates (sensitivity and specificity, respectively). In this sense, most of the output variables of discriminant models can be expressed as a continuous score ($\hat{y}$ values in Eq. (3.1)) that indicates how close the sample is to the positive or negative classes. For example, Figure 3.8(a) depicts the predicted y score of a PLSDA model developed by Mancini *et al.* for leishmaniasis diagnosis in serum using SERS [39]. It can be seen that most of the positive samples hold positive values close to the reference $\hat{y} = 1$ value for the positive class, while negative samples presented a predicted Y closer to the $\hat{y} = 0$ established for the negative samples. From these distributions of predicted $\hat{y}$ values, the probability of being either positive or negative can be calculated. Alternatively, a threshold value can be established to determine the sample class. In Figure 3.8(a) the threshold is depicted as a red dashed line which separates positive from negative samples, creating a few false negatives (green dots below the red line) and false positives (blue dots above the red line).

In principle, 0.5 is the midpoint between 0 and 1 and therefore it can be considered the most logical cut-off value. In contrast, the authors used a Bayesian optimization technique to set the cut-off value slightly above 0.5. The optimal threshold can be indeed altered considering the requirements of a diagnostic methodology in terms of false positive and false negatives and, to that end, the so-called Receiver Operating Characteristic (ROC) curve is used. Figure 3.8(b) shows a ROC curve corresponding to the results of a logistic regression created by Webster *et al.* [40], which aimed to provide a screening method for esophageal adenocarcinoma using biomarkers obtained from SERS analysis of blood (blue line). In the ROC, all the possible threshold values are considered, providing the corresponding true positive and true negative rates which are plotted as a curve in the sensitivity/1 – specificity axes. From this

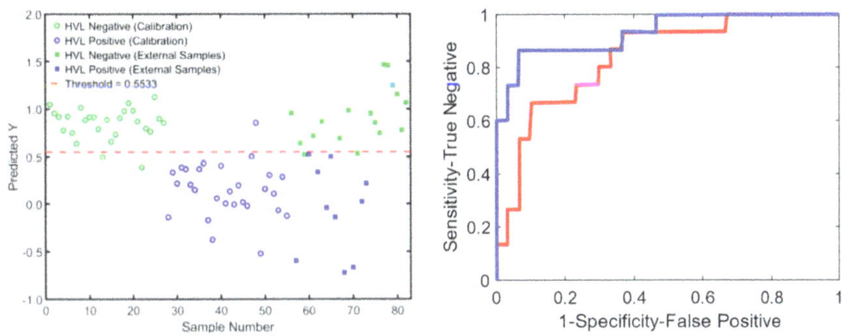

(a) (b)

Figure 3.8. Typical plots used for the creation and evaluation of diagnostic models using Raman spectroscopy and chemometrics. (a) Predicted PLSDA *y* value for calibration and test samples obtained in a PLSDA model created for the diagnosis of leishmaniasis in serum using SERS. The dashed red line indicates the threshold selected in the study. Reproduced from Ref. [39] with permission. (b) ROC curves obtained in logistic models for the screening of esophageal adenocarcinoma using a biomarker panel (blue) and a clinical risk panel (red). Adapted from Ref. [40], CC BY 4.0.

plot one can select the optimal threshold value according to the requirements of the diagnosis. Furthermore, the larger the area under the curve (AUROC), the better the performance of the classification, and therefore this value can be used to compare the methodologies. For example, Figure 3.8(b) also shows the ROC curve for a logistic regression using clinical risk variables such as age and body mass index (red). It can be seen that the biomarker model performed much better with AUROC values of 0.830 and 0.930 for the red and blue ROCs, respectively.

3.3.1.1 *Single-Point Measurements*

One of the most popular Raman approaches employed in diagnostic methods is the measurement of a single spectrum representative of the general composition of a clinical biofluid or tissue. It can be performed in a straightforward and fast way by using inexpensive and portable instrumentation, offering methodologies very suitable for diagnosis within a Point-of-Care testing context [41]. Furthermore, a single spectrum of specific regions of tissue can be recorded, serving as representative Raman variables which can be used for diagnostic purposes [42, 43]. Similarly, a spectrum of a whole cell can be obtained and modeled to classify different classes of cells [44] or bacterium [45].

Table 3.4. The versatility of diagnostic methods based on single-point Raman spectroscopy. Examples of methodologies proposed for the diagnosis of disease using chemometric models and Raman spectra from different samples.

Disease	Markers Targeted	PLS	Sample	Ref.
Malaria	Hemozoin (Resonance)	PLSDA	Red blood cells	[47]
Leukemia	Multiple	PLSDA	Plasma	[46]
Bladder cancer	Multiple	RF	Urine (SERS)	[49]
Oesophagus cancer	Multiple	LDA	Oesophagus tissue (*ex vivo*)	[50]
Nasopharyngeal carcinoma	Multiple	CNN	Nasopharyngeal tissue (*in vivo*)	[43]

Table 3.4 shows some examples of discrimination models based on the Raman spectra of different samples such as red blood cells, plasma, urine, and tissue. This exemplifies the versatility of Raman spectroscopy, which is able to obtain information from a wide range of matrices. Regardless of the sample measured or disease under study, once the single spectrum is recorded, classification models previously created are used to directly predict the condition of the patient. In most cases, the disease under study affects several parts of the sample phenotype, changing the concentration and/or internal structure of several sample biomolecules. This pattern of changes provokes shifts and alterations on the intensity of a lot of Raman bands, which are used by the discriminant models to detect the presence of the disease [46]. In other cases, when the changes due to an individual biomarker dominates the spectrum, a more selective approach can be made by focusing on changes of the bands from the specific biomarker. For example, discriminant models created to identify malaria-infected red blood cells focus on bands of hemozoin crystals, a byproduct of the digestion of hemoglobin by the plasmodium parasite [47, 48].

Finally, due to the tremendous advantages (e.g., point-of-care capability) and diagnostic potential of single-point Raman spectroscopy, the development of classification methods based on single-point Raman is evolving rapidly with the implementation of more sophisticated algorithms. Shu *et al.* [43] has recently proposed a deep learning model featuring CNN for the identification of nasopharyngeal carcinoma from *in vivo* Raman measurements of nasopharyngeal tissue. CNN models outperformed, in most of the cases, classical PLS-LDA models, providing sensitivity values above 80% [43].

Nevertheless, one of the main challenges of using such sophisticated models is the need for a large number of samples for the training step. This is a notable limitation in the case of diagnostic studies, where it is hard to obtain a considerable number of patients with proper diagnosis. In this regard, scientists can include several spectra from the same patient [43], or apply novel data augmentation methodologies [51]. Moreover, the validation can also be adapted to deal with an unbalanced number of data classes [52]. It must be noted that these strategies should be implemented carefully because they can lead to overly optimistic results when replicates of the same sample are included in calibration and testing, providing a "leaky" validation (also called replicate sample trap in the chemometric field) [53].

3.3.1.2 *Imaging*

Hyperspectral Raman images can also be used for creating classification models, which take into account both the composition of the sample (captured by the Raman spectra) and spatial features of the images for the diagnosis. In this case, however, the complexity of the models increases exponentially with the size of the images, as it requires one to deal with a hypercube instead of a single spectrum per sample. In most of the cases, with the use of simple Raman intensity maps or unsupervised analysis such as high content analysis (HCA) or PCA, the sub-micron lateral resolution of Raman spectroscopy enables the spatial allocation of organelles within a cell and the assignment of different kinds of tissue on a tissue biopsy [54].

However, due to the high phenotypic variability among different patients, the creation of robust models that can predict the "positive" and "negative" nature of a sample from the hyperspectral image represents a more challenging task. It generally needs more sophisticated algorithms and a large database of images for representative training and validation. Machine learning-based techniques have been extensively used in regular histopathology for automatized diagnosis by analyzing stained images. This requires the segmentation of images with three channels corresponding to red, green, and blue intensities. The staining can be specific to a biomolecule (e.g., DNA or lipids), providing chemical information which is used to identify spatial features (e.g., size and shape of the nucleus) that are used by advanced algorithms to provide a diagnosis. In contrast, Raman imaging provides label-free chemical information as a set of thousands of variables, which can be included in computing intensive models that combine both spatial and chemical features in tissues [55, 56] and cells [57].

3.3.2 *Use of Regression Methodologies for the Quantification of Clinical Parameters*

The use of Raman spectroscopy for the prediction of clinical parameters in biofluids has been proposed since the early 2000s [58]. Multivariate models aim to predict a continuous clinical parameter which can be used for a wide range of clinical applications including risk assessment, diagnosis, or prognosis. Figures of merit used in regression aim to assess the performance of the model by calculating the prediction error (i.e., the difference between the predicted and actual values). The most popular figure is the RMSEP, which can be normalized using the standard deviation, average or range of the actual values to compare among different validation sets. In the case of biomedical methodologies, it is recommended to always plot the actual versus predicted values to study the performance along the whole range of concentrations, putting special interest on the pathological values.

Again, the versatility of Raman spectroscopy has been exploited to develop quantifications of different parameters in different matrices (see examples in Table 3.5). In general, the complexity of the model depends on the analytical problem under study. For example, if SERS offers enough intrinsic selectivity for a specific analyte, quantifications can be carried out by simple models based on the ratio of bands, which use an internal standard to compensate for the irreproducibility of SERS signals [59]. In other cases, due to the large

Table 3.5. Examples of recent publications on quantitative applications of clinical parameters employing Raman spectroscopy.

Analyte	Raman Technique	Data Analysis Method	Sample	Ref.
GSH	SERS	Ratio of bands	Lysed RBC	[59]
Virus	SERS	SVR	Virus solution	[60]
mRNA	SERS	CNN	Tissue	[61]
Total protein, glucose, urea, uric acid, cholesterol, triglycerides, HDL cholesterol, and LDL cholesterol	Raman	PLS	Oesophagus tissue (*ex vivo*)	[58]
Glucose and lactate	SORS	PLS	Supernatant mixtures of RBC	[62]

complexity of the matrices involved, SERS signals require treatment from machine learning methodologies [60]. Finally, deep learning is also being implemented in biomarker detection for treating signals from multiplexed sensors with different SERS-active "nanorattles" [61].

When the prediction of clinical parameters is performed using non-enhanced Raman spectroscopy, the regression becomes more challenging. The bands of other biomolecules from complex biological matrices overlap with the ones from the target analyte. In these cases, to create robust quantification models, extensive training and testing sets are required, which should be representative of a wide clinical range of both analytes and interferences contained in the sample. For example, a recent study used PLS and SVR for the multiparametric quantification of quality parameters of blood using space-offset Raman spectroscopy (SORS) [62]. The quantification of glucose and lactate allowed the quality control of blood prior to donation through the blood bag, eliminating any potential contamination of blood, which is key in the transfusion process.

3.3.3 *Analysis of Longitudinal Datasets*

One of the key advantages of Raman spectroscopy is that, under well-controlled laser power conditions, it does not destroy the sample. Therefore, it can be used to repeatedly analyze the same sample over time in longitudinal studies. Clinical researchers have taken advantage of this feature to characterize changes in the composition of cells in different time-dependent biological processes [63]. Longitudinal experiments generally require the monitoring of the spectra of cells incubated in the presence of an external agent such as a drug, a toxic molecule or ultraviolet radiation. The outcome is a time-dependent dataset which provides information about subtle changes in the molecular composition over time provoked by the presence of the agent, and offers valuable insights into the underlying mechanisms of drug activity [64] or toxicity [65] involved.

The treatment of such datasets requires specific models that can identify spectral changes over time and relate these changes to specific biomolecules. The most straightforward approach is to apply PCA and look for principal components which capture the variance associated with the effect investigated. In this case, the score values can be used to study the evolution of the uptake of a drug or cellular response to a toxicity source over time. Furthermore, loading values can be used for the biological interpretation of the changes, for example by identifying bands of the drug or changes in bands of the cellular components caused by the cell response.

Unfortunately, in most of the cases, other sources of variation dominate the first principal components, and supervised analysis is needed to investigate subtle changes associated with the inoculation time. To that end, regression models such as PLS can be applied by using inoculation time as a variable to predict ($\hat{y}$ values in Eq. (3.1)) and the Raman spectra as predictors. Then, the regression vector can be used to investigate spectral changes associated with the incubation time [64]. One of the main limitations of using PLS is that it is based on linear assumptions and, in contrast, complex processes such as drug uptake or toxicity are not linear with time [66]. Nonlinear models such as SVR can be used, but unfortunately, they do not provide a regression vector for the investigation of spectral bands involved in the modeling.

Multivariate curve resolution-alternate least squares (MCR-ALS) has been proposed as a suitable alternative in this context [66, 67]. MCR-ALS uses iterative optimization to resolve multiple component responses in mixtures by fitting them to a bilinear model, which relates the dataset to a set of components with specific concentration profiles and reference spectra. It requires the input of a few parameters, such as an estimation of the number of components, an initial guess of concentrations or spectra and a set of constraints to guide the iteration (e.g., non-negativity). Its main advantage is that, while the Raman intensities are still assumed to be linear with the concentration of the components, the evolution of the different components over time can follow any profile.

The differences between PLS and MCR-ALS have been studied using datasets which simulated Raman spectra of A549 cells incubated with doxorubicin (see Figure 3.9) [66]. The simulation included two different effects with two different temporal evolutions (Figure 3.9(a)). The first (blue) simulated the fast uptake of DOX by the cell, and the second (green) simulated the subsequent slower cellular response. The simulated bands of the uptake included (Figure 3.9(b)) bands of doxorubicin (orange spectrum) and changes in DNA conformation associated with the binding of the drug (blue spectrum). The simulated bands of the subsequent cellular response

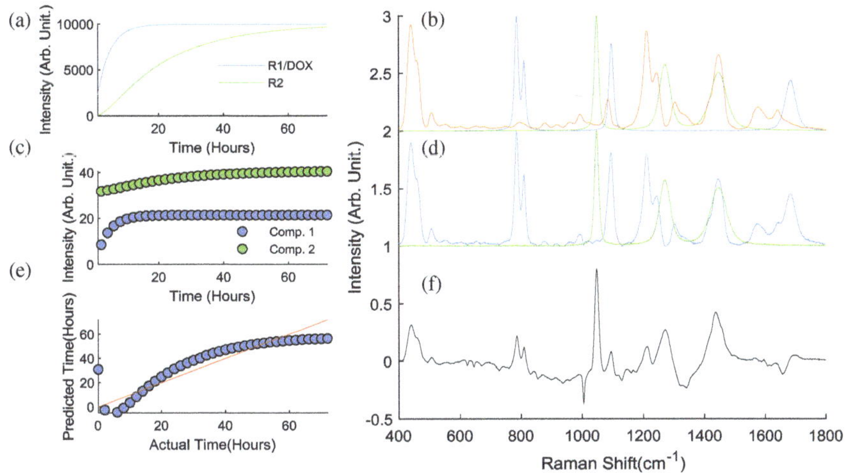

Figure 3.9. MCR-ALS and PLSR analysis of data. (a) Simulated time evolution and (b) simulated spectral signatures employed to build the creation of the Dataset II, which simulated the spectral signatures of the disruption: doxorubicin bonding to DNA (Response 1) and subsequent cellular responses (Response 2). (c) MCR-ALS estimation of the concentration and (d) spectral profiles determined by MCR-ALS. Actual time values. (e) PLSR actual versus predicted (by values obtained by cross-validation) time values and (f) first loading regression vector of the orthogonal PLSR. Reproduced from Ref. [66] with permission.

simulated changes in protein content (green spectrum). The simulated spectra and responses were used to create a dataset which was analyzed using PLS and MCR-ALS. Figure 3.9(e) depicts the actual incubation time values versus PLS predicted values and shows that the model was skewed due to the lack of linearity of the response with time. In addition, the regression vector (see Figure 3.9(f)) showed the bands associated with the incubation time, but it was not able to discriminate between the two responses included in the simulation.

In contrast, MCR-ALS was able to identify the different evolution profiles for both responses in the estimated concentration matrix (Figure 3.9(c)). The spectra matrix (Figure 3.9(d)) showed the computed spectra of the uptake (blue), which included bands of the drug and of the binding, and spectra of the cell response (green). In both cases MCR-ALS was able to successfully predict the spectra and evolution of the responses. Furthermore, kinetic constrains can also be implemented to create hard-soft models which take into account the pharmacokinetics of the drugs within the model, providing an estimation of the constant rates [68].

3.3.4 *Data Fusion and Other Applications*

Raman spectroscopy provides information about a wide range of Raman-active compounds with clinical interest. Nevertheless, sometimes it is necessary to measure the same sample with other complementary techniques (e.g., infrared, X-ray fluorescence) to obtain a more comprehensive picture of the phenotype. The result of these multimodal experiments are extended data matrices (or extended hypercubes in the case of images), which are analyzed with data fusion methodologies that perform an integrated analysis of data obtained from different modalities. Considering the increasing number of spectroscopic modalities used nowadays, low-level or high-level data fusion methodologies have emerged as very suitable tools to acquire information about the sample by investigating relationships among spectral markers from the different methodologies [69].

Since Raman- and infrared-active modes provide complementary information, their integrated analysis could assist in the assignments of bands. Statistical heterospectroscopy, for example, has been applied to study the covariance between Raman and IR signals measured across the same sample set [70]. Besides, 2D correlation analysis has also been used to create plots of synchronous and asynchronous maps in longitudinal studies [67]. In addition, Raman spectra can be fused from data from other molecular techniques such as matrix-assisted laser desorption/ionization [71] or with elemental techniques such as laser-induced breakdown spectroscopy [72].

A more troublesome task is the data fusion of hyperspectral images of cells and tissues, which requires accurate registration of the data cubes obtained by the different modalities. This can be obtained by careful acquisition of the images and by using specific image registration software [73]. On top of that, lateral resolutions of different spectroscopies are generally not the same, requiring the unification of the pixel size before concatenating the images. However, multimodal imaging provides unmatched comprehensive information on the composition of spatial features of the samples. For example, Figure 3.10 shows an HCA of a multimodal image containing fused IR and Raman spectra of an algae from the genus *Micrasterias* [70]. The average spectra of IR (Figure 3.10(d)) and Raman (Figure 3.10(b)) show bands associated with the cell wall, algae lobes, chloroplasts and cytoplasm depicted in blue, yellow, violet and orange, respectively. Interesting correlations among IR and Raman bands can be found, such as the high intensity of C–H bands (2800–3000 cm^{-1}) for the lobe class in both modalities. In fact, the fusion

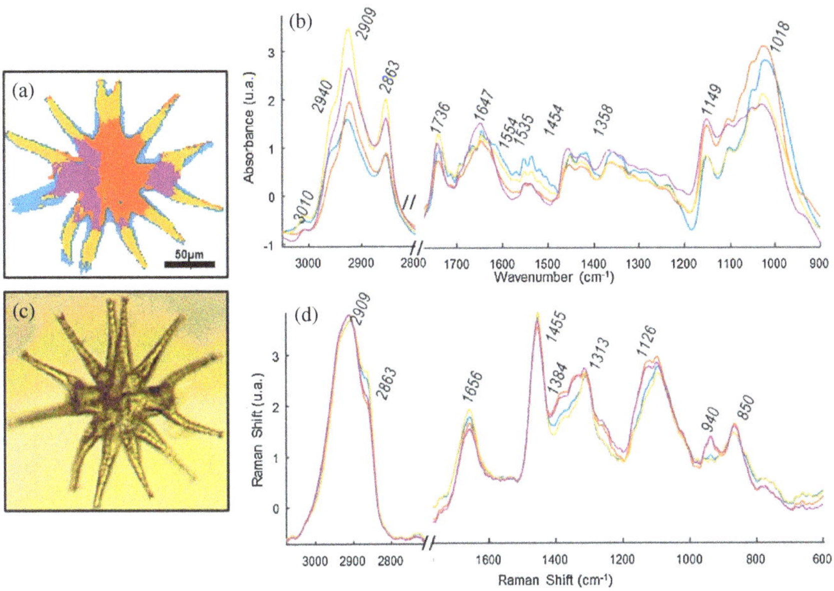

Figure 3.10. Fused IR and Raman images of *Micrasterias* analyzed by HCA. (a) Cluster image. (b) Class averages spectra for Raman variables. (c) Visible image. (d) Class averages spectra for infrared variables. Reproduced from Ref. [70] with permission.

of IR and Raman is nowadays gaining popularity considering the recent development of microscopes which combine optical-photothermal IR and Raman, allowing for simultaneous acquisition of Raman and IR with sub-micron lateral resolution [74].

Acknowledgements

Authors acknowledge the financial support from the projects RYC2019-026556-I and RPID2020-119326RA-I00 funded by MCIN/AEI/ 10.13039/501100011033. Á.S-I. was supported by the Margarita Salas grant (ref. UP2021-044-MS21-084) from the Ministry of Universities of the Government of Spain, financed by the European Union, NextGenerationEU.

References

1. Niaura, G. (2014) Raman Spectroscopy in Analysis of Biomolecules. In *Encyclopedia of Analytical Chemistry*, pp. 1–34, John Wiley & Sons.

2. De Gelder, J., De Gussem, K., Vandenabeele, P. and Moens, L. (2007) Reference database of Raman spectra of biological molecules. J. Raman Spectrosc. **38**, 1133–1147.
3. Diem, M. (2015) Appendix F: Infrared and Raman Spectra of Selected Cellular Components. In *Modern Vibrational Spectroscopy and Micro-Spectroscopy*, pp 399–404, John Wiley & Sons.
4. Morais, C. L. M., Lima, K. M. G., Singh, M. and Martin, F. L. (2020) Tutorial: multivariate classification for vibrational spectroscopy in biological samples. Nat. Protoc. **15**, 2143–2162.
5. Ellis, D. I., Brewster, V. L., Dunn, W. B., Allwood, J. W., Golovanov, A. P. and Goodacre, R. (2012) Fingerprinting food: current technologies for the detection of food adulteration and contamination. Chem. Soc. Rev. **41**, 5706–5727.
6. Goodacre, R., Graham, D. and Faulds, K. (2018) Recent developments in quantitative SERS: Moving towards absolute quantification. Trends Anal. Chem. **102**, 359–368.
7. Wang, J., Chen, Q., Belwal, T., Lin, X. and Luo, Z. (2021) Insights into chemometric algorithms for quality attributes and hazards detection in foodstuffs using Raman/surface enhanced Raman spectroscopy. Compr. Rev. Food Sci. Food Saf. **20**, 2476–2507.
8. Abu-Mostafa, Y. S., Magdon-Ismail, M. and Lin, H.-T. (2012) *Learning from Data: A Short Course*, AMLBook.
9. Houhou, R. and Bocklitz, T. (2021) Trends in artificial intelligence, machine learning, and chemometrics applied to chemical data. Anal. Sci. Adv. **2**, 128–141.
10. Brereton, R. G., Jansen, J., Lopes, J., Marini, F., Pomerantsev, A., Rodionova, O., Roger, J. M., Walczak, B. and Tauler, R. (2018) Chemometrics in analytical chemistry — part II: modeling, validation, and applications. Anal. Bioanal. Chem. **410**, 6691–6704.
11. Bailey, G. F. and Horvat, R. J. (1972) Raman spectroscopic analysis of the cis/trans isomer composition of edible vegetable oils. J. Am. Oil Chem. Soc. **49**, 494–498.
12. Wang, P., Sun, Y., Li, X., Wang, L., Xu, Y., He, L. and Li, G. (2021) Recent advances in dual recognition based surface enhanced Raman scattering for pathogenic bacteria detection: A review. Anal. Chim. Acta **1157**, 338279.
13. Yan, S., Wang, S., Qiu, J., Li, M., Li, D., Xu, D., Li, D. and Liu, Q. (2021) Raman spectroscopy combined with machine learning for rapid detection of food-borne pathogens at the single-cell level. Talanta **226**, 122195.
14. Adejimi, O., Ignat, T., Sadhasivam, G., Zakin, V., Schmilovitch, Z. and Shapiro, O. (2022) Low-resolution Raman spectroscopy for the detection of contaminant species in algal bioreactors. Sci. Total Environ. **809**, 151138.
15. Deng, J., Zhang, X., Li, M., Jiang, H. and Chen, Q. (2022) Feasibility study on Raman spectra-based deep learning models for monitoring the contamination degree and level of aflatoxin B-1 in edible oil. Microchem. J. **180**, 107613.

16. Guo, Z., Wang, M., Wu, J., Tao, F., Chen, Q., Wang, Q., Ouyang, Q., Shi, J. and Zou, X. (2019) Quantitative assessment of zearalenone in maize using multivariate algorithms coupled to Raman spectroscopy. Food Chem. **286**, 282–288.
17. Li, H., Geng, W., Hassan, M. M., Zuo, M., Wei, W., Wu, X., Ouyang, Q. and Chen, Q. (2021) Rapid detection of chloramphenicol in food using SERS flexible sensor coupled artificial intelligent tools. Food Control **128**, 108186.
18. Lee, K., Yarbrough, D., Kozman, M., Herrman, T., Park, J., Wang, R. and Kurouski, D. (2020) Rapid detection and prediction of chlortetracycline and oxytetracycline in animal feed using surface-enhanced Raman spectroscopy (SERS). Food Control **114**, 107243.
19. Pan, H., Ahmad, W., Jiao, T., Zhu, A., Ouyang, Q. and Chen, Q. (2022) Label-free Au NRs-based SERS coupled with chemometrics for rapid quantitative detection of thiabendazole residues in citrus. Food Chem. **375**, 131681.
20. Guo, Z., Barimah, A., Guo, C., Agyekum, A., Annavaram, V., El-Seedi, H., Zou, X. and Chen, Q. (2020) Chemometrics coupled 4-Aminothiophenol labelled Ag-Au alloy SERS off-signal nanosensor for quantitative detection of mercury in black tea. Spectrochim. Acta Part A **242**, 118747.
21. Xiao, X., Liu, X., Mei, T., Xu, M., Lu, Z., Dai, H., Pi, F. and Wang, J. (2022) Estimation of contamination level in microplastic-exposed crayfish by laser confocal micro-Raman imaging. Food Chem. **397**, 133844.
22. Popping, B., Buck, N., Bánáti, D., Brereton, P., Gendel, S., Hristozova, N., Chaves, S. M., Saner, S., Spink, J., Willis, C., *et al.* (2022) Food inauthenticity: Authority activities, guidance for food operators, and mitigation tools. Compr. Rev. Food Sci. Food Saf. **21**, 1–36.
23. Valadés, P. S.-P., Paz, M. P. de la, Copa, P. de A., Ribota, O. G. and Borda, I. A. (2003) Toxic oil syndrome: Survival in the whole cohort between 1981 and 1995. J. Clin. Epidemiol. **56**, 701–708.
24. Sharma, K. and Paradakar, M. (2010) The melamine adulteration scandal. Food Secur. **2**, 97–107.
25. Xu, Y., Zhong, P., Jiang, A., Shen, X., Li, X., Xu, Z., Shen, Y., Sun, Y. and Lei, H. (2020) Raman spectroscopy coupled with chemometrics for food authentication: A review. Trends Anal. Chem. **131**, 116017.
26. Hu, R., He, T., Zhang, Z., Yang, Y. and Liu, M. (2019) Safety analysis of edible oil products via Raman spectroscopy. Talanta **191**, 324–332.
27. Varnasseri, M., Xu, Y. and Goodacre, R. (2022) Rapid detection and quantification of the adulteration of orange juice with grapefruit juice using handheld Raman spectroscopy and multivariate analysis. Anal. Methods **14**, 1663–1670.
28. Joshi, R., Lohumi, S., Joshi, R., Kim, M. S., Qin, J., Baek, I. and Cho, B.-K. (2020) Raman spectral analysis for non-invasive detection of external and internal parameters of fake eggs. Sens. Actuators B Chem. **303**, 127243.
29. Monago-Maraña, O., Eskildsen, C. E., Afseth, N. K., Galeano-Díaz, T., Muñoz de la Peña, A. and Wold, J. P. (2019) Non-destructive Raman spectroscopy as a

tool for measuring ASTA color values and Sudan I content in paprika powder. Food Chem. **274**, 187–193.

30. Li, Y., Fang, T., Zhu, S., Huang, F., Chen, Z. and Wang, Y. (2018) Detection of olive oil adulteration with waste cooking oil via Raman spectroscopy combined with iPLS and SiPLS. Spectrochim. Acta. A **189**, 37–43.
31. Karunathilaka, S. R., Yakes, B. J., He, K., Brückner, L. and Mossoba, M. M. (2018) First use of handheld Raman spectroscopic devices and on-board chemometric analysis for the detection of milk powder adulteration. Food Control **92**, 137–146.
32. Perez-Guaita, D., Richardson, Z., Rajendra, A., Byrne, H. J. and Wood, B. (2021) From bench to worktop: Rapid evaluation of nutritional parameters in liquid foodstuffs by IR spectroscopy. Food Chem. **365**, 130442.
33. Silva, M. G., de Paula, I. L., Stephani, R., Edwards, H. G. M. and de Oliveira, L. F. C. (2021) Raman spectroscopy in the quality analysis of dairy products: A literature review. J. Raman Spectrosc. **52**, 2444–2478.
34. Węglińska, M., Szostak, R., Kita, A., Nemś, A. and Mazurek, S. (2020) Determination of nutritional parameters of bee pollen by Raman and infrared spectroscopy. Talanta **212**, 120790.
35. Wang, X., Esquerre, C., Downey, G., Henihan, L., O'Callaghan, D. and O'Donnell, C. (2018) Assessment of infant formula quality and composition using Vis-NIR, MIR and Raman process analytical technologies. Talanta **183**, 320–328.
36. Pezzotti, G., Zhu, W., Chikaguchi, H., Marin, E., Boschetto, F., Masumura, T., Sato, Y.-I. and Nakazaki, T. (2021) Raman molecular fingerprints of rice nutritional quality and the concept of Raman barcode. Front. Nutr. **8**, 663569.
37. Yazgan, N. N., Genis, H. E., Bulat, T., Topcu, A., Durna, S., Yetisemiyen, A. and Boyaci, I. H. (2020) Discrimination of milk species using Raman spectroscopy coupled with partial least squares discriminant analysis in raw and pasteurized milk. J. Sci. Food Agric. **100**, 4756–4765.
38. Ralbovsky, N. M. and Lednev, I. K. (2020) Towards development of a novel universal medical diagnostic method: Raman spectroscopy and machine learning. Chem. Soc. Rev. **49**, 7428–7453.
39. Mancini, R. S. N., Sabaine, A. E., Castro, C. E., Carnielli, J. B. T., Dietze, R., de Oliveira, V. L., Lanfredi, A. J. C., Kubota, L. T., Mamián-López, M. B. and Alves, W. A. (2022) Development and validation of a SERS-based serological test combined with PLS-DA method for leishmaniasis detection. ACS Appl. Electron. Mater. **4**, 3997–4006.
40. Webster, J. A., Wuethrich, A., Shanmugasundaram, K. B., Richards, R. S., Zelek, W. M., Shah, A. K., Gordon, L. G., Kendall, B. J., Hartel, G., Morgan, B. P., *et al.* (2021) Development of EndoScreen chip, a microfluidic pre-endoscopy triage test for esophageal adenocarcinoma. Cancers **13**, 2865.
41. Pérez-Guaita, D. and de la Guardia, M. (2023) Introductory statement — PoC special issue — Microchemical journal. Microchem. J. **184**, 108153.
42. Kong, K., Kendall, C., Stone, N. and Notingher, I. (2015) Raman spectroscopy for medical diagnostics — From in-vitro biofluid assays to in-vivo cancer detection. Adv. Drug Deliv. Rev. **89**, 121–134.

43. Shu, C., Yan, H., Zheng, W., Lin, K., James, A., Selvarajan, S., Lim, C. M. and Huang, Z. (2021) Deep learning-guided fiberoptic Raman spectroscopy enables real-time in vivo diagnosis and assessment of nasopharyngeal carcinoma and post-treatment efficacy during endoscopy. Anal. Chem. **93**, 10898–10906.
44. Huang, W., Shang, Q., Xiao, X., Zhang, H., Gu, Y., Yang, L., Shi, G., Yang, Y., Hu, Y., Yuan, Y., *et al.* (2022) Raman spectroscopy and machine learning for the classification of esophageal squamous carcinoma. Spectrochim. Acta. A **281**, 121654.
45. Kanno, N., Kato, S., Ohkuma, M., Matsui, M., Iwasaki, W. and Shigeto, S. (2021) Machine learning-assisted single-cell Raman fingerprinting for in situ and nondestructive classification of prokaryotes. iScience **24**, 102975.
46. da Silva, A. M., de Siqueira E Oliveira, F. S. A., de Brito, P. L. and Silveira, L. (2018) Spectral model for diagnosis of acute leukemias in whole blood and plasma through Raman spectroscopy. J. Biomed. Opt. **23**, 1–11.
47. Marzec, K. M., Perez-Guaita, D., De Veij, M., McNaughton, D., Baranska, M., Dixon, M. W., Tilley, L. and Wood, B. R. (2014) Red blood cells polarize green laser light revealing hemoglobin's enhanced non-fundamental Raman modes. ChemPhysChem **15**, 3963–3968.
48. Perez-Guaita, D., Marzec, K. M., Hudson, A., Evans, C., Chernenko, T., Matthäus, C., Miljkovic, M., Diem, M., Heraud, P., Richards, J. S., *et al.* (2018) Parasites under the spotlight: applications of vibrational spectroscopy to malaria research. Chem. Rev. **118**, 5330–5358.
49. Moisoiu, T., Dragomir, M. P., Iancu, S. D., Schallenberg, S., Birolo, G., Ferrero, G., Burghelea, D., Stefancu, A., Cozan, R. G., Licarete, E., *et al.* (2022) Combined miRNA and SERS urine liquid biopsy for the point-of-care diagnosis and molecular stratification of bladder cancer. Mol. Med. **28**, 39.
50. Ishigaki, M., Maeda, Y., Taketani, A., Andriana, B. B., Ishihara, R., Wongravee, K., Ozaki, Y. and Sato, H. (2016) Diagnosis of early-stage esophageal cancer by Raman spectroscopy and chemometric techniques. Analyst **141**, 1027–1033.
51. Zhang, X., Li, H., Tian, X., Chen, C., Su, Y., Li, M., Lv, J., Chen, C. and Lv, X. (2022) Application of spectral small-sample data combined with a method of spectral data augmentation fusion (SDA-Fusion) in cancer diagnosis. Chemom. Intell. Lab. Syst. **231**, 104681.
52. Song, H., Leng, H., Hou, Z., Gao, R., Chen, C., Meng, C., Sun, J., Li, C. and Ma, B. (2022) Grouped-sampling technique to deal with unbalance in Raman spectral data modeling. Photodiagnosis Photodyn. Ther. **40**, 103059.
53. Pérez-Guaita, D., Kuligowski, J., Lendl, B., Wood, B. R. and Quintás, G. (2018) Assessment of discriminant models in infrared imaging using constrained repeated random sampling — Cross validation. Anal. Chim. Acta **1033**, 156–164.
54. Dodo, K., Fujita, K. and Sodeoka, M. (2022) Raman spectroscopy for chemical biology research. J. Am. Chem. Soc. **144**, 19651–19667.
55. Taieb, A., Berkovic, G., Haifler, M., Cheshnovsky, O. and Shaked, N. T. (2022) Classification of tissue biopsies by Raman spectroscopy guided by quantitative

phase imaging and its application to bladder cancer. J. Biophotonics **15**, e202200009.
56. Fung, A. A. and Shi, L. (2020) Mammalian cell and tissue imaging using Raman and coherent Raman microscopy. Wiley Interdiscip. Rev. Syst. Biol. Med. **12**, e1501.
57. Yosef, H. K., Krauß, S. D., Lechtonen, T., Jütte, H., Tannapfel, A., Käfferlein, H. U., Brüning, T., Roghmann, F., Noldus, J., Mosig, A., *et al.* (2017) Noninvasive diagnosis of high-grade urothelial carcinoma in urine by raman spectral imaging. Anal. Chem. **89**, 6893–6899.
58. Rohleder, D., Kiefer, W. and Petrich, W. (2004) Quantitative analysis of serum and serum ultrafiltrate by means of Raman spectroscopy. Analyst **129**, 906–911.
59. Sánchez-Illana, Á., Mayr, F., Cuesta-García, D., Piñeiro-Ramos, J. D., Cantarero, A., Guardia, M. de la, Vento, M., Lendl, B., Quintás, G. and Kuligowski, J. (2018) On-capillary surface-enhanced Raman spectroscopy: determination of glutathione in whole blood microsamples. Anal. Chem. **90**, 9093–9100.
60. Yang, Y., Xu, B., Murray, J., Haverstick, J., Chen, X., Tripp, R. A. and Zhao, Y. (2022) Rapid and quantitative detection of respiratory viruses using surface-enhanced Raman spectroscopy and machine learning. Biosens. Bioelectron. **217**, 114721.
61. Li, J. Q., Dukes, P. V., Lee, W., Sarkis, M. and Vo-Dinh, T. (2022) Machine learning using convolutional neural networks for SERS analysis of biomarkers in medical diagnostics. J. Raman Spectrosc. **53**, 2044–2057.
62. Dybas, J., Wajda, A., Alcicek, F. C., Kaczmarska, M., Bulat, K., Szczesny-Malysiak, E., Martyna, A., Perez-Guaita, D., Sacha, T. and Marzec, K. M. (2022) Label-free testing strategy to evaluate packed red blood cell quality before transfusion to leukemia patients. Sci. Rep. **12**, 21849.
63. Farhane, Z., Nawaz, H., Bonnier, F. and Byrne, H. J. (2018) In vitro label-free screening of chemotherapeutic drugs using Raman microspectroscopy: Towards a new paradigm of spectralomics. J. Biophotonics **11**, e201700258.
64. Farhane, Z., Bonnier, F. and Byrne, H. J. (2017) Monitoring doxorubicin cellular uptake and trafficking using in vitro Raman microspectroscopy: short and long time exposure effects on lung cancer cell lines. Anal. Bioanal. Chem. **409**, 1333–1346.
65. Efeoglu, E., Casey, A. and Byrne, H. J. (2016) In vitro monitoring of time and dose dependent cytotoxicity of aminated nanoparticles using Raman spectroscopy. Analyst **141**, 5417–5431.
66. Perez-Guaita, D., Quintas, G., Farhane, Z., Tauler, R. and Byrne, H. J. (2020) Data mining Raman microspectroscopic responses of cells to drugs in vitro using multivariate curve resolution-alternating least squares. Talanta **208**, 120386.
67. Perez-Guaita, D., Chrabaszcz, K., Malek, K. and Byrne, H. J. (2020) Multimodal vibrational studies of drug uptake in vitro: Is the whole greater than the sum of their parts? J. Biophotonics **13**, e202000264.

68. Pérez-Guaita, D., Quintás, G., Farhane, Z., Tauler, R. and Byrne, H. J. (2022) Combining pharmacokinetics and vibrational spectroscopy: MCR-ALS hard-and-soft modelling of drug uptake in vitro using tailored kinetic constraints. Cells **11**, 1555.
69. Azam, K. S. F., Ryabchykov, O. and Bocklitz, T. (2022) A review on data fusion of multidimensional medical and biomedical data. Molecules **27**, 7448.
70. Pérez-Guaita, D., Kochan, K., Martin, M., Andrew, D. W., Heraud, P., Richards, J. S. and Wood, B. R. (2017) Multimodal vibrational imaging of cells. Vib. Spectrosc. **91**, 46–58.
71. Ryabchykov, O., Popp, J. and Bocklitz, T. (2018) Fusion of MALDI spectrometric imaging and Raman spectroscopic data for the analysis of biological samples. Front. Chem. **6**, 257.
72. Teng, G., Wang, Q., Cui, X., Wei, K., Xiangli, W. and Chen, G. (2021) Feature-level fusion of laser-induced breakdown spectroscopy and Raman spectroscopy for improving support vector machine in clinical bacteria identification. J. Raman Spectrosc. **52**, 805–814.
73. Quintás, G., Wood, B. R., Byrne, H. J. and Perez-Guaita, D. (2021) Multiplexed Fourier Transform Infrared and Raman Imaging. In *Multiplexed Imaging*, pp. 299–312, Humana.
74. Spadea, A., Denbigh, J., Lawrence, M. J., Kansiz, M. and Gardner, P. (2021) Analysis of fixed and live single cells using optical photothermal infrared with concomitant Raman spectroscopy. Anal. Chem. **93**, 3938–3950.

https://doi.org/10.1142/9789811264610_0004

Chapter 4

Raman Spectroscopy and Machine Learning as a Potential Universal Diagnostic Technique*

Nicole M. Ralbovsky,[1,2] Igor K. Lednev[1,2,†]

[1]*Department of Chemistry, University at Albany, SUNY, 1400 Washington Avenue, Albany, NY 12222, USA*
[2]*The RNA Institute, University at Albany, SUNY, 1400 Washington Avenue, Albany, NY 12222, USA*
[†]*Corresponding author: ilednev@albany.edu*

4.1 Introduction

Receiving a diagnosis for an ailment is an event nearly every individual in the world will experience at least once in their lifetime. Whether the illness is a viral infection, blood disorder, or cancer, early and accurate detection is at the heart of properly treating and aiding the afflicted individual. However, just as the diseases a person can contract are diverse, so too are the methods utilized for screening and diagnosing them. Within these various techniques lies significant room for improving measures such as the test's sensitivity and specificity, its access and availability, and its definitiveness, as well as reducing the cost, time to perform, and level of invasiveness associated with the test. To address these needs, there has been a strong push toward developing a novel method which can be applied for universal medical diagnostics; that is, the development of a minimally invasive single test which can simply and accurately screen for as well as diagnose a wide variety of illnesses and diseases early on while also

* Adapted with permission from Ralbovsky, N. M. and Lednev, I. K. (2020) Towards development of a novel universal medical diagnostic method: Raman spectroscopy and machine learning. Chem. Soc. Rev. **49**, 7428–7453. Copyright © RSC Publishing.

being time-efficient and cost-effective. Raman spectroscopy (RS) is proposed here as a method which can satisfy this massively important role.

RS is an exceptional analytical tool used for obtaining very specific information regarding a sample's molecular composition. RS involves the irradiation of a sample by a monochromatic light source. Incident photons of light will interact with the sample, causing excitation and deactivation of molecular vibrations as a result of inelastic, or Raman, scattering. The energy difference between the incident and scattered photons is thus equivalent to the energy of numerous molecular vibrations in the sample. Thus, RS is said to provide a vibrational "fingerprint" of the sample that is known to be the most specific spectroscopic characteristic of the material.

RS provides incredible detail regarding the biochemical composition of a biological sample; due to its specificity, it is expected that RS will be able to determine differences between biological samples collected from healthy and diseased donors. Further, it can collect and process spectral information from multiple positions on a sample with the purpose of providing statistically significant characterization of the sample's heterogeneity and multicomponent composition. This creates the opportunity to detect multiple biomarkers simultaneously, which most diagnostic tests and exams are not capable of doing. In addition to its specificity, RS has considerable advantages over other methods used for diagnostics. The method is inherently non-invasive and can be used *in vivo* due to the advent of handheld instruments and fiber-optic probes. RS is not expensive in comparison to diagnostic imaging tests, and it is objective, which makes it a more desirable tool over diagnostic methods which require human interpretation of the results, such as histopathology. Most importantly, RS is easy to use, fast, reliable, and can simply be adapted for use in clinical settings.

It is important to note that the changes which occur between spectra of different biological samples can oftentimes be small and not easily observable. As a result, chemometrics, or machine learning, is frequently used to interpret the collected spectral data. The application of chemometrics to data which exists as a matrix, such as Raman spectral data, allows the user to generate machine learning prediction algorithms for the purpose of sorting and separating chemical data. Specifically, the prediction algorithms learn similarities and differences between classes of data, such as that obtained from biological samples of healthy donors and donors with a disease. Once the model is built using known data, it can then be applied toward making a classification prediction on new, unknown, data presented to it. In this way, these algorithms can be used for specific and accurate medical screening and diagnostic purposes.

There are many different chemometric methods which exist to answer a variety of scientific questions. Specifically, there are two main types of statistical models that can be built: supervised and unsupervised models. Techniques which are unsupervised do not utilize user-defined information during model construction; these types of methods tend to be exploratory in nature and are sufficient for separating dissimilar sets of data while grouping together data that are similar. Examples of unsupervised methods include principal component analysis and K-means cluster analysis. The other category of models is called supervised methods because these do consider user-defined information, such as class labels. Within supervised methods, regression models and classification models exist. Regression models, such as logistic regression, can compare Raman spectral data to changes in time or concentration, for example, and thus function similarly to the ideas of calibration curves. Classification techniques are known to yield qualitative responses, such as the class of a donor. Examples of supervised classification methods include partial least squares and support vector machine discriminant analyses. Chemometric methods have been applied to solve a variety of issues using RS and its variations [1–3]. Table 4.1 provides a brief overview of commonly used methods discussed herein; for a more detailed review of chemometric methods, including various advantages

Table 4.1. Brief introduction to commonly used chemometric methods.

Method	Function	Description
ANN	Classification and regression analysis	Computing system consisting of a collection of connected units called artificial neurons; input neurons connect to a defined number of hidden layers, which subsequently connect to an output layer which generates the class prediction
GA	Optimization methodology	Generates evolved solutions by relying on biological operators including selection, mutation, and cross-over
KNN	Classification and regression analysis	Determines an unknown case by comparing the distance of the unknown to all stored available cases
LDA	Dimensionality reduction and classification analysis	Recognizes the ideal linear combination of features which characterizes or separates two or more classes of objects

(Continued)

Table 4.1. (*Continued*)

Method	Function	Description
PCA	Unsupervised feature extraction and dimensionality reduction	An orthogonal transformation of the original dataset into a reduced subspace of features with eigenvalues describing their importance in decreasing order of explained variance
PLS-DA	Dimensionality reduction and classification analysis	Linear classification model which projects predicted variables and observable variables into a new space
RF	Classification and regression analysis	Constructs many decision trees during training; the output classification of a new sample is the mean prediction of all trees
SVM	Classification and regression analysis	Determines the hyperplane which maximizes the distance between classes while minimizing misclassifications

and disadvantages of the methods, the reader is referred to other works which go into greater detail [4–7].

Validation of the chemometric model is required after it has been built. Receiver operating characteristic curves are sometimes used for illustrating the ability of a binary classification system to make a correct classification as its discrimination threshold is varied. Further, there are two main variations of validation. Cross-validation (CV) implies a validation scheme where the spectral data that is used to build the model is also used to test its prediction abilities. This can be done in several ways; the most common include leave-one-spectrum-out, leave-one-sample-out, and k-fold CV. The first and second methods involve leaving either a single spectrum or all spectra from one sample out of the model-building process. The left-out data is used to test the performance of the model. This process is then repeated until all data have been left out. Similarly, k-fold CV randomly divides the data set into k groups and builds the model with k−1 groups. The leftover group is again repeatedly used for evaluating its performance. The second type of validation is called independent or external validation. This method evaluates the performance of the model on data that were not used to build it. This type of validation indicates whether a model was over-fit and allows the builder to determine how it may perform in further clinical applications. The results of external validation are crucial to pushing the method toward real-world use.

Due to their significant advantages independently as well as combined, abundant research has been published on screening and diagnosing a wide range of diseases using RS and chemometric techniques. In addition to research articles, reviews have been conducted which address the topic of RS for medical diagnostics. However, an update is necessary. Upon investigating reviews published in 2014 or later, many informative documents were written which emphasized different aspects of the topic at hand. For example, some evaluated analytical techniques beyond RS [8–11]; on the other hand, several others specifically discussed surface-enhanced Raman spectroscopy (SERS) [12–16] or fiber-optic probes, alone [17]. In some, specialized clinical areas are investigated including oncology [18–22], diabetes [23, 24], and regenerative medicine [25]. While some reviews differ in their level of conclusiveness [26, 27], others are comprehensive but are outdated and require an update on the current literature [28–31]. The reader is suggested to investigate these alternative and excellent reviews for further information on the aforementioned specialized topics.

The intention of this review is to fill in the necessary gap in the literature and provide a fully comprehensive review of manuscripts published primarily between 2018 and 2020. A review of this nature is critical and necessary to keep the field moving forward. Because of the immense potential of the Raman method for solving a number of screening and diagnostic issues, it is incredibly important and useful to inform the community of the progress which has already been made to establish the steps leading to future productive work, including fully introducing the methodology into clinical settings. Specifically, articles which utilize RS and chemometric techniques for the purpose of screening or diagnosing any and all illnesses or diseases will be reviewed. Both SERS and spontaneous RS will be considered, as well as any research conducted using fiber-optic probes. Other variations of RS will also be considered if used in conjunction with chemometric techniques. In this regard, only research which incorporates chemometric and machine learning methods will be considered. In order to bring the methodology into clinical settings, it is anticipated that an automatic data analysis procedure will be required to examine Raman spectral data and generate a diagnosis. Chemometrics can be performed using easily available software and can provide rapid, definitive, and accurate diagnosis quickly and cost-effectively, thereby improving significantly upon the current methods used for diagnostics. The goal of this review is to promote and declare RS in combination with chemometrics as being a highly suitable universal method for medical diagnostics and screening applications. A critical evaluation of the benefits and risks of the method as well as comparisons between various studies will be included within the review in an effort to create a platform from which future work can successfully be accomplished.

4.2 Spontaneous Raman Spectroscopy

Spontaneous Raman spectroscopy employs a laser which emits monochromatic light typically in the visible to near-infrared (IR) range. Photons from the laser light interact with the molecules within the irradiated sample and the resultant inelastically scattered photons are detected by the instrument in a quantitative way. The Raman spectrum that is produced is very specific to the sample in a manner similar to the uniqueness and specificity of a human fingerprint. Spontaneous RS permits detection and characterization of the multicomponent composition of a heterogeneous sample, making it useful for studying various biological samples. Typically, multiple spectra are collected from a single sample to better account for this heterogeneity. One of the most notable advantages of RS is its ability to integrate multiple potential biomarkers into one spectroscopic signature, thus improving the sensitivity and specificity of the method. Many different studies have utilized spontaneous RS for assessing its ability to diagnose a variety of diseases including cancers, infectious diseases, blood disorders, neurodegenerative diseases, and more. Those studies which have done so in 2018 and beyond are reviewed here.

4.2.1 *Cancer*

The greatest number of studies have focused on accomplishing the detection of various forms of cancer within biological samples. In one study, the tumor suppressor wild type p53 protein, considered a cancer biomarker, was investigated by Hernández-Vidales *et al.* Principal component analysis (PCA) and support vector machine (SVM) algorithms showed that the wild and mutant types of this biomarker were separated with 94% accuracy after leave-one-out cross-validation (LOOCV); the limit of detection of the wild-type p53 was found to be 0.946 μM, opening the door for applying this method in investigating any cancer using spontaneous RS [32].

Bladder Cancer

In a study led by Bovenkamp *et al.*, optical coherence tomography (OCT) was used in combination with RS for identifying different stages and grades of bladder cancer through the analysis of bladder tissue samples from eight donors. Degenerated tissue was first identified by OCT; RS was then used to determine molecular characteristics at suspicious sites. K-nearest neighbor (KNN) with five-fold CV was used to analyze OCT data, achieving 71% accuracy for staging a tumor; analysis of RS data achieved 93% accuracy for discriminating between low- and high-grade lesions via PCA followed by KNN, indicating RS as a preferred method for identifying the cancer [33].

Brain Cancer

Brain cancer was investigated by several different research groups. Tissue from grade IV medulloblastoma was compared to non-tumor samples from five individuals; results of partial least squares discriminant analysis (PLS-DA) with CV gave a sensitivity and specificity of 96.3% and 92%, respectively. Atomic force microscopy (AFM) was used to further recognize the heterogeneous mechanical properties of the tissue [34]. Mehta *et al.* investigated meningioma, a primary brain and central nervous system tumor. RS was used to classify blood serum from 35 control and 35 meningioma subjects; PCA combined with PC-linear discriminant analysis (PC-LDA) yielded 92% and 80% classification efficiencies for healthy and meningioma subjects, respectively, after leave-one-sample-out cross-validation (LOSOCV) [35]. In a three-tiered study, brain metastases from primary adenocarcinomas of the lung (n = 7) and colorectum (n = 7) were analyzed in comparison to metastatic melanoma (n = 7). PCA in combination with a linear discriminant classifier gave rise to classification accuracies of 69% for colorectal adenocarcinoma, 69% for lung carcinoma, and 72% for melanoma. A comparison to ATR-FTIR spectroscopy was made, where the same statistical analysis method resulted in accuracies of 60% for colorectal adenocarcinoma, 59% for lung carcinoma, and 47% for melanoma. Interestingly, when the two adenocarcinoma groups were combined, the classification accuracies increased to 85% for adenocarcinoma and 75.4% for melanoma using the Raman spectral data. It should be noted, however, that no validation was reported [36]. Depciuch *et al.* also compared the usefulness of FTIR spectroscopy versus RS for investigating chemical changes in brain tissues and glioblastoma tumor tissues. Data collected from cancer and marginal brain tissues using both methods showed significant differences in chemical composition when compared to control brain tissues. PCA indicated these observed changes were significant for differentiating between infected and healthy tissue as well as between adjacent brain tissue and control tissue. This research opens the door for further analysis of the

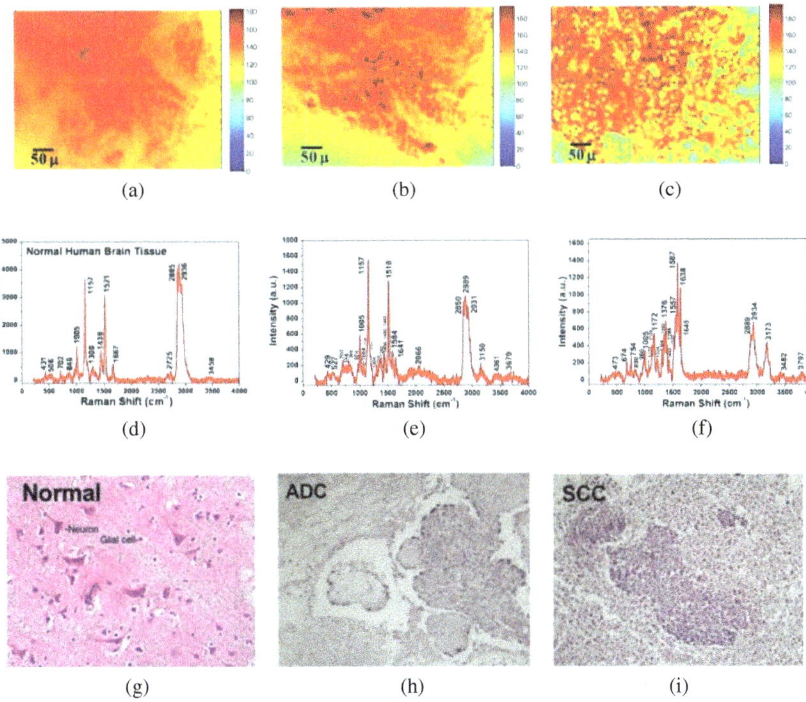

Figure 4.1. Three sets of data from brain metastases of lung cancer and normal tissue. Upper row: A set of typical cropped confocal micrograph images using pseudo color of (a) normal brain tissue, (b) brain metastasis from adenocarcinoma, and (c) brain metastasis from squamous cell carcinoma (SCC). Middle row: A set of resonance Raman spectra of (d) normal brain tissue, (e) brain metastasis from adenocarcinoma, and (f) brain metastasis from SCC. The spectra in (d)–(f) are corresponding to the images in (a)–(c), respectively. Bottom row: H&E-stained images from (g) normal brain tissue, (h) brain metastasis from adenocarcinoma, and (i) brain metastasis from SCC. All the H&E images used 20× objective and correspond to the images in (a)–(c), respectively. Reproduced from Ref. [38] with permission.

data for diagnostic applications as well as for a better understanding of the biochemical changes which occur during cancer progression [37]. Zhou *et al.* utilized RS for differentiating brain metastases of lung cancer adenocarcinoma and squamous cell carcinoma (SCC) from normal tissue (Figure 4.1). The results of optical spatial frequency spectroscopy analysis, which determines the difference in random spatial frequency structures among micrograph images of the tissues, combined with RS was examined using SVM and receiver operating characteristic (ROC) curve analysis. All three types of brain tissue were identified with high levels of accuracy; further, normal and cancerous tissues were discriminated in a binary model with 88.5% sensitivity and 75% specificity with an area under the ROC curve (AUC) of 0.93; validation is needed to further support the results [38]. The best outcomes were obtained when tissue was analyzed using a simple PC-LDA classifier.

Breast Cancer

Attempts to investigate breast cancer were frequent. An ant colony optimization (ACO) algorithm was used to improve the power of breast cancer diagnosis by RS. Spectra from normal (n = 3), benign (n = 5), and cancerous (n = 3) breast tissue were collected. ACO identified five features which were optimum for diagnosis, and quadratic discriminant analysis (QDA) resulted in 87.7% accuracy for differentiating between the three types of tissue after LOOCV [39]. Marro *et al.* compared the ability of multivariate curve resolution (MCR) versus PCA for deconvolution of the meaningful components in the spectral dataset of breast cancer cells. The MCR algorithm combined with alternating least squares (ALS) analysis showed a strong ability to monitor the progression of breast cancer cells to bone metastasis, providing crucial biochemical insights into the molecular progression of cancer cells as compared to PCA. Further, two cell lines (BO2 and MDA-MB-435P) were discriminated from each other using PLS-DA with CV, reaching 100% specificity and 90% specificity, respectively [40]. In another study, the ability of RS to discriminate between benign lesions and cancer tissue of 20 different donors was investigated. Several different chemometric methods were applied to the spectral dataset; PCA-LDA, PCA-QDA, and PLS-DA all achieved >80% sensitivity and specificity for classification whereas PCA-SVM achieved >90% sensitivity and specificity after external validation [41]. In a unique study, white light interference microscopy (WLIM) was combined with RS in an attempt to differentiate between 80 cancerous and normal breast tissue samples collected from 16 patients. WLIM provided quantitative phase information about the samples whereas RS detected the molecular changes occurring during cancer progression. A SVM classifier was built to classify the tissue samples; a ROC curve was used to check the accuracy of the model, which achieved 90.6% accuracy for cancer detection during external validation [42]. Talari *et al.* studied breast cancer tissue using RS in conjunction with PCA and LDA. LDA classified biopsies into luminal A, luminal B, HER2, and triple negative subtypes with an average accuracy of 89.2% after CV [43]. Alternatively, RS and an orthogonal partial least squares (OPLS) discriminant analysis algorithm could successfully separate data obtained from healthy and invasive ductal carcinoma in breast tissue samples based on cluster analysis with a very low root mean square error of CV (0.09) [44]. Of the studies which examined tissue, varying results were achieved, indicating the importance of selecting the optimum chemometric technique for analyzing spontaneous RS data.

The analysis of body fluids was used in additional reports for diagnosing breast cancer. PCA-LDA could discriminate between blood plasma of normal (n = 26) and breast cancer (n = 19) subjects, achieving 100% classification accuracy after LOSOCV. Further, ROC curve analysis of spectral variations of various biomolecules, including phenylalanine, proteins, and lipids, resulted in 100% sensitivity and 83–100% specificity for classification [45]. Blood plasma of breast cancer patients and healthy controls was also investigated by another group; PCA-factorial discriminant analysis (FDA) with CV could classify all blood plasma samples from breast cancer donors (n = 18) with 100% specificity and 99% sensitivity when compared to healthy controls (n = 8). Further, PCA-FDA successfully differentiated stage II and stage III breast cancer with 94% specificity and 95% sensitivity, and stage II and stage IV breast cancer with 100% specificity and 90% sensitivity, indicating the potential of the method for achieving early diagnosis and staging of breast cancer [46]. Interestingly, blood plasma seemed to provide more biochemical information than the tissue samples, resulting in better prediction accuracies.

Cervical Cancer

Several studies were published on efforts to identify cervical cancer. PCA and artificial neural networks (ANN) with CV were used in one study to discriminate between normal (n = 64), neoplastic (n = 36), and malignant (n = 145) cells/tissues with 99% accuracy. PC-LDA with CV was then used to separate well-differentiated, moderately differentiated, and poorly differentiated SCC with 94.0% accuracy, demonstrating the potential of RS to replace histopathology [47]. Cells were again analyzed in a different study; high-grade squamous intraepithelial (HSIL) cells were investigated through analysis of HSIL-associated biochemical changes in normal appearing intermediate and superficial cells using RS. PLS-DA with CV could diagnose HSIL compared to intermediate, superficial, and mixed intermediate/superficial cells with an average sensitivity of 95.6% and specificity of 93.6%, suggesting morphologically normal appearing cells can be used to identify the differences between negative and HSIL cytology [48]. In a different report, 95 total cervical adenocarcinoma and cervical SCC tissues were distinguished from each other with 93.1% accuracy using PCA-SVM with external validation [49]. On the other hand, blood plasma of 30 normal and 18 cervical cancer patients was separated using PCA-LDA with 94.4% sensitivity and 96.7%

specificity after LOOCV; ROC curve analysis yielded 100% accuracy [50]. The aforementioned reports indicate that regardless of the biological sample studied, respectable diagnostic performance can be achieved through analysis of spontaneous RS data for detecting cervical cancer.

Colorectal Cancer

Spontaneous RS was investigated for its potential to diagnose colorectal cancer through analysis of two different colorectal cancer cell lines (SW480 and SW620). PCA with LDA yielded an accuracy of 98.7% for classification. Further, five different cell lines (HL60, HT29, HCT116, SW620, and SW480) were separated using PCA-LDA with 92.4% accuracy, suggesting cells as a preferred biological sample for identifying colorectal cancer. Both analyses were verified using 10-fold CV [51].

Esophageal Cancer

Maitra *et al.* examined whether RS could interrogate various body fluids for the purpose of detecting different stages of esophageal adenocarcinoma, including normal/squamous epithelium, inflammatory, Barrett's, low-grade dysplasia, high-grade dysplasia, and esophageal adenocarcinoma. A combination of genetic algorithm with QDA resulted in 100% separation of all classes using saliva and urine samples after external validation. Plasma and serum samples could be classified with >90% accuracy for all esophageal stages. This study poses an interesting comparison of different body fluids and their potential for diagnosing the same disease [52].

Gastric Cancer

Bahreini *et al.* investigated RS for distinguishing between blood serum samples of 40 healthy controls and 20 patients with gastric cancer using PLS-DA. Results of CV yielded 87.5% classification efficiency, presenting RS analysis of serum as a potential screening tool for gastric cancer [53]. These results were comparable to those reported using SERS.

Head and Neck Cancers

Khan *et al.* studied nasopharyngeal cancer (NPC) via analysis of blood serum from 15 healthy controls and 14 NPC patients. SVM classification resulted in 93% accuracy after CV [54]. Larynx cancer was evaluated through analysis of healthy (n = 13) and cancerous (n = 13) tissues. Raman spectral data was subjected to OPLS with CV, and the generated algorithm successfully clustered healthy and cancerous tissue spectra [55]. Furthermore, inverted papillomas, tumors of the sinonasal tract, were analyzed by RS. Three different types of sinonasal tissues were explored using PCA-LDA; the model effectively distinguished between normal sinonasal mucosa, chronic rhinosinusitis, and inverted papilloma tissue with an average accuracy of 90.2%; a validation scheme was not reported [56].

Leukemia

The diagnosis of leukemia was examined by Managò *et al.* Initially, different leukocyte subpopulations of lymphocytes (B, T, and NK cells) as well as monocytes and granulocytes were identified using PCA and LDA with about 99% accuracy after LOOCV. Secondly, normal B cells and transformed MN60 lymphocyte leukemic cell lines were efficiently separated via the same procedure [57]. In a different study, an attempt was made to differentiate between 7 leukemia, 16 breast cancer, and 22 cervical cancer blood serum donors by superparamagnetic clustering and PCA, which was found to be successful [58]. Lastly, the differences of whole blood (n = 38) and plasma (n = 40) samples taken from healthy controls and leukemic subjects were investigated using RS. PLS was used to build discriminatory models, yielding 91.9% sensitivity and 100% specificity for classifying whole blood spectra. The plasma spectra were separated with 95.7% sensitivity and 98% specificity after LOSOCV, demonstrating the ability of RS to diagnosis acute leukemia in both whole blood and plasma samples with similar levels of success (Figure 4.2) [59].

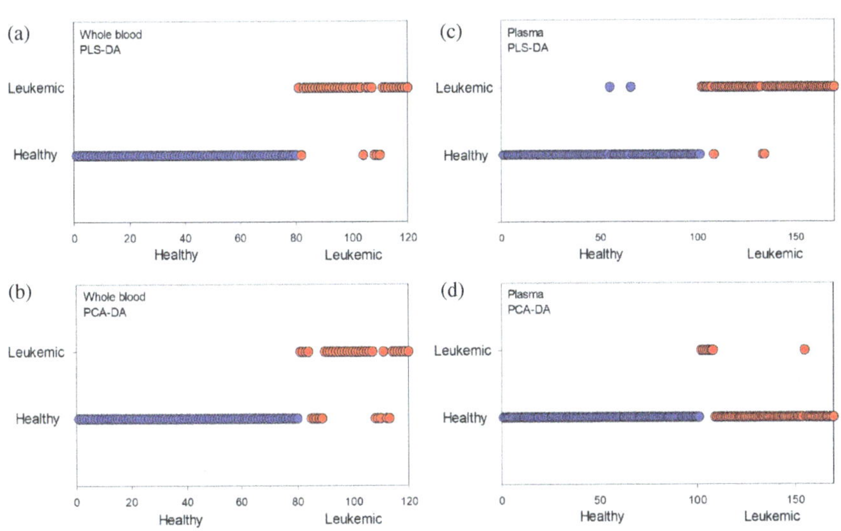

Figure 4.2. Confusion plot with the classifications by healthy and leukemic groups through DA, being (a) PLS-DA (whole blood); (b) PCA-DA (whole blood); (c) PLS-DA (plasma); and (d) PCA-DA (plasma). Reproduced from Ref. [59] with permission.

Lung Cancer

Lung cancer was investigated using spontaneous RS in three recent studies. Wang *et al.* measured Raman spectra from blood serum of healthy volunteers (n = 14) and patients with different stages of non-small cell lung cancer (NSCLC, n – 77). PCA-LDA with CV separated healthy, stage I, stage II, and stage III/IV NSCLC serum samples with an average of 78.3% sensitivity and 92.5% specificity; the overall accuracy was 92% [60]. Alternative research focused on using two different excitation wavelengths for identifying lung cancer in normal, non-cancerous abnormal, and cancerous tissue from 32 patients. LDA with CV showed 84% accuracy for discrimination using FT-Raman (λ_{ex} = 1064 nm) and 100% accuracy with the standard 785 nm excitation after CV, indicating a strong preference for near IR excitation [61]. Zheng *et al.* used SVM and KNN to cytopathologically diagnose lung cancer with almost 99% accuracy; no validation was reported [62]. Generally, the different biological samples employed in these reports provided similar levels of biochemical information which could be used for differentiation.

Lymphatic Cancers

B-cell non-Hodgkin lymphoma was studied through RS for the purpose of distinguishing normal B-cells and B-cell non-Hodgkin lymphoma cells. PCA showed successful clustering of the two different cell types as well as between different types of B-cell non-Hodgkin lymphoma cells, indicating the potential of the method for analyzing tumor cells [63]. In a related work, lymph nodes of 20 patients affected by different conditions including reactive follicular hyperplasia (benign), follicular lymphoma (low-grade primary tumor), diffuse B-cell lymphoma (high-grade primary tumor), and tumor metastasis (secondary tumors) were examined by RS. A PLS-DA classifier for benign versus malignant tissues provided 85.7% accuracy at the donor level for external validation. Other binary classification models reached similar levels of success for discerning different types of lymph nodes [64].

Oral Cancer

The identification of oral cancer was explored using spontaneous RS and chemometrics. Molecular differences between oral cavity SCC and healthy tissue structures in the tongue were investigated by RS analysis of 44 tongue samples from 21 donors. A non-negative least-squares algorithm was used for fitting to determine the spectral contributions of different chemical classes. Carbohydrate, protein, and amino acid content had the strongest capabilities for discriminating between oral cavity SCC and healthy tissue; a classification model of tumor versus healthy tissue was built based on these differences, with results of external validation providing 93% specificity and 100% sensitivity for discrimination [65]. Exfoliated cells from tumor (n = 16) and contralateral-normal appearing mucosa (n = 16) of oral cancer patients and from healthy tobacco users (n = 20) were analyzed via PCA-LDA. A model built to separate contralateral-normal and tumor spectra resulted in 74% sensitivity and 73% specificity for identifying normal spectra during LOOCV. A three-class model, including the healthy tobacco users, displayed an average of 70.2% accuracy after LOOCV [66]. Exfoliated cells were again studied in a different and more successful work, this time using both FTIR spectroscopy and RS for discerning normal, pre-cancerous, and cancerous conditions. PCA-LDA with 10-fold CV of the combined FTIR and RS spectral dataset showed 98% classification accuracy, an improvement upon analysis conducted using only FTIR (85%) or RS (82%) spectral data [67]. Jeng *et al.* investigated 80 tissue samples from the tongue, buccal mucosa, and gingiva of the oral mucosa which represented normal and tumor tissue sites. A PCA-QDA classifier could differentiate the tissues with 90.9% sensitivity and 83.3% specificity after CV, outperforming a PCA-LDA classifier built to achieve the same goal [68]. Lastly, an exploration into both oral and cervical cancer was made using Raman exfoliated cytology. Oral (29 tumor and 15 normal) and cervical (38 tumor and 28 normal) exfoliated cell samples were studied. PCA-LDA with LOSOCV yielded classification efficiencies of 82% and 77% for identifying oral tumor and cervical tumor cells, respectively; these results increased to 86% and 84% classification efficiency for identifying oral tumor and cervical tumor cells at the subject level [69]. These studies show the importance of which classifier is selected for analysis and the effect that the selection of data can have.

Prostate Cancer

RS analysis using a 1064 nm wavelength laser for excitation was proposed as a method for screening prostate cancer. A classifier based on SVM could predict the Gleason scores (benign, or score of 6, 7, or 8) of 37 prostate tissue specimens of eight donors with 95% classification accuracy after LOSOCV [70]. These results are generally better than those reported using SERS.

Skin Cancer

Feng *et al.* investigated relevant Raman biomarkers for guiding basal cell carcinoma (BCC) margin resection; data was collected from skin tissue samples of 30 individuals undergoing Mohs surgery. The data showed that BCC results in different concentrations of nucleus, keratin, collagen, triolein, and ceramide biomolecules compared to normal skin structures. ROC curve analysis and LOSOCV indicated 90% sensitivity and 92% specificity for discriminating between BCC and normal tissue structures [71]. High wavenumber Raman spectra were collected from 174 excised melanocytic lesions suspicious for melanoma; a PCA-LDA model was developed to distinguish melanomas and non-melanoma, achieving 100% sensitivity and 43.8% specificity after external validation, perhaps indicating this spectral region was not necessarily useful for achieving better diagnostic results [72]. Lastly, non-melanoma skin cancer (BCC and SCC), actinic keratosis, and normal tissue of 25 subjects were investigated by Raman spectra collected both *in vivo* and *ex vivo*. DA based on Mahalanobis distances was applied for discriminating lesions and normal tissue, achieving 94.1% sensitivity, 93.6% specificity and 93.8% accuracy for classification of the *in vivo* spectra and 100% sensitivity, specificity, and accuracy for the *ex vivo* tissue spectra. These results were superior to those achieved using DA performed via Euclidean distances, although no validation scheme was mentioned [73]. Not surprisingly, tissue samples were most commonly used for analyzing skin cancer, providing varying levels of success for classification.

Thyroid Cancer

Thyroid cancer was studied by a myriad of researchers using spontaneous RS. In one study, FTIR spectroscopy and RS were combined with statistical analysis to distinguish between thyroid adenomas (n = 17) and carcinomas (n = 15). PCA-LDA with LOOCV showed sensitivities around 62% and 65% and specificities around 70% and 75% for Raman and FTIR spectroscopies, respectively, for distinguishing widely invasive follicular thyroid carcinoma, follicular thyroid adenoma, and normal tissues [74]. In an improvement, Senol *et al.* used an OPLS algorithm to distinguish thyroid tumor and healthy tissue with 81.8% sensitivity and specificity after CV [75]. A different project investigated RS for correctly classifying cell lines which represented benign thyroid cells and various subtypes of thyroid cancer. PCA-LDA, without validation, gave good sensitives (74–85%), specificities (65–93%), and accuracies (71–88%) for identifying thyroid cancer in various binary models [76]. De Oliveira *et al.* obtained Raman hyperspectral images of single cells from benign thyroid (n = 127) and classical papillary carcinoma (n = 121) nodules. PCA and LDA with CV could identify the cells with 97% diagnostic accuracy, which were the best results obtained recently for identifying the cancer. Further, differences in spectral data collected from cells of follicular adenoma (n = 20), follicular carcinoma (n = 25), and the follicular variant of papillary carcinoma (n = 18) nodules indicated the feasibility of the approach for discrimination of further thyroid cancer subtypes [77].

4.2.2 *Bacterial and Viral Infections*

While there is an abundance of literature published on identifying various cancers using spontaneous RS, research has progressed toward investigating other illnesses, such as infectious diseases with bacterial, fungal, and viral origins, as well.

Khan *et al.* analyzed blood serum collected from 60 tuberculosis patients and 14 healthy age matched controls using RS. SVM and PCA with 5-fold CV could diagnose the illness with 92% accuracy, 98% specificity, and 81% sensitivity, illustrating the potential for an early screening mechanism of tuberculosis despite the uneven distribution of sample donors [78]. Another bacterial infection, called *Clostridium difficile* infection (CDI), was also investigated using blood serum. Here, serum was spiked with various concentrations of two different *Clostridium* pathogenic factors (toxin A and toxin B or both). Toxin-spiked serum at various concentrations (1 ng/mL, 1 pg/mL, and 0.1 pg/mL) could be segregated from control serum with 87–100% sensitivity and 77–100% specificity after CV, demonstrating the potential for RS to be used as a sensitive method for detecting clinically relevant concentrations of CDI toxins for diagnostic purposes [79].

Both hepatitis B and hepatitis C, common viral infections, were studied by different research groups using spontaneous RS. Ditta *et al.* studied blood plasma from hepatitis C-infected individuals and healthy donors. The RS data was analyzed using PCA; the differences between spectral features resulted in successful separation of the two groups [80]. In a quantitative study, the hepatitis C infection was explored using RS and a proximity-based machine learning technique (PCA-Prox). The PCA-Prox algorithm separated blood serum from 227 infected and healthy donors with accuracy, sensitivity, and specificity levels of 95%, 97%, and 94%, respectively, after 5-fold CV. The PCA-Prox algorithm was found to perform better than other classifiers, including KNN, random forest (RF), and SVM [81]. In a large study, Tong *et al.* investigated the potential of RS for diagnosing hepatitis B through analysis of 1,000 blood serum samples from healthy and infected donors. The model was built using PCA and SVM; double-blind verification (external validation) of the model's performance showed 87% sensitivity and 92% specificity for the first group and 80% sensitivity and 79% specificity for the second group, showing a potential new method for hepatitis B virus detection [82]. In a smaller study, blood serum from 119 hepatitis B-infected and 84 healthy donors were analyzed by RS. SVM with CV gave a diagnostic accuracy of about 98%, an improvement upon the previous study [83].

RS was used to analyze neutrophils, cells of the immune system responsible for recognizing pathogens, to detect and identity the cause of an infection. Here, neutrophils were isolated from human peripheral blood and stimulated in an *in vitro* infection model with two bacterial pathogens (*Staphylococcus aureus* and *Escherichia coli*) and one viable fungi (*Candida albicans*). A high-throughput screening Raman microscope was used to obtain Raman spectra of greater than 2,000 neutrophils, individually, from three donors in each treatment group, resulting in almost 20,000 total spectra. RF models could distinguish between infected and non-infected neutrophils with 90% accuracy; additionally, the three different pathogens were differentiated with 92% accuracy after CV, thus providing a label-free and time-saving method for bloodstream infection diagnostics [84]. In related work, RS was explored for identifying the pathogenicity of *E. coli* strains. A total of 14 strains were investigated, where half were non-pathogenic, and half were pathogenic. The Raman spectra from these strains was used to build a PCA-SVM model, which was then externally tested using Raman spectra obtained from three additional *E. coli* strains. The three strains were shown to be predicted correctly with 77% sensitivity, which is deemed acceptable for a fast screening method for the pathogenicity of bacterial cells [85].

The dengue virus infection was studied in several recent papers. RS was used to analyze blood plasma from dengue-infected (n = 17) and healthy (n = 17) donors. PCA with FDA and LOOCV yielded 97.9% sensitivity and 95.4% specificity for identifying the infection. Further analysis compared healthy donors to patients who scored low on one of the dengue biomarker tests, but high or medium for two others; the same analysis method was used, resulting in 97.4% sensitivity and 86.2% specificity, fully indicating the method as an unambiguous screening technology [86]. Blood serum of healthy controls was compared to malaria- and dengue-infected donors. PCA-LDA could separate malaria, dengue, and healthy control groups with an average accuracy of about 89% after external validation. These results were complemented with mass spectrometry-based analysis, where metabolites assigned to the predominant RS bands were found to overlap with those trends identified by mass spectrometry [87]. In a related study, typhoid and dengue infections were analyzed together due to their similarities in symptoms. PCA with LDA and 10-fold CV were applied and could successfully separate the two sets of data, illustrating an interesting potential of RS to separate infections with similar symptoms [88]. Blood, including serum and plasma samples, appears to be the most useful biological fluid for identifying the dengue virus. Of great recent interest, preliminary studies show RS as being a viable tool for addressing the COVID-19 pandemic, which is caused by the SARS-CoV-2 viral infection [89]. Indeed, Jacobi *et al.* have already begun investigation into mapping the nanostructure of the COVID-19 virus using low-frequency and regular RS and comparing the structure with that of other coronaviruses and viral materials. This work is vital for laying the foundation for future studies into this disastrous disease [90]. Further, Yeh *et al.* propose a microfluidic platform in conjunction with surface-enhanced RS as a novel method to track and monitor viral outbreaks, such as the COVID-19 outbreak, in real time [91]. Work which employs surface-enhanced RS for diagnostic efforts is discussed further in Section 4.3.

4.2.3 *Blood Disorders and Diabetes*

Beyond infectious diseases, diagnosis of blood disorders and diabetes have frequently been investigated using spontaneous RS. Research led by da Silva investigated iron deficiency anemia and sickle cell disease in comparison to healthy controls. PLS-DA and PCA-DA with LOSOCV were employed; the former resulted in 95.0% and the latter 93.8% diagnostic accuracy [92]. In a related work, detection of type II diabetes was investigated via RS analysis of blood serum from 35 donors. PCA and LDA were used for developing the discrimination method, yielding 96% sensitivity and 99% specificity for classification after LOSOCV [93].

4.2.4 *Kidney, Heart, and Thyroid Diseases*

A variety of biological issues associated with the kidney, heart, and thyroid were examined using spontaneous RS. Chen *et al.* explored the ability of RS to classify urine samples from 48 patients with chronic renal failure and from 44 subjects with normal renal function. Five different classifiers were used for distinguishing between the two groups; the best classifier, a grid search SVM, achieved 84.6% diagnostic accuracy after external validation, indicating the potential of the method as a rapid screening tool of urine samples [94]. In an alternate study, different mineral components within kidney stones were investigated. PCA-KNN and PCA-SVM both gave diagnostic accuracies of 96.3% after CV, showing RS can provide support for generating treatment recommendations for patients with kidney stones [95].

High renin hypertension was explored using serum RS combined with various classification algorithms. Groupings of PCA with SVM, LDA, and KNN plus LOOCV were investigated for generating a prediction algorithm. Both PCA-SVM and PCA-LDA achieved 93.5% diagnostic accuracy whereas the PCA-KNN algorithm demonstrated 89.1% accuracy, indicating the importance of exploring multiple machine learning techniques for achieving optimal results [96]. The same research group continued on to successfully detect thyroid dysfunction using serum RS and SVM, attaining a diagnostic accuracy of 82.7% for external validation [97]. Du *et al.* explored blood samples from 29 people with normal thyroid function and 38 individuals with hyperthyroidism and 32 with hypothyroidism. PLS-SVM was used for data classification, and the results of external validation indicated discriminatory specificity was 88.8%, sensitivity was 100%, and accuracy was 96.7%, an improvement on the previous study [98]. RS was then used to discriminate between healthy parathyroid tissue and parathyroid adenoma from 18 donors. A PLS-DA model could correctly classify all samples in the calibration and external validation datasets with 100% prediction accuracy. Chief cell adenoma and oxyphil cell adenoma were additionally classified using PLS-DA with 99.8% and 100% accuracy, respectively, after external validation [99].

4.2.5 *Autoimmune and Neurodegenerative Diseases*

Abundant research has been published recently on identifying various autoimmune disorders and neurodegenerative diseases. Fornasaro *et al.* utilized Raman hyperspectral imaging to characterize colon tissues from patients with Celiac disease (CD). Using MCR-ALS, k-means cluster analysis, and hierarchical clustering methods, biochemical differences between CD patients and healthy controls were identified which allowed for separation of the two groups. The algorithm was successfully externally validated using samples from patients with Crohn's disease, opening the door for future work to be conducted using an automated algorithm for classification [100]. In a quantitative study, red blood cells (RBCs) from CD patients and healthy donors on a gluten-free diet were analyzed using RS, PLS-DA and ROC curve analysis. Results showed 100% classification accuracy after external validation for correctly predicting the class of a donor [101].

Two groups focused strongly on investigating Alzheimer's disease (AD) using RS. Ralbovsky *et al.* successfully investigated AD and mild cognitive impairment through the analysis of saliva. Using genetic algorithm and ANN, 100% accuracy was achieved during external validation for differentiating between the three groups [102]. Blood serum was then successfully investigated by the same group for the identification of AD and other related forms of dementia, achieving high levels of success after external validation [103, 104]. Further, RS and machine learning showed success for identifying AD in cerebrospinal fluid. Here, Raman spectra were measured from 21 AD patients and 16 healthy controls. Subsequent ANN and SVM-DA models were able to differentiate between the subjects with 84% sensitivity and specificity after CV [105]. Most recent work by this group focused on using RS for identifying AD in its early stages using rat models. Although successful — the PLS-DA model with ROC curve analysis achieved 100% accuracy at the donor level after external validation — this work falls beyond the scope of the review due to the use of an animal model in lieu of human donors [106]. On the other hand, Paraskevaidi *et al.* focused on identifying AD and dementia with Lewy bodies in blood plasma. Various binary algorithms were built using SVM to differentiate between healthy controls, early-stage AD donors, late-stage AD donors, and donors with dementia with Lewy bodies. The classification algorithms achieved an average sensitivity of 81.3% and specificity of 85.7% after CV, suggesting the significance of selecting the best combination of biological sample with statistical method for analysis.

4.2.6 *Other Diseases*

An assortment of other diseases was also investigated using spontaneous RS. Parlatan *et al.* utilized RS for non-invasive diagnosis of endometriosis in a large study (Figure 4.3). 94 blood serum samples from healthy and diseased donors were investigated using PCA, KNN, and SVM. The best results were obtained using KNN, achieving 80.5% sensitivity and 89.7% specificity; further verification of the model using unseen data for external validation yielded 100% sensitivity and specificity values [108]. Another research group studied asthma via blood serum RS combined with PLS-DA. The classification model attained 100% sensitivity and specificity for correctly predicting the class of a

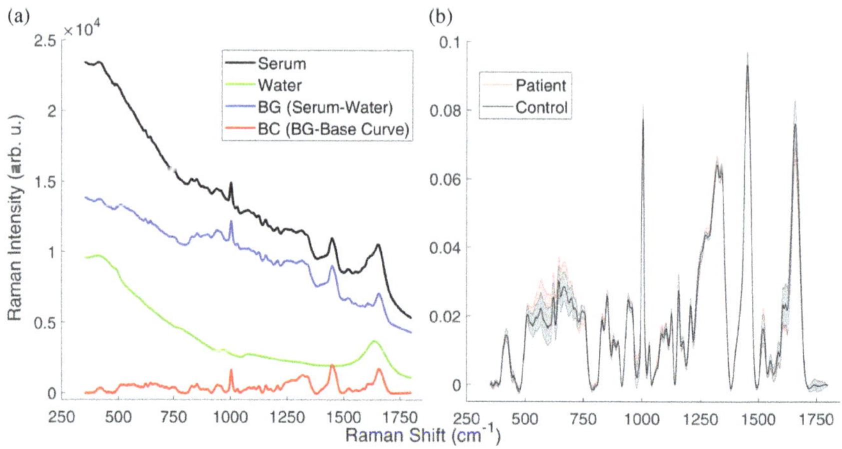

Figure 4.3. (a) Background (BG) and baseline-corrected (BC) Raman spectra of a serum sample. (b) Normalized BC mean Raman spectra of the control and patient groups. Standard deviations of each group were plotted and overlaid as shaded curves. Reproduced from Ref. [108] with permission.

donor in the external validation dataset [109]. Ochronotic and non-ochronotic cartilage was studied by RS for the purpose of monitoring the progress of ochronosis in patients with alkaptonuria, an inherited disorder of tyrosine metabolism. Analysis by PCA-LDA showed effective separation of the groups; further validation of the method is required [110]. Although out of scope for this review, Duchenne muscular dystrophy was investigated with great success by one group using a mouse model. Here, Raman spectra of diseased and control mice were differentiated using PLS-DA with 95.2% sensitivity and 94.6% specificity after CV and with 100% accuracy at the donor level after external validation. Further work could benefit from translating the results to human studies [111, 112].

Ulcerative colitis was studied using RS for identifying colonic inflammation. 42 colon biopsy samples taken from individuals across the four-level Mayo subscore for endoscopic disease severity were examined. A one-dimensional convolutional neural network (CNN) was developed, reaching 78% sensitivity and 93% specificity after LOSOCV for predicting the disease severity of ulcerative colitis [113]. In a final study, Sun *et al.* inspected the ability of RS to identify ocular diseases through analysis of tear samples. 69 patients with various ocular diseases (including conjunctivitis, blepharitis, meibomian gland cyst, cataracts, and glaucoma) and 48 healthy donors donated tears; a PLS-SVM algorithm could diagnose with 85.7% accuracy, 100% specificity, and 76.2% sensitivity after external validation, indicating the potential of RS analysis of tears for identifying different ocular diseases [114].

As these studies so clearly show, the potential of spontaneous RS is vast and can be applied toward investigating any disease which exhibits pathophysiological changes during its progression. Regardless of the biological sample used, the chemometric technique applied, or the disease studied, the promise of the method for medical diagnostics is clear. Spontaneous RS has the advantage of being the most straightforward variation of RS, requiring the least amount of effort to set up, learn, and understand (that is, in comparison to other methods to be further reviewed). Although the results are promising, more research is necessary to investigate the potential of spontaneous RS for *in vivo* and statistically significant validated trials, which are crucial for bringing the methodology into clinical settings.

4.3 Surface-Enhanced Raman Spectroscopy

Current efforts in disease diagnostics often focus on the detection of biomarkers which are present at low average concentrations. Many medical diagnostic tests lack either the sensitivity or the specificity, and sometimes both, to detect these crucial biomolecules. In this section, we review the potential of SERS to address this need. SERS combines the specificity of RS with the ability to detect biomolecules present at ultra-low concentrations. Typically, the interaction of the laser with the substrate (which are typically nano-sized metal structures) creates a plasmonic light field; molecules that are adsorbed in or near this enhanced field at the surface of the substrate experience enhanced Raman scattering, thus enhancing the produced Raman signal, as well. This enhancement ideally allows for a much more sensitive detection of biomolecules present within a biological sample. This can result in improved discrimination between two similar biological samples, such as those obtained from healthy and diseased donors. While sounding ideal, the SERS method does have a number of potential drawbacks, including the requirement of close contact between the enhancing surface and the sample, limited reusability of the substrate, and most importantly, potential problems with reproducing the SERS signal from a substrate [115]. Both the benefits and the limitations of the method are crucial to consider when moving toward the goal of creating a successful universal diagnostic method. In this section we discuss recent papers which utilized SERS for detecting various diseases within human biological samples.

4.3.1 Cancer

Bladder Cancer

Jin *et al.* used SERS to study bladder cancer. Here, tissue from individuals with both luminal (n = 24) and basal (n = 26) subtypes of bladder cancer were investigated; using PCA-LDA, the two subtypes were classified with 86% accuracy after CV [116]. In a different paper, non-muscle-invasive and muscle-invasive bladder cancer blood serum samples were compared to healthy controls. In a three-group modeling system, PLS-LDA with LOOCV provided an overall diagnostic accuracy of 93.3%. In two different binary models, the same analysis yielded accuracies of 97.8% and 93.2% for considering healthy controls versus all bladder cancer groups and for differentiating non-muscle-invasive and muscle-invasive bladder cancer, respectively [117]. Blood serum was also analyzed from 23 low- and 25 high-grade bladder cancer patients as well as 40 healthy volunteers using SERS and SVM. The resultant model gave 96.4% and 95.4% accuracy for separating all bladder cancer samples from normal subjects and for discriminating low- and high-grade bladder cancer serum, respectively, after 10-fold CV [118]. The performance results of these reports are comparable to those conducted using spontaneous RS.

Breast Cancer

Breast cancer was investigated using SERS by Moisoiu *et al.* in two separate studies. First, urine from 53 breast cancer patients and 22 healthy controls was studied; a PCA-LDA algorithm, with no validation scheme reported, showed the SERS spectra could be differentiated with 81% sensitivity, 95% specificity, and an overall accuracy of 88%, highlighting the ability of the method to be used as a novel screening strategy for breast cancer with no invasive collection procedure [119]. Following this, serum was collected from 253 donors total with either breast, colorectal, lung, ovarian, or oral cancer and healthy controls. PCA-LDA was again used for analysis, this time with 5-fold CV, giving 98% sensitivity and 91% specificity for distinguishing between cancer patients and controls. When comparing each cancer to healthy controls, SERS spectra from each type were correctly assigned with accuracies of 76% for breast cancer, 88% for oral cancer, 86% for colorectal cancer, 80% for ovarian cancer, and 59% for lung cancer after CV, importantly indicating the potential of the developed method for successfully investigating multiple cancers at the same time [120].

Colorectal Cancer

Králová *et al.* used SERS for studying colorectal cancer via analysis of blood plasma from 15 oncological patients and 15 healthy volunteers. PCA could successfully differentiate between the two groups based on biochemical differences, including those due to tyrosine and adenine [121]. While useful, other studies conducted using spontaneous RS were able to further achieve useful quantitative prediction capabilities for diagnostics.

Gastric Cancer

Investigation of 68 serum samples from gastric cancer patients and healthy controls was conducted by Guo *et al.* Using PCA, biological differences between donors due to nucleic acids, amino acids and carbohydrates were found to be sufficient for separating the two groups [122]. In an alternative study, a detection method based on identifying a modified nucleoside in urine was used for gastric cancer and breast cancer diagnosis. Affinity chromatography was used to purify the modified nucleoside from the cancer patient's urine; SERS spectra of the urinary modified nucleoside were collected from 50 gastric cancer patients, 43 breast cancer patients, and 48 healthy volunteers. PCA-LDA with LOOCV could identify each group in three different binary models with an average sensitivity of 80.9% and specificity of 91.3% [123].

Head and Neck Cancers

NPC was studied by Wu *et al.* via SERS analysis of plasma samples from 40 pre-treatment and post-treatment NPC cases as well as 30 healthy volunteers. Binary PCA-LDA models achieved classification with sensitives of 83.3%, 61.8% and 95.1%, and specificities of 91.2%, 67.4% and 93% for separating pre- and post-treatment samples, post-treatment and normal samples, and pre-treatment and normal samples, respectively, after LOSOCV [124]. Similar results were achieved in a related study using spontaneous RS.

Leukemia

Leukemia cell lines were studied using SERS and SVM with leave-one-batch-out CV. Classification yielded sensitivity, specificity, and accuracy levels greater than 99% for differentiating Jurkat, THP-1, and MONO-MAC-6 leukemia cell lysates [125]. Interestingly, these results are comparable to those achieved in several aforementioned studies which employed spontaneous RS.

Liver Cancer

Liver cancer was exclusively studied using SERS by several different research groups. First, SERS was used to obtain spectra from hepatocellular carcinoma (HCC) tissue; spectra were analyzed using PCA-LDA and LOOCV, giving 93.8% sensitivity and 100% specificity for discriminating between healthy and HCC groups. HCC tissue and adjacent HCC tissue were separated with 79.2% sensitivity and 93.8% specificity [126]. In one large and successful study, serum protein samples were obtained from 104 liver cancer patients and 100 NPC patients as well as 95 healthy volunteers. PLS with SVM could classify the three groups with 95.1% and 90.7% accuracy using training and unknown testing (external validation) datasets, respectively. Further, PLS was found to be a better dimensionality reduction method than PCA [127]. In an even larger combination study, SERS spectra of serum from 304 normal individuals, 333 patients with hepatopathy, and 99 patients with esophageal cancer were studied. OPLS-DA with ROC curve analysis and 10-fold CV could differentiate between the various groups with AUC values all greater than 0.97, indicating excellent classification [128]. Zhang *et al.* studied cancerous and normal liver tissue slices from 56 patients with liver cancer; PCA-LDA was used for classification, giving 100% sensitivity and specificity, each, after ROC curve analysis. No additional validation was reported [129]. Based on the successful results of all reports, the efficacy of SERS for detecting liver cancer is unquestionable.

Lung Cancer

Lung cancer was heavily studied using SERS. Qian *et al.* analyzed saliva samples from 127 healthy and lung cancer patients; SVM and RF were used for generating prediction algorithms. Using SVM with LOOCV, 95.1% sensitivity and 100% specificity was achieved. RF with LOOCV reached 96.7% sensitivity and 100% specificity, indicating both statistical analysis methods were successful for identifying the cancer [130]. Zhang *et al.* used PCA-LDA to interrogate SERS serum spectra of 50 lung cancer donors and 50 healthy controls. With ROC curve analysis, 100% sensitivity and 90% specificity was accomplished [131]. In further research by the same group, tissue slices from a smaller set of donors was studied using PCA-LDA and ROC curve analysis, resulting in 95.7% sensitivity and specificity, each, of the method, comparable to their study performed using serum [132]. Interestingly, validation was not reported in either study. Cao *et al.* developed a serum-based SERS test for diagnosing NSCLC. Here, PCA could distinguish between different types of NSCLC due to intrinsic differences in biochemical composition [133]. NSCLC was also studied in a different project via exosomes from normal and NSCLC cells. The unique peaks of cancerous exosomes were extracted using PCA, allowing for decent separation of the two groups [134]. In a quantitative study by Liu *et al.*, human serum from normal individuals (n = 82) and individuals with lung adenocarcinoma (n = 108) were analyzed using SERS (Figure 4.4).

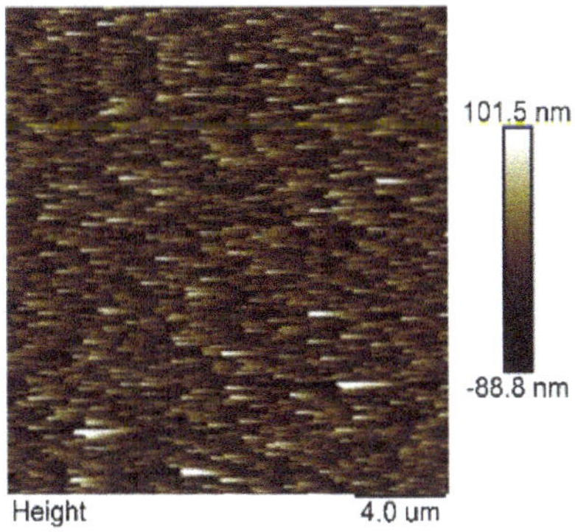

(a)

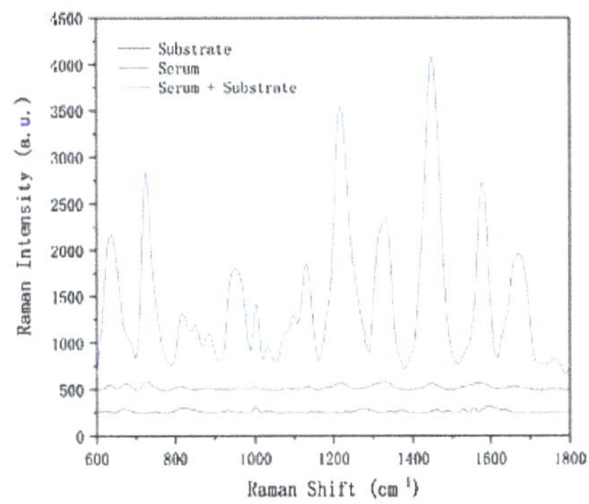

(b)

Figure 4.4. Characterization of Ag nanorods wrapped with Al_2O_3 layer. (a) AFM image of the prepared substrate. (b) Raman spectra of Ag nanorods wrapped with Al_2O_3 layer, serum, and serum with the substrate. Reproduced from Ref. [135] with permission.

OPLS-DA could separate the two groups with 97.6% specificity and 98.1% sensitivity after LOSOCV. Staging lung adenocarcinoma was also successful; accuracies of screening for stage I, stage II, and stage III/IV reached 84.3%, 93.3%, and 86.5%, respectively [135]. Malignant pleural effusion (PE) was studied by the same group via SERS analysis of 83 PE samples, including 32 benign PE and 51 malignant PE. OPLS-DA was again used, providing 92.2% sensitivity and 93.8% specificity for diagnoses based on LOOCV [136]. Although a variety of biological samples were analyzed and machine learning methods were used, the results of SERS analysis for identifying lung cancer are generally comparable to each other, demonstrating extreme strength and utility of the method; nevertheless, several studies which did not report validation require further investigation to verify the true strength of the method.

Oral Cancer

Recently, two different groups investigated the diagnosis of oral cancer using SERS. One group analyzed serum samples from 135 oral SCC patients at various tumor stages and histologic grades; PCA with LDA could accurately detect oral SCC based on tumor size, lymph node metastasis, and histologic grades all with accuracies of detection greater than 85% after LOOCV [137]. In the second smaller study, oral tissue samples from 37 patients were examined. Oral tissues consisting of oral SCC, verrucous carcinoma, premalignant leukoplakia, and disease-free conditions were classified with an accuracy of 97.2% using PCA-DA with CV. Three grades of oral SCC tumors were further classified with 97.8% accuracy, indicating the potential of SERS for use as a point-of-care tool [138]. These two reports are generally more successful than the studies conducted using spontaneous RS.

Ovarian Cancer

Ovarian cancer was exclusively analyzed using SERS technology in recent years. SERS was first used to evaluate the potential of haptoglobin in ovarian cyst fluid as a potential diagnostic biomarker for epithelial ovarian cancers. In comparison with histology, measurements of haptoglobin resulted in 94% sensitivity and 91% specificity of detection after CV. Logistic regression with ROC curve analysis gave an AUC of 0.966 [139]. Zermeño-Nava *et al.* used SERS to determine the sialic acid levels in saliva for the purpose of comparing benign tumor and ovarian cancer patients. ROC curve analysis established a cut-off value of sialic acid (15.5 mg/dL), which yielded 80% sensitivity and 100% specificity for distinguishing between the two cases. No validation was reported [140]. In a comparison study, Paraskevaidi *et al.* used both SERS and spontaneous RS to probe blood plasma samples from 27 patients with ovarian cancer, including 17 early cases, and 28 donors with benign gynecological conditions (Figure 4.5). Analysis of SERS data by SVM with CV could detect ovarian cancer with 87% sensitivity and 89% specificity; early ovarian cancer was identified with 80% sensitivity and 94% specificity. Interestingly, these results were not an improvement compared to spontaneous RS, which could detect ovarian cancer with 94% sensitivity and 96% specificity and early ovarian cancer with 93% sensitivity and 97% specificity [141]. It should be noted that these studies show a wide variety of biological fluids are useful for identifying ovarian cancer with similar levels of success.

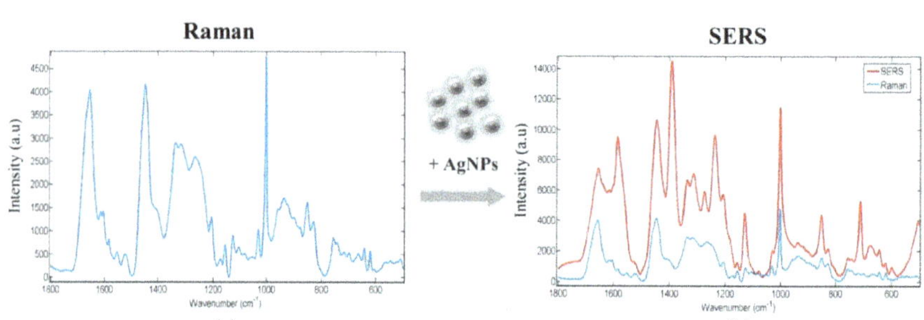

Figure 4.5. Enhancement effect of SERS after the addition of silver nanoparticles (AgNPs) in blood samples. Reproduced from Ref. [141] with permission.

Pancreatic Cancer

Two reports were made on studying pancreatic cancer using SERS. Li *et al.* used ROC curve analysis to show that a migration inhibitor factor SERS-based immunoassay could discriminate between 71 pancreatic cancer patients and 32 healthy individuals as well as distinguish metastasized tumors from metastasis-free tumors, and Tumor Node Metastasis P1–2 stages from the P3 stage with 95.7% discriminatory sensitivity; however, no validation was reported [142]. In the second study, exosomes purified from normal and pancreatic cancer cell lines were studied via SERS and PCA-FDA; the origin of the exosomes could be identified with 90% accuracy after external validation. Interestingly, the cell-line trained model could also differentiate serum-purified exosomes with 87% and 90% accuracy after external validation for healthy control and prostate cancer samples, respectively, depicting the universality of the technique [143].

Prostate Cancer

The last cancer recently studied using SERS was prostate cancer. In one publication, PCA and ROC curve analysis could score the risk of developing prostate cancer through analysis of urine with 87% sensitivity and 90% specificity after external validation and an AUC of 0.84, providing a risk stratification approach to diagnosing prostate cancer [144]. Stefancu *et al.* combined SERS serum spectra with serum prostate-specific antigen levels of prostate cancer and non-malignant pathologies to build a discriminatory algorithm using PCA-LDA. The model yielded 94% accuracy for discriminating between 30 cancerous and 24 control serum samples, though no validation scheme was mentioned [145]. SERS with PCA-LDA was used in a large study to evaluate early biochemical recurrence after radical prostatectomy. 306 preoperative plasma spectra from 102 patients were collected and a comparison was made between those who developed early biochemical recurrence and those who remained biochemical recurrence-free. Using PCA-LDA with LOOCV, the model revealed 65.8% sensitivity, 87.5% specificity, and 79.4% accuracy, suggesting a novel method for predicting early biochemical recurrence in prostate cancer [146].

4.3.2 *Bacterial, Parasitic, and Viral Infections*

Outside of cancer, infections from various sources are commonly studied using SERS. The bacterial infection methicillin-resistant *Staphylococcus aureus* (MRSA) was investigated in comparison to methicillin-sensitive *Staphylococcus aureus* (MSSA); 52 MSSA isolates and 215 MRSA isolates from clinical samples were discriminated by PLS-DA with 10-fold CV, achieving almost 100% diagnostic accuracy, indicating SERS as a potential tool for studying antibiotic resistance [147]. Pérez *et al.* investigated Chagas disease, a parasitic infectious disease, in blood serum samples. A total of 110 samples were collected from healthy donors and infected donors, who were split into asymptomatic and symptomatic groups. PCA and LDA was used for analysis, generating 96.3% accuracy for correctly classifying the samples into one of the three groups after external validation [148]. In a different study, sialic acid levels in saliva among 93 total periodontitis-affected, gingivitis, and control patients were measured using SERS. ROC curve analysis was used to determine the optimum threshold of sialic acid concentration for discrimination; threshold concentrations were found to be 5.98, 7.32, and 17.12 mg/dL for control, gingivitis, and periodontitis patients, respectively, confirming the possibility of SERS as a diagnostic tool for frequent bacteria-causing oral diseases; further validation of the method is necessary [149]. A diagnostic assay for identifying Ebola and malaria was developed using SERS to detect antigens from each within a single blood sample. 190 clinical samples collected from the 2014 West African Ebola outbreak were studied in addition to 163 malaria-positive and 233 negative controls. After ROC curve analysis, Ebola was detected with 90.0% sensitivity and 97.9% specificity and malaria with 100% sensitivity and 99.6% specificity, showcasing SERS as an important tool for outbreak detection in low-resource areas. Again, validation of the method will be required to move it forward [150]. The analysis of various biological samples using SERS is clearly useful for identifying a variety of different infectious diseases, regardless of their origin.

4.3.3 *Kidney and Heart Diseases*

SERS was used in one study to investigate the diagnosis of chronic kidney diseases. SERS spectra were collected from 50 normal and 60 afflicted individuals; PCA with LDA was used for statistical analysis, showing 100% sensitivity and specificity for classification after external validation [151]. In a different study, a prospective diagnostic method for coronary heart disease was investigated using SERS spectra of urine samples. Urine from 87 patients with the disease, including those with percutaneous coronary intervention (PCI) before operation and those without PCI, and 20 healthy controls was measured. PCA-LDA and LOSOCV could correctly classify the SERS spectra with 90% sensitivity and 78.9% specificity, showcasing the ability of the method to detect the disease with minimal invasiveness [152].

4.3.4 *Autoimmune and Neurodegenerative Diseases*

Analysis of the autoimmune disorder Sjogren's syndrome (SjS) was studied by Stefancu *et al.* Here, saliva and blood serum from 21 healthy donors and 29 SjS patients were collected and analyzed using SERS. PCA-LDA models with LOOCV built using each body fluid yielded classification accuracies of 94% for saliva and 98% for serum, suggesting SERS analysis as a potential novel point-of-care diagnostic method [153]. The neurodegenerative disorder, amyotrophic lateral sclerosis (ALS), was explored via SERS analysis of blood plasma from 138 sporadic ALS cases (Figure 4.6). PCA, ROC curve, and CV analysis showed spectral differences between the short-duration group and long-duration group of sporadic ALS cases, which could be classified with an AUC of 0.972 [154].

Two studies were published which used SERS for diagnosing AD. The first study focused on optimizing a protocol for analyzing blood serum of AD and healthy control donors. PCA and LDA were used for statistical analysis; LOOCV gave diagnostic accuracy, precision, and specificity values of 83%, 86%, and 86%. A direct comparison of the SERS spectra was made to hippocampus degeneration, indicating a promising potential instrument for monitoring AD progression [155]. Ryzhikova *et al.* also used SERS for studying blood serum, here of 48 AD, healthy controls, and donors with other forms of dementia. ANN achieved diagnostic accuracies of 96% for differentiating AD and healthy controls and 98% for identifying AD, healthy control, and donors with other forms of dementia in a tertiary model after external validation [156].

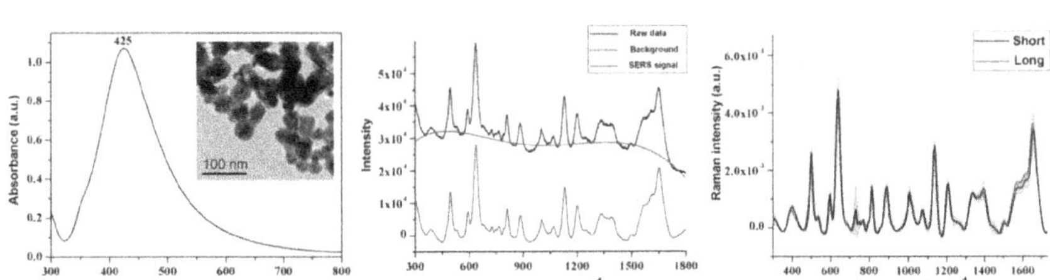

(a) (b) (c)

Figure 4.6. The spectral characteristics of blood plasma analyzed using SERS. (a) The UV/visible absorption curve and micrograph of silver colloid obtained using an electron microscope. The absorption maximum is located at 425 nm. (b) Typical raw spectra and the effect of autofluorescence subtraction applied during SERS data preprocessing. (c) Comparison of the mean spectrum of the short-duration group (black line, n = 62) vs that of the long-duration group (red line, n = 76). The shaded areas represent the standard deviations of the means. Reproduced from Ref. [154] with permission.

Interestingly, these results are comparable to those which were achieved using spontaneous RS for AD detection.

4.3.5 *Other Diseases*

An assortment of other diseases has additionally been studied using SERS analysis of various biological samples. Kim *et al.* used SERS to investigate amniotic fluids of individuals with subclinical intra-amniotic infection and preterm delivery; these prenatal diseases could be identified using PCA-SVM with greater than 92% clinical sensitivity and specificity; unfortunately, no validation was reported [157]. Knee osteoarthritis was studied via SERS analysis of synovial fluid combined with PCA-LDA and LOSOCV. The classification algorithm provided a diagnostic accuracy of 91% for distinguishing between low-grade and high-grade osteoarthritis. Resonant RS data was also collected from the same samples, reaching a diagnostic accuracy of 74%. Interestingly, combining the two sets of spectral data gave a classification accuracy of 100% [158]. SERS spectra of saliva from 26 children with asthma and 18 healthy children was investigated using PCA-LDA with LOOCV; the method resulted in a sensitivity of 85%, specificity of 82%, and accuracy of 84% for separating asthmatic saliva from control saliva [159]. Lin *et al.* performed research on type II diabetes using SERS of blood plasma from 35 diabetic and 45 healthy individuals. PCA and LDA could identify diabetic SERS spectra with a specificity of 100% and sensitivity of 80% during external validation. ROC curve analysis showed an optimal AUC of 1.00 [160], which is comparable to the study performed using spontaneous RS. Lastly, causative pathogens for the two most common sexually transmitted diseases, *Chlamydia trahomatis* (elementary bodies) and *Neisseria gonorrheoae*, were studied. SERS signatures were collected *in vitro* for both and showed obvious differences between the two. PLS-DA could discriminate SERS spectra of *Chlamydia trahomatis* from spectra of avidin and human serum albumin proteins with 99%/97% sensitivity and 98%/96% specificity for Au/Ag substrates after CV [161].

Using SERS for examining a wide variety of diseases is shown here to be just as successful, if not more so in some cases, than the previously reviewed spontaneous RS studies. While more time is required to prepare the substrates used in SERS analysis, the potential of the method for achieving positive results with greater sensitivity is apparent. It is necessary to contemplate both the benefits and the limitations of the technique as effort is made toward achieving a singular universal diagnostic method based on RS.

4.4 Other Variations of Raman Spectroscopy

While SERS and spontaneous RS account for the majority of the research articles written in the past few years, there still remain other variations of RS which were used for the similar purpose of developing novel medical diagnostic methods. These techniques are briefly described herein and are organized by the specific approach used.

4.4.1 *Deep-Ultraviolet Raman Spectroscopy*

Deep-ultraviolet Raman spectroscopy (DUVRS) was used in two recent studies. DUVRS utilizes an excitation wavelength in the deep ultraviolet range of light, which increases the inelastic scattering produced by biological samples composed of aromatic amino acids and nucleic acids due to their absorption of light in the same range. Generally, less fluorescence interference is also known to occur at wavelengths shorter than 250 nm, thus resulting in a Raman spectrum with an improved signal-to-noise ratio.

In one study, DUVRS was used to investigate the spores of eight different fungal species implicated in respiratory diseases. PCA-LDA generated classification models built at the genus, species, and strain levels. After leave-one-batch-out CV, an accuracy of 97.5% at the genus level was achieved, the four different *Aspergillus* species were classified with 100% accuracy, and the three different *Aspergillus fumigatus* strains were classified with 89.4% accuracy, demonstrating DUVRS as an innovative approach for fast identification of fungal spores related to respiratory diseases [162]. Ralbovsky *et al.* similarly used DUVRS for diagnostic purposes, showing in a proof-of-concept study that both cancerous and control brain tissue and normal and cancerous prostate cells could be easily discriminated, setting the stage for a quantitative study to be performed in the future [163].

4.4.2 *Raman Spectroscopy Combined with Optical Tweezers*

The combination of RS with optical tweezers is a powerful tool used for characterizing and evaluating cells in a non-invasive and sterile way. The cells are captured by optical force, preventing random motion. Further, the laser tweezer RS (LTRS) system can collect Raman spectra from single living cells without interference from substrates or their liquid environment.

LTRS was used by Liu *et al.* to examine colon cancer cells with single-base mutations in the KRAS gene. The different cell lines include DKS-8 (KRAS wild-type (WT)), DLD-1 (KRAS mutant-type (MT)), HKE-3 (KRAS WT), and HCT-116 (KRAS MT). When using PCA-LDA statistical analysis, DKS-8 and DLD 1 cells were classified with 97.5% accuracy, HKE 3 and HCT 116 cells were classified with 97% accuracy, and classification efficiency of WT versus MT cells reached 81.2%. Although no validation was reported, these results are comparable to similar studies which used spontaneous RS and SERS, thus providing promising results for further development of a successful detection method for circulating tumor cells in a liquid biopsy [164]. Extracellular vesicles (EV) released by mammalian cells was explored in a different paper as a potential prostate cancer biomarker. LTRS was used to collect the Raman signatures of four different samples which consisted of RBC- and platelet-derived EVs of healthy and prostate cancer cell lines (Figure 4.7). PCA could easily separate and classify the groups, setting the stage for future work to use EVs for monitoring prostate cancer [165].

RBCs were explored to identify β-thalassemia, an inherited blood disorder, using a LTRS system. Raman spectra of RBCs from 33 patients with β-thalassemia-major, 49 with β-thalassemia-minor, and 65 healthy controls were collected. Once again, it was found that PCA could successfully distinguish between RBCs of β-thalassemia-major patients and healthy controls. Further improvement to the recognition of β-thalassemia-minor is required [166]. In a final study utilizing LTRS, RBCs were again analyzed, this time for detecting type II diabetes. An algorithm built using PCA-LDA could differentiate between RBCs of healthy donors and those with diabetes with 100% sensitivity and 90% specificity after external validation [167],

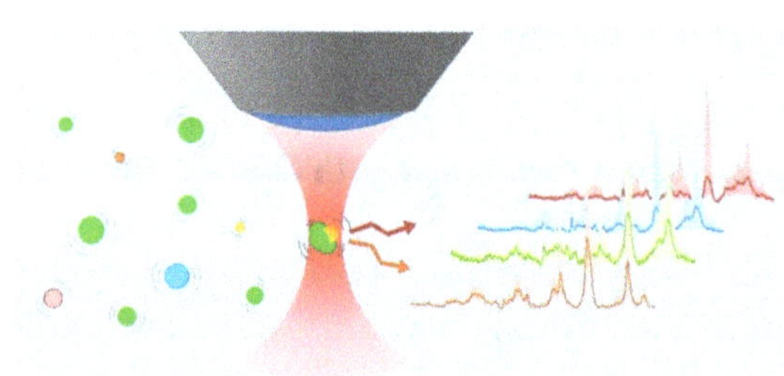

Figure 4.7. Schematic depiction of Raman optical tweezer system used to obtain the Raman signatures of four different extracellular vesicle samples. Reproduced from Ref. [165] with permission.

which is similar to results obtained using both spontaneous RS and SERS for identifying type II diabetes. The LTRS system provides a great capacity for studying cells for diagnostic purposes, but it should be noted that it does not apply for studying other biological samples, thus making it difficult for universal medical diagnostics.

4.4.3 *Shifted-Excitation Raman Difference Spectroscopy and Dual Excitation Raman Spectroscopy*

Shifted-excitation Raman difference spectroscopy (SERDS) was used in one study to classify eight breast tissue samples as healthy, fibroadenoma, or invasive carcinoma. SERDS involves the collection of spectra using two slightly different excitation wavelengths; when the difference of the two spectra is taken, the contribution of fluorescence is ideally removed, resulting in better interpretability of the obtained spectra. Here, the excitation wavelengths used were 784 nm and 785 nm. The differences in spectra were examined using PCA and LDA, which gave excellent classification after LOOCV. Specifically, invasive breast carcinoma and the absence of it were identified with 99.2% and 90.4% sensitivity and specificity, respectively. Tumor tissue in tumor-containing tissue could be recognized with 100% sensitivity and the absence of tumor in the no-tumor containing tissue was recognized with 100% specificity. This study shows SERDS has a strong potential for supporting histopathological diagnoses of various breast pathologies, with results comparable to those obtained using spontaneous RS.

Two different studies employed dual excitation RS for the identification of prostate cancer in biological samples. Pinto *et al.* utilized a dual-wavelength laser source (680 nm and 785 nm excitation) for collecting spectra from 20 whole prostates following prostatectomy. Dual excitation captures both the fingerprint and the high wavenumber region of Raman spectral data at the same time. The obtained spectral data from the prostate and the extra prostatic tissue were distinguished with 91% accuracy, 90.5% sensitivity, and 96% specificity after ROC curve analysis with external validation. *In vivo* spectra were also collected from four patients, showing similarities to the spectra collected *ex vivo*, indicating the potential for future expansion of the work [169]. In a second study, dual-wavelength RS (671 nm and 785 nm excitation) was used to collect data simultaneously from fingerprint and high wavenumber Raman spectra. 18 prostate slices obtained post-prostatectomy were analyzed; SVM with LOOCV and ROC curve analysis could differentiate between normal and cancerous spectra with an AUC of 0.91 when data from both excitation wavelengths were combined, which was an improvement upon results obtained from each considered separately [170]. Interestingly, these methods show great potential for studying two different types of cancer with similar levels of success as those obtained by means of more well-used variations of RS; supplementary research would be necessary to understand any further benefit of the methods toward investigating other diseases.

4.4.4 *Fiber-Optic Probes and Handheld Instruments*

Raman spectroscopic systems which employ the use of fiber-optic probes are beginning to gain popularity for medical diagnostic studies. The use of probe systems is a transition to the ultimate goal of reaching *in vivo* detection of various maladies. Typically, the system consists of the laser source, the handheld fiber-optic Raman probe itself, a compact spectrometer, and a detector. The entire system is small, portable, and easy to use within clinical settings. The fiber-optic probes are less expensive than benchtop Raman spectrometers, take up less space and, most importantly, can be used intraoperatively, preventing the need for any additional testing or surgeries to obtain biological samples. The analysis time is short but still sufficient for capturing useful biochemical information about a sample.

Fiber-optic probes have been employed in a variety of research endeavors for medical diagnostic purposes. In two different studies, Chen *et al.* investigated their use for identifying bladder cancer. First, a low-resolution fiber-optic Raman sensing system (Figure 4.8) was used to evaluate a total of

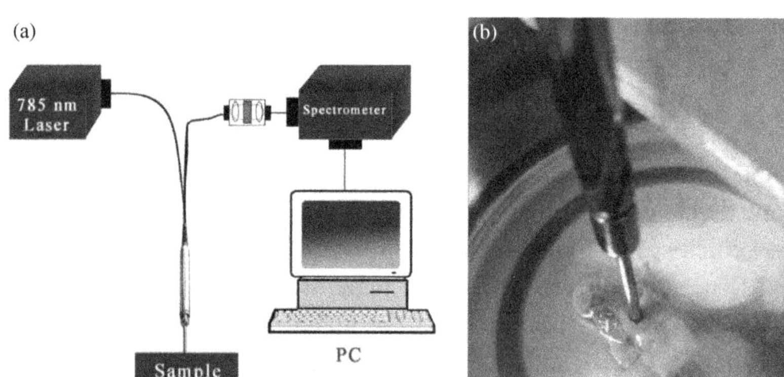

Figure 4.8. (a) The low-resolution fiber-optic Raman sensing system used in this study (an additional long-pass filter stage is added before the collected signal goes into the spectrometer); (b) probe placement during measurement. Reproduced from Ref. [171] with permission.

32 different *ex vivo* bladder specimens which were considered either normal bladder tissues, low-grade bladder tumors, or high-grade bladder tumors. PCA-ANN with CV successfully discriminated the groups with an overall accuracy of 93.1% and an average sensitivity and specificity of 91.3% and 97.3%, respectively [171]. In a follow-up study, a variety of experimental conditions as well as chemometric techniques were considered for optimizing the method for clinical applications. Here, spectral data were collected from 42 bladder tissue specimens from 10 patients who were either healthy or had high- or low-grade bladder cancer. It was found that increasing the integration time had the greatest improvement on prediction accuracy. The best results were obtained using PCA-ANN with a laser power of 150 mW and integration time of five seconds; the overall accuracy of the tertiary classification system under these parameters was 95.4% with an average sensitivity of 94.9% and specificity of 97.6% after CV [172]. This study further confirms the ability of the low-resolution Raman fiber-optic system for identifying bladder cancer pathologies with similar, if not better, levels of success as SERS and spontaneous RS.

Li *et al.* used their own fiber-optic RS system to collect data from 16 breast tissue samples from healthy controls and individuals with breast cancer. A novel algorithm of entropy-weighted local-hyperplane KNN was used for identifying spectra, yielding 92.3% accuracy, 93.8% sensitivity, and 87.8% specificity during randomized grouping CV. These results were an improvement over KNN alone as well as the adaptive weighted k-local hyperplane algorithm [173].

A custom-made microprobe was used for collecting *in vivo* Raman spectra from 13 cancerous and 17 healthy lung tissues for the detection of lung cancer. A novel variational classifier based on SVM with hierarchical CV yielded 93% accuracy for differentiation between the samples [174].

NPC was also studied via fiber-optic RS. In one study, *in vivo* fingerprint and high wavenumber region spectra were collected from 14 NPC patients and 48 healthy subjects during nasopharyngeal endoscopic examinations. GA-PLS-LDA was used for classifying the spectra; after LOSOCV, the algorithm achieved 98.2% diagnostic accuracy, 93.3% sensitivity, and 100% specificity. The research suggests a strong potential for the fiber-optic system to improve real-time *in vivo* detection of NPC over other methods such as SERS [175]. In a slightly alternative approach, Desroches *et al.* investigated the high wavenumber region of Raman spectral data using a core needle biopsy probe system for detection of human dense cancer of brain tissue *in situ* during surgery. The method achieved 80% sensitivity and 90% specificity using SVM with LOOCV [176].

Prostate cancer was investigated using a handheld contact RS probe system. Here, 32 post-prostatectomy specimens were analyzed; spectra were collected from areas characterized by tissue type (extraprostatic or prostatic), tissue malignancy (benign or malignant), cancer grade (grade groups I–V), and tissue glandular level. Neural networks with LOOCV and ROC curve analysis were used for determining the diagnostic abilities of the RS method. Extraprostatic and prostatic tissue were distinguished with 82% sensitivity and 83% specificity; benign and malignant tissue with 87% sensitivity and 86% specificity; and benign versus each grade group were compared in several binary models, achieving an average sensitivity of 81.8% and specificity of 85.2%, demonstrating the potential of the method for allowing RS studies to move into clinical settings for identifying prostate cancer [177]. The same group of researchers showed in a previous study that they could also use their handheld contact probe for accomplishing *in vivo* detection of cancer cells within the brain. Using the probe, normal brain, dense cancer, and normal brain invaded by cancer cells were differentiated with 93% sensitivity and 91% specificity using a boosted trees algorithm with CV [178].

Feng *et al.* investigated the use of a fiber-optic RS system for identifying biophysical markers for skin cancer diagnosis. An inverse biophysical skin cancer model was developed to better understand the biophysical changes which occur and allow for diagnoses. Spectra were collected *in vivo* from 65 patients who were diagnosed with either malignant melanoma, dysplastic nevi, BCC, SCC, or actinic keratosis. A logistic regression model with LOSOCV identified diagnostically relevant model components. Interestingly, the biophysical model could capture the diagnostic power of the previously developed statistical classification model while additionally providing information about the skin's biophysical composition [179]. In a different study, a non-classical logic called paraconsistent logic was used to differentiate between various cutaneous tissue samples analyzed by RS. Spectra from four histopathological groups, including 115 spectra of BCC, 21 of SCC, 57 of actinic keratosis, and 30 of normal skin were collected. The normal skin group was compared to the group of non-melanoma cancer lesions (BCC+SCC) and the actinic keratosis tumor lesion; the paraconsistent algorithm achieved 75.8% efficiency after CV, which was superior to the classification system built using PCA-DA [180].

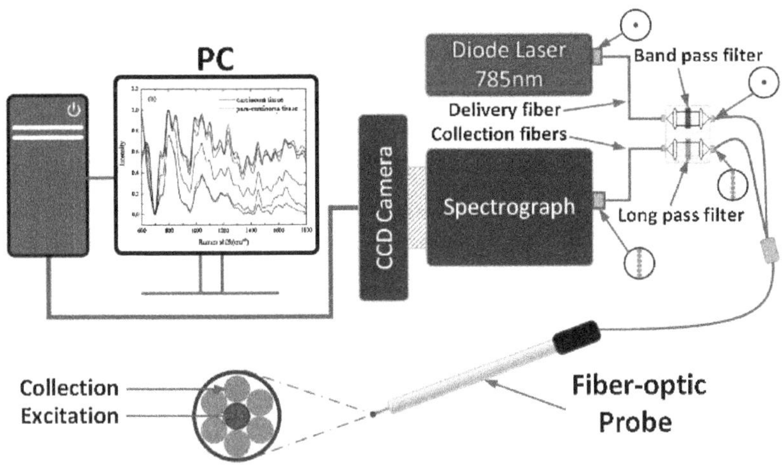

Figure 4.9. Schematic description of fiber-optic Raman spectroscopy system. Reproduced from Ref. [181] with permission.

Two different articles focused on investigating tongue SCC using fiber-optic RS. Yu *et al.* collected spectral data from tumorous and non-tumorous tissue of 12 patients who had undergone a surgical resection due to tongue SCC (Figure 4.9). Deep CNN could classify the data with 99.3% sensitivity and 94.4% specificity after 5-fold CV [181]. Similarly, Yan *et al.* also used CNN to discriminate tongue SCC from non-tumorous tissue. Here, the model yielded 99.1% sensitivity and 95.4% specificity; despite no validation reported, the study indicates the strong potential of CNN with fiber-optic RS to evaluate tongue SCC intraoperatively [182]. Interestingly, tongue cancer was not studied using other variations of RS, suggesting the advantage of fiber-optic RS probes for studying a less frequently examined cancer.

Handheld Raman spectrometers were likewise investigated for a variety of diagnostic purposes. Handheld spectrometers, while similarly advantageous to probes, have different features. The handheld instruments can also make *in vivo* diagnoses, are smaller and less cumbersome than a desktop instrument, and are less expensive. Handheld Raman spectrometers function more under the idea of "point-and-shoot", making them incredibly user-friendly and plausible for both clinical and at-home measurements. While the handheld instrument is much smaller and more cost-effective than a benchtop instrument, the resolution is not always comparable. However, the continuous improvement of these instruments and their specifications has allowed for some recent successful studies.

Guevara *et al.* used a handheld Raman spectrometer for investigating type II diabetes. Here, *in vivo* spectra were collected from afflicted individuals and healthy controls from four different sites (ear lobe, inner arm, thumbnail, and median cubital vein). ANN with CV could discriminate between the groups with 88.9–90.9% accuracy. PCA with SVM with CV did not perform as well, achieving only 76–82.5% diagnostic accuracy. With the success of the ANN algorithm, the method showed to be a promising tool for non-invasive and automated detection of type II diabetes [183].

A portable and cost-effective spectroscopic system (Figure 4.10) was employed by Khristoforova *et al.* to study skin cancer. Skin tumors including malignant melanoma, BCC and various benign neoplasms were studied *in vivo*; in addition, autofluorescence spectra were also collected. PLS-DA analysis with LOOCV of both Raman and autofluorescence spectra gave specificity and sensitivity levels between 78.9% and 100% for identifying the various pathologies [184].

Cancerous and non-cancerous tissues from 12 patients undergoing surgery for colorectal cancer were analyzed using a handheld RS system. PCA and

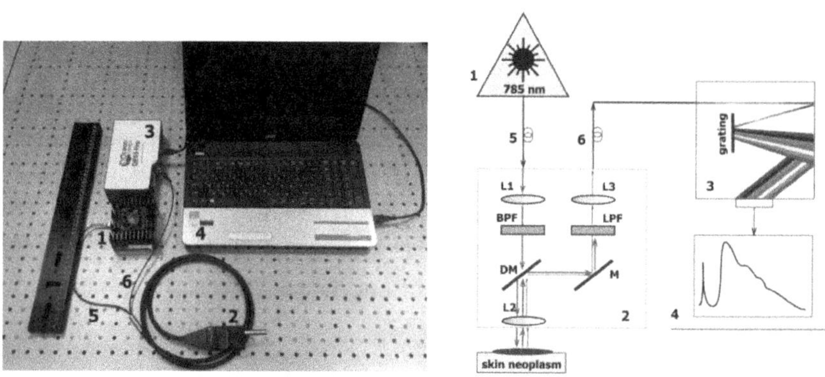

(a) (b)

Figure 4.10. Details of the portable Raman system: (a) photo, (b) experimental scheme. 1 — laser module, 2 — optical Raman probe, 3 — spectrometer, 4 — PC, 5 — excitation fiber, 6 — collection fiber; 785 nm laser radiation is delivered to the optical detector by excitation fibers 5 (100 μm diameter, 0.22 NA) and collimating lens L1, passes through the bandpass filter (BPF) to cut off unwanted fluorescence and Raman signal generated inside the optical fiber. The dichroic mirror (DM) transmits laser radiation to lens L2, which focuses exciting radiation onto the sample. The same lens L2 collects Raman, autofluorescence, and backscattered radiation. DM and mirror (M) transmit collected radiation on longpass filter (LPF) to cut off exciting laser radiation. The scattered radiation transmits to multichannel spectrograph by matching lens L3, and collection fibers 6 (200 μm diameter, 0.22 NA). Reproduced from Ref. [184] with permission.

LDA resulted in 87.5% sensitivity, 82.6% specificity, and 85.1% accuracy for discrimination. Early cancer and advanced cancer tissue samples could also be differentiated with 85.7% sensitivity, 83.3% specificity, and 85.4% accuracy [185]. A final study performed using a handheld instrument involved analysis of tissue samples from 20 patients who underwent surgery for colorectal cancer. PCA with ROC curve analysis could identify colorectal cancer with 85.1% accuracy [186]. Validation was not reported in either study. However, while only few diseases were recently explored using handheld RS instruments, the potential they hold is limitless and deserves further exploration in the future.

4.4.5 *Other Variations of Raman Spectroscopy*

In addition to the aforementioned variations of RS, there remain several others which were used recently in only a very few number of studies. For example, coherent anti-Stokes Raman scattering (CARS) was used for the fast and non-invasive diagnosis of cervical cancer. CARS utilizes multiple photons to produce a coherent effect, thus producing a stronger anti-Stokes Raman signal. In addition to CARS, second-harmonic generation/two-photon fluorescence (SHG/TPF) imaging was performed on Pap smears from patients with specimens negative for intraepithelial lesions or malignancy and low-grade and high-grade squamous intraepithelial lesions. Deep CNNs were trained with CARS, SHG/TPR, and Raman imaging independently. Each method could most advantageously categorize the normal and cancerous Pap smears with 100% accuracy after LOSOCV [187].

An alternative approach was used for studying colorectal cancer based on a high-throughput RS system. The high-throughput analysis of blood serum from 30 cancer patients and 30 healthy controls combined with PLS-DA gave a diagnostic sensitivity and specificity of 83% each after CV for classifying colorectal cancer [188]. These results are not necessarily an improvement on other studies but do importantly allow for many samples to be probed quickly, saving time and effort for generating diagnoses.

Finally, short-wave infrared (SWIR) dispersive RS was used for differentiating normal and malignant renal samples. SWIR RS dramatically reduces background fluorescence in specific bulk tissue specimens. A sparse multinomial logistic regression with ROC curve analysis achieved 95.8%

sensitivity and 88.8% specificity for diagnosis after LOSOCV, indicating the advantages of SWIR RS for detecting the renal malignancies [189].

Many different variations of RS have been employed for reaching the same goal of successful medical diagnostic applications. While some systems perform better than others, it remains that the most successful results tend to be achieved with spontaneous RS. This is an interesting observation, as it indicates that the more complicated and laborious Raman spectroscopic set-ups are not necessary for achieving better and more accurate screening and diagnostic results.

4.5 Critical Evaluation

Many of the accomplishments made recently represent minor, but important, victories for the field of medical diagnostics. Numerous research articles capitalize on basic chemometric methods to address complicated issues in small, proof-of-concept studies. Despite the lack of complexity, some of the most successful work were done using these basic methods. Importantly, these experiments are crucial for laying the groundwork from which researchers can build upon before spending costly time and resources to investigate larger *in vivo* applications of the method. Furthermore, as the method continues to develop, the variety of diseases which are examined continuously expand, opening new doors for future research. Within the last few years alone, a vast amount of research has been conducted which capitalizes on the advantages of RS and machine learning for screening and diagnosing a wide assortment of ailments and diseases. It is clear the method of RS itself is incredibly advantageous for being a diagnostic tool. It is specific, objective, inexpensive and easy to use, and can be sensitive and non-invasive. The aforementioned summarized articles aim to support the conclusion that RS has extreme potential to be used in clinical settings for real-time accurate and definitive universal medical diagnostics.

However, it is important to acknowledge the pitfalls as well as the advantages of the herein described studies. Firstly, some use a very small sample pool; while this by itself is a non-issue, larger, statistically significant, trials are absolutely necessary to perform so that scientists can fully evaluate the method and its reliability. Those studies which do not provide quantitative results, and instead are qualitative in nature (e.g., utilize unsupervised machine learning methods), require further validation to ensure that objective results and diagnoses can be achieved, instead of subjective results based on clustering of data.

Along that line, not all studies reported validation of the machine learning methods. That is, data of samples from donors which were not used to build the statistical algorithms were not consistently used to then test the performance of the model. This validation, referred to as external validation, is absolutely crucial for establishing the trustworthiness of a statistical method. External validation functions to ensure there are no other factors which may be influencing differentiation. In fact, successful external validation is an indication that unlabeled spectra can accurately be predicted as belonging to a class based on the spectral changes that result from differences in disease state alone, thus indicating that the method will not be affected by other biological factors. Successful external validation further indicates that the developed method does not suffer from being over-fit to the data used to build it, and suggests the model is not biased and can be deemed both statistically and realistically ready for use in clinical settings. However, external validation cannot always be easily performed. Additional samples (from new donors) are required for this validation step; these additional samples may not be easily attainable due to problems with funding, donor participation, and/or lack of collaboration. These can prevent researchers from performing this crucial step, leading to potentially overestimating the capability of the method. This is an area of major concern which needs to be addressed in future progression of this line of work, as it is vital to apply unseen data to the prediction models to determine whether they perform adequately.

Lastly, the majority of the studies discussed herein are considered *ex vivo* experiments. To bring this work into clinical settings, additional progress toward *in vivo* research is absolutely crucial. The overarching goal is to apply the method directly into medical settings; it is thus necessary to continue advancing the research using fiber-optic probes and handheld instruments which are better equipped for *in vivo* analysis but which have not been used to investigate all illnesses.

A summary of the types of diseases analyzed, the validation used, and whether the study was performed *in vivo* or *ex vivo* for cancer and all other diseases is provided in Tables 4.2 and 4.3, respectively.

Table 4.2. Summary of types of studies related to diagnosing cancer using RS and chemometrics since 2018.

Type of Cancer	# of Studies	# of *in vivo* vs. *ex vivo*	Validation Used
Bladder	6	*ex vivo* — 6	Cross-validation — 6
Brain	8	*ex vivo* — 6 *in situ* — 1 *in vivo* — 1	Cross-validation — 4 NVR — 4
Breast	12	*ex vivo* — 12	Cross-validation — 9 External Validation — 2 NVR — 1
Cervical	5	*ex vivo* — 5	Cross-validation — 4 External Validation — 1
Colorectal	6	*ex vivo* — 6	Cross-validation — 2 NVR — 4
Esophageal	1	*ex vivo* — 1	External Validation — 1
Gastric	3	*ex vivo* — 3	Cross-validation — 2 NVR — 1
Head and Neck	5	*ex vivo* — 4 *in vivo* — 1	Cross-validation — 4 NVR — 1
Leukemia	4	*ex vivo* — 4	Cross-validation — 3 NVR — 1
Liver	4	*ex vivo* — 4	Cross-validation — 2 External Validation — 1 NVR — 1
Lung	11	*ex vivo* — 10 *in vivo* — 1	Cross-validation — 6 NVR — 5
Lymphatic	2	*ex vivo* — 2	External Validation — 1 NVR — 1
Oral	7	*ex vivo* — 7	Cross-validation — 6 External Validation — 1
Ovarian	3	*ex vivo* — 3	Cross-validation — 2 NVR — 1
Pancreatic	2	*ex vivo* — 2	External Validation — 1 NVR — 1
Prostate	8	*ex vivo* — 8	Cross-validation — 4 External Validation — 2 NVR — 2
Renal	1	*ex vivo* — 1	Cross-validation — 1

(*Continued*)

Table 4.2. (*Continued*)

Type of Cancer	# of Studies	# of *in vivo* vs. *ex vivo*	Validation Used
Skin	6	*ex vivo* — 3 *in vivo* — 3	Cross-validation — 4 External Validation — 1 NVR — 1
Thyroid	4	*ex vivo* — 4	Cross-validation — 3 NVR — 1
Tongue	2	*ex vivo* — 2	Cross-validation — 1 NVR — 1
p53 biomarker	1	*ex vivo* — 1	Cross-validation — 1

*NVR = no validation reported.

Table 4.3. Summary of types of studies related to diagnosing all other diseases using RS and chemometrics since 2018.

Disease Category	# of Studies	# of *in vivo* vs. *ex vivo*	Validation Used
Bacterial and Fungal Infections	6	*ex vivo* — 5 *in vitro* — 1	Cross-validation — 4 External Validation — 1 NVR — 1
Parasitic Infections	1	*ex vivo* — 1	External Validation — 1
Viral Infections	8	*ex vivo* — 8	Cross-validation — 4 External Validation — 2 NVR — 2
Blood Disorders	2	*ex vivo* — 2	Cross-validation — 1 NVR — 1
Diabetes	4	*ex vivo* — 3 *in vivo* — 1	Cross-validation — 2 External Validation — 2
Kidney Diseases and related	3	*ex vivo* — 3	Cross-validation — 1 External Validation — 2
Heart Diseases and related	2	*ex vivo* — 2	Cross-validation — 2
Thyroid Diseases and related	3	*ex vivo* — 3	External Validation — 3
Autoimmune Diseases	3	*ex vivo* — 3	Cross-validation — 1 External Validation — 2
Neurodegenerative Diseases	7	*ex vivo* — 7	Cross-validation — 4 External Validation — 3
Ochronosis	1	*ex vivo* — 1	NVR — 1
Ocular Diseases	1	*ex vivo* — 1	External Validation — 1
Osteoarthritis	1	*ex vivo* — 1	Cross-validation — 1

Table 4.3. (*Continued*)

Disease Category	# of Studies	# of *in vivo* vs. *ex vivo*	Validation Used
Endometriosis	1	*ex vivo* — 1	External Validation — 1
Prenatal Diseases	1	*ex vivo* — 1	NVR — 1
Respiratory Diseases and related	3	*ex vivo* — 3	Cross-validation — 2 External Validation — 1
Sexually Transmitted Diseases	1	*in vitro* — 1	Cross-validation — 1
Ulcerative Colitis	1	*ex vivo* — 1	Cross-validation — 1

*NVR = no validation reported

While not all studies are perfect, there are many which demonstrate ideal scenarios. The epitome of a successful study would be one in which a statistically significant number of donors is analyzed, and optimal performance of the model is achieved during both CV and external validation steps. Several studies reviewed here satisfy these requirements and are considered reliable, and the potential exists for further expansion on those studies which need it.

It is interesting to note the prediction performance results of studies which were accomplished using data from spontaneous RS versus SERS or other variations of RS. In most cases, the performance results of the machine learning models are comparable; some studies performed using SERS or other forms of RS achieve better results than those performed using spontaneous RS, although only marginally. It can thus be hypothesized that spontaneous RS is sufficient for achieving just as successful results, and the complicated and sometimes time-consuming set-ups and procedures involved in other variations of RS are not necessary for generating accurate diagnoses. However, it should still be noted that there are some situations where it is suggested that spontaneous RS is not optimally suitable, such as for conducting deep tissue analysis. In this scenario, spatially offset Raman spectroscopy (SORS) is a preferred method. While research has progressed significantly using SORS, a combination of the method with chemometrics has seldom been recently reported. For more information on SORS, the reader is referred to external works [190–192]. Further, CARS can be seen as a preferred alternative method due to the lack of fluorescence interference, allowing for measurements to be made more rapidly as compared to spontaneous RS. Unfortunately, this is another method which is rarely used by scientists due to its more complicated and time-consuming nature, as illustrated by only one publication which used CARS for medical diagnostics in the last few years.

With that being said, the application of devices such as fiber-optic probes and handheld instruments are areas which require further exploration. To one day bring the technology into clinical settings, smaller, portable RS instruments are required. Those studies reported in this review which utilize probes and handheld instruments, while successful, require their own further expansion and improvement. Interestingly, probes and portable instruments have already found themselves at the patients' bedside, as is evident from the aforementioned studies and as reviewed by others [193, 194]. As these technologies continue to advance, additional research may be accomplished to support the introduction of these methods to clinical settings.

Two remaining challenges exist for establishing RS within medical settings for screening and diagnostic purposes. First is the need to standardize the instrument across all users, which includes developing regulations regarding factors such as laser power and excitation wavelength, which instruments to use, and the parameters needed to analyze the data. Additionally, a unification of machine learning analysis will be required. To make the method as simple as possible, it would be ideal to consolidate the techniques which are employed for making classification decisions. An automatic and user-friendly system will be the most useful for high-throughput, rapid, and accurate diagnoses.

The second, and equally important, issue is the need to bridge the gap in trust between medical professionals and analytical chemists and, specifically, spectroscopists. It is vital for the medical community to understand the Raman methodology and its dramatic advantages to begin to trust the process and allow for it to make life-altering diagnoses. This will only happen if increasingly more scientists continue to advance the field forward, spreading the word at conferences and professional meetings, and encouraging collaborations with those in the medical community. It is expected that by sharing information, the medical community may learn more about this technique and be encouraged to practice it in their own settings. Further, large-scale multi-center trials between spectroscopists and medical communities will need to occur to demonstrate the feasibility of the method for full-time clinical introduction. If these prove successful, the pathway toward revolutionizing medical diagnostics becomes clear.

Both of these issues will require tremendous collaboration and willingness of experts in both fields to accomplish; ideally, the potential of the Raman method and its ability to transform the field of medical diagnostics will be enough to encourage those brilliant minds to take on such a grueling, but rewarding, task. Several prominent researchers delve further into the considerations required for translating RS into clinical settings [8, 18, 21, 31, 195, 196]. Although there is much work to be done, it remains that RS in combination with machine learning methods has shown incredible potential to be used as a novel universal screening and disease detection method which is non-invasive, objective, accurate and definitive.

4.6 Conclusions

Receiving a medical diagnosis for a condition an individual has should be a simple, definitive, and straightforward process. Unfortunately, for many people around the world, a diagnosis is either impossible to make due to insufficient diagnostic tests or resources, unreliability of the diagnostic test, or inability to generate a diagnosis until a disease has progressed too far. Raman spectroscopy in combination with machine learning techniques is proposed here as a universal method for medical diagnostics which is fast, accurate, objective, and definitive. The method itself is inherently non-invasive, easy to use, and has the potential to easily be implemented into clinical settings. This review highlights momentous works which have primarily been conducted between 2018 and 2020 by researchers around the world who have utilized Raman spectroscopy for screening and diagnosing a wide range of ailments and diseases. Although there remains room for improvement and hurdles to overcome before bringing the method into clinical settings, there is a great and promising potential for Raman spectroscopy in combination with chemometrics to become the first universal method for medical diagnostics.

References

1. Lussier, F., Thibault, V., Charron, B., Wallace, G. Q. and Masson, J.-F. (2020) Deep learning and artificial intelligence methods for Raman and surface-enhanced Raman scattering. Trends in Analytical Chemistry **124**, 115796.
2. Fikiet, M. A., Khandasammy, S. R., Mistek, E., Ahmed, Y., Halámková, L., Bueno, J. and Lednev, I. K. (2018) Surface-enhanced Raman spectroscopy: A review of recent applications in forensic science. Spectrochimica Acta Part A: Molecular and Biomolecular Spectroscopy **197**, 255–260.
3. Mazivila, S. J. and Olivieri, A. C. (2018) Chemometrics coupled to vibrational spectroscopy and spectroscopic imaging for the analysis of solid-phase pharmaceutical products: A brief review on non-destructive analytical methods. Trends in Analytical Chemistry **108**, 74–87.

4. DePaoli, D., Lemoine, É., Ember, K., Parent, M., Prud'homme, M., Cantin, L., Petrecca, K., Leblond, F. and Côté, D. C. (2020) Rise of Raman spectroscopy in neurosurgery: a review. Journal of Biomedical Optics **25**, 050901.
5. Binkhonain, M. and Zhao, L. (2019) A review of machine learning algorithms for identification and classification of non-functional requirements. Expert Systems with Applications: X **1**, 100001.
6. Carvalho, T. P., Soares, F. A. A. M. N., Vita, R., Francisco, R. d. P., Basto, J. P. and Alcalá, S. G. S. (2019) A systematic literature review of machine learning methods applied to predictive maintenance. Computers and Industrial Engineering **137**, 106024.
7. Zantalis, F., Koulouras, G., Karabetsos, S. and Kandris, D. (2019) A review of machine learning and IoT in smart transportation. Future Internet **11**, 94.
8. Baker, M. J., Byrne, H. J., Chalmers, J., Gardner, P., Goodacre, R., Henderson, A., Kazarian, S. G., Martin, F. L., Moger, J., Stone, N. and Sulé-Suso, J. (2018) Clinical applications of infrared and Raman spectroscopy: state of play and future challenges. Analyst **143**, 1735–1757.
9. Baker, M. J., Hussain, S. R., Lovergne, L., Untereiner, V., Hughes, C., Lukaszewski, R. A., Thiéfin, G. and Sockalingum, G. D. (2016) Developing and understanding biofluid vibrational spectroscopy: a critical review. Chemical Society Reviews **45**, 1803–1818.
10. Leal, L. B., Nogueira, M. S., Canevari, R. A. and Carvalho, L. F. C. S. (2018) Vibration spectroscopy and body biofluids: Literature review for clinical applications. Photodiagnosis and Photodynamic Therapy **24**, 237–244.
11. Pahlow, S., Weber, K., Popp, J., Bayden, R. W., Kochan, K., Rüther, A., Perez-Guaita, D., Heraud, P., Stone, N., Dudgeon, A., Gardner, B., Reddy, R., Mayerich, D. and Bhargava, R. (2018) Application of vibrational spectroscopy and imaging to point-of-care medicine: A review. Applied Spectroscopy **72**, 52–84.
12. Henry, A.-I., Sharma, B., Cardinal, M. F., Kurouski, D. and Van Duyne, R. P. (2016) Surface-enhanced Raman spectroscopy biosensing: in vivo diagnostics and multimodal imaging. Analytical Chemistry **88**, 6638–6647.
13. McAughtrie, S., Faulds, K. and Graham, D. (2014) Surface-enhanced Raman spectroscopy (SERS): potential applications for disease detection and treatment. Journal of Photochemistry and Photobiology C: Photochemistry Reviews **21**, 40–53.
14. Laing, S., Jamieson, L. E., Faulds, K. and Graham, D. (2017) Surface-enhanced Raman spectroscopy for in vivo biosensing. Nature Reviews Chemistry **1**, 60.
15. Moore, T. J., Moody, A. S., Payne, T. D., Sarabia, G. M., Daniel, A. R. and Sharma, B. (2018) In vitro and in vivo SERS biosensing for disease diagnosis. Biosensors **8**, 46.
16. Masson, J.-F. and McKeating, K. S. (2017) Surface spectroscopy of nanomaterials for detection of diseases. In *Nanopatterned and Nanoparticle-Modified Electrodes*

(Alkire, R. C., Bartlett, P. N. and Lipkowski, J., Eds.), pp. 271–294, John Wiley & Sons.
17. Cordero, E., Latka, I., Matthäus, C., Schie, I. W. and Popp, J. (2018) In-vivo Raman spectroscopy: from basics to applications. Journal of Biomedical Optics **23**, 071210.
18. Jermyn, M., Desroches, J., Aubertin, K., St-Arnaud, K., Madore, W.-J., De Montigny, E., Guiot, M.-C., Trudel, D., Wilson, B. C., Petrecca, K. and Leblond, F. (2016) A review of Raman spectroscopy advances with an emphasis on clinical translation challenges in oncology. Physics in Medicine and Biology **61**, R370.
19. Auner, G. W., Koya, S. K., Huang, C., Broadbent, B., Trexler, M., Auner, Z., Elias, A., Mehne, K. C. and Brusatori, M. A. (2018) Applications of Raman spectroscopy in cancer diagnosis. Cancer and Metastasis Reviews **37**, 691–717.
20. Ralbovsky, N. M. and Lednev, I. K. (2019) Raman spectroscopy and chemometrics: A potential universal method for diagnosing cancer. Spectrochimica Acta Part A: Molecular and Biomolecular Spectroscopy **219**, 463–487.
21. Santos, I. P., Barroso, E. M., Bakker Schut, T. C., Caspers, P. J., van Lanschot, C. G. F., Choi, D.-H., van der Kamp, M. F., Smits, R. W. H., van Doorn, R., Verdijk, R. M., Noordhoek Hegt, V., von der Thüsen, J. H., van Deurzen, C. H. M., Koppert, L. B., van Leenders, G. J. L. H., Ewing-Graham, P. C., van Doorn, H. C., Dirven, C. M. F., Busstra, M. B., Hardillo, J., Sewnaik, A., ten Hove, I., Mast, H., Monserez, D. A., Meeuwis, C., Nijsten, T., Wolvius, E. B., Baatenburg de Jong, R. J., Puppels, G. J. and Koljenović, S. (2017) Raman spectroscopy for cancer detection and cancer surgery guidance: translation to the clinics. Analyst **142**, 3025–3047.
22. Upchurch, E., Isabelle, M., Lloyd, G. R., Kendall, C. and Barr, H. (2018) An update on the use of Raman spectroscopy in molecular cancer diagnostics: current challenges and further prospects. Expert Review of Molecular Diagnostics **18**, 245–258.
23. Ralbovsky, N. M. and Lednev, I. K. (2021) Vibrational spectroscopy for detection of diabetes: a review. Applied Spectroscopy **75**, 929–946.
24. Ralbovsky, N. M. and Lednev, I. K. (2022) Infrared and Raman Spectroscopy Assisted Diagnosis of Diabetics. In *Advanced Bioscience and Biosystems for Detection and Management of Diabetes* (Sadasivuni, K. K., Cabibihan, J.-J., Al-Ali, A. K. A. M and Malik, R. A., Eds.), pp. 133–164, Springer.
25. Ember, K. J. I., Hoeve, M. A., McAughtrie, S. L., Bergholt, M. S., Dwyer, B. J., Stevens, M. M., Faulds, K., Forbes, S. J. and Campbell, C. J. (2017) Raman spectroscopy and regenerative medicine: a review. NPJ Regener. Med. **2**, 12.
26. Krafft, C. and Popp, J. (2019) Medical needs for translational biophotonics with the focus on Raman-based methods. Translational Biophotonics **1**, e201900018.
27. Krafft, C. and Popp, J. (2015) The many facets of Raman spectroscopy for biomedical analysis. Analytical and Bioanalytical Chemistry **407**, 699–717.

28. Eberhardt, K., Stiebing, C., Matthäus, C., Schmitt, M. and Popp, J. (2015) Advantages and limitations of Raman spectroscopy for molecular diagnostics: an update. Expert Review of Molecular Diagnostics **15**, 773–787.
29. Kong, K., Kendall, C., Stone, N. and Notingher, I. (2015) Raman spectroscopy for medical diagnostics—From in-vitro biofluid assays to in-vivo cancer detection. Advanced Drug Delivery Reviews **89**, 121–134.
30. Mitchell, A. L., Gajjar, K. B., Theophilou, G., Martin, F. L. and Martin-Hirsch, P. L. (2014) Vibrational spectroscopy of biofluids for disease screening or diagnosis: translation from the laboratory to a clinical setting. Journal of Biophotonics **7**, 153–165.
31. Pence, I. and Mahadevan-Jansen, A. (2016) Clinical instrumentation and applications of Raman spectroscopy. Chemical Society Reviews **45**, 1958–1979.
32. Hernández-Vidales, K., Guevara, E., Olivares-Illana, V. and González, F. J. (2019) Characterization of wild-type and mutant p53 protein by Raman spectroscopy and multivariate methods. Journal of Raman Spectroscopy **50**, 1388–1394.
33. Bovenkamp, D., Sentosa, R., Rank, E., Erkkilä, M. T., Placzek, F., Püls, J., Drexler, W., Leitgeb, R. A., Garstka, N., Shariat, S. F., Stiebing, C., Schie, I. W., Popp, J., Andreana, M. and Unterhuber, A. (2018) Combination of high-resolution optical coherence tomography and Raman spectroscopy for improved staging and grading in bladder cancer. Applied Sciences **8**, 2371.
34. Abramczyk, H. and Imiela, A. (2018) The biochemical, nanomechanical and chemometric signatures of brain cancer. Spectrochimica Acta Part A: Molecular and Biomolecular Spectroscopy **188**, 8–19.
35. Mehta, K., Atak, A., Sahu, A., Srivastava, S. and Krishna, C. M. (2018) An early investigative serum Raman spectroscopy study of meningioma. Analyst **143**, 1916–1923.
36. Bury, D., Faust, G., Paraskevaidi, M., Ashton, K. M., Dawson, T. P. and Martin, F. L. (2018) Phenotyping metastatic brain tumors applying spectrochemical analyses: segregation of different cancer types. Analytical Letters **52**, 575–587.
37. Depciuch, J., Tołpa, B., Witek, P., Szmuc, K., Kaznowska, E., Osuchowski, M., Król, P. and Cebulski, J. (2020) Raman and FTIR spectroscopy in determining the chemical changes in healthy brain tissues and glioblastoma tumor tissues. Spectrochimica Acta Part A: Molecular and Biomolecular Spectroscopy **225**, 117526.
38. Zhou, Y., Liu, C.-H., Pu, Y., Wu, B., Nguyen, T. A., Cheng, G., Zhou, L., Zhu, K., Chen, J., Li, Q. and Alfano, R. R. (2019) Combined spatial frequency spectroscopy analysis with visible resonance Raman for optical biopsy of human brain metastases of lung cancers. Journal of Innovative Optical Heath Sciences **12**, 1950010.
39. Fallahzadeh, O., Dehghani-Bidgoli, Z. and Assarian, M. (2018) Raman spectral feature selection using ant colony optimization for breast cancer diagnosis. Lasers in Medical Science **33**, 1799–1806.

40. Marro, M., Nieva, C., de Juan, A. and Sierra, A. (2018) Unravelling the metabolic progression of breast cancer cells to bone metastasis by coupling Raman spectroscopy and a novel use of MCR-ALS algorithm. Analytical Chemistry **90**, 5594–5602.
41. Lyng, F. M., Traynor, D., Nguyen, T. N. Q., Meade, A. D., Rakib, F., Al-Saady, R., Goormaghtigh, E., Al-Saad, K. and Ali, M. H. (2019) Discrimination of breast cancer from benign tumours using Raman spectroscopy. PloS One **14**, e0212376.
42. Dubey, V., Ahmad, A., Butola, A., Qaiser, D., Srivastava, A. and Mehta, D. S. (2019) Low coherence quantitative phase microscopy with machine learning model and Raman spectroscopy for the study of breast cancer cells and their classification. Applied Optics **58**, A112–A119.
43. Talari, A. C. S., Rehman, S. and Rehman, I. U. (2019) Advancing cancer diagnostics with artificial intelligence and spectroscopy: identifying chemical changes associated with breast cancer. Expert Review of Molecular Diagnostics **19**, 929–940.
44. Albayrak, M., Senol, O., Demirkaya-Miloglu, F., Calik, M. and Kadioglu, Y. (2019) Novel chemometrics-assisted spectroscopic methods for diagnosis and monitoring of invasive ductal carcinoma in breast tissue. Bratislavske Lekarske Listy **120**, 184–187.
45. Chithra, K., Aruna, P., Vijayaraghavan, S., Prasad, S. G. and Ganesan, S. (2019) Monitoring of breast cancer patients under pre and post treated conditions using Raman spectroscopic analysis of blood plasma. Vibrational Spectroscopy **105**, 102982.
46. Nargis, H. F., Nawaz, H., Ditta, A., Mahmood, T., Majeed, M. I., Rashid, N., Muddassar, M., Bhatti, H. N., Saleem, M., Jilani, K., Bonnier, F. and Byrne, H. J. (2019) Raman spectroscopy of blood plasma samples from breast cancer patients at different stages. Spectrochimica Acta Part A: Molecular and Biomolecular Spectroscopy **222**, 117210.
47. Daniel, A., Prakasarao, A. and Ganesan, S. (2018) Near-infrared Raman spectroscopy for estimating biochemical changes associated with different pathological conditions of cervix. Spectrochimica Acta Part A: Molecular and Biomolecular Spectroscopy **190**, 409–416.
48. Duraipandian, S., Traynor, D., Kearney, P., Martin, C., O'Leary, J. J. and Lyng, F. M. (2018) Raman spectroscopic detection of high-grade cervical cytology: Using morphologically normal appearing cells. Scientific Reports **8**, 15048.
49. Zheng, C., Qing, S., Wang, J., Lü, G., Li, H., Lü, X., Ma, C., Tang, J. and Yue, X. (2019) Diagnosis of cervical squamous cell carcinoma and cervical adenocarcinoma based on Raman spectroscopy and support vector machine. Photodiagnosis and Photodynamic Therapy **27**, 156–161.

50. Raja, P., Aruna, P., Koteeswaran, D. and Ganesan, S. (2019) Characterization of blood plasma of normal and cervical cancer patients using NIR raman spectroscopy. Vibrational Spectroscopy **102**, 1–7.
51. Gala de Pablo, J., Armistead, F. J., Peyman, S. A., Bonthron, D., Lones, M., Smith, S. and Evans, S. D. (2018) Biochemical fingerprint of colorectal cancer cell lines using label-free live single-cell Raman spectroscopy. Journal of Raman Spectroscopy **49**, 1323–1332.
52. Maitra, I., Morais, C. L. M., Lima, K. M. G., Ashton, K. M., Date, R. S. and Martin, F. L. (2020) Raman spectral discrimination in human liquid biopsies of oesophageal transformation to adenocarcinoma. Journal of Biophotonics **13**, e201960132.
53. Bahreini, M., Hosseinzadegan, A., Rashidi, A., Miri, S. R., Mirzaei, H. R. and Hajian, P. (2019) A Raman-based serum constituents' analysis for gastric cancer diagnosis: In vitro study. Talanta **204**, 826–832.
54. Singh, S. P., Mukherjee, S., Galindo, L. H., So, P. T., Dasari, R. R., Khan, U. Z., Kannan, R., Upendran, A. and Kang, J. W. (2018) Evaluation of accuracy dependence of Raman spectroscopic models on the ratio of calibration and validation points for non-invasive glucose sensing. Anal. Bioanal. Chem. **410**, 6469–6475.
55. Senol, O. and Albayrak, M. (2019) Evaluation of larynx cancer via chemometrics assisted Raman spectroscopy. Current Optics and Photonics **3**, 150–153.
56. Mascarella, M. A., Alrasheed, A., Fnais, N., Gourgas, O., Jalani, G., Cerruti, M. and Tewfik, M. A. (2018) Raman spectroscopy for inverted papilloma: a proof-of-concept study. Otolaryngology–Head and Neck Surgery **159**, 587–589.
57. Managò, S., Mirabelli, P., Napolitano, M., Zito, G. and De Luca, A. C. (2018) Raman detection and identification of normal and leukemic hematopoietic cells. Journal of Biophotonics **11**, e201700265.
58. González-Solís, J. L. (2019) Discrimination of different cancer types clustering Raman spectra by a super paramagnetic stochastic network approach. PloS One **14**, e0213621.
59. da Silva, A. M., de Siqueira e Oliveira, F. S. A., de Brito, P. L. and Silveira Jr, L. (2018) Spectral model for diagnosis of acute leukemias in whole blood and plasma through Raman spectroscopy. Journal of Biomedical Optics **23**, 107002.
60. Wang, H., Zhang, S., Wan, L., Sun, H., Tan, J. and Su, Q. (2018) Screening and staging for non-small cell lung cancer by serum laser Raman spectroscopy. Spectrochimica Acta Part A: Molecular and Biomolecular Spectroscopy **201**, 34–38.
61. Sinica, A., Brožáková, K., Brůha, T. and Votruba, J. (2019) Raman spectroscopic discrimination of normal and cancerous lung tissues. Spectrochimica Acta Part A: Molecular and Biomolecular Spectroscopy **219**, 257–266.

62. Zheng, Q., Li, J., Yang, L., Zheng, B., Wang, J., Lv, N., Luo, J., Martin, F. L., Liu, D. and He, J. (2020) Raman spectroscopy as a potential diagnostic tool to analyse biochemical alterations in lung cancer. Analyst **145**, 385–392.
63. Shiramizu, B., Oda, R., Kamada, N., Garcia, M. A., Shieh, T., Maeda, T. A., Choi, S. Y., Lim, E. and Misra, A. (2018) Unique Raman spectroscopic fingerprints of B-cell non-Hodgkin lymphoma: Implications for diagnosis, prognosis and new therapies. Journal of Biological and Medical Sciences **2**, 105.
64. Rau, J. V., Marini, F., Fosca, M., Cippitelli, C., Rocchia, M. and Di Napoli, A. (2019) Raman spectroscopy discriminates malignant follicular lymphoma from benign follicular hyperplasia and from tumour metastasis. Talanta **194**, 763–770.
65. Cals, F. L. J., Schut, T. C. B., Caspers, P. J., Baatenburg de Jong, R. J., Koljenović, S. and Puppels, G. J. (2018) Raman spectroscopic analysis of the molecular composition of oral cavity squamous cell carcinoma and healthy tongue tissue. Analyst **143**, 4090–4102.
66. Sahu, A., Gera, P., Malik, A., Nair, S., Chaturvedi, P. and Krishna, C. M. (2019) Raman exfoliative cytology for prognosis prediction in oral cancers: A proof of concept study. Journal of Biophotonics **12**, e201800334x.
67. Ghosh, A., Raha, S., Dey, S., Chatterjee, K., Chowdhury, A. R. and Barui, A. (2019) Chemometric analysis of integrated FTIR and Raman spectra obtained by non-invasive exfoliative cytology for the screening of oral cancer. Analyst **144**, 1309–1325.
68. Jeng, M.-J., Sharma, M., Sharma, L., Chao, T.-Y., Huang, S.-F., Chang, L.-B., Wu, S.-L. and Chow, L. (2019) Raman spectroscopy analysis for optical diagnosis of oral cancer detection. Journal of Clinical Medicine **8**, 1313.
69. Hole, A., Tyagi, G., Sahu, A., Shaikh, R. and Krishna, C. M. (2018) Exploration of Raman exfoliated cytology for oral and cervical cancers. Vibrational Spectroscopy **98**, 35–40.
70. Magalhães, F. L., Machado, A. M. C., Paulino, E., Sahoo, S. K., de Paula, A. M., Garcia, A. M., Barman, I., Soares, J. S. and Mamede, M. (2018) Raman spectroscopy with a 1064-nm wavelength laser as a potential molecular tool for prostate cancer diagnosis: a pilot study. Journal of Biomedical Optics **23**, 121613.
71. Feng, X., Fox, M. C., Reichenberg, J. S., Lopes, F. C. P. S., Sebastian, K. R., Markey, M. K. and Tunnell, J. W. (2019) Biophysical basis of skin cancer margin assessment using Raman spectroscopy. Biomedical Optics Express **10**, 104–118.
72. Santos, I. P., van Doorn, R., Caspers, P. J., Schut, T. C. B., Barroso, E. M., Nijsten, T. E. C., Hegt, V. N., Koljenović, S. and Puppels, G. J. (2018) Improving clinical diagnosis of early-stage cutaneous melanoma based on Raman spectroscopy. British Journal of Cancer **119**, 1339–1346.
73. Ferreira Lima, A. M., Daniel, C. R., Navarro, R. S., Bodanese, B., Pasqualucci, C. A., Pacheco, M. T. T., Zângaro, R. A. and Silveira Jr, L. (2019) Discrimination

of non-melanoma skin cancer and keratosis from normal skin tissue in vivo and ex vivo by Raman spectroscopy. Vibrational Spectroscopy **100**, 131–141.
74. Depciuch, J., Stanek-Widera, A., Skrzypiec, D., Lange, D., Biskup-Frużyńska, M., Kiper, K., Stanek-Tarkowska, J., Kula, M. and Cebulski, J. (2019) Spectroscopic identification of benign (follicular adenoma) and cancerous lesions (follicular thyroid carcinoma) in thyroid tissues. Journal of Pharmaceutical and Biomedical Analysis **170**, 321–326.
75. Senol, O., Albayrak, M., Demirkaya Miloglu, F., Kadioglu, Y. and Calik, M. (2018) Application of photonics in diagnosis of papillary thyroid carcinoma tissues through Raman spectroscopy-assisted with chemometrics. Analytical Letters **51**, 229–235.
76. O'Dea, D., Bongiovanni, M., Sykiotis, G. P., Ziros, P. G., Meade, A. D., Lyng, F. M. and Malkin, A. (2019) Raman spectroscopy for the preoperative diagnosis of thyroid cancer and its subtypes: An in vitro proof-of-concept study. Cytopathology **30**, 51–60.
77. De Oliveira, M. A. S., Campbell, M., Afify, A. M., Huang, E. C. and Chan, J. W. (2019) Hyperspectral Raman microscopy can accurately differentiate single cells of different human thyroid nodules. Biomedical Optics Express **10**, 4411–4421.
78. Khan, S., Ullah, R., Shahzad, S., Anbreen, N., Bilal, M. and Khan, A. (2018) Analysis of tuberculosis disease through Raman spectroscopy and machine learning. Photodiagnosis and Photodynamic Therapy **24**, 286–291.
79. Koya, S. K., Brusatori, M., Martin, J. V., Yurgelevic, S., Huang, C., Liberati, D. M., Auner, G. W. and Diebel, L. N. (2018) Rapid detection of Clostridium difficile toxins in serum by Raman spectroscopy. Journal of Surgical Research **232**, 195–201.
80. Ditta, A., Nawaz, H., Mahmood, T., Majeed, M. I., Tahir, M., Rashid, N., Muddassar, M., Al-Saadi, A. A. and Byrne, H. J. (2019) Principal components analysis of Raman spectral data for screening of Hepatitis C infection. Spectrochimica Acta Part A: Molecular and Biomolecular Spectroscopy **221**, 117173.
81. Sohail, A., Khan, S., Ullah, R., Qureshi, S. A., Bilal, M. and Khan, A. (2018) Analysis of hepatitis C infection using Raman spectroscopy and proximity based classification in the transformed domain. Biomedical Optics Express **9**, 2041–2055.
82. Tong, D., Chen, C., Zhang, J., Lv, G., Zheng, X., Zhang, Z. and Lv, X. (2019) Application of Raman spectroscopy in the detection of hepatitis B virus infection. Photodiagnosis and Photodynamic Therapy **28**, 248–252.
83. Khan, S., Ullah, R., Khan, A., Ashraf, R., Ali, H., Bilal, M. and Saleem, M. (2018) Analysis of hepatitis B virus infection in blood sera using Raman spectroscopy and machine learning. Photodiagnosis and Photodynamic Therapy **23**, 89–93.
84. Arend, N., Pittner, A., Ramoji, A., Mondol, A. S., Dahms, M., Rüger, J., Kurzai, O., Schie, I. W., Bauer, M., Popp, J. and Neugebauer, U. (2020) Detection and

differentiation of bacterial and fungal infection of neutrophils from peripheral blood using Raman spectroscopy. Analytical Chemistry **92**, 10560–10568.

85. Lorenz, B., Ali, N., Bocklitz, T., Rösch, P. and Popp, J. (2020) Discrimination between pathogenic and non-pathogenic E. coli strains by means of Raman microspectroscopy. Analytical and Bioanalytical Chemistry **412**, 8241–8247.
86. Mahmood, T., Nawaz, H., Ditta, A., Majeed, M. I., Hanif, M. A., Rashid, N., Bhatti, H. N., Nargis, H. F., Saleem, M., Bonnier, F. and Byrne, H. J. (2018) Raman spectral analysis for rapid screening of dengue infection. Spectrochimica Acta Part A: Molecular and Biomolecular Spectroscopy **200**, 136–142.
87. Patel, S. K., Rajora, N., Kumar, S., Sahu, A., Kochar, S. K., Krishna, C. M. and Srivastava, S. (2019) Rapid discrimination of malaria-and dengue-infected patients sera using Raman spectroscopy. Analytical Chemistry **91**, 7054–7062.
88. Naseer, K., Amin, A., Saleem, M. and Qazi, J. (2019) Raman spectroscopy based differentiation of typhoid and dengue fever in infected human sera. Spectrochimica Acta Part A: Molecular and Biomolecular Spectroscopy **206**, 197–201.
89. de Carvalho, L. F. d. C. e. S. and Nogueira, M. S. (2020) Optical techniques for fast screening–towards prevention of the coronavirus COVID-19 outbreak. Photodiagnosis Photodynamic Therapy **30**, 101765.
90. Jacobi, L., Damle, V. H., Rajeswaran, B. and Tischler, Y. R. (2020) Low-frequency Raman spectroscopy as a diagnostic tool for COVID-19 and other coronaviruses. Royal Society Open Science.
91. Yeh, Y.-T., Gulino, K., Zhang, Y., Sabestien, A., Chou, T.-W., Zhou, B., Lin, Z., Albert, I., Lu, H., Swaminathan, V., Ghedin, E. and Terrones, M. (2020) A rapid and label-free platform for virus capture and identification from clinical samples. Proceedings of the National Academy of Sciences **117**, 895–901.
92. da Silva, W. R., Silveira Jr, L. and Fernandes, A. B. (2020) Diagnosing sickle cell disease and iron deficiency anemia in human blood by Raman spectroscopy. Lasers in Medical Science **35**, 1065–1074.
93. González-Solís, J. L., Villafan-Bernal, J. R., Martínez-Zérega, B. E. and Sánchez-Enríquez, S. (2018) Type 2 diabetes detection based on serum sample Raman spectroscopy. Lasers in Medical Science **33**, 1791–1797.
94. Chen, C., Yang, L., Zhao, J., Yuan, Y., Chen, C., Tang, J., Yang, H., Yan, Z., Wang, H. and Lv, X. (2020) Urine Raman spectroscopy for rapid and inexpensive diagnosis of chronic renal failure (CRF) using multiple classification algorithms. Optik **203**, 164043.
95. Cui, X., Zhao, Z., Zhang, G., Chen, S., Zhao, Y. and Lu, J. (2018) Analysis and classification of kidney stones based on Raman spectroscopy. Biomedical Optics Express **9**, 4175–4183.
96. Zheng, X., Lv, G., Zhang, Y., Lv, X., Gao, Z., Tang, J. and Mo, J. (2019) Rapid and non-invasive screening of high renin hypertension using Raman spectroscopy

and different classification algorithms. Spectrochimica Acta Part A: Molecular and Biomolecular Spectroscopy **215**, 244–248.

97. Zheng, X., Lv, G., Du, G., Zhai, Z., Mo, J. and Lv, X. (2018) Rapid and low-cost detection of thyroid dysfunction using raman spectroscopy and an improved support vector machine. IEEE Photonics Journal **10**, 1–12.
98. Du, Y., Lü, G., Du, G., Lü, X., Tang, J., Liu, J., Yue, X., Mo, J. and Sun, T. (2019) Diagnosis of hyperthyroidism and hypothyroidism serum by SVM-based Raman spectroscopy. Laser Physics Letters **16**, 065602.
99. Palermo, A., Fosca, M., Tabacco, G., Marini, F., Graziani, V., Santarsia, M. C., Longo, F., Lauria, A., Cesareo, R., Giovannoni, I., Taffon, C., Rocchia, M., Manfrini, S., Crucitti, P., Pozzilli, P., Crescenzi, A. and Rau, J. V. (2018) Raman spectroscopy applied to parathyroid tissues: a new diagnostic tool to discriminate normal tissue from adenoma. Analytical Chemistry **90**, 847–854.
100. Fornasaro, S., Vicario, A., De Leo, L., Bonifacio, A., Not, T. and Sergo, V. (2018) Potential use of MCR-ALS for the identification of coeliac-related biochemical changes in hyperspectral Raman maps from pediatric intestinal biopsies. Integrative Biology **10**, 356–363.
101. Ralbovsky, N. M. and Lednev, I. K. (2021) Analysis of individual red blood cells for Celiac disease diagnosis. Talanta **221**, 121642.
102. Ralbovsky, N. M., Halámková, L., Wall, K., Anderson-Hanley, C. and Lednev, I. K. (2019) Screening for Alzheimer's disease using saliva: a new approach based on machine learning and Raman hyperspectroscopy. Journal of Alzheimer's Disease **71**, 1351–1359.
103. Ralbovsky, N. M. and Lednev, I. K. (2019) Raman hyperspectroscopy shows promise for diagnosis of Alzheimer's. Biophotonics **4**, 33–37.
104. Ryzhikova, E., Kazakov, O., Halamkova, L., Celmins, D., Malone, P., Molho, E., Zimmerman, E. A. and Lednev, I. K. (2015) Raman spectroscopy of blood serum for Alzheimer's disease diagnostics: specificity relative to other types of dementia. Journal of Biophotonics **8**, 584–596.
105. Ryzhikova, E., Ralbovsky, N. M., Sikirzhytski, V., Kazakov, O., Halamkova, L., Quinn, J., Zimmerman, E. A. and Lednev, I. K. (2021) Raman spectroscopy and machine learning for biomedical applications: Alzheimer's disease diagnosis based on the analysis of cerebrospinal fluid. Spectrochimica Acta Part A: Molecular and Biomolecular Spectroscopy **248**, 119188.
106. Ralbovsky, N. M., Fitzgerald, G. S., McNay, E. C. and Lednev, I. K. (2021) Towards development of a novel screening method for identifying Alzheimer's disease risk: Raman spectroscopy of blood serum and machine learning. Spectrochimica Acta Part A: Molecular and Biomolecular Spectroscopy **254**, 119603.
107. Paraskevaidi, M., Morais, C. L. M., Halliwell, D. E., Mann, D. M. A., Allsop, D., Martin-Hirsch, P. L. and Martin, F. L. (2018) Raman spectroscopy to diagnose Alzheimer's disease and dementia with Lewy bodies in blood. ACS Chemical Neuroscience **9**, 2786–2794.

108. Parlatan, U., Inanc, M. T., Ozgor, B. Y., Oral, E., Bastu, E., Unlu, M. B. and Basar, G. (2019) Raman spectroscopy as a non-invasive diagnostic technique for endometriosis. Scientific Reports **9**, 19795.
109. Ullah, R., Khan, S., Farman, F., Bilal, M., Krafft, C. and Shahzad, S. (2019) Demonstrating the application of Raman spectroscopy together with chemometric technique for screening of asthma disease. Biomedical Optics Express **10**, 600–609.
110. Taylor, A. M., Jenks, D. D., Kammath, V. D., Norman, B. P., Dillon, J. P., Gallagher, J. A., Ranganath, L. R. and Kerns, J. G. (2019) Raman spectroscopy identifies differences in ochronotic and non-ochronotic cartilage; a potential novel technique for monitoring ochronosis. Osteoarthritis and Cartilage **27**, 1244–1251.
111. Ralbovsky, N. M., Dey, P., Galfano, A., Dey, B. K. and Lednev, I. K. (2020) Diagnosis of a model of Duchenne muscular dystrophy in blood serum of mdx mice using Raman hyperspectroscopy. Scientific Reports **10**, 11734.
112. Ralbovsky, N. M., Dey, P., Galfano, A., Dey, B. K. and Lednev, I. K. (2022) A novel method for detecting Duchenne muscular dystrophy in blood serum of mdx mice. Genes **13**, 1342.
113. Kirchberger-Tolstik, T., Pradhan, P., Vieth, M., Grunert, P., Popp, J., Bocklitz, T. W. and Stallmach, A. (2020) Towards an interpretable classifier for characterization of endoscopic mayo scores in ulcerative colitis using Raman spectroscopy. Analytical Chemistry **92**, 13776–13784.
114. Sun, T., Xie, X., Li, H., Lv, G., Lv, X., Tang, J., Yue, X. and Mo, J. (2019) Rapid, noninvasive screening of ocular diseases using tear raman spectroscopy and different classification algorithms. Laser Physics **30**, 015701.
115. Mosier-Boss, P. A. (2017) Review of SERS substrates for chemical sensing. Nanomaterials **7**, 142.
116. Jin, D., Wang, X., Fu, B., Li, T., Chen, N., Chen, Z., Chen, H. and Liu, S. (2019) Raman spectroscopy of luminal subtype and basal subtype muscle invasive bladder cancer. International Journal of Clinical and Experimental Medicine **12**, 5447–5453.
117. Chen, S., Zhu, S., Cui, X., Xu, W., Kong, C., Zhang, Z. and Qian, W. (2019) Identifying non-muscle-invasive and muscle-invasive bladder cancer based on blood serum surface-enhanced Raman spectroscopy. Biomedical Optics Express **10**, 3533–3544.
118. Zhang, Y., Lai, X., Zeng, Q., Li, L., Lin, L., Li, S., Liu, Z., Su, C., Qi, M. and Guo, Z. (2018) Classifying low-grade and high-grade bladder cancer using label-free serum surface-enhanced Raman spectroscopy and support vector machine. Laser Physics **28**, 035603.
119. Moisoiu, V., Socaciu, A., Stefancu, A., Iancu, S. D., Boros, I., Alecsa, C. D., Rachieriu, C., Chiorean, A. R., Eniu, D., Leopold, N., Socaciu, C. and Eniu, D.

T. (2019) Breast cancer diagnosis by surface-enhanced raman scattering (SERS) of urine. Applied Sciences **9**, 806.

120. Moisoiu, V., Stefancu, A., Gulei, D., Boitor, R., Magdo, L., Raduly, L., Pasca, S., Kubelac, P., Mehterov, N., Chiş, V., Simon, M., Muresan, M., Irimie, A. I., Baciut, M., Stiufiuc, R., Pavcl, I. E., Achimas-Cadariu, P., Ionescu, C., Lazar, V., Sarafian, V., Notingher, I., Leopold, N. and Berindan-Neagoe, I. (2019) SERS-based differential diagnosis between multiple solid malignancies: breast, colorectal, lung, ovarian and oral cancer. International Journal of Nanomedicine **14**, 6165–6178.
121. Králová, Z. O., Oriňak, A., Oriňaková, R., Petruš, O., Macko, J., Radoňak, J., Lakyová, L. S., Jurašeková, Z., Smith, R. M., Strečková, M. and Koval, K. (2018) Electrochemically deposited silver detection substrate for surface-enhanced Raman spectroscopy cancer diagnostics. Journal of Biomedical Optics **23**, 075002.
122. Guo, L., Li, Y., Huang, F., Dong, J., Li, F., Yang, X., Zhu, S. and Yang, M. (2019) Identification and analysis of serum samples by surface-enhanced Raman spectroscopy combined with characteristic ratio method and PCA for gastric cancer detection. Journal of Innovative Optical Health Sciences **12**, 1950003.
123. Lin, X., Wang, L., Lin, H., Lin, D., Lin, J., Liu, X., Qiu, S., Xu, Y., Chen, G. and Feng, S. (2019) A novel urine analysis technique combining affinity chromatography with Au nanoparticle based surface-enhanced Raman spectroscopy for potential applications in non-invasive cancer screening. Journal of Biophotonics **12**, e201800327.
124. Wu, Q., Qiu, S., Yu, Y., Chen, W., Lin, H., Lin, D., Feng, S. and Chen, R. (2018) Assessment of the radiotherapy effect for nasopharyngeal cancer using plasma surface-enhanced Raman spectroscopy technology. Biomedical Optics Express **9**, 3413-3423.
125. Hassoun, M., Rüger, J., Kirchberger-Tolstik, T., Schie, I. W., Henkel, T., Weber, K., Cialla-May, D., Krafft, C. and Popp, J. (2018) A droplet-based microfluidic chip as a platform for leukemia cell lysate identification using surface-enhanced Raman scattering. Analytical and Bioanalytical Chemistry **410**, 999–1006.
126. Lin, K., Xu, J., Li, L., Liao, F., Dong, X. and Lin, J. (2018) Label-free detection of liver cancer based on silver nanoparticles coated tissue surface-enhanced Raman spectroscopy. Laser Physics Letters **15**, 125601.
127. Yu, Y., Lin, Y., Xu, C., Lin, K., Ye, Q., Wang, X., Xie, S., Chen, R. and Lin, J. (2018) Label-free detection of nasopharyngeal and liver cancer using surface-enhanced Raman spectroscopy and partial lease squares combined with support vector machine. Biomedical Optics Express **9**, 6053–6066.
128. Shao, L., Zhang, A., Rong, Z., Wang, C., Jia, X., Zhang, K., Xiao, R. and Wang, S. (2018) Fast and non-invasive serum detection technology based on surface-enhanced Raman spectroscopy and multivariate statistical analysis for liver disease. Nanomedicine: Nanotechnology, Biology and Medicine **14**, 451–459.

129. Zhang, K., Hao, C., Man, B., Zhang, C., Yang, C., Liu, M., Peng, Q. and Chen, C. (2018) Diagnosis of liver cancer based on tissue slice surface-enhanced Raman spectroscopy and multivariate analysis. Vibrational Spectroscopy **98**, 82–87.
130. Qian, K., Wang, Y., Hua, L., Chen, A. and Zhang, Y. (2018) New method of lung cancer detection by saliva test using surface-enhanced Raman spectroscopy. Thoracic Cancer **9**, 1556–1561.
131. Zhang, K., Liu, X., Man, B., Yang, C., Zhang, C., Liu, M., Zhang, Y., Liu, L. and Chen, C. (2018) Label-free and stable serum analysis based on Ag-NPs/PSi surface-enhanced Raman scattering for noninvasive lung cancer detection. Biomedical Optics Express **9**, 4345–4358.
132. Zhang, K., Hao, C., Huo, Y., Man, B., Zhang, C., Yang, C., Liu, M. and Chen, C. (2019) Label-free diagnosis of lung cancer with tissue-slice surface-enhanced Raman spectroscopy and statistical analysis. Lasers in Medical Science **34**, 1849–1855.
133. Cao, X., Wang, Z., Bi, L. and Zheng, J. (2018) Label-free detection of human serum using surface-enhanced Raman spectroscopy based on highly branched gold nanoparticle substrates for discrimination of non-small cell lung cancer. Journal of Chemistry **2018**, 9012645.
134. Shin, H., Jeong, H., Park, J., Hong, S. and Choi, Y. (2018) Correlation between cancerous exosomes and protein markers based on surface-enhanced Raman spectroscopy (SERS) and principal component analysis (PCA). ACS Sensors **3**, 2637–2643.
135. Liu, K., Jin, S., Song, Z., Jiang, L., Ma, L. and Zhang, Z. (2019) Label-free surface-enhanced Raman spectroscopy of serum based on multivariate statistical analysis for the diagnosis and staging of lung adenocarcinoma. Vibrational Spectroscopy **100**, 177–184.
136. Liu, K., Jin, S., Song, Z. and Jiang, L. (2020) High accuracy detection of malignant pleural effusion based on label-free surface-enhanced Raman spectroscopy and multivariate statistical analysis. Spectrochimica Acta Part A: Molecular and Biomolecular Spectroscopy **226**, 117632.
137. Xue, L., Yan, B., Li, Y., Tan, Y., Luo, X. and Wang, M. (2018) Surface-enhanced Raman spectroscopy of blood serum based on gold nanoparticles for tumor stages detection and histologic grades classification of oral squamous cell carcinoma. International Journal of Nanomedicine **13**, 4977–4986.
138. Chundayil Madathil, G., Iyer, S., Thankappan, K., Gowd, G. S., Nair, S. and Koyakutty, M. (2019) A novel surface-enhanced Raman catheter for rapid detection, classification, and grading of oral cancer. Advanced Healthcare Materials **8**, 1801557.
139. Perumal, J., Mahyuddin, A. P., Balasundaram, G., Goh, D., Fu, C. Y., Kazakeviciute, A., Dinish, U., Choolani, M. and Olivo, M. (2019) SERS-based detection of haptoglobin in ovarian cyst fluid as a point-of-care diagnostic assay for epithelial ovarian cancer. Cancer Management and Research **11**, 1115–1124.

140. Zermeño-Nava, J. d. J., Martínez-Martínez, M. U., Rámirez-de-Ávila, A. L., Hernández-Arteaga, A. C., García-Valdivieso, M. G., Hernández-Cedillo, A., José-Yacamán, M. and Navarro-Contreras, H. R. (2018) Determination of sialic acid in saliva by means of surface-enhanced Raman spectroscopy as a marker in adnexal mass patients: ovarian cancer vs benign cases. Journal of Ovarian Research **11**, 61.
141. Paraskevaidi, M., Ashton, K. M., Stringfellow, H. F., Wood, N. J., Keating, P. J., Rowbottom, A. W., Martin-Hirsch, P. L. and Martin, F. L. (2018) Raman spectroscopic techniques to detect ovarian cancer biomarkers in blood plasma. Talanta **189**, 281–288.
142. Li, T.-D., Zhang, R., Chen, H., Huang, Z.-P., Ye, X., Wang, H., Deng, A.-M. and Kong, J.-L. (2018) An ultrasensitive polydopamine bi-functionalized SERS immunoassay for exosome-based diagnosis and classification of pancreatic cancer. Chemical Science **9**, 5372–5382.
143. Carmicheal, J., Hayashi, C., Huang, X., Liu, L., Lu, Y., Krasnoslobodtsev, A., Lushnikov, A., Kshirsagar, P. G., Patel, A., Jain, M., Lyubchenko, Y. L., Lu, Y., Batra, S. K. and Kaur, S. (2019) Label-free characterization of exosome via surface-enhanced Raman spectroscopy for the early detection of pancreatic cancer. Nanomedicine: Nanotechnology, Biology and Medicine **16**, 88–96
144. Koo, K. M., Wang, J., Richards, R. e. S., Farrell, A., Yaxley, J. W., Samaratunga, H., Teloken, P. E., Roberts, M. J., Coughlin, G. D., Lavin, M. F., Mainwaring, P. N., Wang, Y., Gardiner, R. A. and Trau, M. (2018) Design and clinical verification of surface-enhanced Raman spectroscopy diagnostic technology for individual cancer risk prediction. ACS Nano **12**, 8362–8371.
145. Stefancu, A., Moisoiu, V., Couti, R., Andras, I., Rahota, R., Crisan, D., Pavel, I. E., Socaciu, C., Leopold, N. and Crisan, N. (2018) Combining SERS analysis of serum with PSA levels for improving the detection of prostate cancer. Nanomedicine **13**, 2455–2467.
146. Pan, J., Shao, X., Zhu, Y., Dong, B., Wang, Y., Kang, X., Chen, N., Chen, Z., Liu, S. and Xue, W. (2019) Surface-enhanced Raman spectroscopy before radical prostatectomy predicts biochemical recurrence better than CAPRA-S. International Journal of Nanomedicine **14**, 431–440.
147. Chen, X., Tang, M., Liu, Y., Huang, J., Liu, Z., Tian, H., Zheng, Y., de la Chapelle, M. L., Zhang, Y. and Fu, W. (2019) Surface-enhanced Raman scattering method for the identification of methicillin-resistant Staphylococcus aureus using positively charged silver nanoparticles. Microchimica Acta **186**, 102.
148. Pérez, A., Prada, Y. A., Cabanzo, R., González, C. I. and Mejía-Ospino, E. (2018) Diagnosis of chagas disease from human blood serum using surface-enhanced Raman scattering (SERS) spectroscopy and chemometric methods. Sensing and Bio-Sensing Research **21**, 40–45.
149. Hernández-Cedillo, A., García-Valdivieso, M. G., Hernández-Arteaga, A. C., Patiño-Marín, N., Vértiz-Hernández, Á. A., José-Yacamán, M. and Navarro-

Contreras, H. R. (2019) Determination of sialic acid levels by using surface-enhanced Raman spectroscopy in periodontitis and gingivitis. Oral Diseases **25**, 1627–1633.

150. Sebba, D., Lastovich, A. G., Kuroda, M., Fallows, E., Johnson, J., Ahouidi, A., Honko, A. N., Fu, H., Nielson, R., Carruthers, E., Diédhiou, C., Ahmadou, D., Soropogui, B., Ruedas, J., Peters, K., Bartkowiak, M., Magassouba, N. F., Mboup, S., Amor, Y. B., Connor, J. H. and Weidemaier, K. (2018) A point-of-care diagnostic for differentiating Ebola from endemic febrile diseases. Science Translational Medicine **10**, eaat0944.
151. Guo, J., Rong, Z., Li, Y., Wang, S., Zhang, W. and Xiao, R. (2018) Diagnosis of chronic kidney diseases based on surface-enhanced Raman spectroscopy and multivariate analysis. Laser Physics **28**, 075603.
152. Yang, H., Zhao, C., Li, R., Shen, C., Cai, X., Sun, L., Luo, C. and Yin, Y. (2018) Noninvasive and prospective diagnosis of coronary heart disease with urine using surface-enhanced Raman spectroscopy. Analyst **143**, 2235–2242.
153. Stefancu, A., Badarinza, M., Moisoiu, V., Iancu, S. D., Serban, O., Leopold, N. and Fodor, D. (2019) SERS-based liquid biopsy of saliva and serum from patients with Sjögren's syndrome. Analytical and Bioanalytical Chemistry **411**, 5877–5883.
154. Zhang, Q.-J., Chen, Y., Zou, X.-H., Hu, W., Lin, X.-L., Feng, S.-Y., Chen, F., Xu, L.-Q., Chen, W.-J. and Wang, N. (2019) Prognostic analysis of amyotrophic lateral sclerosis based on clinical features and plasma surface-enhanced Raman spectroscopy. Journal of Biophotonics **12**, e201900012.
155. Carlomagno, C., Cabinio, M., Picciolini, S., Gualerzi, A., Baglio, F. and Bedoni, M. (2019) SERS-based biosensor for Alzheimer disease evaluation through the fast analysis of human serum. Journal of Biophotonics **13**, e201960033.
156. Ryzhikova, E., Ralbovsky, N. M., Halámková, L., Celmins, D., Malone, P., Molho, E., Quinn, J., Zimmerman, E. A. and Lednev, I. K. (2019) Multivariate statistical analysis of surface-enhanced Raman spectra of human serum for Alzheimer's disease diagnosis. Applied Sciences **9**, 3256.
157. Kim, W., Lee, S. H., Kim, J. H., Ahn, Y. J., Kim, Y.-H., Yu, J. S. and Choi, S. (2018) Paper-based surface-enhanced Raman spectroscopy for diagnosing prenatal diseases in women. ACS Nano **12**, 7100–7108.
158. Bocsa, C. D., Moisoiu, V., Stefancu, A., Leopold, L. F., Leopold, N. and Fodor, D. (2019) Knee osteoarthritis grading by resonant Raman and surface-enhanced Raman scattering (SERS) analysis of synovial fluid. Nanomedicine: Nanotechnology, Biology and Medicine **20**, 102012.
159. Zamora-Mendoza, B. N., Espinosa-Tanguma, R., Ramirez-Elias, M. G., Cabrera-Alonso, R., Montero-Moran, G., Portales-Perez, D., Rosales-Romo, J. A., Gonzalez, J. F. and Gonzalez, C. (2019) Surface-enhanced Raman spectroscopy: A non invasive alternative procedure for early detection in childhood asthma biomarkers in saliva. Photodiagnosis and Photodynamic Therapy **27**, 85–91.

160. Lin, J., Lin, X., Hu, C., Bai, P., Yang, H., Dai, Y., Qiu, H., Lin, M., Feng, S. and Pan, J. (2018) Silver nanoparticle based surface-enhanced Raman spectroscopy for label-free discrimination of diabetic albumin under near-infrared laser excitation. Laser Physics Letters **15**, 095703.
161. Chen, Y., Premasiri, W. R. and Ziegler, L. D. (2018) Surface-enhanced Raman spectroscopy of Chlamydia trachomatis and Neisseria gonorrhoeae for diagnostics, and extra-cellular metabolomics and biochemical monitoring. Scientific Reports **8**, 5163.
162. Žukovskaja, O., Kloß, S., Blango, M. G., Ryabchykov, O., Kniemeyer, O., Brakhage, A. A., Bocklitz, T. W., Cialla-May, D., Weber, K. and Popp, J. (2018) UV-Raman spectroscopic identification of fungal spores important for respiratory diseases. Analytical Chemistry **90**, 8912–8918.
163. Ralbovsky, N. M., Egorov, V., Moskovets, E., Dey, P., Dey, B. K. and Lednev, I. K. (2019) Deep-ultraviolet Raman spectroscopy for cancer diagnostics: a feasibility study with cell lines and tissues. Cancer Studies and Molecular Medicine: Open Journal **5**, 1–10.
164. Liu, M., Liu, X., Huang, Z., Tang, X., Lin, X., Xu, Y., Chen, G., Kwok, H. F., Lin, Y. and Feng, S. (2019) Rapid discrimination of colon cancer cells with single base mutation in KRAS gene segment using laser tweezers Raman spectroscopy. Journal of Biophotonics **12**, e201800332.
165. Lee, W., Nanou, A., Rikkert, L., Coumans, F. A. W., Otto, C., Terstappen, L. W. M. M. and Offerhaus, H. L. (2018) Label-free prostate cancer detection by characterization of extracellular vesicles using Raman spectroscopy. Analytical Chemistry **90**, 11290–11296.
166. Jia, W., Chen, P., Chen, W. and Li, Y. (2018) Raman characterizations of red blood cells with β-thalassemia using laser tweezers Raman spectroscopy. Medicine **97**, e12611.
167. Lin, J., Shao, L., Qiu, S., Huang, X., Liu, M., Zheng, Z., Lin, D., Xu, Y., Li, Z., Lin, Y., Chen, R. and Feng, S. (2018) Application of a near-infrared laser tweezers Raman spectroscopy system for label-free analysis and differentiation of diabetic red blood cells. Biomedical Optics Express **9**, 984–993
168. Gebrekidan, M. T., Erber, R., Hartmann, A., Fasching, P. A., Emons, J., Beckmann, M. W. and Braeuer, A. (2018) Breast tumor analysis using shifted-excitation Raman Difference Spectroscopy (SERDS). Technology in Cancer Research and Treatment **17**, 1–11.
169. Pinto, M., Zorn, K. C., Tremblay, J.-P., Desroches, J., Dallaire, F., Aubertin, K., Marple, E. T., Kent, C., Leblond, F., Trudel, D. and Lesage, F. (2019) Integration of a Raman spectroscopy system to a robotic-assisted surgical system for real-time tissue characterization during radical prostatectomy procedures. Journal of Biomedical Optics **24**, 025001.
170. Aubertin, K., Desroches, J., Jermyn, M., Trinh, V. Q., Saad, F., Trudel, D. and Leblond, F. (2018) Combining high wavenumber and fingerprint Raman

spectroscopy for the detection of prostate cancer during radical prostatectomy. Biomedical Optics Express **9**, 4294–4305.

171. Chen, H., Li, X., Broderick, N., Liu, Y., Zhou, Y., Han, J. and Xu, W. (2018) Identification and characterization of bladder cancer by low-resolution fiber-optic Raman spectroscopy. Journal of Biophotonics **11**, e201800016.
172. Chen, H., Li, X., Broderick, N. G. R. and Xu, W. (2019) Low-resolution fiber-optic Raman spectroscopy for bladder cancer diagnosis: A comparison study of varying laser power, integration time, and classification methods. Journal of Raman Spectroscopy **51**, 323–334.
173. Li, Q., Li, W., Zhang, J. and Xu, Z. (2018) An improved k-nearest neighbour method to diagnose breast cancer. Analyst **143**, 2807–2811.
174. Krbcova, Z., Kukal, J., Mares, J., Habartova, L. and Setnicka, V. (2019) Variational approach to cancerous tissue identification from in vivo Raman spectra. Biomedical Signal Processing and Control **49**, 520–527.
175. Zuvela, P., Lin, K., Shu, C., Zheng, W., Lim, C. M. and Huang, Z. (2019) Fiber-optic Raman spectroscopy with nature-inspired genetic algorithms enhances real-time in vivo detection and diagnosis of nasopharyngeal carcinoma. Analytical Chemistry **91**, 8101–8108.
176. Desroches, J., Jermyn, M., Pinto, M., Picot, F., Tremblay, M.-A., Obaid, S., Marple, E., Urmey, K., Trudel, D., Soulez, G., Guiot, M.-C., Wilson, B. C., Petrecca, K. and Leblond, F. (2018) A new method using Raman spectroscopy for in vivo targeted brain cancer tissue biopsy. Scientific Reports **8**, 1792.
177. Aubertin, K., Trinh, V. Q., Jermyn, M., Baksic, P., Grosset, A.-A., Desroches, J., St-Arnaud, K., Birlea, M., Vladoiu, M. C., Latour, M., Albadine, R., Saad, F., Leblond, F. and Trudel, D. (2018) Mesoscopic characterization of prostate cancer using Raman spectroscopy: potential for diagnostics and therapeutics. BJU International **122**, 326–336.
178. Jermyn, M., Mok, K., Mercier, J., Desroches, J., Pichette, J., Saint-Arnaud, K., Bernstein, L., Guiot, M.-C., Petrecca, K. and Leblond, F. (2015) Intraoperative brain cancer detection with Raman spectroscopy in humans. Science Translational Medicine **7**, 274ra219.
179. Feng, X., Moy, A. J., Nguyen, H. T. M., Zhang, Y., Zhang, J., Fox, M. C., Sebastian, K. R., Reichenberg, J. S., Markey, M. K. and Tunnell, J. W. (2018) Raman biophysical markers in skin cancer diagnosis. Journal of Biomedical Optics **23**, 057002.
180. Garcia, D. V., da Silva Filho, J. I., Silveira Jr, L., Pacheco, M. T. T., Abe, J. M., Carvalho Jr, A., Blos, M. F., Pasqualucci, C. A. G. and Mario, M. C. (2019) Analysis of Raman spectroscopy data with algorithms based on paraconsistent logic for characterization of skin cancer lesions. Vibrational Spectroscopy **103**, 102929.
181. Yu, M., Yan, H., Xia, J., Zhu, L., Zhang, T., Zhu, Z., Lou, X., Sun, G. and Dong, M. (2019) Deep convolutional neural networks for tongue squamous cell carcinoma

classification using Raman spectroscopy. Photodiagnosis and Photodynamic Therapy **26**, 430–435.

182. Yan, H., Yu, M., Xia, J., Zhu, L., Zhang, T. and Zhu, Z. (2019) Tongue squamous cell carcinoma discrimination with Raman spectroscopy and convolutional neural networks. Vibrational Spectroscopy **103**, 102938.
183. Guevara, E., Torres-Galván, J. C., Ramírez-Elías, M. G., Luevano-Contreras, C. and González, F. J. (2018) Use of Raman spectroscopy to screen diabetes mellitus with machine learning tools. Biomedical Optics Express **9**, 4998–5010.
184. Khristoforova, Y. A., Bratchenko, I. A., Myakinin, O. O., Artemyev, D. N., Moryatov, A. A., Orlov, A. E., Kozlov, S. V. and Zakharov, V. P. (2019) Portable spectroscopic system for in vivo skin neoplasms diagnostics by Raman and autofluorescence analysis. Journal of Biophotonics **12**, e201800400.
185. Sekine, R., Sato, S., Tanaka, J.-i., Kagoshima, H., Aoki, T. and Murakami, M. (2018) Potential application of Raman spectroscopy for real-time diagnosis and classification of colorectal cancer. The Showa University Journal of Medical Sciences **30**, 381–389.
186. Sato, S., Sekine, R., Kagoshima, H., Kazama, K., Kato, A., Shiozawa, M. and Tanaka, J.-i. (2019) All-in-one Raman spectroscopy approach to diagnosis of colorectal cancer: analysis of spectra in the fingerprint regions. Journal of the Anus, Rectum and Colon **3**, 84–90.
187. Aljakouch, K., Hilal, Z., Daho, I., Schuler, M., Krauß, S. D., Yosef, H. K., Dierks, J., Mosig, A., Gerwert, K. and El-Mashtoly, S. F. (2019) Fast and noninvasive diagnosis of cervical cancer by coherent anti-stokes Raman scattering. Analytical Chemistry **91**, 13900–13906.
188. Jenkins, C. A., Jenkins, R. A., Pryse, M. M., Welsby, K. A., Jitsumura, M., Thornton, C. A., Dunstan, P. R. and Harris, D. A. (2018) A high-throughput serum Raman spectroscopy platform and methodology for colorectal cancer diagnostics. Analyst **143**, 6014–6024.
189. Haifler, M., Pence, I., Sun, Y., Kutikov, A., Uzzo, R. G., Mahadevan-Jansen, A. and Patil, C. A. (2018) Discrimination of malignant and normal kidney tissue with short wave infrared dispersive Raman spectroscopy. Journal of Biophotonics **11**, e201700188.
190. Stone, N., Faulds, K., Graham, D. and Matousek, P. (2010) Prospects of deep Raman spectroscopy for noninvasive detection of conjugated surface-enhanced resonance Raman scattering nanoparticles buried within 25 mm of mammalian tissue. Analytical Chemistry **82**, 3969–3973.
191. Stone, N., Kerssens, M., Lloyd, G. R., Faulds, K., Graham, D. and Matousek, P. (2011) Surface-enhanced spatially offset Raman spectroscopic (SESORS) imaging–the next dimension. Chemical Science **2**, 776–780.
192. Nicolson, F., Andreiuk, B., Andreou, C., Hsu, H.-T., Rudder, S. and Kircher, M. F. (2019) Non-invasive in vivo imaging of cancer using surface-enhanced spatially offset Raman spectroscopy (SESORS). Theranostics **9**, 5899–5913.

193. Wang, W., Zhao, J., Short, M. and Zeng, H. (2015) Real-time in vivo cancer diagnosis using Raman spectroscopy. Journal of Biophotonics **8**, 527–545.
194. Kallaway, C., Almond, L. M., Barr, H., Wood, J., Hutchings, J., Kendall, C. and Stone, N. (2013) Advances in the clinical application of Raman spectroscopy for cancer diagnostics. Photodiagnosis and Photodynamic Therapy **10**, 207–219.
195. Wilson, B. C., Jermyn, M. and Leblond, F. (2018) Challenges and opportunities in clinical translation of biomedical optical spectroscopy and imaging. Journal of Biomedical Optics **23**, 030901.
196. Panikar, S. S., Cialla-May, D., De la Rosa, E., Salas, P. and Popp, J. (2021) Towards translation of surface-enhanced Raman spectroscopy (SERS) to clinical practice: Progress and trends. Trends in Analytical Chemistry **134**, 116122.

https://doi.org/10.1142/9789811264610_0005

Chapter 5

Raman Spectroscopy for Health Science

Mariko Egawa

MIRAI Technology Institute
Shiseido Co., Ltd.,
Yokohama, 220-0011, Japan
mariko.egawa@shiseido.com

5.1 Introduction

Because of lifestyle changes in response to the recent COVID-19 pandemic, there has been a noticeable shift in people's interest in their daily lives to valuing their own "health" more. The WHO constitution states that "health is a state of complete physical, mental and social well-being and not merely the absence of disease or infirmity" and that "health science" comprises three elements: science to prevent illness from pre-symptomatic disease, science to prevent pre-symptomatic disease from pre-symptomatic disease, and science to promote healthy conditions [1]. There are various causes and factors that lead to a state of health impairment, and the changes in the body because of them are also manifested in the skin [2, 3].

The skin is an organ located in the outermost layer of the body, and its properties can easily change depending on the body condition and external environment; as a result, it is easy for us to perceive changes from the pre-disease stage on a daily basis. For example, psychological stress is a major health issue in daily life because of its involvement in multiple physiological and psychological illnesses, particularly in industrialized societies [4–6]. Several studies have examined the effects of psychological stress on the skin, indicating that stress exacerbates several skin disorders. Specifically, interview stress (Trier Social Stress Test [7]), which applies acute stress to participants through mock interviews, caused delayed recovery of the barrier function of the skin, increased plasma cortisol levels, and activated several inflammation and immune systems in the blood, including IL-1β and IL-10 [4]. The mechanisms contributing to acute psychological stress-induced exacerbation of inflammatory skin disorders, including psoriasis, eczema, atopic dermatitis, and aggravated contact dermatitis, have been suggested to be stress-induced impairments of skin permeability barrier homeostasis [4, 8, 9]. Even for healthy subjects, it was reported that final examination stress on students [10] or marital difficulty [11] delayed skin barrier recovery. Thus, the stress in daily life affects the body and the skin, even in systems where the experimental conditions are not strictly controlled. Even in the pre-disease stage, changes in the body condition are thought to be reflected in the skin condition from an early stage, and the skin is like a mirror that reflects the body condition.

In this chapter, I introduce our application of Raman microscopies for skin evaluation, as well as include the research trends in skin measurements. Specifically, spontaneous Raman scattering microscopy that is applied to *in vivo* skin measurements and coherent Raman scattering microscopy that enables high-speed imaging are described in evaluating skin major components such as water, proteins, and lipids [12].

5.2 Skin

5.2.1 *Structure and Function of Skin*

Skin is the largest organ in the body and acts as a protective barrier, separating the body from the outside environment [13]. Epidermis, dermis, and subcutaneous fat form an integrated structure with skin appendages, sweat glands, sebaceous glands, and hair follicles [14]. The foremost physical barrier of the skin is the outermost epidermis, which comprises the stratum corneum with its brick and mortar-like structure and tight junctions that regulate the passage of fluid and electrolytes in and out of the skin [13, 15]. The skin has developed complex protective functions against constant exposure to various environmental stresses such as solar radiation, pollutants, bacteria, viruses, and allergens [16, 17]. The immune system contributes to this first line of defense against external foreign matter [14].

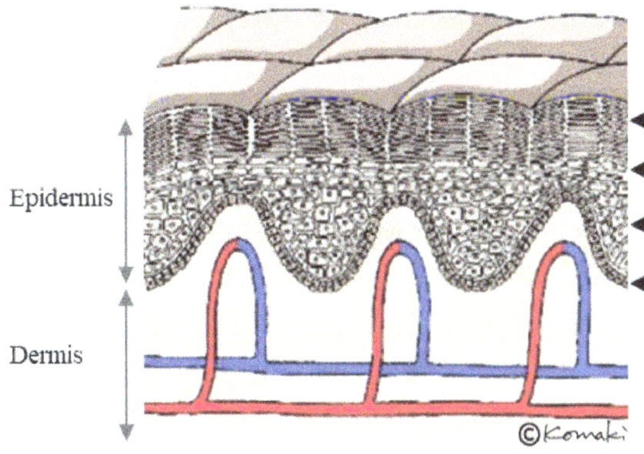

Figure 5.1. Image of the vertical structure of human skin.

The skin is classified into three layers; from top to bottom, the epidermis, dermis, and subcutaneous layers [18]. The epidermis is most important because of its barrier function. The epidermis has four distinct sub-layers; from outer to inner, the stratum corneum, stratum granulosum, stratum spinosum, and stratum basale (Figure 5.1). Epidermal differentiation is particularly important in the dermatology and cosmetology fields because it is considered to be related to the condition of the skin [19]. Specifically, smooth enucleation in the upper part of the epidermis results in the generation of a healthy and strong stratum corneum that maintains the skin's proper protective barrier function. Dermatological studies using immunostaining with fluorescent dyes or proteins have had limited success in revealing skin functions as these methods are known to affect the main components of the epidermis, including the water, lipids, and proteins.

In dermatology, histological methods, such as electron microscopy [20] and immunostaining [21], are widely used to elucidate the properties of the epidermis. However, conventional histological methods require chemical pretreatment processes, such as slicing, fixation, and labeling, which change the morphology and function of the skin. Because chemical treatment has a large effect on proteins and lipids, and water cannot be fixed, what is observed as a stained image is thought to be different than the actual *in vivo* skin. In addition, the labeling of proteins at the genetic level cannot be applied experimentally *in vivo* in humans. With these limitations, it is impossible to observe the condition of skin as it is *in vivo* in humans.

5.2.2 Non-invasive Measurement of Skin

Light generally refers to electromagnetic waves with wavelengths from 1 nm to 1 mm, and it is classified into ultraviolet, visible, and infrared rays according to the wavelength band (Figure 5.2) [22]. Spectroscopy is a technique that treats the spectrum of light that is transmitted, reflected, and absorbed by a substance by dividing it into wavelengths or frequencies. It is a useful technique for identifying and understanding the molecular structure of the constituents invisible to the human eye, and is an indispensable analytical method in basic research and many fields such as materials and life science. Furthermore, in the industrial field, analytical techniques based on spectroscopy are playing an active role in many industries, such as semiconductors, electronic equipment, food, pharmaceuticals, cosmetics, medical, and energy, helping to improve the quality of life.

Recent progress in optical imaging techniques, such as confocal microscopy [23] and optical coherence tomography [24], enable the evaluation of the skin structure *in vivo*. However, it remains difficult to identify individual skin components using the above optical methods because they detect the morphological differences in the refractive index at the cell boundary.

Alternatively, molecular vibrational signatures can be obtained using spectroscopic techniques such as Raman scattering microscopy. The most advantageous characteristic of non-labeling and non-invasive spectroscopic techniques is that they can detect the skin condition in humans *in vivo* and *ex vivo*. In addition, it is a time-lapse measurement. Among the components of skin, water is a very suitable target for spectroscopic measurement. The amount of water in the skin changes when the skin is removed from the body because water is continuously supplied from the inside of the skin. Therefore,

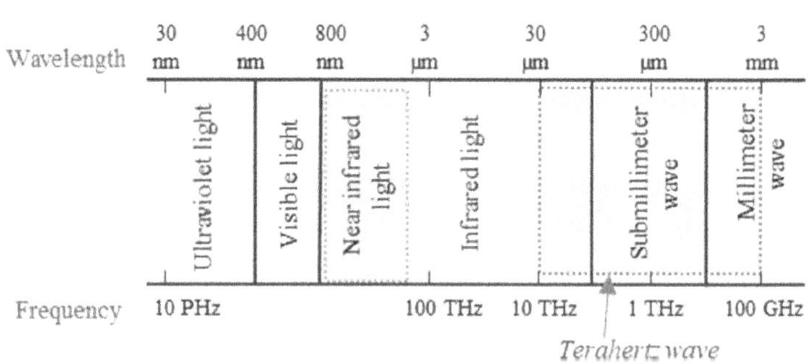

Figure 5.2. Types of electromagnetic waves. Reproduced from Ref. [22] with permission.

water is a measurement target that can make the most of the merits of non-invasive spectroscopy. Regarding proteins and lipids in the skin, even if there are difficulties in identifying their type using spectroscopy, non-invasive spectroscopy can be applied to visualize their morphology with molecular vibrational signatures. As a result, their detected changes could allow for Raman spectroscopy to be used in the medical and industrial fields.

5.3 Spontaneous Raman Scattering Microscopy

5.3.1 *In Vivo Human Skin Measurement*

Spontaneous Raman scattering spectroscopy is a useful technique that enables molecular sensing of skin components without a chemical pretreatment process. The spontaneous Raman spectra of human skin measured *in vivo*, especially in a high wavenumber region targeting water, was reported in 2000 by Puppels *et al.* [25]. In 2001, the same group reported a calculation algorithm of the depth distribution of components, including water, lipids, and amino acids [26], for wide use in dermatology and cosmetology.

Figures 5.3 and 5.4 respectively show the spontaneous Raman scattering spectra of the high wavenumber region and fingerprint region measured by

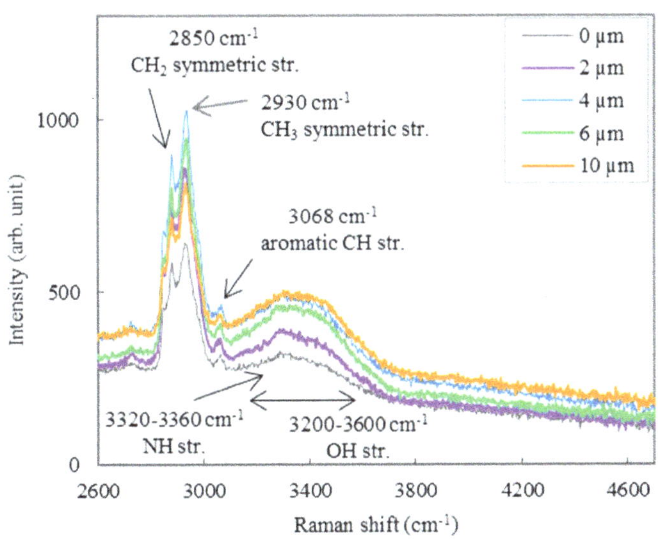

Figure 5.3. Spontaneous Raman scattering spectra of human skin in the high wavenumber region. The spectra are obtained at different depths in the skin: 0 to 10 μm from the skin surface. Reproduced from Ref. [12] with permission.

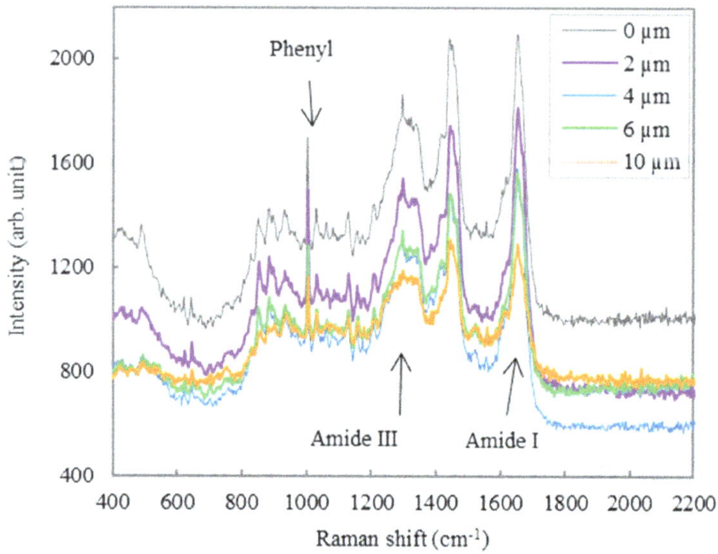

Figure 5.4. Spontaneous Raman scattering spectra of human skin in the fingerprint region. The spectra are obtained at different depths in the skin: 0 to 10 μm from the skin surface. Reproduced from Ref. [12] with permission.

backscattered light of human skin *in vivo* at depths of 0–10 μm from the skin's surface with the auto-fluorescence offset. As the skin is a highly scattering material, accurate quantification of a component cannot be determined without considering the attenuation of the irradiating and scattered light in the skin. Therefore, in conventional biochemical methods, component quantification is often calculated as a relative amount per unit protein. The calculation in spontaneous Raman scattering spectroscopy according to the relative amount of the CH_3 band (mainly protein) of 2930 cm^{-1} can also be used for consideration with biochemical methods. The calibration formula [26], obtained by dividing the OH band of 3350–3550 cm^{-1} by the CH_3 band of 2910–2965 cm^{-1} in the high frequency region and multiplying it by a coefficient, is still commonly used to calculate the water content of the skin in dermatology and cosmetology. For the semi-quantitative analysis of lipids and free amino acids, the particular band of the functional group of each skin component in the fingerprint region is calculated using a fitting model as a relative amount to the amide I band at 1650 cm^{-1} or the entire spectrum of keratin [26].

Note that even though the irradiating laser is near-infrared, the signal/noise ratio (S/N) of the fingerprint spectrum is often poor because autofluorescence from the skin contributes to interference. Thus, the measurement time for a fingerprint region spectrum is usually longer than that for a high wavenumber region to obtain a high S/N. Especially during *in vivo* skin measurements, there are many factors affecting the variability of the obtained data, such as multidirectional movements of the measurement area because of the heartbeat, breathing, posture, and blinking. Additionally, there are selection criteria for the measurement spots, variations between subjects, parts of the body, amount of melanin pigment, plane location of skin microstructures, and influence of contact measurement. Furthermore, results with inappropriate data would result in misinterpretation. Therefore, it is important to acquire the data by devising ways to control these variations during measurement.

5.3.2 *In Vivo* Water and Water-binding Component Evaluation

There are various studies [27–29] reporting the depth distribution of skin components using spontaneous Raman scattering microscopy *in vivo* with the algorithm proposed by Caspers and Puppels *et al.* We have also reported results on the depth distribution of skin components in the stratum corneum obtained *in vivo*, especially targeting water and water-related components [30–32]. Specifically, we measured the site difference in the water depth distribution from the skin surface (Figure 5.5) [30] and the change in the water depth distribution in the skin after applying water to the skin surface using cotton (Figure 5.6) [31]. Regarding the water depth distribution in each part of the body, Figure 5.5 shows the flexion side of the forearm and the palm as examples [30]. Each individual plot in the graph shows the individual data of 15 subjects. We were unable to fully control skin fixation and it took a long time to start

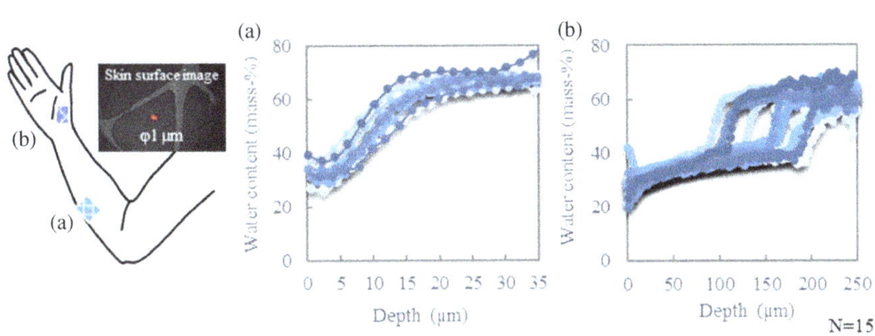

Figure 5.5. Regional difference in the depth distribution of water content. The Raman spectra at 1 μm diameter spot were obtained at (a) forearm and (b) palm (base of the thumb) from 15 subjects, and water content in the skin was calculated by dividing the OH band of 3350–3550 cm^{-1} by the CH_3 band of 2910–2965 cm^{-1} using the calibration formula shown in [26]. Reproduced from Ref. [30] with permission.

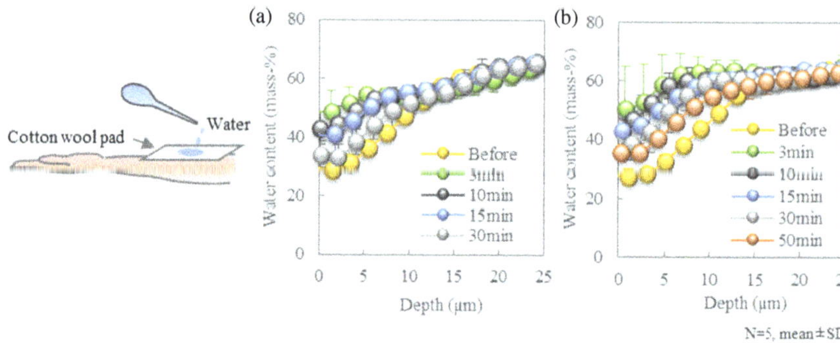

Figure 5.6. Differences in the depth distribution of water content in the forearm skin before and after the forced hydration procedure with water-soaked cotton wool for (a) 50 min and (b) 90 min. Raman spectra of the skin were obtained before and 3, 10, 15, 30, and 50 min after the hydration procedure. Reproduced from Ref. [31] with permission.

measurement; as a result, increasing water was observed near the skin surface. The water content of the skin was 20 to 30 mass-% at the skin surface, and the content gradually increased with depth. The water content was approximately 65 to 70 mass-% in the viable epidermal layer from the granular layer to the basal layer. The depth distribution pattern of water differed in the stratum corneum according to location such as thin at the forearm (Figure 5.5(a)) and upper arm, and thick at the palm (Figure 5.5(b)) and heel. In the middle of the thick stratum corneum, there was a region where the gradient of water content was low. Notably, individual differences in the depth distribution of water content and differences within the body may affect the variation in the absorption coefficient of the skin, which is a prerequisite for other optical measurements.

Furthermore, when water was applied from the skin surface, it had more difficulty entering the inner part of the stratum corneum than previously expected. Figure 5.6 shows the changes in the depth distribution of water content when water was applied with occlusion for 50 min and 90 min [31]. Each plot in the graph is the elapsed time after the skin was exposed to air after the water application, before, and 3–50 min after. The water content slightly increased in the upper part of the stratum corneum with the 15-min water application (data not shown here [31]). Alternatively, with a 50-min application (Figure 5.6(a)), an increase in water content was observed up to a depth of 12 μm, which corresponds to the first inflection point of the water distribution curve. The point is suggested to be the bottom of the stratum corneum layer, which is clarified by comparing the depth distribution of amino acids contained only in the stratum corneum with the amount of

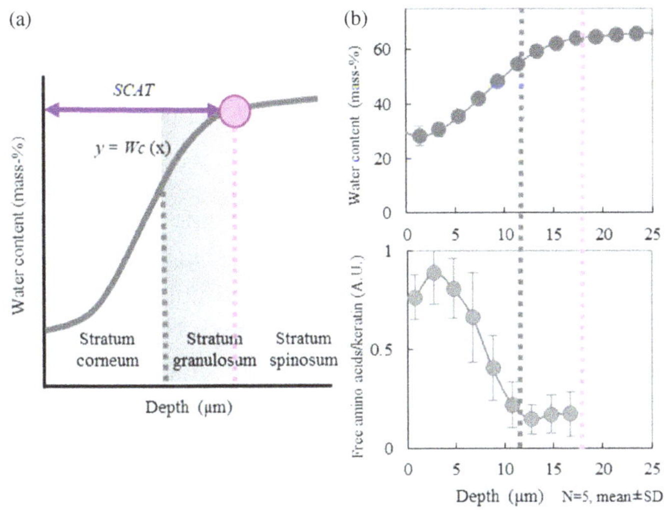

Figure 5.7. Definition of stratum corneum apparent thickness (SCAT). (a) Definition of SCAT, (b) depth distribution of water and free amino acid content calculated according to the method of Caspers *et al.* [26] in forearms of five female subjects in their 20s and 30s.

water [26, 30, 31]. Interestingly, water applied from the outside did not enter the stratum granulosum located just below the stratum corneum considering its strong barrier function [33, 34]; however, water did reach the stratum granulosum at around a depth of 20 μm, where the distribution curve of the water content levelled (Figure 5.6(b)). The depth at which the slope of the water content becomes flat is considered to be the region at or below the stratum granulosum on the basis of other research comparing the distribution curve of water with the morphology of the same measurement spot using confocal microscopy [35]. Our report was the first showing the possibility of water permeation to the living cell layer in the epidermis *in vivo*.

Moreover, using the depth distribution curve of water content, we defined the depth at which the increase in water content reached a plateau as the stratum corneum apparent thickness (SCAT) (Figure 5.7(a)) including viable cell layers, such as the granular layer and stratum corneum, for a simple comparison index for stratum corneum thickness in human studies. Compared with the depth distribution of amino acids measured at the same time (Figure 5.7(b)), the change in water depth distribution after applying water (Figure 5.6), and the result of the same field of view measurement by combining confocal microscopy and confocal Raman spectrometry [35], the true stratum corneum is presumed to be the inflection point during the increase before the curve reaches a constant. However, the calculation of this inflection point may not be possible because of the movement of the subject during measurement; therefore, we proposed SCAT for practical use.

5.3.3 *In Vivo* Skin Disease Evaluation

In vivo evaluation of skin components using spontaneous Raman microscopy has also introduced the possibility of evaluating skin diseases, such as atopic dermatitis [36–39] and skin cancer [40], taking advantage of the non-invasive measurement. In particular, Raman microscopy is used for researching differences in water content depending on the atopic dermatitis severity because it affects the water content of the skin.

We have evaluated the characteristics of psoriatic skin using Raman spectroscopy [41]. Psoriasis is a chronic, immuno-inflammatory disorder characterized by acanthosis with disturbed keratinocyte differentiation. We compared the depth distribution of water and water-related components. Figure 5.8 shows the depth distribution of the water content in the areas affected and unaffected by psoriasis. The water content was lower in the affected areas than the unaffected areas, especially in the high severity score group. Including other skin components, changes in the distribution of each component were observed depending on the differences in the

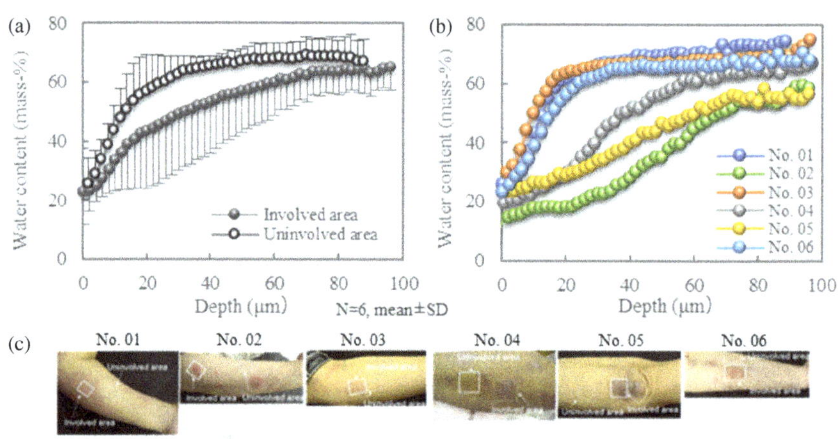

Figure 5.8. Depth distribution of water content in the affected and unaffected areas of psoriasis skin. (a) Mean plot, (b) individual subject plot, and (c) photographs of the measurement areas. Affected areas were defined as lesions in the active phase and unaffected areas were apparently healthy-looking skin near the affected areas. The water content was less in the affected area than in the unaffected areas, especially in the high severity score group. Reproduced from Ref. [41] with permission.

dermatologist's severity score. The clinical use of Raman spectroscopy for psoriasis evaluation will increase if a less expensive and easier-to-operate microscope is developed.

5.3.4 *In Vivo Ultraviolet Light Damage Evaluation*

By evaluating the fingerprint area, spontaneous Raman microscopy can also be applied to the change in the epidermis composition because of the influence of the external environment. We applied spontaneous Raman microscopy to evaluate ultraviolet (UV) light damage to skin by calculating the amount of *cis*- and *trans*-urocanic acid (Figure 5.9) in the stratum corneum [42, 43].

Urocanic acid [44] is a major component in the epidermis that absorbs UV and is isomerized from the *trans* to the *cis* form upon UV exposure. Figure 5.10 shows the average amounts of (a) *cis*- and (b) *trans*-urocanic acid in the stratum corneum of the volar forearms of 10 healthy Japanese subjects before and after UV exposure without and with sunscreen, and without UV exposure with sunscreen. Our approach showed that the concentrations of *cis*- and *trans*-urocanic acid could be measured at the same time *in vivo*,

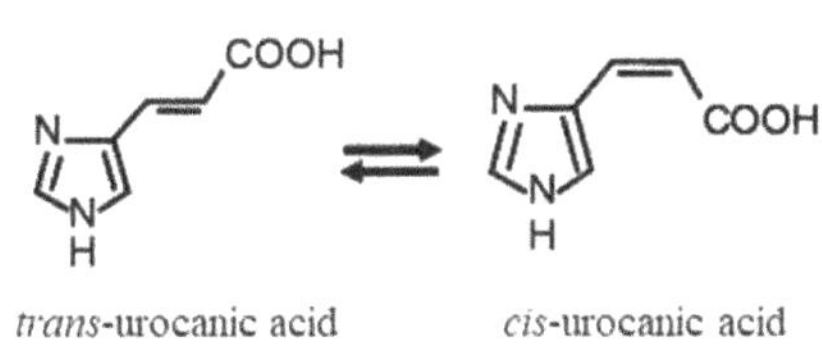

Figure 5.9. The structures of urocanic acid isomers. Reproduced from Ref. [43] with permission.

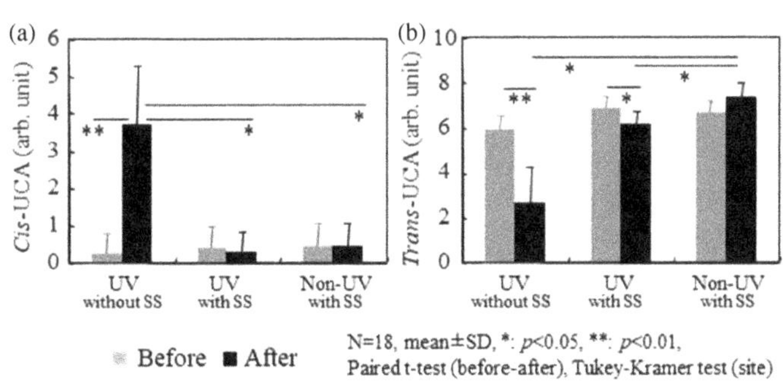

Figure 5.10. The average amount of (a) *cis*- and (b) *trans*-urocanic acid (UCA) between 0 and 12 μm in the stratum corneum, before and after UV exposure without and with sunscreen (SS), and without UV exposure with SS. Reproduced from Ref. [43] with permission.

and the protective capacity of sunscreen could be evaluated by monitoring the amount of urocanic acid isomers, even at sub-erythemal doses of UV light.

5.3.5 *In Vivo* Transdermal Absorption Evaluation

Spontaneous Raman microscopy is also an attractive technique for evaluating the behavior of transdermal absorption of external agents *in vivo*. Therefore, spontaneous Raman microscopy has been used as an evaluation method in drug delivery research [45–54]. We also demonstrated that the depth distribution of the two forms of urea in skin could be monitored *in vivo* [55]. Because urea is a natural moisturizing factor in the stratum corneum, it has been used in topical moisturizing products to improve the skin's condition. Figure 5.11 shows typical Raman spectra of the skin before and after the application of two creams containing urea to volar forearm skin. The characteristic band of urea in a water solution was observed at 1004 cm^{-1} and that of the solid state at 1010 cm^{-1} after application of either cream. Spontaneous Raman microscopy would be useful in evaluating the characteristics of the penetration behavior of urea in the skin *in vivo* (Figure 5.12). However, because the detection sensitivity is greater when a large amount of skin is collected by tape stripping or similar, the use of spontaneous Raman microscopy is limited to practical evaluations of transdermal absorption.

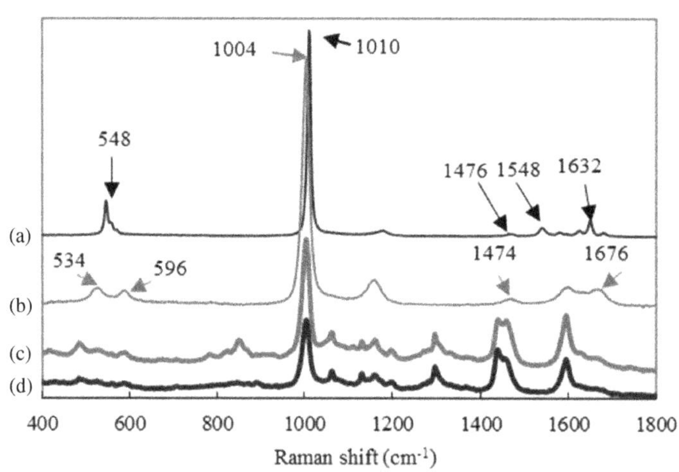

Figure 5.11. Raman spectra of urea and urea-containing cream. (a) Urea in solid type, (b) urea in soluble type, (c) cream formulation R, and (d) cream formulation F. Reproduced from Ref. [55] with permission.

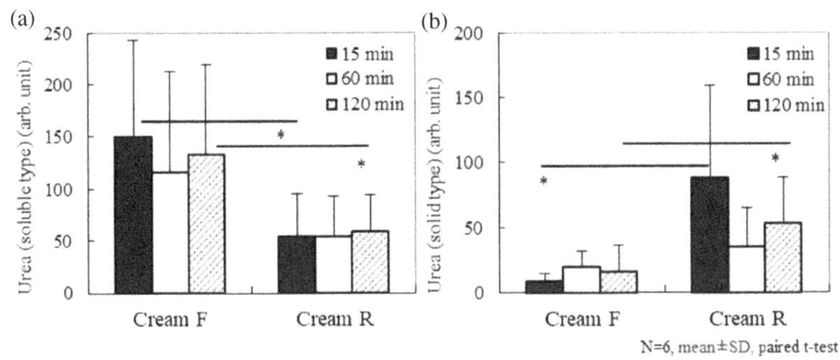

Figure 5.12. Comparison of urea penetration amount into stratum corneum, 0 to 12 μm from the skin surface. (a) Urea in soluble type and (b) urea in solid type. Each bar shows 15, 60, and 120 min after application of urea-containing moisturizing cream formulation F and R. Reproduced from Ref. [55] with permission.

5.3.6 *Further Perspectives*

Another issue in skin measurements with spontaneous Raman scattering microscopy is the high level of scattering at the stratum corneum. Autofluorescence from substances in the skin and absorbed dyes also influence the evaluation. Therefore, evaluations up to a depth of approximately 100 μm are the practical limit when measuring the skin in a confocal system using a light intensity that does not adversely affect the skin. Furthermore, because it takes approximately 1–20 s per spectrum to obtain a Raman spectrum with high S/N *in vivo*, molecular imaging of the skin using spontaneous Raman scattering microscopy has been limited.

Raman imaging with line lighting [56] and light sheet direct Raman imaging [57] have been reported in areas not specializing in skin measurement. For skin measurement, it is necessary to select an excitation laser whose Raman spectra are less affected by autofluorescence of the skin and to modify the attachment for contact with the skin. These Raman imaging methods have great potential in skin research in the near future. Development of a handheld probe aimed at wide application to human measurements has also been reported [58]. However, spontaneous Raman currently requires long acquisition times and is rarely applied to skin imaging, especially *in vivo*. Therefore, other techniques with shorter measurement times are required to obtain 2D and 3D molecular imaging of the various functional groups of molecules in the skin.

5.4 Coherent Raman Scattering Microscopy

5.4.1 *Molecular Imaging of Skin*

Coherent Raman scattering microscopy is a possible option for molecular imaging of skin because it enables faster measurement than spontaneous Raman scattering microscopy. Coherent anti-Stokes Raman scattering (CARS) microscopy and stimulated Raman scattering (SRS) microscopy may be used for non-labeling measurements of *in vivo* human skin.

In 2005, the application of coherent Raman to skin measurements on the CH_2 band of lipids at 2845 cm^{-1} in mouse skin *in vivo* using CARS microscopy was reported by Xie *et al.* [59]. Molecular imaging of the 2120 cm^{-1} band unique to dimethylsulfoxide applied to the skin surface was also reported [60]. Furthermore, in 2014, clear molecular images of the CD band of d_{34}-oleic acid at 2105 cm^{-1}, the CH_2 band of lipids at 2850 cm^{-1}, the CH_3 band of proteins at 2950 cm^{-1}, and the OH band of water at 3340 cm^{-1} in pig skin were reported using SRS microscopy [61]. Given the high-speed imaging by coherent Raman microscopy, such as CARS and SRS, its application has been used for the measurement of transdermal absorption materials applied to the skin surface using *ex vivo* skin or a 3D skin tissue model [62–66]. Research on the discrimination of cancer cells has also been performed as an example of use in the medical field [67, 68].

5.4.2 *Ex Vivo Molecular Imaging of the High Wavenumber Region of Human Skin Using SRS Microscopy*

We applied SRS microscopy to visualize changes in the intracellular morphology during the epidermal differentiation process in each of the four layers of the epidermis, not just the outermost stratum corneum, by focusing on skin components such as proteins and lipids. In 2012, Ozeki *et al.* showed SRS imaging of the sebaceous glands of mice ears *in vivo* using forward-scattering SRS microscopy [69]. We visualized changes in the intracellular morphology of the human epidermis by molecular imaging over the wavenumber range of 2800 cm^{-1} to 3100 cm^{-1} corresponding to the CH stretching region [70, 71], using the optical system [72]. As shown in Figure 5.13, characteristic bands related to lipids were observed near 2850 cm^{-1} and 2880 cm^{-1} only in the stratum corneum where intercellular lipids exist by comparing the SRS spectra in each layer of the epidermis. Figure 5.14 shows an example of spectroscopic

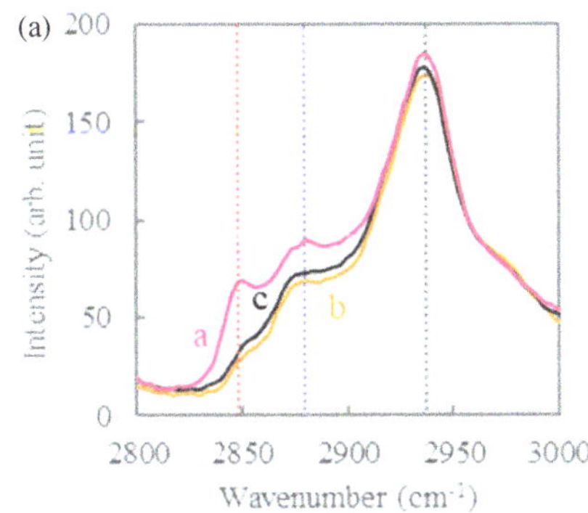

Figure 5.13. The high wavenumber region spectra at each epidermal layer of the abdominal skin of a 64-year-old Caucasian female. (a) SRS spectra, (b) spectrum acquisition position in the protein image at 2930 cm^{-1}. Reproduced from Ref. [71] with permission.

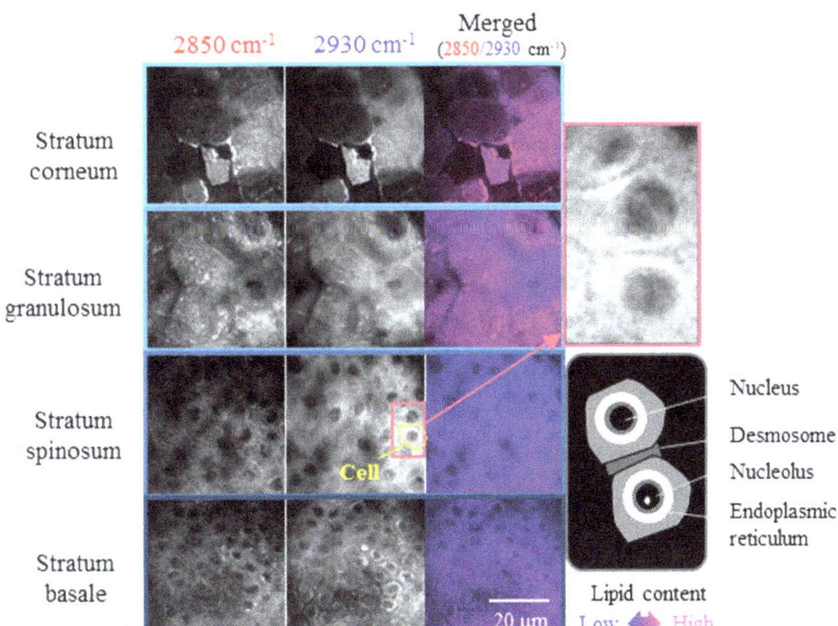

Figure 5.14. Typical SRS spectral image of each epidermal layer. Reproduced from Ref. [71], public domain.

images of the CH_3 band at 2930 cm^{-1} and CH_2 band at 2850 cm^{-1} acquired at 1 μm intervals in the depth direction of the four epidermal layers [71]. The greater the brightness value (white color in the image), the greater the amount of each component. We clarified and visualized intracellular morphologies

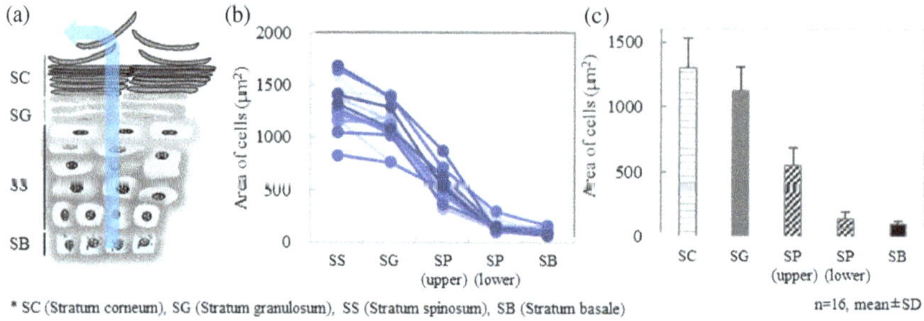

Figure 5.15. Changes in keratinocyte size during differentiation. (a) Structure of epidermis, (b) average area of keratinocyte in each epidermal layer, and (c) individual data of (b). Reproduced from Ref. [71], public domain.

such as intracellular nuclei and cell-to-cell adhesive desmosomes. In addition, the characteristics of the intracellular morphology of each layer, such as the nucleoli observed only in the 2930 cm^{-1} (mainly reflects protein) image, granular structures in the stratum granulosum observed only in the 2850 cm^{-1} (mainly reflects lipid) image, and differences in the thickness of each layer using merged images of protein and lipids, were evaluated.

From both the 2930 cm^{-1} (mainly reflects protein) band and 2850 cm^{-1} (mainly reflects lipid) band images, the size of the epidermal cells were approximately 10 times larger from the stratum basale to the stratum corneum during epidermal differentiation (Figure 5.15).

Thus, we showed that SRS microscopy made it possible to non-invasively visualize changes in the intracellular morphology with skin component information during the epidermal differentiation process, which is important in dermatological research. This achievement is because nonlinear spectroscopic techniques enable high-speed measurements without fixing or labeling, which was not previously achievable using conventional histological methods.

Another advantage of nonlinear spectroscopic techniques is the ability to obtain time-lapse images of the components without damaging the tissue. It has been difficult to observe time-dependent changes in the distribution of components in skin tissue using histological techniques. Nonlinear Raman spectroscopy made it possible. Figure 5.16 shows an example of changes in intracellular morphology during the enucleation process in the epidermis from the spinous layer to the granular layer [71]. The greater the brightness value, the greater the amount of each component. Specifically, after obtaining

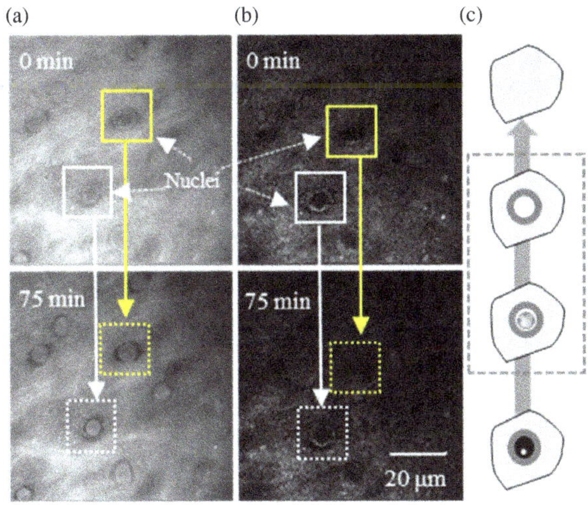

Figure 5.16. Time-lapse SRS spectral image of abdominal skin of a 49-year-old female subject. (a) 2930 cm^{-1}, (b) 2850 cm^{-1}, and (c) expected image of the enucleation process. The images in the top row show the initial observation and the images in the bottom row show the skin 75 min later. Reproduced from Ref. [71], public domain.

the initial image, the skin was maintained for 75 min, and the same area was observed again at 2930 cm^{-1} (Figure 5.16(a)) and 2850 cm^{-1} (Figure 5.16(b)). Different changes in intracellular morphology near the nucleus were observed. Specifically, there was a white circular area with a high brightness value in the cell nucleus after only 75 min in the protein image at 2930 cm^{-1}, as shown in the square areas in Figure 5.16. In dermatology, the type of changes cell nuclei undergo during the enucleation process when they eventually disappear have not been clarified. Our time-lapse observation acquired without fixing or staining using spectroscopy indicates the potential of nonlinear Raman microscopy in dermatological research. Continuous spectroscopic images in the depth direction could detect changes in the nucleus in the enucleation process at the upper part of the stratum corneum.

We also observed holes in the SC in horizontal cross-section images, whereby the intensity at both 2850 cm^{-1} and 2930 cm^{-1} was quite low (Figure 5.17). Our observations suggest that the nuclear membrane would remain intact, such that keratin fibres did not fill the inside remnant of the nuclear membrane, thus leaving a distinct hole after digestion of the nucleus. These information can be applied to clarify which differentiation processes are important in forming healthy skin with a strong barrier function.

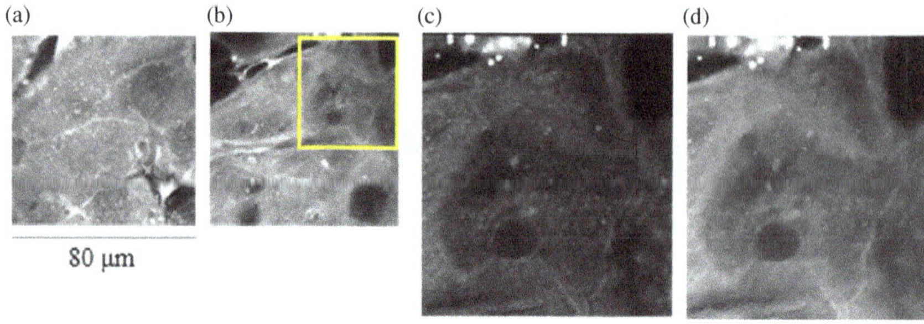

Figure 5.17. Existence of holes in the stratum corneum of abdominal skin of a 31-year-old female subject. SRS images of upper part of the stratum corneum (a) without, (b) with the halls at 2930 cm^{-1}, and (c) spectroscopic image of yellow square area in (b) at 2850 cm^{-1} and (d) at 2930 cm^{-1} of abdomen from a 31-year-old female subject. Reproduced from Ref. [71], public domain.

5.4.3 *Ex Vivo Molecular Imaging of the Fingerprint Region of Human Skin Using CARS Microscopy*

We are also conducting molecular imaging of the fingerprint region using CARS microscopy [73], and have studied human hair [74]. Hair is an appendage of the skin, and analysis of the properties of the hair shaft leads to consideration of the properties of the stratum corneum in the epidermis because both are end products of differentiation and do not contain living cells. Intra-medulla lipids were clearly visualized by CARS spectroscopic imaging. Two groups of intra-medulla lipids were found, active and inactive second harmonic generation (SHG), and the two groups were identified as free fatty acids and wax esters, respectively.

Furthermore, CARS spectroscopic imaging was used to visualize the distribution of water concentration in human skin *ex vivo* [75]. The CARS signal of the OH stretching vibrational mode of water was found to coexist with the signal of intercellular lipids, such as ceramides, which were visualized by a sharp vibrational band at 2882 cm^{-1} (Figure 5.18). These findings demonstrate the powerful potential of CARS spectroscopic imaging for probing pathological changes caused by anomalous water concentration distribution in human skin.

Currently, in molecular imaging at the practical level, SRS is capable of high-speed, three-dimensional molecular imaging; however, it is limited to imaging in the high wavenumber region. Alternatively, CARS does not have enough measurement speed for time-lapse measurements; however, it can measure the entire Raman shift. Therefore, complementing and using both methods would be the fastest way to apply them in life science research.

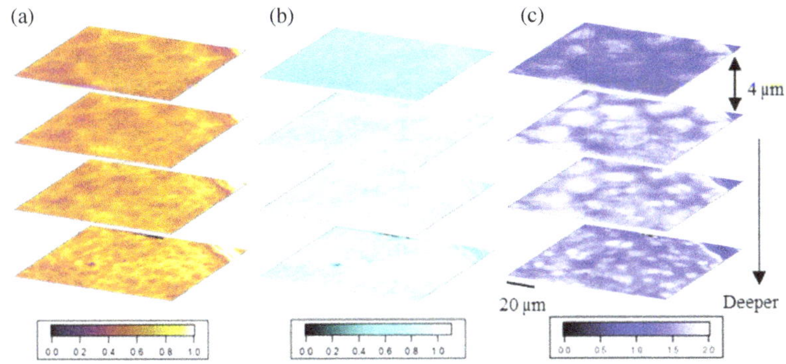

Figure 5.18. Depth-resolved water imaging of skin using CARS. CARS images of upper part of epidermis at (a) 2930 cm^{-1}, (b) 3476 cm^{-1}, and (c) 3476 cm^{-1}/2930 cm^{-1}. Reproduced from Ref. [75] with permission.

5.4.4 *In Vivo Molecular Imaging of Human Skin*

We can visualize, non-invasively and at high speed, changes in intracellular morphology containing component information, such as protein, lipids, and water, during the epidermal differentiation process, which is expected to be used in the field of dermatology via SRS and CARS microscopy. Application to *in vivo* human skin measurements has been reported from other research groups, although the measurement conditions are limited.

Molecular imaging of the CH_3 band at 2950 cm^{-1} of proteins and the CH_2 band at 2845 cm^{-1} of lipids in the human stratum corneum *in vivo* using SRS microscopy were reported in 2010 [76]. In 2011 and 2012, two-photon fluorescence imaging and CARS imaging of the CH_2 band of lipids at 2845 cm^{-1} in healthy and psoriatic skin *in vivo*, and water imaging of the OH band at 3295 cm^{-1}, were reported by König *et al.* [77–79]. In 2019, Sarri *et al.* reported the *in vivo* CARS imaging of transdermal absorption into the stratum corneum using a glycerol-specific band at 2100 cm^{-1} [80]. Thus, there has been *in vivo* skin research by multiple groups using SRS and CARS microscopy. However, the measurable depth for *in vivo* human skin measurements was near the skin surface, mainly in the stratum corneum.

5.4.5 *Further Perspectives*

The advantage of SRS and CARS compared with spontaneous Raman is high-speed measurements, which are very important for *in vivo*/*ex vivo* measurements of biological samples, such as skin, whose conditions change from moment to moment. Furthermore, if the final target is *in vivo* human measurement, imaging in the shortest possible time is a top priority because humans cannot stop moving for long. In this respect, coherent Raman has an advantage over spontaneous Raman. However, it is not sufficient for *in vivo* measurement in terms of the strong light intensity at the sample point, spectrum accuracy, and the narrowness of the measurable wavenumber region. With current back-scattering coherent Raman scattering microscopy for skin measurement, molecular vibrational images up to approximately 100 μm are attainable [81]. The depth is similar to that of spontaneous Raman scattering microscopy, although it depends on the intensity of the skin's autofluorescence. To extend the measurement depth while maintaining a weak light intensity at the sample point, it is necessary to increase the efficiency of light to the detector or improve the sensitivity of the detector. Furthermore, miniaturization is important for practical use of coherent Raman in the healthcare fields, and the development of handheld SRS microscopes for *in vivo* skin measurements had been reported [82, 83]. Even if current applications of coherent Raman scattering microscopy to *in vivo* measurements remain limited, the possibility of skin spectral imaging *in vivo* is expected to contribute to healthcare fields.

5.5 Conclusion

In this chapter, the application of Raman microscopy to health science, especially skin measurements, was introduced. As *in vivo* measurement in humans is often the final target for skin analysis, non-invasive, high-speed and highly sensitive techniques are required, and thus Raman spectroscopy has been rapidly used in skin research [84]. Because the skin is a layered, heterogeneous, and highly scattering organ, it is difficult to make a quantitative comparison between data at different positions in the depth direction without correcting for changes in light intensity. Therefore, relative amounts with keratin proteins are suitable for quantitative comparison with the precondition that the protein is homogeneous in the depth direction of each layer of the skin.

Furthermore, because of recent advances in optical techniques, the target has changed from numerical measurement at one point to 2D or 3D imaging. Even in the evaluation of skin components using spectroscopy, the needs have changed from simple spectral measurement to component imaging. Our results using coherent Raman scattering microscopy show the potential of Raman microscopy in the field of health science. The components in the skin that can be measured by Raman cannot always be measured by conventional histological methods used in biology, i.e., there is sometimes no previous comparison data for water, protein, and lipid content in human skin *in situ*. Therefore, validating the obtained data should be performed by observing the changing behaviors of the skin, such as site differences, age differences, environmental changes, and time-lapse measurements, to check whether the changed behavior is appropriate compared with established dermatology knowledge.

Some Raman instruments targeting *in vivo* human skin are already commercially available, such as gen2-SCA (RiverD International B.V., Rotterdam, the Netherlands) [25, 26] and MPTflex-CARS (JenLab GmbH, Berlin, Germany) [79]. However, spectroscopy has not been widely used in practical fields, such as health science, compared with confocal microscopy [23] and optical coherence tomography [24]. In addition to the commercially available instruments described above, it will be important to provide algorithms that calculate the evaluation components. The advantages of each Raman microscopy should be maximized depending on whether spectrum accuracy is needed for quantitative evaluation or measurement speed for imaging.

Furthermore, measurement of changes in skin conditions because of diseases of organs other than skin or the state of the whole body have been reported recently as a medical application of Raman spectroscopy [85–88]. These are attempts to perceive the skin as a sensor that indicates the state of the whole body, and show the possibility of using the skin as a sensor for disease detection in daily life.

Raman spectroscopy has the advantage of being able to specify functional groups and estimate the components, as well as being able to acquire the data in three dimensions non-invasively and without labeling. In research using Raman spectroscopy, the target is the evaluation of skin properties and application to the evaluation of the whole-body condition through the skin. In the future, Raman spectroscopy will become a more useful measurement method for healthcare science and human society.

References

1. https://www.who.int/data/gho/data/major-themes/health-and-well-being.
2. Ortiz, A. and Grando, S. A. (2012) Smoking and the skin. Int. J. Dermatol. **51**(3), 250–262.
3. Bensadoun, R. J., Humbert, P., Krutman, J., Luger, T., Triller, R., Rougier, A., Seite, S. and Dreno, B. (2013) Daily baseline skin care in the prevention, treatment, and supportive care of skin toxicity in oncology patients: recommendations from a multinational expert panel. Cancer Manag. Res. **5**, 401–408.
4. Altemus, M., Rao, B., Dhabhar, F. S., Ding, W. and Granstein, R. D. (2001) Stress-induced changes in skin barrier function in healthy women. J. Invest. Dermatol. **117**, 309–317.
5. Chrousos, G. P. (2009) Stress and disorders of the stress system. Nat. Rev. Endocrinol. **5**, 374–381.
6. González-Cabrera, C., Fernández-Prada, M., Iribar-Irabe, C. and Peinado, M. (2014) Acute and chronic stress increase salivary cortisol: A study in the real-life setting of a national examination undertaken by medical graduates. Stress **17**(2), 149–156.
7. Kirschbaum, C., Pirke, K. M. and Hellhammer, D. H. (1993) The 'Trier Social Stress Test'--a tool for investigating psychobiological stress responses in a laboratory setting. Neuropsychobiology **28**(1–2), 76–81.
8. Hosoi, J., Tanida, M. and Tsuchiya, T. (2001) Mitigation of stress-induced suppression of contact hypersensitivity by odorant inhalation. Br. J. Dermatol. **145**, 716–719.
9. Chen, Y. and Lyga, J. (2014) Brain–skin connection: Stress, inflammation and skin aging. Inflamm. Allergy Drug Targets **13**(3), 177–190.
10. Garg, A., Chren, M. M., Sands, L. P., Matsui, M. S., Marenus, K. D., Feingold, K. R. and Elias, P. M. (2001) Psychological stress perturbs epidermal permeability barrier homeostasis: Implications for the pathogenesis of stress-associated skin disorders. Arch. Dermatol. **37**(1), 53–59.
11. Muizzuddin, N., Matsui, M. S., Marenus, K.D. and Maes, D. H. (2003) Impact of stress of marital dissolution on skin barrier recovery: Tape stripping and measurement of trans-epidermal water loss (TEWL). Skin Res. Technol. **9**(1), 34–38.
12. Egawa, M. (2021) Raman microscopy for skin evaluation. Analyst **146**, 1142–1150.
13. Elias, P. M. (2005) Stratum corneum defensive functions: An integrated view. J. Invest. Dermatol. **125**(2) PP. 183–200.
14. Kabashima, K., Honda, T., Ginhoux, F. and Egawa, G. (2019) The immunological anatomy of the skin. Nat. Rev. Immunol. **19**(1), 19–30.
15. Simpson, C. L., Patel, D. M. and Green, K. J. (2011) Deconstructing the skin: Cytoarchitectural determinants of epidermal morphogenesis. Nat. Rev. Mol. Cell. Biol. **12**(9), 565–580.

16. Suwanpradid, J., Holcomb, Z. E. and MacLeod, A. S. (2017) Emerging skin T-Cell functions in response to environmental insults. J. Invest. Dermatol. **137**(2), 288–294.
17. Suzuki, T., Hidaka, T., Kumagai, Y. and Yamamoto, M. (2020) Environmental pollutants and the immune response. Nat. Immunol. **21**(12), 1486–1495.
18. Griffiths, C., Barker, J., Bleiker, T., Chalmers, R. and Creamer, D. (2016) *Rook's Textbook of Dermatology* 9th ed, John Wiley & Sons.
19. Rawlings, A. V. (2014) Molecular basis for stratum corneum maturation and moisturization. Br. J. Dermatol. **171**(S3), 19–28.
20. Yamanishi, H., Soma, T., Kishimoto, J., Hibino, T. and Ishida-Yamamoto, A. (2019) Marked changes in lamellar granule and trans-golgi network structure occur during epidermal keratinocyte differentiation. J. Invest. Dermatol. **139**(2), 352–359.
21. Kubo, A., Ishizaki, I., Kubo, A., Kawasaki, H., Nagao, K., Ohashi, Y. and Amagai, M. (2013) The stratum corneum comprises three layers with distinct metal-ion barrier properties. Sci. Rep. **3**, 1731.
22. Egawa, M. (2021) Application of spectroscopy to dermatology and cosmetic science (in Japanese). Bunko-kenkyu **70**(4), 104–113.
23. Freeman, E. E., Semeere, A., Osman, H., Peterson, G., Rajadhyaksha, M., González, S., Martin, J. N. anderson, R. R., Tearney, G. J. and Kang, D. (2018) Smartphone confocal microscopy for imaging cellular structures in human skin *in vivo*. Opt. Express. **9**(4), 1906–1915.
24. Wan, B., Ganier, C., Du-Harpur, X., Harun, N., Watt, F. M., Patalay, R. and Lynch, M. D. (2021) Applications and future directions for optical coherence tomography in dermatology. Br. J. Dermatol. **184**(6), 1014–1022.
25. Caspers, P. J., Lucassen, G. W., Bruining, H. A. and Puppels, G. J. (2000) Automated depth-scanning confocal Raman microspectrometer for rapid *in vivo* determination of water concentration profiles in human skin. J. Raman Spectrosc. **31**, 813–818.
26. Caspers, P. J., Lucassen, G. W., Carter, E. A., Bruining, H. A. and Puppels, G. J. (2001) *In vivo* confocal Raman microspectroscopy of the skin: Noninvasive determination of molecular concentration profiles. J. Invest. Dermatol. **116**(3), 434–442.
27. Pudney, P. D. A., Bonnist, E. Y. M., Caspers, P. J., Gorce, J.-P., Marriot, C., Puppels, G. J., Singleton, S. and van der Wolf, M. J. G. (2012) A new *in vivo* Raman probe for enhanced applicability to the body. Appl. Spectrosc. **66**(8), 882–891.
28. Franzen, L. and Windbergs, M. (2015) Applications of Raman spectroscopy in skin research — From skin physiology and diagnosis up to risk assessment and dermal drug delivery. Adv. Drug Deliv. Rev. **89**, 91–104.
29. Richters, R. J. H., Falcone, D., Uzunbajakava, N. E., Varghese, B., Caspers, P. J., Puppels, G. J., van Erp, P. E. and van de Kerkhof, P. C. (2017) Sensitive skin: Assessment of the skin barrier using confocal Raman microspectroscopy. Skin Pharmacol. Physiol. **30**(1), 1–12.

30. Egawa, M., Hirao, T. and Takahashi, M. (2007) *In vivo* estimation of stratum corneum thickness from water concentration profiles obtained with Raman spectroscopy. Acta. Derm. Venereol. **87**, 4–8.
31. Egawa, M. and Tagami, H. (2008) Comparison of the depth profiles of water and water-binding substances in the stratum corneum determined *in vivo* by Raman spectroscopy between the cheek and volar forearm skin: Effects of age, seasonal changes and artificial forced hydration. Br. J. Dermatol. **158**, 251–260.
32. Egawa, M. and Kajikawa, T. (2009) Changes in the depth profile of water in the stratum corneum treated with water. Skin Res. Tech. **15**(2), 242–249.
33. Magunusson, B. M., Runn, P. and Koskinen, L. O. (1997) Terpene-enhanced transdermal permeation of water and ethanol in human epidermis. Acta. Derm. Venereol. **77**(4), 264–267.
34. Squier, C. A. and Hall, B. K. (1985) The permeability of skin and oral mucosa to water and horseradish peroxidase as related to the thickness of the permeability barrier. J. Invest. Dermatol. **84**, 176–179.
35. Caspers, P. J., Lucassen, G. W. and Puppels, G. J. (2003) Combined *in vivo* confocal Raman spectroscopy and confocal microscopy of human skin. Biophys. J. **85**, 572–580.
36. van Smeden, J., Janssens, M., Kaye, E. C. J., Caspers, P. J., Lavrijsen, A. P., Vreeken, R. J. and Bouwstra, J. A. (2013) The importance of free fatty acid chain length for the skin barrier function in atopic eczema patients. Exp. Dermatol. **23**(1), 45–52.
37. van Logtestijn M. D. A., Caspers, P. J., Kezic, S., Hoffman, D. R., Koenig, D. W., Ono, M., Stamatas, G. N. and Tanaka, R. J. (2016) Water resistance profile as a marker of skin barrier damage in atopic dermatitis patients. Dermatol. Sci. **81**(2), 126–128.
38. Verzeaux, L., Vyumvuhore, R., Boudier, D., Le Guillou, M., Bordes, S., Essendoubi, M., Manfait, M. and Closs, B. (2018) Atopic skin: *In vivo* Raman identification of global molecular signature, a comparative study with healthy skin. Exp. Dermatol. **27**(4), 403–408.
39. Nouwen, A. E. M., Karadavut, D., Pasmans, S. G. M. A., Elbert, N. J., Bos, L. D. N., Nijsten, T. E. C., Arends, N. J. T., Pijnenburg, M. W. H., Koljenović, S., Puppels, G. J. and Caspers, P. J. (2020) Natural moisturizing factor as a clinical marker in atopic dermatitis. Allergy **75**(1), 188–190.
40. Bratchenko, I. A., Bratchenko, L. A., Moryatov, A. A., Khristoforova, Y. A., Artemyev, D. N., Myakinin, O. O., Orlov, A. E., Kozlov, S. V. and Zakharov, V. P. (2021) *In vivo* diagnosis of skin cancer with a portable Raman spectroscopic device. Exp. Dermatol. **30**(5), 652–663.
41. Egawa, M., Yamamoto, T., Sakamoto, K., Kunizawa, N., Tagami, H., Hirao, T. and Terui, T. (2010) *In vivo* characterization of the structure and components of lesional psoriatic skin from the observation with Raman spectroscopy and optical coherence tomography: A pilot study. J. Dermatol. Sci. **57**, 66–69.

42. Egawa, M. and Iwaki, H. (2008) *In vivo* evaluation of protective capacity of sunscreen by monitoring urocanic acid isomer in the stratum corneum using Raman spectroscopy. Skin Res. Tech. **14**(4), 410–417.
43. Egawa, M., Nomura, J. and Iwaki, H. (2015) The evaluation of the amount of cis- and trans-urocanic acid in the stratum corneum by Raman spectroscopy. Photochem. Photobiol. Sci. **9**(5), 730–733.
44. Lima, F. V., Martins, T. E. A., Morocho-Jácome, A. L., Almeida, I. F., Rosado, C. F., Velasco, M. V. R. and Baby, A. R. (2021) Analytical tools for urocanic acid determination in human samples: A review. J. Sep. Sci. **44**(1), 438–447.
45. Caspers, P. J., Williams, A. C., Carter, E. A., Edwards, H. G. M., Barry, B. W., Bruining, H. A. and Puppels, G. J. (2002) Monitoring the penetration enhancer dimethyl sulfoxide in human stratum corneum *in vivo* by confocal Raman spectroscopy. Pharm. Res. **19**, 1577–1580.
46. Pudney, P. D. A., Mélot, M., Caspers, P. J., van der Pol, A. and Puppels, G. J. (2007) An *in vivo* confocal Raman study of the delivery of trans retinol to the skin. Appl. Spec. **61**, 804–811.
47. Stamatas, G. N., de Sterke, J., Hauser, M., von Stetten, O. and van der Pol A. (2008) Lipid uptake and skin occlusion following topical application of oils on adult and infant skin. J. Dermatol. Sci. **50**(2), 135–142.
48. Franzen, L. anderski, J. and Windbergs, M. (2015) Quantitative detection of caffeine in human skin by confocal Raman spectroscopy — A systematic in vitro validation study. Eur. J. Pharm. Biopharm. **95**(Pt A), 110–116.
49. Caspers, P. J., Nico, C., Schut, T. C. B., de Sterke, J., Pudney, P. D. A., Curto, P. R., Illand, A. and Puppels, G. J. (2019) Method to quantify the *in vivo* skin penetration of topically applied materials based on confocal Raman spectroscopy. Transl. Biophotonics **1**, e201900004.
50. Krombholz, R., Liu, Y. and Lunter, D. J. (2021) In-line and off-line monitoring of skin penetration profiles using confocal Raman spectroscopy. Pharmaceutics **13**(1), 67.
51. Liu, Y. and Lunter, D. J. (2021) Profiling skin penetration using PEGylated emulsifiers as penetration enhancers via confocal Raman spectroscopy and fluorescence spectroscopy. Eur. J. Pharm. Biopharm. **166**, 1–9.
52. Meng, H., Yin, Y., Wu, W., Liu, Y., Li, L., Dong, Y., Fan, Y., Li, Y. and He, Y. (2021) Raman spectroscopic analysis of skin penetration and moisturizing effects of Bionics vernix caseosa cream compared with Vaseline. Technol. Health Care **29**(S1), 327–334.
53. Essendoubi, M., Alsamad, F., Noël, P., Meunier, M., Scandolera, A., Sandré, J., Manfait, M., Gobinet, C., Reynaud, R. and Piot, O. (2021) Combining Raman imaging and MCR-ALS analysis for monitoring retinol permeation in human skin. Skin Res. Technol. **27**(6), 1100–1109.

54. Liu, Y. and Lunter, D. J. (2021) Optimal configuration of confocal Raman spectroscopy for precisely determining stratum corneum thickness: Evaluation of the effects of polyoxyethylene stearyl ethers on skin. Int. J. Pharm. **597**, 120308.
55. Egawa, M. and Sato, Y. (2015) *In vivo* evaluation of two forms of urea in the skin by Raman spectroscopy after application of urea-containing cream. Skin Res. Tech. **21**(3), 259–264.
56. Watanabe, K., Palonpon, A. F., Smith, N. I., Chiu, L. D., Kasai, A., Hashimoto, H., Kawata, S. and Fujita, K. (2015) Structured line illumination Raman microscopy. Nat. Commun. **6**, 10095.
57. Oshima, Y., Sato, H., Kajiura-Kobayashi, H., Kimura, T., Naruse, K. and Nonaka, S. (2012) Light sheet-excited spontaneous Raman imaging of a living fish by optical sectioning in a wide field Raman microscope. Opt. Express **20**(15), 16195–16204.
58. Zhang, R., Bi, R., Ho Jun Hui, C., Rajarahm, P., Dinish, U. S. and Olivo, M. (2021) A portable ultrawideband confocal Raman spectroscopy system with a handheld probe for skin studies. ACS Sens. **6**(8), 2960–2966.
59. Evans, C. L., Potma, E. O., Puoris'haag, M., Côté, D., Lin, C. P. and Xie, X. S. (2005) Chemical imaging of tissue *in vivo* with video-rate coherent anti-Stokes Raman scattering microscopy. Proc. Natl. Acad. Sci. **102**(46), 16807–16812.
60. Freudiger, C. W., Min, W., Saar, B. G., Lu, S., Holtom, G. R., He, C., Tsai, J. C., Kang, J. X. and Xie, X. S. (2008) Label-free biomedical imaging with high sensitivity by stimulated Raman scattering microscopy. Science **322**, 1857–1861.
61. Drutis, D. M., Hancewicz, T. M., Pashkovski, E., Feng, L., Mihalov, D., Holtom, G. R., Ananthapadmanabhan, K. P., Xie, X. S. and Misra, M. (2014) Three-dimensional chemical imaging of skin using stimulated Raman scattering microscopy. J. Biomed. Opt. **19**(11), 111604.
62. Saar, B. G., Contreras-Rojas, L. R., Xie, X. S. and Guy, R. H. (2011) Imaging drug delivery to skin with stimulated Raman scattering microscopy. Mol. Pharmaceutics. **8**(3), 969–975.
63. Tipping, W. J., Lee, M., Serrels, A., Brunton, V. G. and Hulme, A. N. (2016) Stimulated Raman scattering microscopy: An emerging tool for drug discovery. Chem. Soc. Rev. **45**(8), 2075–2089.
64. Garrett, N. L., Singh, B., Jones, A. and Moger, J. (2017) Imaging microscopic distribution of antifungal agents in dandruff treatments with stimulated Raman scattering microscopy. J. Biomed. Opt. **22**(6), 66003.
65. Ito, T., Iguchi, R., Matsuoka, F., Nishi, Y., Ogihara, T. and Misawa, K. (2021) Label-free skin penetration analysis using time-resolved, phase-modulated stimulated Raman scattering microscopy. Biomed. Opt. Express **12**(10), 6545–6557.
66. Feizpour, A., Marstrand, T., Bastholm, L., Eirefelt, S. and Evans, C. L. (2021) Label-free quantification of pharmacokinetics in skin with stimulated Raman scattering microscopy and deep learning. J. Invest. Dermatol. **141**(2), 395–403.

67. Mittal, R., Balu, M., Krasieva, T., Potma, E. O., Elkeeb, L., Zachary, C. B. and Wilder-Smith, P. (2013) Evaluation of stimulated Raman scattering microscopy for identifying squamous cell carcinoma in human skin. Lasers Surg. Med. **45**(8), 496–502.
68. Lu, F.-K., Basu, S., Igras, V., Hoang, M. P., Ji, M., Fu, D., Holtom, G. R., Neel, V. A., Freudiger, C. W., Fisher, D. E. and Xie, X. S. (2015) Label-free DNA imaging *in vivo* with stimulated Raman scattering microscopy. Proc. Natl. Acad. Sci. **112**(37), 11624–11629.
69. Ozeki, Y., Umemura, W., Otsuka, Y., Satoh, S., Hashimoto, H., Sumimura, K., Nishizawa, N., Fukui, K. and Itoh, K. (2012) High-speed molecular spectral imaging of tissue with stimulated Raman scattering. Nature Photonics **6**, 845– 851.
70. Egawa, M., Tokunaga, K., Hosoi, J. and Ozeki, Y. (2016) In situ visualization of intracellular morphology of epidermal cells using stimulated Raman scattering microscopy. J. Biomed. Opt. **21**(8), 086017.
71. Egawa, M., Iwanaga, S., Hosoi, J., Goto, M., Yamanishi, H., Miyai, M., Katagiri, C., Tokunaga, K., Asai, T. and Ozeki, Y. (2019) Label-free stimulated Raman scattering microscopy visualizes changes in intracellular morphology during human epidermal keratinocyte differentiation. Sci. Rep. **9**, 12601.
72. Ozeki, Y., Asai, T., Shou, J. and Yoshimi, H. (2019) Multicolor stimulated Raman scattering microscopy with fast wavelength-tunable Yb fiber laser. IEEE J. Sel. Top. Quantum Electron. **25**(1), 7100211.
73. Kano, H., Segawa, H., Okuno, M., Leproux, P. and Couderc, V. (2016) Hyperspectral coherent Raman imaging –principle, theory, instrumentation and applications to life sciences. J. Raman Spectrosc. **47**(1), 116– 123.
74. Kaneta, D., Makiko, G., Hagiharam M., Leproux, P., Couderc, V., Egawa, M. and Kano, H. (2021) Visualizing intra-medulla lipids in human hair using ultra-multiplex CARS, SHG and THG microscopy. Analyst **146**, 1163–1168.
75. Kaneta, D., Leproux, P., Couderc, V., Goto, M., Egawa, M. and Kano, H. (2021) Visualization of water concentration distribution in human skin by ultra-multiplex coherent anti-Stokes Raman scattering (CARS) microscopy. Appl. Phys. Express **14**, 042010.
76. Saar, B. G., Freudiger, C. W., Reichman, J., Stanley, C. M., Holtom, G. R. and Xie, X. S. (2010) Video-rate molecular imaging *in vivo* with stimulated Raman scattering. Science **330**(6009), 1368–1370.
77. König, K., Breunig, H.G., Bückle, R., Kellner-Höfer, M., Weinigel, M., Büttner, E., Sterry, W. and Lademann, J. (2011) Optical skin biopsies by clinical CARS and multiphoton fluorescence/SHG tomography. Laser Phys. Lett. **8**(6), 465–468.
78. Breunig, H. G., Bückle, R., Kellner-Höfer, M., Weinigel, M., Lademann, J., Sterry, W. and König, K. (2012) Combined *in vivo* multiphoton and CARS imaging of healthy and disease-affected human skin. Microsc. Res. Tech. **75**(4), 492–498.

79. König, K., Breunig, H. G., Batista, A., Schindele, A., Zieger, M. and Martin, K. (2020) Translation of two-photon microscopy to the clinic: Multimodal multiphoton CARS tomography of *in vivo* human skin. J. Biomed. Opt. **25**(1), 014515.
80. Sarri, B., Chen, X., Canonge, R., Grégoire, S., Formanek, F., Galey, J. B., Potter, A., Bornschlögl, T. and Rigneault, H. (2019) *In vivo* quantitative molecular absorption of glycerol in human skin using coherent anti-Stokes Raman scattering (CARS) and two-photon auto-fluorescence. J. Control. Release **308**, 190–196.
81. Hill, A. H., Manifold, B. and Fu, D. (2020) Tissue imaging depth limit of stimulated Raman scattering microscopy. Biomed. Opt. Express **11**(2), 762–774.
82. Liao, C. S., Wang, P., Huang, C. Y., Lin, P., Eakins, G., Bentley, R. T., Liang, R. and Cheng, J. X. (2018) *In vivo* and in situ spectroscopic imaging by a handheld stimulated Raman scattering microscope. ACS Photonics **5**(3), 947– 954.
83. Lin, P., Ni, H., Li, H., Vickers, N. A., Tan, Y., Gong, R., Bifano, T. and Cheng, J. X. (2020) Volumetric chemical imaging *in vivo* by a remote-focusing stimulated Raman scattering microscope. Opt. Express **28**(20), 30210–30221.
84. Lunter, D., Klang, V., Kocsis, D., Varga-Medveczky, Z., Berkó, S. and Erdő, F. (2022) Novel aspects of Raman spectroscopy in skin research. Exp. Dermatol. **31**(9), 1311–1329.
85. Pahlow, S., Weber, K., Popp, J., Wood, B. R., Kochan. K., Rüther, A., Perez-Guaita, D., Heraud. P., Stone, N., Dudgeon, A., Gardner, B., Reddy, R., Mayerich, D. and Bhargava, R. (2018) Application of vibrational spectroscopy and imaging to point-of-care medicine: A review. Appl. Spectrosc. **72**(Suppl-1), 52–84.
86. Bratchenko, L. A., Bratchenko, I. A., Khristoforova, Y. A., Artemyev, D. N., Konovalova, D. Y., Lebedev, P. A. and Zakharov, V. P. (2021) Raman spectroscopy of human skin for kidney failure detection. J. Biophotonics **14**(2), e202000360.
87. Miyamori, D., Uemura, T., Zhu, W., Fujikawa, K., Nakaya, T., Teramukai, S., Pezzotti, G. and Ikegaya, H. (2021) A Raman algorithm to estimate human age from protein structural variations in autopsy skin samples: A protein biological clock. Sci. Rep. **11**(1), 5949.
88. León-Bejarano, F., Méndez, M. O., Alba, A., Rodríguez-Leyva, I., González, F. J., Rodríguez-Aranda, M. D. C., Guevara, E., Guirado-López, R. A. and Ramírez-Elías, M. G. (2022) Raman spectroscopy study of skin biopsies from patients with Parkinson's disease: Trends in alpha-synuclein aggregation from the amide I region. Appl. Spectrosc. **76**(11), 1317–1328.

https://doi.org/10.1142/9789811264610_0006

Chapter 6

Non-destructive Analytical and Structural Studies of Lipids in Food, Health, and Biomedical Sciences by Raman Spectroscopy

Hidetoshi Sato[1,*] and Yukihiro Ozaki[1,2]

[1]*School of Biological and Environmental Sciences, Kwansei Gakuin University, Sanda, Hyogo 669-1330, Japan*
[2]*Toyota Physical and Chemical Research Institute, Nagakute, Aichi 480-1192, Japan*
**Corresponding author: hidesato@kwansei.ac.jp*

6.1 Introduction

Lipids exist ubiquitously in organisms and foods, and they play very important roles in metabolism as well as tastes and functions of foods [1–3]. Therefore, investigations of the structures and functions of lipids are very important in food, pharmaceutical, health, and biomedical sciences. The structures of lipids have been investigated by various techniques such as infrared (IR) [4, 5], Raman [4–8] and nuclear magnetic resonance (NMR) [9] spectroscopies and mass spectrometry [10]. Among them, Raman spectroscopy is a powerful tool for non-destructive and label-free structural and analytical studies of lipids and related materials. Raman spectroscopic studies of lipids and fatty acids have a history of more than 50 years. Even in the early 1970s, band assignments of simple lipids and fatty acids were proposed by several groups [11, 12]. Using temperature-dependent spectra of lipids, their thermal behaviors and phase transitions were actively studied. Studies of various structures of phospholipids in water such as monolayer, liposome, multilayer, micelle, and emulsion, as well as natural membranes containing lipids, lipid-lipid interaction, lipid-protein interaction, effects of cholesterol on structure and phase transition of lipids, and deuterated lipids as specific and selective probes also started in the 1970s [11, 12].

Lipids have, in general, long non-polar acyl groups, and thus they give strong Raman scattering [5–8, 11, 12]. Their Raman spectra are less complicated compared with those of proteins and carbohydrates, so band assignments and spectra analysis are not too difficult. Raman spectra of lipids have long been investigated, and accordingly the band assignments are well established for simple lipids and fatty acids [5–7, 11, 12]. However, some unresolved problems in band assignments remain for complex lipids and newly synthesized lipids and fatty acids.

Raman spectroscopy studies of lipids have recently been extended in various directions. First, a variety of Raman techniques such as coherent anti-Stokes Raman scattering (CARS) including CARS imaging [13, 14], Raman microscopy and imaging [15], surface-enhanced Raman spectroscopy (SERS) [16], low-frequency Raman, and hand-held Raman spectroscopy have been used extensively. Second, Raman studies of lipids have become more and more active in food [17–26], pharmaceutical, cosmetic (Chapter 5), health (Chapter 5), and medical sciences (Chapters 9 and 16). Thus, Raman studies of lipids have become deeper and wider.

This chapter introduces Raman spectra of fatty acids and lipids first and then outlines the application of Raman spectroscopy to food, health, and biomedical sciences. Particularly, some emphasis is placed on lipid analysis in subcutaneous tissue and accumulation of lipids in cells.

6.2 Raman Spectra of Fatty Acids and Lipids

Figure 6.1 shows Raman spectra of 10 kinds of fatty acids. The following fatty acids were investigated: myristic acid (MA), palmitic acid (PA), stearic acid (SA), arachidic acid (ARA), palmitoleic acid (POA), oleic acid (OA), elaidic acid (EA), linoleic acid (LA), α-linolenic acid (ALA) and arachidonic acid (AA) [7]. According to Czamara *et al.* the Raman spectra of fatty acids can be divided into seven regions I–VII. Region I (3200–2800 cm^{-1}) is the region for the C–H stretching vibrations. Bands in the region of 3000–2800 cm^{-1} are due to the CH stretching modes of CH_3 and CH_2 groups. Unsaturated fatty acids

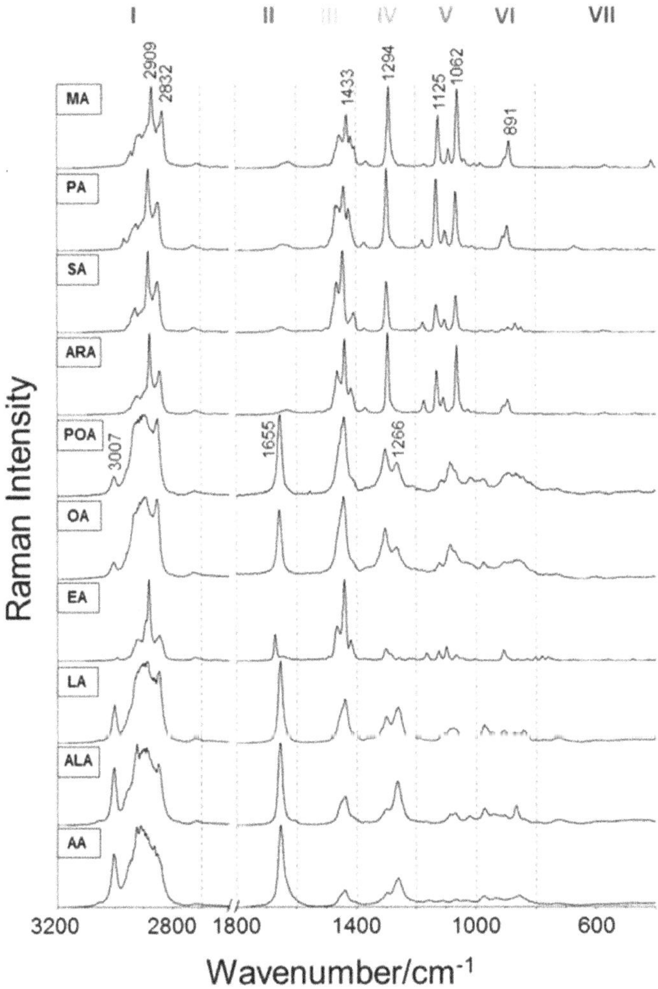

Figure 6.1. Raman spectra of 10 kinds of fatty acids (myristic acid (MA), palmitic acid (PA), stearic acid (SA), arachidic acid (ARA), palmitoleic acid (POA), oleic acid (OA), elaidic acid (EA), linoleic acid (LA), α-linolenic acid (ALA) and arachidonic acid (AA)). Reproduced from Ref. [7] with permission.

have an additional band above 3000 cm^{-1} derived from the stretching mode of the =C–H moieties. Region II (1800–1600 cm^{-1}) contains bands due to C=C stretching modes (1670–1655 cm^{-1}). The position of this band changes with *trans* (~1670 cm^{-1}) and *cis* (~1655 cm^{-1}) conformations, so that one can use this as a marker band for *trans-cis* isomerism. In Figure 6.1 only EA shows a band at 1670 cm^{-1}, revealing that it has *trans* conformation. Saturated and unsaturated fatty acids can be distinguished clearly by the =C–H stretching band in the vicinity of 3005 cm^{-1} region and the band due to the C=C stretching mode in the region of 1670–1655 cm^{-1} [7]. Regions III–V which contain bands due to CH_3 and CH_2 deformation, CH_2 twisting, and C–C stretching modes, respectively, are also clearly different between saturated and unsaturated fatty acids. It is well known that the relative intensity of the two bands at 1655 (C=C stretch) and 1444 cm^{-1} (CH_2 bend) provides information about the degree of unsaturation of fatty acids and lipids [6, 17–19]. In the 1150–1000 cm^{-1} region (Region V), bands arising from vibrations where alternate carbon atoms move in opposite directions along the chain length are included. Below 600 cm^{-1}, bands due to accordion-like modes appear [11, 12]. These bands are very important to investigate conformational changes in alkyl chains in fatty acids and lipids, but they are not discussed in this chapter.

Raman spectra of 17 kinds of triacylglycerols (TAGs) are shown in Figure 6.2 [7]: tricaproin, tricaprylin, tricaprin, trilaurin, trimyristin, tripalmitin, tristearin, triarachidin, tribehenin, tripalmitolein, tripetroselinin, triolein, trielaidin, trilinolein, trilinolenin, tri-11-eicosenoin and trierucin. As in the case with fatty acids, the Raman spectra of TAGs are also divided into seven regions. In Region II, in addition to a band due to C=C stretching , a band arising from a C=O stretching mode is observed near 1745 cm^{-1} for all TAGs. Regions III–V contain bands derived from CH_3 and CH_2 deformation, CH_2 twisting, and C–C stretching modes, respectively. The Raman spectra of TAGs reflect the number of double bonds; with the increase in the number, the relative intensity of the two bands at 1300 and 1260 cm^{-1} increases and the =C–H band shifts to a higher wavenumber [7].

6.3 Non-destructive Analysis of Lipids in Foods by Raman Spectra

6.3.1 *Non-destructive Determination of Iodine Values of Lipids by Raman Spectroscopy and Discrimination of Lipids*

Figure 6.3 presents 1064-nm excited Raman spectra of (a) peanut, (b) beef tallow, and (c) butter [17]. Since the content of lipids is high in these foodstuffs and lipids yields intense Raman bands, all three are practically Raman spectra of lipids. A Raman band due to the C=C stretching band appears at around 1660 cm^{-1}, indicating that lipids in peanut, beef tallow, and butter have *cis* conformation. The relative intensity of the bands at 1660 and 1444 cm^{-1} and that of the two bands at 1305 and 1267 cm^{-1} change significantly among the three spectra, showing that the iodine values for these three foodstuffs are in

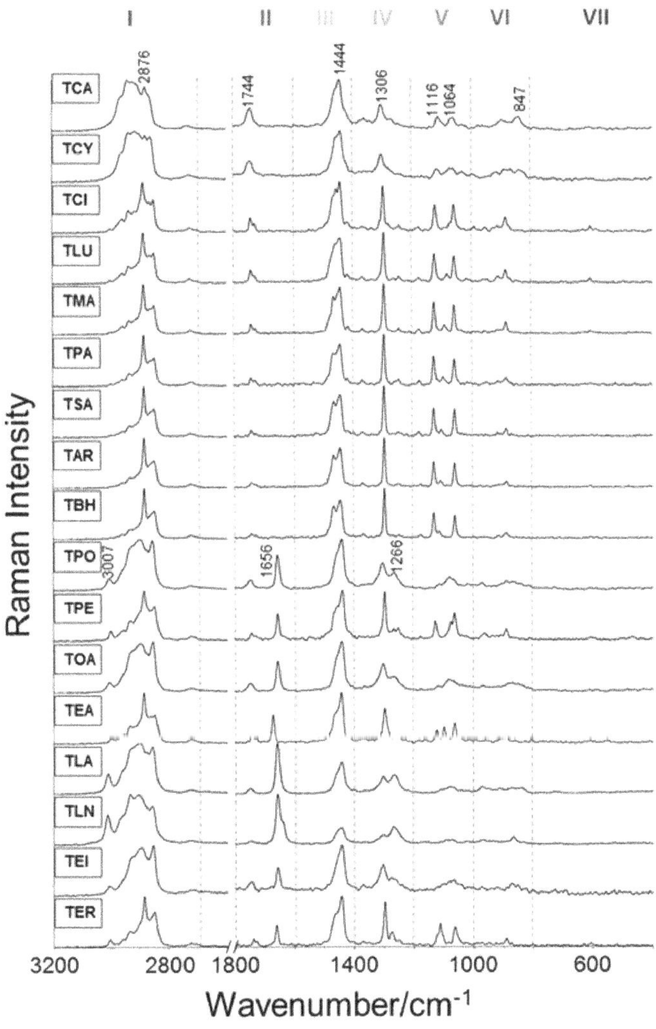

Figure 6.2. Raman spectra of 17 kinds of triacylglycerols (tricaproin (TCA), tricaprylin (TCY), tricaprin (TCI), trilaurin (TLU), trimyristin (TMA), tripalmitin (TPA), tristearin (TSA), triarachidin (TAR), tribehenin (TBH), tripalmitolein (TPO), tripetroselinin (TPE), triolein (TOA), trielaidin (TEA), trilinolein (TLA), trilinolenin (TLN), tri-11-eicosenoin (TEI) and trierucin (TER)). Reproduced from Ref. [7] with permission.

the order of peanut, beef tallow, and butter. The results are in good agreement with the measured iodine values. In this way one can estimate iodine values of foodstuffs non-destructively by Raman spectroscopy [17].

Raman spectra of (a) sunflower, (b) corn, (c) sesame, (d) rapeseed, and (e) olive oils are shown in Figure 6.4 [17]. The relative intensity of the bands

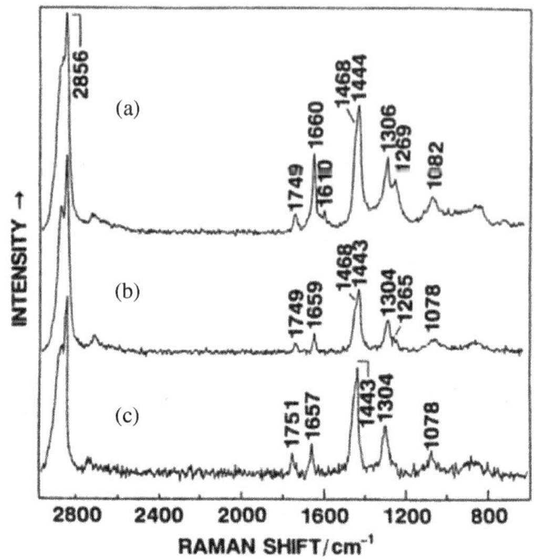

Figure 6.3. 1064-nm excited Raman spectra of (a) peanut, (b) beef tallow, and (c) butter. Reproduced from Ref. [17] with permission.

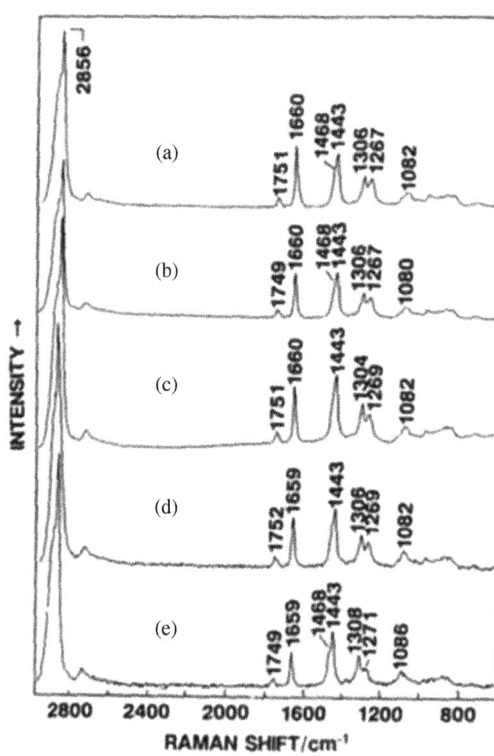

Figure 6.4. 1064-nm excited Raman spectra of (a) sunflower, (b) corn, (c) sesame, (d) rapeseed, and (e) olive oil. Reproduced from Ref. [17] with permission.

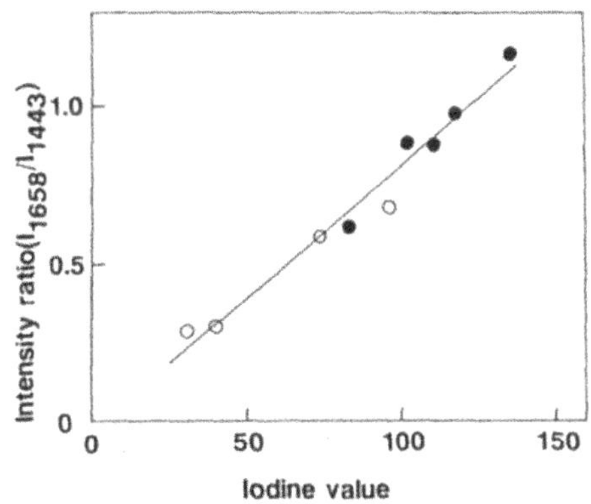

Figure 6.5. The relative intensity of the two bands at 1658 and 1443 cm^{-1} versus iodine value for various fat-containing foodstuffs. Reproduced from Ref. [17] with permission.

at 1660 and 1444 cm^{-1} (I_{1660}/I_{1444}) decreases and that of the two bands at 1305 and 1267 cm^{-1} (I_{1305}/I_{1267}) increases upon going from sunflower to olive oil. The iodine values of sunflower, corn, sesame, rapeseed, and olive oil are 136, 118, 111, 102, and 83, respectively. Therefore, the intensity changes are in good agreement with the measured iodine values.

Figure 6.5 represents the relative intensity of the two bands at 1658 and 1443 cm^{-1} versus iodine value for various fat-containing foodstuffs [17]. Note that there is a linear correlation for a variety of foods. In this way Raman spectroscopy can determine the iodine value non-destructively.

There has been increased attention towards the composition of feeding fats. Assessment of the discrimination of animal fats is very important from the point of food safety. Abbas *et al.* [20]. investigated non-destructive discrimination of animal fats by Raman spectroscopy and chemometrics. Figure 6.6 displays FT-Raman spectra of animal fats from different sources [20]. Note that the relative intensities of the =C–H, C=C, and CH_2 twisting become stronger in the Raman spectra of fish and poultry fats. To separate well different classes of animal fats, Abbas *et al.* [20] employed PCA (Principal Component Analysis) and PLS-DA (Partial Least Square-Discriminant Analysis). The PLS-DA yielded a good result of sensitivity of 0.958 and specificity of 0.914.

6.3.2 *Various Studies of Lipids in Foods by Raman Spectroscopy*

Raman spectroscopy has been used for various studies of lipids in food: discrimination of various animal fats, qualitative analysis of small amounts

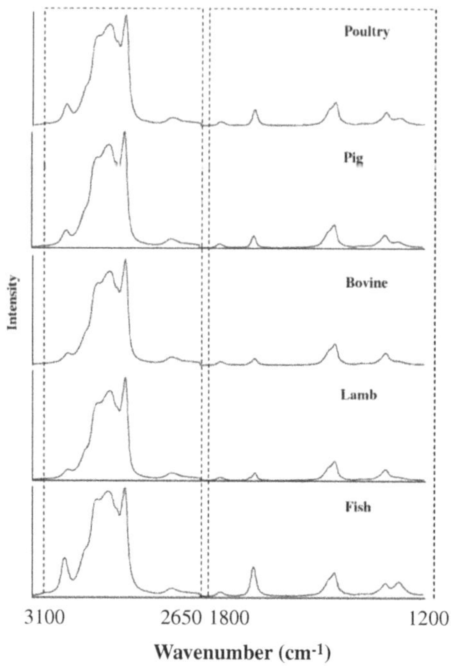

Figure 6.6. 1064-nm excited Raman spectra of animal fats from poultry, pig, bovine, lamb, and fish. Reproduced from Ref. [20] with permission.

of lipids, distribution of lipids in foods, lipid alteration, lipid oxidation, and crystal morphism of lipids. Stefanov *et al.* [21] investigated the potential of Raman spectroscopy combined with PLS regression for the determination of individual or grouped *trans*-monosaturated fatty acids (*trans*-MUFA) and conjugated linoleic acid (CLA) in milk fat. PLA results demonstrated the potential of direct semiroutine quantification of several individual CLA (*cis*-9, *trans*-11, *trans*-10, *cis*-12 C18:2) and trans-MUFA (*trans*-4-15 C18:1) in minor concentrations (below 1.0 g/100 g of milk fat). Distinct bands for *trans*-MUFA (1674 cm^{-1}) and CLA (1653 cm^{-1}) from the *trans*-isolated and *cis, trans*-conjugated C=C bonds were identified [21].

Raman studies of lipid adulteration have been carried out by several groups. Li-Chen [22] investigated the degree of adulteration of olive oil and canola oil by Raman spectra and multivariate analysis. With the increase in canola oil, clear changes were observed for the intensity and shape of the 1445 cm^{-1} band. Their PLS results gave the R^2 (correlation coefficient), 0.99 for all samples and 0.96 for cross-validation and SEP (standard error of prediction), 6.5 for all samples, 7.0 for cross-validation. It has turned out that

Raman-PLS analysis is powerful for non-destructive analysis of adulteration of lipids. Beaten and Aparicio [23] examined the adulteration of virgin olive oil by use of Raman-PCA.

Guzman *et al.* [24] estimated the degree of oxidation of olive oil using a portable Raman spectrometer and PLS. For the indicators, they used peroxide value, K_{232}, and K_{270}. For the peroxide value, $R^2 = 0.91$, PMSEP = 2.57; for K_{232}, $R^2 = 0.88$, RMSEP = 0.37; and for K_{270}, $R^2 = 0.90$, RMSEP = 0.08. This result showed that portable Raman spectrometers can determine the main parameters for evaluating the oxidation of lipids.

Muik *et al.* [25] reported direct monitoring of lipid oxidation in inedible oils by FT-Raman spectroscopy. Raman imaging was also used for the visualization of distributions of components including lipids in foods; for example, lipids in cheese. CARS microscopy studies in Chapter 9 by Kano *et al.* described some lipid research.

Motoyama *et al.* [26] developed a simple discrimination method of beef tallow and pork tallow using Raman spectroscopy. It has been well known that beef tallow and pork tallow have a significant difference in the content of TAG. This difference induces the formation of β'-type crystal polymorphism. Raman spectra of lipids reflect sensitively the differences in crystal polymorphism. For example, a weak band at 1417 cm^{-1} is characteristic of β'-type crystal. The method proposed by Motoyama is based on this band.

6.4 Lipid Analysis in Subcutaneous Tissues by Raman Spectroscopy

6.4.1 *Development of Raman Probes*

Raman scattered light is so weak that a Raman instrument must efficiently collect scattered light coming from the focal point of an excitation laser. The shorter the distance from a sample to a collection lens, the higher the collection efficiency, if the diameter of an objective lens is the same. Therefore, a Raman measurement using a telescope is not feasible especially for biological samples because their Raman scattered light is usually very weak. In contrast, samples such as face skin and inner side of body are not able to be laid in the sampling space of a Raman microscope. Consequently, it is necessary to use a Raman probe to bring the optical sampling point on the surface of a measuring point.

A usual Raman probe is made of optical fibers of which materials are usually normal glass and/or quartz glass. Since the strong excitation light is delivered in a core of the glass fiber, it generates Raman scattered and fluorescent lights due to the glass material, which overwhelms weak Raman signals. Consequently, a Raman probe equips a distal head with a band-pass filter on the optical fiber to deliver the excitation laser light and a long-pass filter on the collection fibers for Raman scattered light. It indicates that the fibers for excitation light must be spatially separated from those for Raman scattered light collection. Moreover, the glass fibers have relatively large numerical aperture near 0.2. Because of these optical properties, it is relatively difficult to make an optimum optical design and control its working distance (WD) and focal depth.

Instead of the glass fiber probes, we developed a miniaturized Raman probe made of a hollow optical fiber (BHRP), of which a ball lens was attached on the distal end [27]. As the hollow optical fiber had no core material, only one fiber without filters was able to be used both for sending and receiving the excitation and Raman scattered lights, respectively. The WD of BHRP was tuned easily by selecting the material and diameter of the ball lens on the distal end. Since the optical axes for the illumination and collection were identical, the optical design was simple and its WD easy to control. Numerical aperture of the hollow optical fiber was small, about 0.07, which gave confocal-like effect to BHRP. We have developed BHRP with a ball lens of 800 μm diameter made of quartz, of which sensitive excitation volume reaches down to 800 μm from the probe head. The types and properties of miniaturized Raman probes are discussed in Chapter 16 in detail.

6.4.2 *Non-invasive Analysis of Subcutaneous Fats*

Our laboratory is in the Kobe-Sanda campus of Kwansei Gakuin University, which is located in Sanda city, Hyogo prefecture, Japan. The area around Sanda is famous for its various and qualified agricultural products, especially Sanda-beef, and is also one of the origins for Kobe-beef. The cow meats with the highest quality among the products are selected and sold as Kobe-beef. There are several large wholesale meat stores in Sanda which deal with farms, markets, and companies all over Japan as well as those in Sanda, and they open retail meat stores also for consumers at their factories. In such a store, it is possible to have detailed information about each type of meat, such as produced area, body part, and quality. In our opinion, the taste of beef is largely influenced by that of fat in the meat. A manager of one of those wholesale stores said that the taste of fat is attributed to feedstuff fed to the cow during the final fattening procedure. As it is known that olive oil is rich in TAG-containing

OA chains, the taste of oil depends on its component of fatty acid chains. This fact strongly suggests that the feed affects the composition of fatty acid chains in cow body fat, and it would be similar in humans. It is an attractive idea to analyze the composition of body fat for food control. We have developed the techniques for fatty acid chain analysis in the body and studied the properties of different fatty acid chains.

A hamster has sebaceous glands and a fat-rich layer relatively close to the skin surface. We fed trilinolein (TL) and tricaprin (TC) to hamsters for six weeks and analyzed the rate of their accumulation in their bodies with Raman spectroscopy [28, 29]. TL has three LA chains (18:2) and TC three decanoic acids (10:0). The Raman spectra of subcutaneous fat layers were measured with a BHRP having a 800 μm-diameter quartz ball lens on the back of the hamster in a totally non-invasive manner. Then, the hamster was sacrificed and its fat tissues were collected from the abdomen and skin. Figure 6.7 exhibits Raman spectra of (a) visceral adipose tissue (VAT) and subcutaneous adipose tissue (SAT) and (b) those obtained by non-invasive skin measurements [28]. The spectra measured directly and over skin, of which signal-to-noise ratios were considerably high, looked similar. Raman bands of skin materials, such as keratin, collagen, blood, and so on, were quite weak in the skin spectra. Since skin spectra measured with a usual BHRP having a 500 μm-diameter sapphire glass ball lens showed spectra of keratin and collagen strongly, the

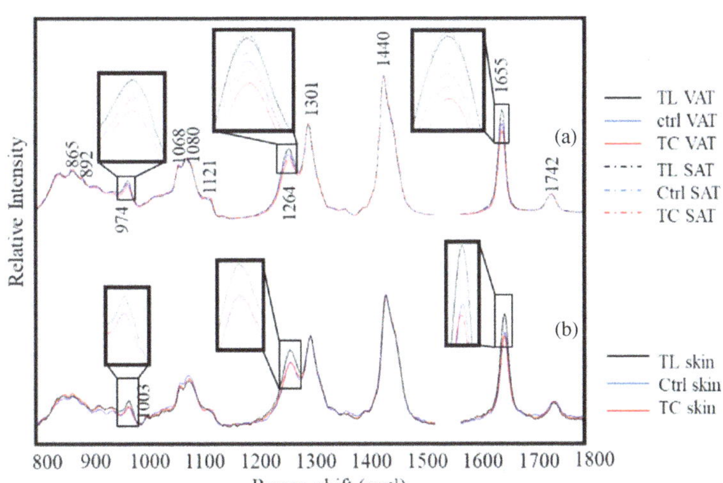

Figure 6.7. Raman spectra of (a) visceral adipose tissue (VAT) and subcutaneous adipose tissue (SAT) and (b) those obtained by non-invasive skin measurements. Reproduced from Ref. [28] with permission.

result revealed that the BHRP with the 800 μm-diameter quartz ball lens had suitable WD to measure the subcutaneous fat of hamster. Moreover, the Raman signal of fat is usually stronger than other hydrophilic materials in a tissue because fat forms droplets in adipocytes in which the fat concentration is extremely high. Appearance of the Raman spectra of VAT and SAT resembled each other, as the GC results indicated that their fat chain compositions were almost identical.

Some bands showed different intensities among the samples that were fed different diets [28, 29]. Bands near 1655 and 1264 cm^{-1} due to the C=C stretching and CH_2 twisting modes, respectively, have strong contributions to the spectra, suggesting that linoleic fatty acid chain component increased in the samples fed TL. Bands below 1100 cm^{-1} showing small spectral changes were important for analysis of fats with different chain lengths. The hamsters in the experiment had normal feedstuff with the fat diets and synthesized fats also in their bodies from sugars and amino acids. Since the adipose tissue of the hamsters contained various fatty acid chains other than linoleic and decanoic acids, it is difficult to estimate the composition correctly only from the intensity changes of major Raman bands.

After measuring Raman spectra of the samples, fat components were extracted from the samples and analyzed with gas chromatography (GC). Partial least square regression (PLSR) analysis was applied to build the quantitative analytical models of Raman spectra for linoleic and decanoic chains with their concentration values obtained by GC [28]. When the composition of fatty acid chains is known, it may be possible to apply classical least square (CLS) analysis which uses pure spectra of the fat components to obtain concentrations of all elements at once [30]. However, PLSR is more robust than CLS when the data includes noise and/or unknown components. The PLSR analytical models built for hamster body fat were applied to the non-invasive skin data to estimate concentrations of linoleic and decanoic fatty acid chains in the subcutaneous fat. The rates of accumulation for linoleic and decanoic acids in the hamster body every two weeks were compared in Table 6.1 [28]. Since the body weight of hamster had increased during the experiment, the values indicated merely relative rates. It should be noted that the values estimated with non-invasive Raman analyses agreed well with those by invasive analysis of VAT and SAT. The accumulation rate of linoleic chain was almost 10 times higher than that of decanoic chain, indicating that adipocytes preferred to keep TL than other fats. The decanoic fatty acid seemed to be consumed to synthesize other fats.

Table 6.1. Accumulation rates for linoleic and decanoic chains in the hamster body every two weeks. Reproduced from Ref. [28] with permission.

Average accumulation rate (%) per 2 weeks		
Linoleic chain in TL-treated group	Visceral adipose tissue (VAT)	4.45 ± 1.6
	Subcutaneous adipose tissue (SAT)	4.37 ± 2.4
	Skin-subcutaneous (skin-SAT)	4.57 ± 3.41
Decanoic chain in TC-treated group	Visceral adipose tissue (VAT)	0.58 ± 0.4
	Subcutaneous adipose tissue (SAT)	0.52 ± 0.38
	Skin-subcutaneous (skin-SAT)	0.63 ± 0.3

As human skin is much thicker than that of a hamster, it may not be possible to apply directly the same techniques to estimate the fatty acid chain compositions in the human skin. Although it would be difficult to extend the WD of BHRP to be more than 1 mm, the procedure can be improved to fit the thickness of human skin, for example, by focusing the probe on the sebaceous gland or by other types of Raman probe which have longer WD. The results introduced above demonstrate that Raman spectroscopy is a powerful tool to analyze fatty acid chain compositions in subcutaneous adipose tissue in a totally non-invasive manner [28, 29]. It can herald a new era for fatty acid chain control in health and dermatologic sciences.

6.4.3 *Analysis of Fatty Acid Effects in Live Cells*

It is well known that adiposity confers negative effects on human health. However, it is not simple how the fat causes health problems, except mechanical damages due to weight. We have studied the effect of fatty acids on a liver model cell [31]. TAGs accumulated in adipose tissues are converted into fatty acids and secreted into blood vessels to be transferred to body parts, when the body needs energy to consume. Liver cells uptake the fatty acids and reconvert them into TAGs to store in the cells. Although the liver cells synthesize fat by themselves, it is assumed that the uptake of the blood fatty acids also causes fatty liver disease, such as non-alcoholic fatty liver disease (NAFLD) and non-alcoholic steatohepatitis (NASH). NAFLD/NASH includes chronic inflammation of liver. It means that liver cells are injured and destroyed by fat that they accumulated by themselves. Previous studies using liver cell models indicated that the cells induced apoptosis by adding PA (16:0) or SA (18:0) that are saturated fatty acids but not OA (18:1). In contrast, an adipocyte can

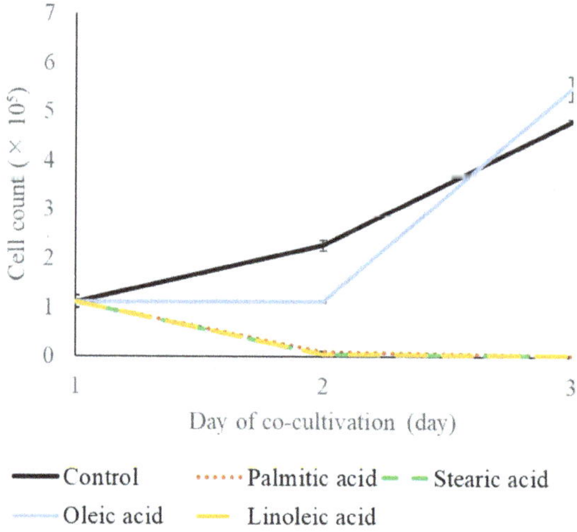

Figure 6.8. Cell count vs day of co-cultivation for control and four kinds of fatty acids. Reproduced from Ref. [31] with permission.

store PA and SA without problems. This fact reveals that the response to a specific fatty acid depends on cell type.

We employed HepG2 cell for a liver cell model to study its uptake and reactions to fatty acids PA, SA, OA and LA. The fatty acids were mixed with albumin that was a typical fatty acid carrier in blood and were dissolved into the culture media. As the culture medium itself had already included necessary materials for cell growth, the fatty acid added to the medium was excess amount for the cell. Their growth curves are shown in Figure 6.8 [31]. The control cell and the cell cultured with OA increased their populations but the cells cultured with PA and SA decreased quickly, agreeing with the results in previous reports. Despite our assumption for LA that the liver cell could accept unsaturated fatty acids, the cell cultured with LA reduced its population quickly as well as that of the cells cultured with saturated fatty acids. The transmission electron microscopic observation showed large vacuoles in the cells cultured with PA, SA and LA, strongly suggesting that the cells had induced apoptosis. Since LA is one of the essential fatty acids that human cannot synthesize in the body, it was assumed that liver cells would prefer it.

The survived cells in the dishes often accumulated multiple lipid droplets in their cytoplasm, according to the microscopic observation. The compositions of

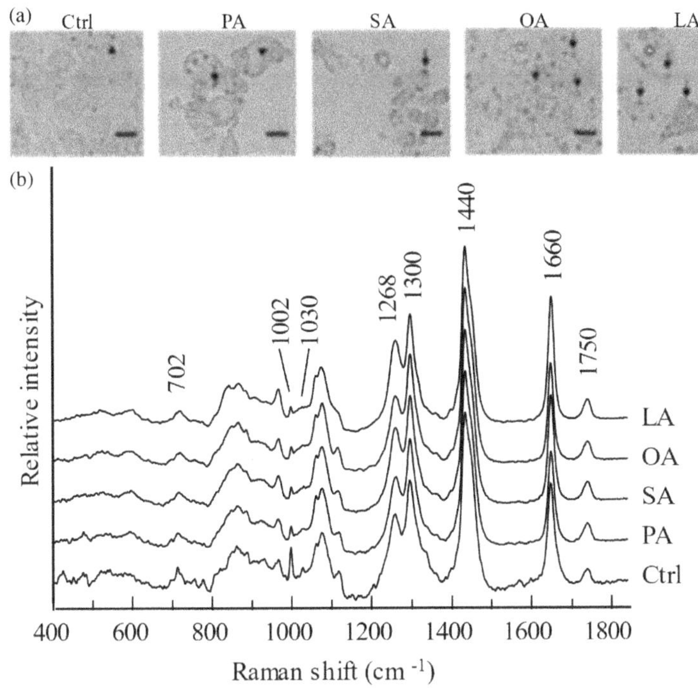

Figure 6.9. (a) Microscopic images of the survived cells and (b) Raman spectra of droplets in them. Reproduced from Ref. [31] with permission.

the lipid droplets in the cells were studied with Raman spectroscopy. Figure 6.9 depicts (a) microscopic images of the survived cells and (b) Raman spectra of droplets in them [31]. The microscopic observations showed that the number of droplets were from 3 to 20 times higher in all the survived cells cultured with fatty acids than that of the control cell. There were very few cells which survived without lipid droplets, because there was no choice for them to stop the uptake of fatty acids. The spectral features resembled a typical spectrum of TAG but a few bands, such as those observed at 1002 and 1030 cm^{-1} assignable to phenylalanine ring modes, suggested the coexistence of proteins. Since the droplets are too small to pick up and the cell includes plenty of different types of lipids such as phospholipids in their membranes, it is too difficult to apply GC for analysis of fat contents in the droplets. Consequently, the PLSR technique which requires many training datasets to build a calibration model cannot be applied for this case, although it is robust to the data with noise and unknown components. Since the cell itself synthesizes several types of

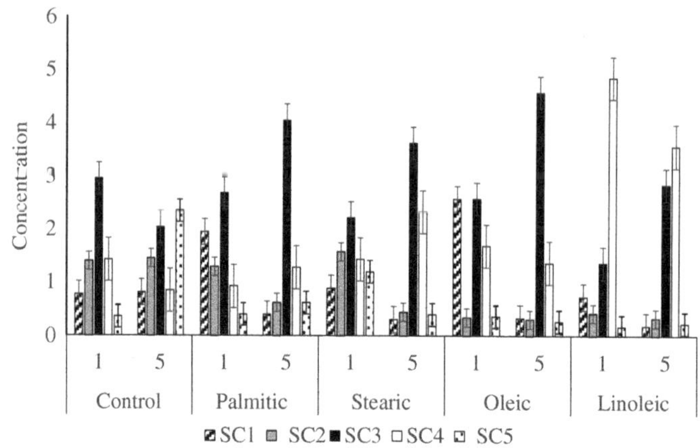

Figure 6.10. The result of MCR-ALS applied for analysis of the fatty acid chain compositions of the lipid droplets. Reproduced from Ref. [31] with permission.

fatty acids, CLS is not be suitable because it requires pure spectra of all major elements included in the sample. Hence, multicurve resolution alternative least square (MCR-ALS) analysis was applied for analysis of the fatty acid chain composition of the lipid droplets.

The results of MCR-ALS are exhibited in Figure 6.10 [31]. Relative concentrations of five components, SC 1–5, are indicated with bars. According to the retrieved spectra of the components, it was suggested that SC3 and SC4 reflected OA and LA well, respectively [31]. In contrast, SC1 and SC2 had contributions of protein species mixed during the MCR analysis, and were not accurate enough for estimation of PA and SA. The concentration of OA was relatively high in all cells, showing that OA was a safe fatty acid for liver cells. The concentration of LA was very high in the survived cell cultured with LA for 1 day, but it subsequently decreased in the cell for five days; instead, the concentration of OA increased. This result suggested that cells expressing more enzymes that modify one of the double bonds of LA to generate OA could survive for five days. HepG2 cell appears to take up fatty acids indiscriminately and its uptake reaction is out of control. The signal pathway to induce apoptosis seems to be totally separated from the uptake control.

As was discussed in the previous section, adipocytes prefer to accumulate LA. In contrast, the liver model cell induces apoptosis with excess LA, as well as saturated fatty acids. The inconsistency in the response between adipocytes and liver cells to fatty acids, especially to LA, may be attributed to hepatic inflammation. It is almost impossible to analyze the liver fat composition in a healthy person, but it may be possible to make a non-invasive analysis of subcutaneous fat with Raman spectroscopy, as was demonstrated in the hamster study. Moreover, the analysis of fatty acid chain composition contained in food would be easier. The studies introduced in this chapter are not enough at this point to cover various fat metabolisms of the total body system. However, they demonstrate that the coupled technology of Raman spectroscopy, its instruments and multivariate analysis has strong feasibility and potential for non-invasive and quantitative analysis of fatty acid chain compositions in the human body, which will lead fat science into health control and medical applications.

6.5 Summary and Prospects

This chapter has introduced non-destructive fat analysis by Raman spectroscopy; it has described representative Raman spectra of fatty acids and triacylglycerols, and then outlined the applications of Raman spectroscopy to the studies of foods, live tissues and cells. Raman spectroscopy is one of the few techniques that can be applied to quantitative and qualitative analysis of lipids in a non-destructive and non-invasive manner, and it can also provide information about their molecular structure and function. Moreover, evolutions in instrumentation and information technologies promise to bring the application of Raman spectroscopy of lipids into a new stage of analysis. There is no doubt that Raman studies and analysis of lipids will develop strongly in various aspects and in various research fields.

For basic and food research, the mechanism of oxidation and degradation and physical properties of lipids will be studied in more detail by use of Raman spectroscopy. Moreover, non-destructive, highly sensitive, and rapid analysis such as those of peroxide value, conjugated value, carboxy value and anisidine value by Raman spectroscopy are expected. For health and biomedical sciences a variety of investigations such as those on lipid metabolism in the body, subcutaneous fats, lipid research in relation to health care and cosmetic science, lipid analysis in relation to diseases such as cancer, and accumulation of lipids in a cell will be carried out actively.

Various state-of-the-art Raman techniques such as Raman imaging including three-dimensional imaging, CARS and CARS imaging, SERS and tip-enhanced Raman spectroscopy will be used more extensively for lipid studies. Moreover, combined uses of Raman spectroscopy and other methods will become more and more important. Particularly, combined use with mass spectrometry or NMR spectroscopy will be valuable.

Last but not least, further development of spectral data analysis methods such as chemometrics, machine learning, and artificial intelligence will become essential for lipid research in the near future (Chapters 3 and 4). Particularly, new methods of big data analysis will become important.

References

1. Sato, K. (Ed.). (2018) *Crystallization of Lipids: Fundamentals and Applications in Food, Cosmetics, and Pharmaceuticals*, John Wiley & Sons.
2. Gurr, M. I., Harwood, J. L., Frayn, K. N., Murphy, D. J. and Michell, R. H. (2016) *Lipids: Biochemistry, Biotechnology and Health*, John Wiley & Sons.
3. Grundy, M. M.-L. and Wilde, P. J. (Eds.). (2022) *Bioaccessibility and Digestibility of Lipids from Food*, Springer.
4. Mossoba, M. M. (Ed.). (1999) *Spectral Methods in Food Analysis*, Marcel Dekker.
5. Lewis, R. N. A. H. and McElhaney, R. N. (2001) Vibrational Spectroscopy of Lipids. In *Handbook of Vibrational Spectroscopy* (Chalmers, J. M. and Griffiths, P. R., Eds.), pp. 3447–3464, John Wiley & Sons.
6. Ozaki, Y. (1999) Raman Spectroscopy. In *Spectral Methods in Food Analysis* (Mossoba, M. M., Ed.), pp. 427–462, Marcel Dekker.
7. Czamara, K., Majzner, K., Pacia, M. Z., Kochan, K., Kaczor, A. and Baranska, M. (2015) Raman spectroscopy of lipids: a review. J. Raman Spectrosc. **46**, 4–20.
8. Baeten, V. (2010) Raman spectroscopy in lipid analysis. Lipid Technol. **22**, 36–38.
9. Pikula, S., Bandorowicz-Pikula, J. and Groves, P. (2015) Chapter Five — Recent Advances in NMR Studies of Lipids. In *Annual Reports on NMR Spectroscopy*, pp. 195–246, Elsevier.
10. Li, L., Han, J., Wang, Z., Liu, J., Wei, J., Xiong, S. and Zhao, Z. (2014) Mass spectrometry methodology in lipid analysis. Int. J. Mol. Sci. **11**, 10492–10507.
11. Carey, P. R. (1982) *Biomedical Applications of Raman and Resonance Raman Spectroscopies*, Academic Press.
12. Tu, A. T. (1982) *Raman Spectroscopy in Biology*, John Wiley & Sons.
13. Hashimoto, M., Ichimura, T., and Fujita, K. (2012) CARS microscopy: Implementation of nonlinear vibrational spectroscopy for far-field and near-field imaging. In *Raman Imaging* (Zoubir, A., Ed.), pp. 317–346, Springer.
14. Rigneault, H. and Gachet, D. (2012) Background-free coherent Raman imaging: The CARS and SRS contrast mechanisms. In *Raman Imaging* (Zoubir, A., Ed.), pp. 347–372, Springer.

15. McGarvey, J. J. and Beattie, J. R. (2012) Raman microscopy: versatile approach to bio-imaging. In *Raman Imaging* (Zoubir, A., Ed.), pp. 219–242, Springer.
16. Prochazka, M. (2015) *Surface-Enhanced Raman Spectroscopy: Bioanalytical, Biomolecular and Medical Applications*, Springer.
17. Ozaki, Y., Cho, R., Ikegaya, K., Muraishi, S. and Kawauchi, K. (1992) Potential of near-infrared Fourier transform Raman spectroscopy in food analysis. Appl. Spectrosc. **46**, 1503–1507.
18. Sadeghi-Jorabchi, H., Hendra, P. J., Wilson, R. H. and Belton, P. S. (1990) Determination of the total unsaturation in oils and margarines by Fourier transform Raman spectroscopy. J. Am. Oil. Chem. Soc. **67**, 483–486.
19. Sadeghi-Jorabchi, H., Wilson, R. H., Belton, P. S., Edwards-Web, J. D. and Coxon, D. T. (1991) Quantitative analysis of oils and fats by Fourier transform Raman spectroscopy. Spectrochim. Acta **47A**, 1449–1458.
20. Abbas, O., Fernandez, J. A., Codony, R., vo Holst, C. and Baeten, V. (2009) Assessment of the discrimination of animal fat by FT-Raman spectroscopy. J. Mol. Struct. **924–926**, 294–300.
21. Stefanov, I., Baeten, V., Abbas, O., Colman, E., Vlaeminck, B., De Baets, B. and Fievez, V. (2011) Determining milk isolated and conjugated trans-unsaturated fatty acids using Fourier Transform Raman Spectroscopy. J. Agri. Food Chem. **59**, 12771–12783.
22. Li-Chan, E. C. Y. (1996) The applications of Raman spectroscopy in food science. Trends in Food Sci. Tech. 7, 361–370.
23. Baeten, V., and Aparicio, R. (2000) Edible oils and fats authentication by Fourier transform Raman spectroscopy. Biotechnologie, Agronomie, Societe et Environement (BASE) **4**, 196–203.
24. Guzman, E., Baeten, V., Pierna, J. A. F. and Garcia-Mesa, J. A. (2011) Application of low-resolution Raman spectroscopy for the analysis of oxidized olive oil. Food Control **22**, 2036–2040.
25. Muik, B., Lendl, B., Molina-Diaz, B. A. and Ayora-Canada, M. J. (2005) Direct monitoring of lipid oxidation in edible oils by Fourier transform Raman spectroscopy. Chem. Phys. Lipids **134**, 173–182.
26. Motoyama, M., Nakajima, I., Ohmori, H., Watanabe, G. and Sasaki, K. (2018) A Raman spectroscopic method of evaluating fat crystalline states and its application in detecting pork fat. JARQ-JAPAN Agri. Res. Quarterly **52**, 17–22.
27. Katagiri, T., Yamamoto, Y. S., Ozaki, Y., Matsuura, Y. and Sato, H. (2009) High axial resolution Raman probe made of a single hollow optical fiber. Appl. Spectrosc. **63**, 103–107.
28. Meksiarun, P., Andriana, B. B., Matsuyoshi, H. and Sato, H. (2016) Non-invasive quantitative analysis of specific fat accumulation in subcutaneous adipose tissues using Raman spectroscopy. Sci. Rep. **6**, 37068-1-8.

29. Meksiarun, P., Maeda, Y., Hiroi, T., Andriana, B. B. and Sato, H. (2015) Analysis of the effects of dietary fat on body and skin lipids of hamsters by Raman spectroscopy. Analyst **140**, 4238–4244.
30. Meksiarun, P., Spegazzini, N., Matsui, H., Nakajima, K., Matsuda, Y. and Sato, H. (2015) In vivo study of lipid accumulation in the microalgae marine diatom Thalassiosira pseudonana using Raman spectroscopy. Appl. Spectrosc. **69**, 45–51.
31. Paramitha, P. N., Zakaria, R., Maryani, A., Kusaka, Y., Andriana, B. B., Hashimoto, K., Nakazawa, H., Kato, S. and Sato, H. (2021) Raman study on lipid droplets in hepatic cells co-cultured with fatty acids. Int. J. Mol. Sci. **22**, 7378–7391.

https://doi.org/10.1142/9789811264610_0007

Chapter 7

Point-of-Care Detection Strategies Aligned to Human Health Using Surface-Enhanced Raman Spectroscopy

Sian Sloan-Dennison, Hayleigh Kearns, Waleed Hassanain, Karen Faulds, Duncan Graham*

Department of Pure and Applied Chemistry, University of Strathclyde, Technology and Innovation Centre, 99 George Street, Glasgow, G1 1RD, UK
**Corresponding author: duncan.graham@strath.ac.uk*

7.1 Introduction

Point-of-care (POC) diagnostics are tests which can be performed at or near the site of a patient to produce results in a timely manner, improving on conventional tests which are mostly confined to a central laboratory. They are used in many different applications including diagnosing highly infectious diseases [1], providing routine daily monitoring of diseases such as diabetes [2], to assess the impact of treatments which includes oral anticoagulants [3] and for at home-testing to determine pregnancy [4]. There are many different types of POC devices and platforms. Due to the COVID-19 pandemic, paper-based lateral flows have become one of the most well known [5]. Microfluidic devices are also routinely used to provide on-the-spot answers [6]. The test also does not necessarily have to use a device and could be as simple as mixing of reagents and samples to produce a solution-based platform. It is usually designed to detect the presence of a biomarker using different chemistries such as the polymerase chain reaction (PCR), immunoassays or enzymatic tests. Labeling molecules are also used which can then be detected visually or with a read-out instrument, to give either a simple yes/no answer or provide a quantitative result.

To be seen as a viable POC diagnostic, the World Health Organization (WHO) has set a list of objectives to which the test should adhere. By following the WHO ASSURED criteria, the test must be 'Affordable, Sensitive, Specific, User-friendly, Rapid and Robust, Equipment-free and Deliverable' [7]. The hardest criteria to achieve is 'equipment-free' as many POC tests depend on a read-out instrument to quantify the concentration of analyte present. Although the read-out instrument is usually unavoidable, when selecting it, it should be portable, provide decision support, connect to other information systems and have a simple interface between the POC test and the instrument to retain a straightforward, easy-to-use POC diagnostic test [8]. A variety of read-out instruments are used to detect the labeling entity including fluorescence readers [9], ultraviolet-visible spectrometers [10] and potentiostats [11]. If nanoparticles are used to label, Raman spectrometers can be used as the read-out instrument to provide sensitive detection of biomarkers by assessing the surface-enhanced Raman scattering (SERS) signal from the device [12]. This chapter will review how SERS has been combined with POC diagnostic tests, the efforts being made to change the opinion of SERS being a lab-based technique and how it can become one of the gold standard methods used in POC testing.

SERS is an ultra-sensitive and selective analytical technique that has been employed in a wide range of biological and chemical applications [13, 14]. SERS substrates exist in the form of colloidal suspensions, electrodes, metal films, specially designed solid surfaces plus shaped and spherical nanoparticles [15]. To date, noble metal nanoparticles, commonly silver and gold, have been used as suspension-based SERS substrates as the bottom-up synthetic approaches are simple, cost-effective, highly reproducible, and the frequency of their surface plasmons fall within the visible region, which coincides with the laser wavelengths commonly used for Raman analysis [16–18]. In recent years, researchers have shown that it is possible to manipulate the size, shape, surface chemistry and/or metal composition and in doing so, it allows fine tuning of the optical properties, which can be exploited to make them application specific, viable in different environments and applicable to many analytes [13, 19–21]. Moreover, immense efforts have been implemented into the design, fabrication and synthesis of reproducible and reliable SERS substrates with finely tuned surface plasmon resonances, ranging from the visible to the near-infrared region (NIR). It is because of this that SERS-based approaches have been realized for many chemical and biomedical systems including the quantitative detection of trace materials, biomarkers, nucleic acids, proteins, pathogenic organisms plus cells associated with cancers and infectious diseases [13, 22–26].

Another area of SERS research that has gained significant attention, since its discovery 50 years ago, is the development of SERS tags. These are *in situ* probes which consist of metallic nanoparticles and organic reporter molecules. To date, most of the research has focused on designing SERS tags for use with visible laser excitations, as there is an abundance of Raman reporters and dye labels available as well as being compatible with POC diagnostics to provide quantitative assessment of biomarkers [15, 27–31]. More recently, however, as well as continuing to develop tags that operate in the visible region, there has also been a drive to develop SERS tags that operate in the NIR. Thus, with laser excitations between 950 and 1700 nm, there is greater depth of light penetration into biological samples, such as blood and tissue samples, compared to the visible region; plus fluorescence can be significantly reduced [32–35]. In addition, there is limited photobleaching and the infrared region provides an uncongested spectral window for optical analysis due to the absorption and scattering backgrounds of many molecules (in particular biomolecules) being at a minimum [35–38]. The drawbacks, however, are the limited availability of instrumentation and the fact that the intensity of Raman scattering is dependent on the fourth power of the excitation frequency. Thus, the scattering effect is weaker at these longer wavelengths [18]. Advancements in instrumentation and the design of NIR-active SERS substrates are making it possible for SERS to be conducted at these longer wavelengths. Hence, research has begun to emerge on the use of SERS combined with 1064 nm laser excitations and more recently with 1280 nm and 1550 nm [19, 39–45]. The groundbreaking work by Kearns *et al.* showed that it was possible to obtain femtomolar detection limits at 1064 nm and picomolar levels at 1280 nm and 1550 nm laser excitations, all using portable Raman spectrometers, by designing a new class of SERS nanotag [19, 42, 46]. Hence, continuing to develop SERS tags that are optically active at these longer wavelengths will be critical for future advancements in biomedical and optical applications, such as for use with photothermal ablation therapy and optical coherence tomography [47, 48]. Moreover, having SERS tags that can operate anywhere in the visible to NIR range provides researchers, scientists and medical professionals with the ability to choose the best detection system for their particular application.

To date, SERS tags have been demonstrated in a wide range of applications where both sensitivity and selectivity have been key requirements, such as in biomedical, forensic, and geological applications plus for homeland security [15, 22, 24, 25, 49–53].

Another important factor when discussing SERS systems is the multiplexing capabilities [22]. Raman-based techniques provide sharp, molecularly specific spectra making it possible to easily discriminate between individual components in a sample mixture, therefore making it an ideal technique for the detection of multiple analytes [18]. The ability to detect multiple targets simultaneously significantly reduces time and cost, whilst allowing for more information to be obtained in a single test. Additional benefits include minimal sample preparation, the ability to detect analytes in aqueous samples, small sample volumes and short analysis times [27]. An excellent example of SERS multiplexing was demonstrated by Faulds *et al.* when they successfully identified six labeled DNA sequences in a single sample [54]. Furthermore, the group has since published several papers in the area of multiplexing relating to human health, from the detection and quantification of meningitis-specific bacterial strains; the simultaneous identification of antimicrobial-resistant pathogens in a single sample at clinically relevant concentrations; and *in vivo* imaging of multiple vascular biomarkers to also multiplex imaging of three SERS tags at a depth of 10 mm within breast cancer tumor models [55–58].

To coincide with the research into fabricating reproducible SERS substrates, SERS tags and nanosensors with multiplexing capabilities, advancements in instrumentation has also been essential. It is the combination of practical and sensitive methods which are cost effective and portable that will be fundamental in SERS being widely accepted as a read-out instrument in POC diagnostic tests [59]. Prior to the turn of the century, most commercially available Raman spectrometers were either dispersive benchtop systems (commonly used with visible laser excitations) or Fourier transform Raman systems (commonly used with infrared laser excitations) [45, 60–62]. These systems are bulky, heavy units that require a connection to a power supply and computer, and therefore cannot easily be employed in a 'realistic field' setting such as at a patient's bedside [42]. This has led to an enormous drive towards developing low-cost, high-quality, handheld and portable Raman spectrometers that are still able to detect trace amounts of materials. This has been made possible thanks to advancements in microfabrication, diode lasers and collection optics [59]. Handheld instruments, especially, are unique in that they are small, light, battery operated (if required), cost effective and can be easily used by a single operator in diverse and challenging environments [46]. Thus, the widespread availability of these portable spectrometers is enabling on-site Raman analysis to become a reality.

The following sections will discuss how SERS can be used to detect clinically relevant biomarkers in a variety of POC platforms. Solution, microfluidics and paper-based platforms have all been combined with SERS to rapidly, sensitively and quantitatively detect a myriad of biomarkers. Conventionally confined to the lab with analysis performed on large, bulky spectrometers, the analysis is now being moved to portable Raman spectrometers to create a truly portable SERS-POC diagnostic test.

7.2 Solution-Based Systems

This section will focus on solution-based SERS approaches, both label-free and labeled systems with early work being discussed first, before providing some examples of research that has been conducted in a laboratory but with potential for use in POC settings. The future work that needs to be conducted so that these platforms can be implemented at the POC will also be highlighted. Following that, we will discuss a solution-based SERS assay that is ready for use, and at scale, in healthcare settings.

SERS-based strategies can be either label-free or label-mediated SERS systems, involving direct or indirect detection of a molecule/analyte respectively. Direct detection involves recording the spectral fingerprint of analytes adsorbed onto or in close proximity to the enhancing metal surface. Important information such as the nature of the analyte, suspension matrix and information regarding the enhancing material can be obtained using this approach; however, the challenge lies with the low Raman cross-section of many molecules, in particular biomolecules. Moreover, indirect strategies use the SERS response of a secondary molecule, such as a label or reporter molecule that has a very high Raman cross-section, that changes in the presence of the analyte and it is the SERS signal of the reporter molecule that is detected in this instance. Labeled SERS approaches are commonly used in more complex systems, for example when quantitative information regarding analytes in biofluids is required [13].

7.2.1 *Label-Free Detection by SERS*

SERS is a technique that has evolved considerably since its discovery, and found a variety of applications in biological and medical applications [63]. As mentioned previously, label-free SERS systems allow the intrinsic vibrational fingerprint of the analyte of interest to be detected and they have been reported in countless applications, including the detection of DNA, microorganisms and biomarkers [13]. These strategies are highly desirable for use in POC settings, because the sampling methodologies tend to be simpler, cost effective and the detection range is not subject to the quantity, reliability, and specificity of bio-recognition molecules such as antibodies or aptamers, hence they have the potential for shorter analysis times.

The first report of bacterial discrimination using a label-free approach was by Jarvis and Goodacre in 2004 [64]. In this report, bacteria were mixed with aggregated silver colloid and multivariate analysis was used to identify and discriminate between clinical bacterial isolates associated with urinary tract infections. The spectroscopic analysis was conducted using a 785 nm confocal Raman microscope and the bacterial mixture was dried onto a calcium fluoride disk. It took almost a decade before Wu *et al.* demonstrated the adaptability of a label-free system to a portable device, but the analysis took four hours and required two filtrations steps which would not be easily conducted in a POC setting [65]. Moreover, in 2015 Chen *et al.* demonstrated the first, fully *in situ* assay for the identification and discrimination of bacterial species in drinking water, namely *Escherichia coli (E. coli)*, *Pseudomonas aeruginosa (P. aeruginosa)* and methicillin-resistant *Staphylococcus aureus* (MRSA). Analysis was conducted in just five minutes with clinically relevant concentrations (10^3 CFU/mL) being obtained; however, it was conducted using a 785 nm benchtop Raman system, making this approach challenging for use in POC settings [66]. In 2016, Kamińska *et al.* detected and discriminated between three meningitis pathogens, *Neisseria meningitides (N. meningitides)*, *Haemophilus influenza (H. influenza)* and *Streptococcus pneumonia (S. pneumonia)*, in clinical cerebrospinal fluid (CSF) samples using a label-free SERS detection system and multivariate analysis [67]. The assay involved the combination of two types of colloids; gold- and silver-coated nucleopore track-etched polycarbonate membranes that allow for simultaneous filtration of CSF, immobilization of CSF components and the enhancement of their Raman signals. 48 clinical samples were analyzed, 38 of which were from patients who had tested positive for meningococcal meningitis and 10 control patients without meningitis.

This work demonstrated the isolation and simultaneous discrimination of multiple bacterial strains in a highly complex matrix. The analysis was conducted on a Raman microscope system making it incompatible with a POC setting; however, the detection platform for injecting the clinical fluids into the SERS-active membranes was portable and could easily be adapted for on-site testing. Moreover, modifying the filtration system and incorporating a portable spectrometer plus demonstrating the quantitative capabilities at clinically relevant concentrations would be beneficial for bringing this label-free detection platform to the clinic. In the same report, Kamińska *et al.* also demonstrated that it was possible to monitor the levels of the biomarker, neopterin, to determine if a patient had meningococcal meningitis. The results of the study confirmed that bacterial meningitis was associated with elevated CSF neopterin levels and thus could be used to predict meningitis, but that it was not possible to determine the bacterial strain causing the meningitis infection.

In addition to infectious disease detection, cancer has been a target for detection using SERS. MicroRNAs (miRNAs) have shown great promise as a biomarker for the early detection of various cancers. In 2016, Vo-Dinh *et al.* developed a new label-free detection strategy for the multiplexed detection of miRNAs [68]. This new sensing technology, called inverse molecular sentinel (iMS), can be used as a homogenous bioassay in solution. The iMS sensing mechanism employs plasmonic-active nanostars functionalized with stem-loop (hairpin) oligonucleotide probes that change conformation in the presence of target sequences, thus exploiting the distance dependence of SERS as the signal is switched from 'OFF to ON' upon binding to a specific bio-target. The platform allows for single-step detection without labeling or any subsequent wash steps, thus rendering the technique simple, inexpensive and user-friendly, all requirements for use in POC settings. The initial work by Wu and Vo-Dinh demonstrated the exciting new concept and the multiplexing capabilities by discriminating between two miRNA biomarkers associated with breast cancer [68]. Following on from this, Crawford *et al.* extended the work to directly detect biomarker miR-21, associated with esophageal cancer (see Figure 7.1), and then demonstrated the potential clinical capabilities by successfully detecting the esophageal biomarker in RNA extracted from endoscopic tissue biopsies [69]. This strategy is particularly advantageous as it uses only one probe and does not rely on aggregation between two nanoparticles, which could lead to instability in the SERS signal. The SERS enhancement of the hairpin formation is actually from the increased electromagnetic field

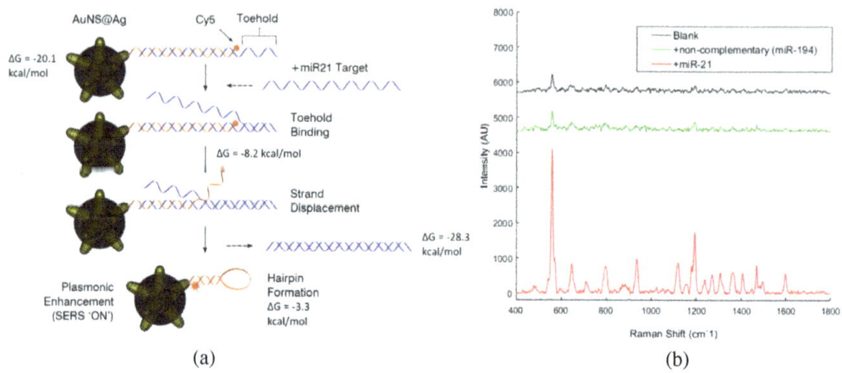

Figure 7.1. (a) Detection scheme of the SERS iMS nanoprobe. The "OFF-to-ON" signal switch is based on a non-enzymatic strand-displacement process and the conformational change of stem-loop (hairpin) oligonucleotide probes upon target binding. (b) SERS measurements of the iMS nanoprobe designed for the detection of miR21 in the absence of the target (black spectrum), in the presence of 1 μM non-complementary DNA with sequences corresponding to miR-194 miRNA (green spectrum), and in the presence of 1 μM miR-21 synthetic DNA targets (red spectrum). Reproduced from Ref. [69] with permission.

produced by single gold nanostar probes. The technique was validated against the gold standard, TaqMan quantitative reverse transcription PCR, with comparative results but it should be noted that this technique does not require target amplification, thus shortening the analysis time and making it a simpler approach to employ in clinical settings. The main drawback to this technique currently is that it utilizes a confocal Raman microscope system for analysis; however, if this SERS platform was integrated with a portable device and the quantitative capabilities demonstrated then it could potentially be employed as an alternative, simpler diagnostic tool to histopathology and a step-change in cancer diagnostics.

Furthermore, the ability to directly detect DNA has long been regarded as a valuable diagnostic indicator to monitor the presence and progression of various diseases. Label-free strategies have been applied to the direct SERS detection of DNA nucleotides, single-base mismatches plus single- and double-stranded DNA [22]. In 2012, Papadopoulou *et al.* demonstrated the direct detection of single- and double-stranded DNA at nanomolar concentrations as well as being able to discriminate between five DNA sequences, each corresponding to a different *E. coli* strain [70], thus demonstrating the sensitivity and multiplexing capabilities which can be achieved. However, in order for quantification to be determined, most DNA approaches utilize indirect detection strategies and often require target amplification; these modes of detection will be discussed further in the next section. Whilst label-free approaches do not depend on the efficacy of bio-recognition molecules and can produce sensitive and specific pathogen detection, there are several challenges associated with their use: i) it is difficult to obtain strong and reproducible Raman signals from analytes of interest due to the low Raman cross-section of many biomolecules, ii) most label-free systems require benchtop systems in order to achieve high levels of sensitivity, iii) generally additional handling steps are required such as target amplification or filtration, leading to longer analysis times, especially when portable instrumentation is employed and iv) often complex SERS spectra are obtained that require advanced data processing such as multivariate analysis and chemometric approaches to be utilized, adding another layer of complexity to the detection strategy [13]. To overcome some of these issues, labeled systems have been extensively investigated as discussed next.

7.2.2 *Indirect Detection by SERS*

An important branch of diagnostics for disease and pathogen detection lies with the indirect detection of nucleic acid sequences. PCR is commonly employed in combination with fluorescence as it enables sensitive and quantifiable detection of target analytes. However, it produces broad spectra, meaning fluorescence-based techniques cannot be used to detect multiple disease targets simultaneously. This is in contrast to SERS which, as described previously, is able to detect multiple bio-targets in a single complex matrix, sensitively and quantitatively [14]. Early research by Graham *et al.* demonstrated that nanoparticles functionalized with DNA could significantly enhance SERS signals through controlled aggregation following a specific biological recognition event such as DNA-DNA hybridization [71]. Feng *et al.* developed a sensitive and highly selective dual-mode nanosensor for the detection of telomerase activity, a biomarker associated with multiple cancers [72]. They demonstrated a wide detection range ($100–10^6$ cells/mL) and low detection limit (1 cell). Furthermore, they proved clinical capabilities by successfully detecting telomerase activity in 12 urine specimens from patients with bladder cancer with a detection limit down to 6.1×10^{-15} IU within one hour. This concept has since been extended to the identification of multiple targets; Mabbot *et al.* was able to discriminate between four DNA sequences, each corresponding to a different fungi species [73]. In the same study they successfully detected a single-stranded PCR product, relating to *Candida krusei*, to demonstrate that the methodology could be employed for the detection and diagnosis of invasive fungal infections. Furthermore, Gracie *et al.* developed a multiplex SERS assay for the detection and quantification of three bacterial strains associated with meningitis, with picomolar detection limits being obtained [55]. In an extension of this work, the authors demonstrated the detection of *S. pneumoniae* and *N. meningitidis* genomic DNA extracted from the CSF and blood of 28 patients admitted for sepsis and meningitis and confirmed its potential for use in a clinical setting [74]. The analysis was performed on a 532 nm benchtop Raman system with a total time, from preparing samples to obtaining the result, of five hours. The ability to easily change the sequences of the capture and reporter probes means this approach is not limited to bacterial meningitis detection and could be adapted for other infectious pathogens. Furthermore, the assay time is significantly quicker than culture-based methods which take ~36 hours. Nevertheless, to be truly used at the POC, additional improvements would need to be made such as integrating the platform with a portable spectrometer, significantly reducing the analysis time and clinical testing would need to be conducted on a greater scale. Moreover, magnetic nanoparticles have also been incorporated into DNA detection systems as they enable the benefit of applying magnetic separation to capture and isolate target analytes in complex matrices. This allows for concentration of samples and removal of unbound materials through wash or filtration steps, ultimately reducing the background signals and the chance of false positives, hence leading to improved sample quality and sensitivities [75]. This was first demonstrated by Zhang and Johnson in 2012, where they used gold-coated paramagnetic nanoparticles as both a SERS substrate and bio-separation reagent [76]. Two target DNA sequences complementary to Rift Valley Fever virus (RVFV) and West Nile virus (WNV) were isolated and detected at nanomolar concentrations in just one hour. Another report by Donnelly *et al.* describes a multi-target molecular diagnostic assay for fungal infections [77]. This time, two separate colloidal solutions were prepared; DNA-functionalized silver nanoparticles with probe one and a second complementary DNA probe functionalized on silver-coated magnetic nanoparticles, in a sandwich-type approach. By applying magnetic separation and washing away unbound materials, it led to improved sample quality with the signal enhancement, from 20 femtomoles of target DNA (sample) over the control, being 10 times. They also demonstrated the multiplexing capabilities of this platform with detection of two targets at a target DNA concentration of 100 femtomoles. These two separate nanoparticle approaches, one for the optical read-out and a second for magnetic capture, in a sandwich type assay tends to be the most commonly utilized magnetic separation strategy.

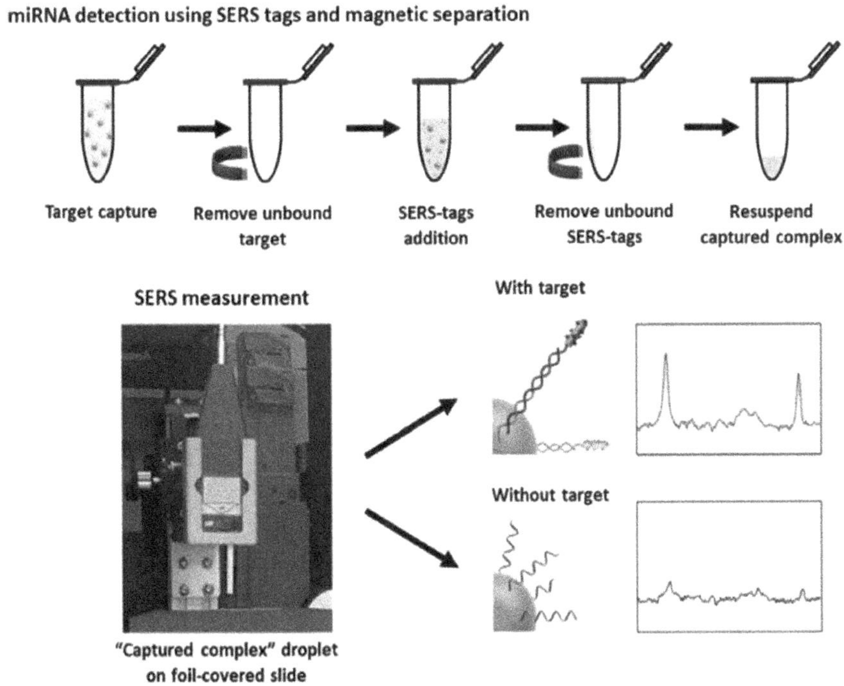

Figure 7.2. Schematic of magnetic capture-SERS platform for miRNA detection. SERS tags and magnetic nanoparticles are functionalized with complementary DNA probes specific to the target miRNA. Upon addition of magnetic nanoparticles conjugated with complementary DNA probes, the target miRNA is captured and then labeled with SERS tags conjugated with complementary reporter DNA through specific hybridization. The resultant hybridization complexes are magnetically concentrated and separated for the SERS measurement. The SERS tags assembly creates multiple 'hotspots' that enhance electromagnetic radiation of Raman molecules coated on the gold nanorods. Thus, an intense SERS signal occurred in the presence of the target. When there is no target, the hybridization complex cannot be formed, and the SERS tags will be washed away after magnetic separation, resulting in the absence of the SERS signal. Reproduced from Ref. [78] with permission.

Treerattrakoon *et al.* demonstrated a miRNA-based platform (Figure 7.2) for the detection of the cancer biomarker, miRNA29a, incorporating SERS-active gold nanorods functionalized with DNA detection probes and DNA-functionalized magnetic nanoparticles which enabled magnetic capture and separation. A purpose-built, SERS system was developed and analysis was conducted by focusing on a sample droplet. Analysis time was 1.5 hours and the detection limit was 10 pM without the need for amplification [78]. Moreoever, Zhang *et al.* reported the simultaneous detection of the foodborne pathogens *Salmonella typhimurium* (*S. typhimurium*) and *Staphylococcus aureus* (*S. aureus*) at concentrations of 15 and 35 CFU/mL respectively [79].

Díaz-Amaya *et al.* [80] detected and quantified whole cell *E. coli* in just 20 minutes in both pure culture and ground beef samples at concentrations of 10^1 and 10^2 CFU/mL respectively. Furthermore, Zhang *et al.* reported a dual-recognition sandwich assay utilizing vanocymin-functionalized gold-coated magnetic nanoparticles, a broad-spectrum glycopeptide to capture and isolate the bacterial pathogens, and *E. coli* and *S. aureus* at concentrations of 50 and 20 CFU/mL, respectively, in just 15 minutes [81]. In addition, they demonstrated the specificity and sensitivity of this assay in clinical samples, by detecting and quantifying *E. coli* in urine samples down to 50 CFU/mL in 1.5 hours. In order for this type of SERS platform to be considered for use in a POC setting it would need to be further optimized, hence the analysis time would need to be reduced to less than 30 minutes and the detection platform would need to be optimized, as a microscope-based system is not user friendly or ideal for use in a clinic.

Another area of significant interest for disease and pathogen detection is the development of SERS-based immunoassays. These are quantitative tests that utilize the specific binding between antigens and antibodies and have been exploited in a wide range of areas, from foodborne diseases to cancer detection due to the high specificity, sensitivity and ability to detect multiple biomarkers simultaneously [22]. This type of platform has been employed to detect protein biomarkers such as immunoglobulin G (IgG) and prostate-specific antigen (PSA) at very low limits of detection (approximately 1 pg/mL) [82]. Since then, a vast number of papers have emerged on the detection of protein biomarkers and their applicability in clinical samples demonstrated [23]. In 2013, Neng *et al.* employed antibody-functionalized paramagnetic nanoparticles in conjunction with SERS-active gold nanoparticles for the detection of antigens specific to WNV and RVFV, with detection limits as low as 5 fg/mL when the assay was performed in salt buffer and 25 pg/mL in buffer spiked with fetal bovine serum [83]. This assay was further optimized with silica-encapsulated gold nanoparticles being utilized for SERS detection, improving the stability, reproducibility and signal capabilities of the SERS tags and also the assay was adapted for use with portable instrumentation. In this work, three antigens were detected simultaneously, namely, WNV, RVFV and *Yersinia pestis*, at a concentration of ~10 pg/mL in 20% fetal bovine serum [84]. Kearns *et al.* demonstrated a similar magnetic separation approach for the capture and isolation of three bacterial pathogens, *E. coli*, *S. typhimurium* and MRSA in a single sample within one hour, at the clinically relevant concentration of 10^3 CFU/mL and 10^1 CFU/mL in each of the single pathogen tests [56]. However, in this work a legume lectin (concanavalin A) was used as the capture biomolecule of choice as it binds specifically to terminal α-*D*-mannosyl and α-*D*-glucosyl groups present on the surface of bacteria, thus enabling broadband capture of multiple pathogens. The use of a biomolecule, such as a lectin, makes this approach easily adaptable for use with other pathogenic species. Further, pathogen verification could be done by eye without the need for complex data processing, thus simplifying the technique significantly. Since then the SERS platform has been transferred to a portable system, demonstrating its potential as a sensitive and reliable on-site diagnostic tool for bacterial pathogens [85]. Future work would involve reducing the analysis time, simplifying the sample preparation for non-technical end-users and testing the assay in complex biofluids, such as urine or blood taken from patients. Moreover, biomarkers enabling cancer detection have also gained extensive interest. In 2017, Cheng *et al.* reported a SERS-based immunoassay using magnetic beads and SERS tags for the determination of free to total (f/t) PSA ratio in clinical serum. In addition, they demonstrated the simultaneous detection of two PSA markers, free PSA and complexed PSA, with limits of detection at 0.012 ng/mL and 0.15 ng/mL, respectively. Small sample volumes were used (10 μL) and the analysis time was short (less than one hour), but a confocal microscope was employed [86]. Moreover in 2021, Zhang *et al.* simultaneously detected multiple protein biomarkers expressed on cancer-derived small extracellular vesicles (EVs) [87]. Specifically, they detected three receptors specific to pancreatic cancer using a magnetic sandwich assay approach with detection down to 2.3×10^6 particles/mL using a portable Raman spectrometer. They were also able to phenotype the profiles of small EVs from pancreatic cancer, colorectal cancer, and bladder cancer cell lines in both serum and PBS by SERS. Another promising and non-invasive approach for cancer detection in liquid, circumventing the need for invasive practices such as biopsies, was demonstrated by Sorina-Tater *et al.* In this approach, the authors use a sandwich-type SERS immunosensor to detect and quantify the tumor marker, carcinoembryonic antigen-related cell adhesion molecule 5, at a concentration of ~3 ng/mL using a portable spectrometer [88]. These approaches show great promise for detecting and monitoring clinically relevant biomarkers in complex biofluids. The next steps for these types of SERS platforms to be considered for non-invasive cancer diagnosis and drug monitoring would be quantitative studies in patient samples and at scale. Additionally, the sampling process would need to be made less labor intensive as currently only trained personnel would be able to conduct the analysis.

7.2.3 *Solution-Based SERS Systems in POC*

As discussed already, huge efforts are being made in the design and development of solution-based platforms for facilitating the use of SERS in POC settings. As directed by the WHO, a POC system or device has to meet the following requirements: it must be robust, rapid, sensitive, specific, cost effective, reproducible, user friendly, adaptable and field deployable [89]. The previous examples all show promise for use in the clinic, but the limitations which have been discussed throughout must first be overcome. Nevertheless, very recently there has been a report where a solution-based SERS platform is ready for use at the POC. It is a rapid and ultra-sensitive SERS immunoassay for the detection of the severe acute respiratory syndrome coronavirus 2 virus (SARS-CoV-2), better known as the COVID-19 virus, which caused the 2019 pandemic. The detection assay reported by Mohammadi *et al.*, and shown in Figure 7.3, involves the use of a single-chain Fv (scFv) recombinant antibody

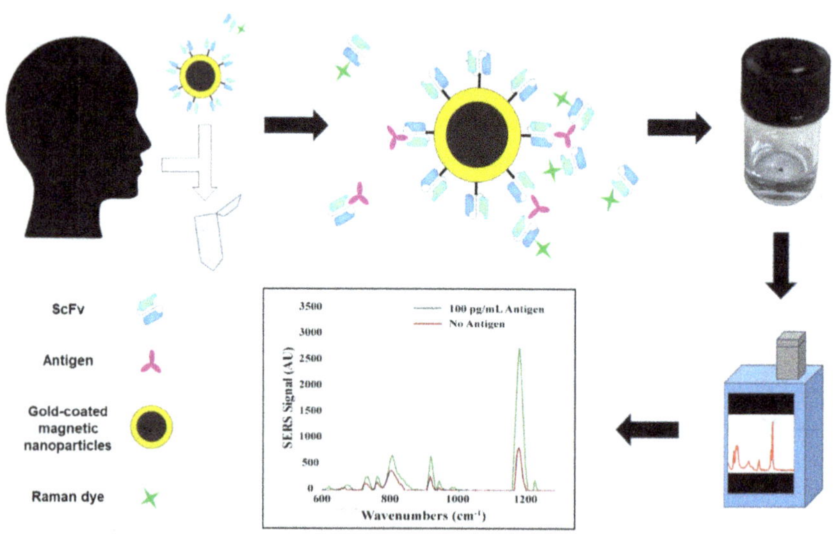

Figure 7.3. Schematic of the single-particle SERS immunoassay. Virus-binding scFv antibody fragments labeled with the Raman-active dye malachite green and scFv-conjugated magnetic gold nanoshells are mixed with saliva samples. In the presence of antigen, immunocomplexes form. An external magnet is used to pellet any immunocomplexes, and the SERS spectrum and signal intensity of that pellet is measured. Reproduced from Ref. [90] with permission.

labeled with a SERS active dye, plus unlabeled scFv-conjugated gold-coated magnetic nanoparticles; in the presence of the target analyte, SARS-CoV-2 spike protein, an immunocomplex forms and an increase in SERS signal is observed [90]. An external magnet is used to pellet the immunocomplex, and the SERS spectrum and signal intensity of that pellet is measured. The assay detects inactivated SARS-CoV-2 virus and spike protein in saliva at concentrations of 1.94×10^3 genomes/mL and 4.7 fg/mL, respectively, giving limits of detection in the range comparable to that of the gold standard PCR test. Further, the assay was able to detect all SARS-CoV-2 spike proteins of concern, i.e., alpha, beta, gamma, delta, and omicron variants, without recognizing the closely related SARS-CoV and MERS-CoV spike proteins, demonstrating the specificity of the test. In addition, the total analysis time from sampling to result is just 30 minutes, comparable to lateral flow assays (LFAs) and significantly faster than PCR tests. The test uses a handheld, battery-powered Raman spectrometer and does not require any wash steps — only sample mixing and a simple magnetic separation step. Thus, the simplicity of the technique means that it can be conducted by persons with minimum scientific knowledge, ultimately making the technique user friendly.

As it stands, this rapid, low-cost, solution-based SERS assay is ready for use and could be implemented immediately in healthcare settings, as well as workplaces, schools, airports, etc., actually anywhere large-scale screening is required to reduce transmission. The simplicity of the approach can also be adapted for a number of different biomarkers, creating the opportunity for solution-based SERS-POC platforms that can be used in many environments.

Solution-based SERS systems produce a simple 'one-pot' detection platform; however, it is difficult to make these platforms automated and errors in handling the reagents when pipetting and mixing can occur. To address this, biomarker detection assays can take place in microfluidic devices which eliminate human error. Their applications in POC and combination with SERS will be discussed next.

7.3 Microfludic-Based Systems

Microfluidic devices take a sample in a fluid and process it by manipulating the flow of the fluid through a series of channels in an automated fashion. Known as a 'lab on a chip,' they are designed to have the ability to carry out pre-treatment, dilution, mixing, chemical reactions, detection and product abstraction on the nano- or microscale. They are considered to be portable devices due to their small size and have seen increasing use in POC applications, especially in resource-limited settings, due to the low sample volume needed, low associated costs with reagents and chip material, being easily reusable or disposable and have a rapid processing time while still maintaining sensitivity and selectivity [91].

A simplistic view of a microfluidic device is shown in Figure 7.4. It is comprised of a series of microchannels etched or molded into a material such as glass, silicon or polymer. The dominant fluid regime is laminar flow which moves and delivers flow. Laminar flow patterns allow two or more fluids to move side by side in a channel without interference and is governed by the Reynolds number, a term which relates the density, velocity, and viscosity of a fluid [92]. A large Reynolds number corresponds to a turbulent flow but, if low, laminar flow regime occurs as is the case in the microchannels. Capillary-driven flow is another flow which uses capillary action to manipulate fluids, therefore not relying on external forces such as pressure controllers or syringe pumps. The action takes into account the surface tension of a liquid and the geometry and surface chemistry of its solid support [93]. The design of the channels is used to manipulate the fluid in a certain way such as pumping, sorting and mixing. The channels are confined to the chip which is connected to the outside by inlet or outlet ports, serving as the interface between the macro and micro world. The sample is injected (using a syringe or peristaltic pump) into the inlet and moved to the sample preparation chamber. Preparation of the sample can include mixing, conjugation and separation. After this, the solution is moved into the detection chamber. What happens here is dependent on the application of the device. The result is usually detected here but a separate analysis zone is also an option.

There are a number of biochemical reactions which have been performed on microfluidic devices. These include PCR [94], loop-mediated isothermal

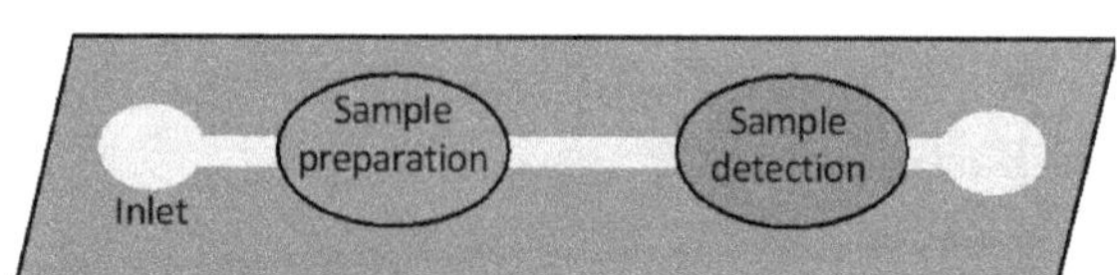

Figure 7.4. Simplistic view of a microfluidic device showing the inlet, sample preparation chamber, detection chamber and outlet.

amplification [95] and immunoassays based on aptamer- or antibody-to-antigen recognition [96]. To detect and quantify, a variety of methods have been applied including fluorescence, mass spectrometry and SERS.

PCR has been routinely used in nucleic acid diagnostics; however, it has been restricted to the lab due to the complex sample preparation required which includes thermocycling. Using microfluidic chips, reaction conditions such as temperature and time can be carefully controlled providing rapid analysis for a number of infectious pathogens including COVID-19 [97], influenza A (H1N1) [98] and human papillomavirus [99]. The PCR products are detected using fluorescence. Generally, this involves sliding the chip into a fluorescence reader where real-time analysis can take place [100]. However, expensive, bulky readers severely limit the portability aspect of the device as a whole. To overcome this, real-time *in situ* fluorescence monitoring of the reaction has been achieved using a smartphone camera developed to analyze the fluorescence signal intensity of the collected images [101]. Smartphone-based imaging is becoming a massive component in moving devices from the lab to the POC, allowing faster and cheaper analysis on-site. As this broadens the situations that devices can be used in, it also has great potential to study epidemiology of diseases as accurate geographic and demographic data can now be stored [102].

Microfluidic devices can also be coupled with mass spectrometry instruments, generally electrospray ionization and matrix-assisted laser desorption/ionization. The microfluidic devices usually have the role of pre-treating a sample, separating it or protein digestion [103]. Although this coupling may not be fruitful in terms of POC applications, due to the large, expensive mass spectrometry equipment, it has shown advantages in food analysis [104], cell metabolism [105] and elemental analysis [106].

As discussed, a very common POC application is the detection of biomarkers using immunoassays. In POC situations, they are used to detect the presence and concentration of a biomarker in a complex matrix with little sample preparation. The rapid result will give quick feedback for the user and can lead to better patient stratification or isolation if infectious, to stop the risk of spreading. Immunoassays in a microfluidic device can adopt numerous formats and labels. A conventional format injects the sample and captures antibody labeled with a fluorescent microsphere into the inlets. The two are introduced together and bind to form an immunocomplex, which flows to a section of the device where the detection antibody has been immobilized.

The sandwich immunoassay is formed and analyzed by placing the chip into a fluorescence reader to measure the amount of label present. This format has been used to detect SARS-CoV-2-IgM/IgG/Antigen in serum with an associated cost of only 0.71 dollar [107]. Using a similar immunoassay format, alternariol monomethyl ether antigens have been detected using antibodies labeled with gold nanoparticles via UV spectroscopy. In this example, the antibody-antigen interaction took place in a micro-mixing channel and was then introduced to the immobilized detection antibody. When analyzed, alternariol monomethyl ether was detected at 12.5 pg/mL. A smartphone reading was also performed on the device which detected as low as 200 pg/mL of alternariol monomethyl in less than 15 minutes, creating a truly portable system [108]. Another possible immunoassay format utilizes a 'lab-on-disk' device to assess the formation of nanoclusters that form in a solution when the antigen is present. Using magnetic nanoparticles, the amount and size of the nanoclusters was quantified using an optomagnetic readout. This approach has been used to detect dengue fever in 8 minutes, with only 6 mL of serum with a limit of detection of 25 ng/mL [109]. Fluorescence, UV, mass spectrometry and optomagnetic read-outs all show promise for microfluidic devices; however, they lack sensitivity and multiplexing capabilities. To achieve this, SERS can be used.

7.3.1 *SERS and Microfluidics*

The combination of SERS and microfluidics has huge benefit in various applications, particularly reaction monitoring, food analysis, environmental samples and bio-analysis. This is due to a number of advantages, first being that water is a very weak Raman scatterer and easily integrated with the aqueous solvents used in microfluidics. SERS can provide fingerprint data about a variety of biomolecules when trapped and sorted in microfluidic devices. Real-time detection of chemical and biological processes can be followed. Most importantly, in terms of POC aspect, SERS is also quantitative and can lead to the detection of very low concentrations of biomarkers of interest. However, this advantage comes with a caveat, as quantitative SERS is challenging due to poor reproducibility [110]. It is entirely dependent on the quality of the metal nanostructures being used and the measurement conditions. Their synthesis has to be expertly characterized in order to provide a platform for quantitative detection in the POC devices and their analysis should produce stable SERS signals with little fluctuation. Nanostructures in microfluidic devices can either be nanoparticle solutions injected into the device which react along the channels, or stationary substrates which are integrated or *in situ*. To produce strong, reproducible SERS signals, SERS microfluidics uses two different methods: continuous flow and droplet-based platforms. Each type has its own advantages and disadvantages. For example, continuous flow-based systems use small sample volumes, are easy to manipulate and control, have no liquid modification and allow rapid diffusion of analytes towards the substrate. However, it suffers from memory effects and poor reproducibility. Droplet-based platforms have very good reproducibility, high-throughput and rapid reactions but the droplets can become unstable [111]. It is important that the device has a high degree of control in order to produce the most reproducible SERS signal possible.

If continuous flow and homogenous mixing conditions are maintained, a reproducible SERS signal can be achieved. This has been demonstrated by Lee *et al.* who built a gradient microfluidic device with gold-patterned microarray wells for the detection of alpha-fetoprotein model protein biomarker in an immunoassay [112]. The layout of the chip is shown in Figure 7.5(a) and consists of three layers. In the top layer, capture antibodies labeled with hollow gold nanoparticles are coated in a Raman reporter and antibody, buffer and the antigen are injected. The injected flow then splits into six streams initially at the same concentration. This is connected to the middle layer which is capable of generating antigen gradients with six diluted concentrations. This was possible using a cascade-mixing stage which removes tedious manual dilution that can

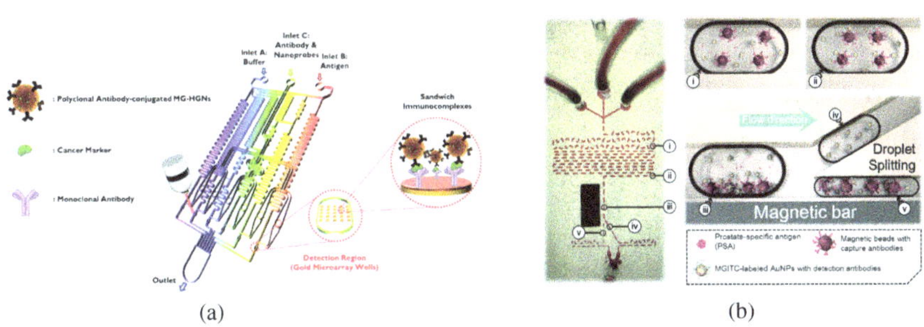

Figure 7.5. (a) Image of gold array-embedded gradient microfluidic device. Layer 1 contains the inlets, layer 2 has the N cascade-mixing channels and layer 3 consists of the gold microarray detection region. A schematic of the sandwich immunocomplex formed on the arrays is also shown. (b) Optical image of SERS-based microdroplet sensor for wash-free magnetic assay showing channels filled with red ink and schematic of immunoassay showing droplet-spilling mechanism: i) Mixing of reagents. ii) Formation of immunocomplex. iii) Isolation of magnetic immunocomplexes. iv) Supernatum including unbound gold nanoparticles. v) Separated magnetic immunocomplexes. Reproduced from Refs. [112] and [122], respectively, with permission.

lead to serious experimental error. The bottom layer has six gold-patterned microarrays coated in detection antibodies. The sandwich immunoassay is formed here. A large SERS signal is generated when the immunoassay formed, first from the hollow gold nanoparticles, second from the hotspots emerging between the aggregates formed on the array, and third from the hotspots formed between the edge of the nanoparticles and the gold substrate. The fully automatic and programmable microfluidic device was capable of producing consistent and stable SERS signals with a low limit of detection. Similar continuous flow immunoassay microfluidic devices have been used to detect hepatitis B in human blood plasma [113]. Another approach used a self-referencing continuous dielectrophoretic microfluidic device to detect and characterize *E. coli* at high sensitivity in water [114]. The duplex detection of *Entamoeba histolytica (E. histoytica)* pathogens using nano-yeast single-chain variable fragments instead of antibodies to reduce the overall cost of the assay and nanoclusters coated in silica to produce stable SERS signals have also been applied to a continuous microfluidic device [115].

Many SERS-microfluidic immunoassays use magnetic nanoparticles coated in antibodies to trap the sandwich immunocomplex, using an external magnet underneath the device. The immunocomplex will contain a nanoparticle coated in a Raman reporter, which will be present at the trapping zone, leading to the formation of hotspots which produce a strong SERS signal when analyzed. This was first shown by Li *et al.* for the detection of carcinoembryonic antigen [116]. Another approach is to use a 'SERS-based optofluidic sensor' with integrated solenoids. The antigen to be detected and buffer are added to the inlets at the top which serial dilutes the antigen using the groove structure region. Hollow gold nanoparticles functionalized with a Raman reporter and polyclonal antibody, and magnetic nanoparticles functionalized with a monoclonal antibody, are then added and the immunocomplex forms. The immunocomplex is trapped in the microfluidic channel by the selonids where the SERS analysis takes place. Using rabbit IgG as a proof of concept, a good linear response was observed from 0–100 ng/mL with low error in the SERS measurements. Similar designs have been used to detect the anthrax biomarker poly-y-d-glutamic acid [117], immunoglobulin [118] and influenza A [119].

Microdroplets offer significant advantages in microfluidic devices in terms of lower sample volumes and high-throughput analysis. When combined with optical detection, careful control over the pump and analysis parameters needs to be taken into account to create a system which can be quantitative. Syme *et al.* demonstrated this by combining SERS detection with microdroplets for the quantitative real-time spectral characterization of variable analyte mixtures within individual microdroplets [120]. In this design, the device had three inlets, one for oil and two for aqueous analytes. Droplet formation occurred at the T-junction where the oil meets the aqueous solution, and the dimensions were carefully controlled by the selected flow rate. Real-time SERS of the flowing droplets was measured using fast acquisition time (20 ms) and it was possible to measure two different Raman reporters' signals titrated at different concentrations from the droplets over five minutes. This demonstrated the novel combination of SERS multiplexing and real-time microdroplet detection. Gao *et al.* devised a SERS-based microdroplet sensor for the detection of diaquat dibromide monohydrate (DQ) in water [121]. The device was composed of two different segmented flow regimes, one with fresh silver nanoparticles and the other which merged them with DQ for label-free SERS detection. They proposed that by synthesizing the silver nanoparticles in the device the reaction conditions could be controlled to obtain various sizes with little contamination.

SERS microfluidic, microdroplet-based systems have also been used for the detection of biomarkers using immunoassays. In order to increase sensitivity and improve control, magnetic nanoparticles have also been incorporated. This combination reduces washing unbound reagents and the need for complicated solenoid fabrications which have been used to trap magnetic immunocomplexes. An example of this by Gao *et al.* uses magnetic nanoparticles coated in capture antibody and gold nanoparticles coated in Raman reporter and detection antibodies [122]. The system has four distinct components which generate microdroplets, separate the immunocomplexes and supernatum, isolate magnetic complex droplets and collect unbound SERS droplets for SERS detection. An optical image of the device is shown in Figure 7.5(b), highlighting the key areas and depicting how the droplets are split once the immunoassays are formed due to magnetic separation. The SERS signal of the supernatant droplets were measured with a frequency of 174 droplets per minute, an integration time of 10 seconds, and quantitative analysis of PSA was achieved with an excellent linear response between 0.05–200 ng/mL, which is consistent with the requirements in clinical applications [122]. This group advanced on this work by creating a parallel droplet-based microfluidic device which was designed and fabricated to automatically perform dual immunoassays for the quantitative analysis of free PSA and total PSA, with a good linear response achieved for both [123].

7.3.2 *Microfluidic-Based SERS Platforms in POC*

Microfluidic devices are small and portable. However, if the read-out technique is bulky and expensive, the device is left in the lab. Large, expensive Raman microscope instruments are conventionally used to analyze microfluidic devices, by focusing on the detection zone using a microscope. The majority of the examples given before uses this methodology. This inevitably leads to SERS microfluidics being left out of POC uses. However, handheld Raman readers are being integrated with microfluidics to create a truly portable system that can be used at the POC. This has recently been reported by coupling SERS microfluidic device with a portable fiber-based setup. A roughened gold nanoparticle surface embedded into the device was tested by flowing rhodamine 6G samples as a proof of concept and then an Alzheimer biomarker in a label-free approach [124]. Another label-free SERS approach identified four different pathogens on an *in situ* silver nanostructure with a portable Raman spectrometer [125]. A portable Raman system has also been coupled to a microfluidic electrophoresis device for the detection of *E. coli* [126]. The authors noted that the probe diameter at the focal point of the portable system was larger than the benchtop Raman system. This allowed signal to be collected from more bacteria yielding better statistics; however, the laser intensity was lower as it was spread over a larger area. The results demonstrate a compact portable system for rapid and highly sensitive detection of specific pathogens in the field. Although not related to health care, portable SERS microfluidics has also been used to detect the contaminant crystal violet in water [127].

POC is usually thought of as detecting biomarkers to diagnose an illness more quickly in order to lead to earlier intervention, and the immunoassay examples given here have all focused on faster detection of biomarkers related to disease with very high sensitivity. However, recently personal health and wellbeing have become of huge importance. Personal health technology includes portable devices with sensors linked to smartphones and cloud-based servers. The sensors can be environmental and capture a user's environment, behavioral such as counting steps, and physiological which will capture the user's bodily state [128]. Physiological devices use flexible microfluidics which are 'stuck' to the wearer and provide information about their health immediately by enabling cognition of molecular-level signatures related to physiological information in sweat [129]. Colorimetric, fluorescent and electrochemical sensors have all been widely adopted but have issues with poor sensitivity, are susceptible to external lighting, and require sophisticated

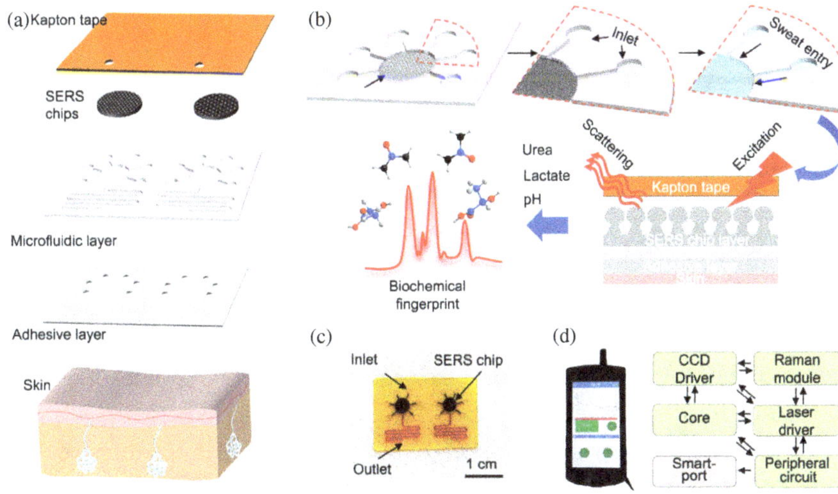

Figure 7.6. (a) Stacked view showing each layer of the microfluidic device. (b) Schematic of all-in-one biofluid flowing, store, and SERS analysis. (c) Actual image of as-prepared microfluidic SERS sensor attached to the skin. (d) System-level block diagram showing the internal functional modules of the portable Raman analyzer. Reproduced from Ref. [129]. with permission.

electrode and circuit design, respectively. These issues have been overcome by combining wearable, microfluidic, nanoplasmonic sensors with portable SERS measurements to detect urea, lactate and pH in sweat. The design of the microfluidic design, shown in Figure 7.6, allows sweat to be driven to the plasmonic metasurface which is then analyzed using a portable handheld Raman reader. In contrast to the heavy desktop instruments, this method allows sweat to be tracked on the go.

The combination of SERS with microfluidic devices have produced an ultra-sensitive platform allowing for complex reactions to be automated. Many of the examples given concentrate the SERS signal, allowing for very sensitive detection limits of clinically relevant biomarkers to be achieved. However, the sophisticated design of many of these devices will lead to increased cost, a hindrance when trying to produce POC devices. The last section will review cheaper, paper-based alternatives.

7.4 Paper-Based SERS Devices

Paper is widely used in our daily life as a cheap, multipurpose and flexible material. The advance in modern and innovative technology promoted the use of paper-based platforms, as the material of choice, in many scientific and biomedical applications such as pH testing paper, pregnancy testing strips, blood glucose dipsticks, and lateral flow strips for disease biomarker diagnosis, etc. [130]. This could be attributed to the ease of use, low cost of production, and most importantly the intrinsic capacity of paper to transport fluid [131], which make the paper-based platforms compatible with different biological matrices.

Due to the fundamental characteristics of paper-based platforms such as flexibility, lightweight, biocompatibility, biodegradability and availability [132], different interesting paper-based substrate designs have been widely integrated with SERS for various applications, such as POC clinical diagnosis [133, 134], food safety [135], forensics [136], pharmaceuticals [137] and environmental monitoring [138]. The paper-based substrates offer several advantageous properties over other solid-based platforms, such as uniformity, reproducibility and inherent low cost [132], which participate in improving the overall performance of the SERS detection. Additionally, the physical properties of paper-based substrates enable the loading of hotspots onto their surface easily, which increases the SERS detection sensitivity. Moreover, the paper surface is rich with cellulose and hence the hydroxyl functional group, which enables the easy functionalization of the paper surface with different functional groups and with a variety of metallic nanostructures of different shapes and sizes [139]. Furthermore, paper-based substrates possess high compatibility with multiplexed detection, and samples can be easily separated and concentrated. Therefore, due to all these properties, paper-based platforms are currently considered as a promising choice for SERS-based immunoassays [130].

The first use of paper-based substrates in SERS measurement can be traced back to 1984 when Vo-Dinh *et al.* [140] and Tran [141] reported the use of paper substrates for the SERS detection of different organic components and dyes, respectively, with detection limits of sub-nanogram levels. Since then, the number of publications reporting the use of paper-based substrates in SERS-based detection methods has increased tremendously as per Figure 7.7, which demonstrates an upward trend within the last 20 years. Generally, paper-based platforms for SERS could be classified into three main categories: (1) lateral flow test strips, (2) microfluidics paper-based analytical devices and (3) plasmonic nanostructured paper SERS substrates. In the next sections, the fabrication methods for each category and their potential use for POC purposes will be highlighted.

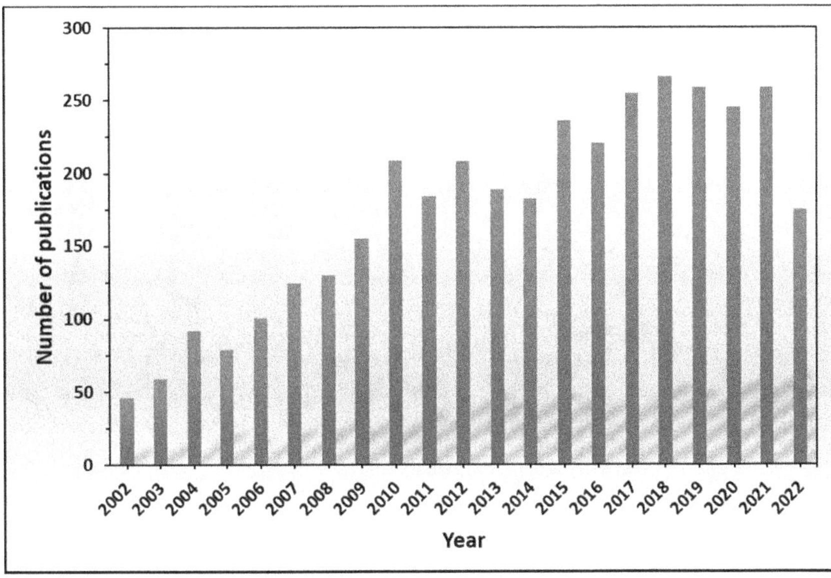

Figure 7.7. Number of publications per year that reported the use of paper-based substrates for SERS-based detection methods in the last 20 years as per the Web of Science database search in December 2022.

7.4.1 *Lateral Flow Test Strips*

Conventional lateral flow strips are simple paper-based devices that are used to indicate the presence of a target analyte in a given sample. They are currently used as well-established, commercially available, rapid diagnostic tests for many POC and home applications such as in the screening of infectious diseases [142], drugs of abuse [143] and pregnancy tests [144]. They are used successfully in different matrices such as blood, urine and saliva. They are often used as qualitative screening tests to indicate a yes/no answer, through the visual interpretation of the results via monitoring the color change of the test lines by the naked eye within a short time (10–20 minutes) [144].

The lateral flow strips are usually made of four main components: (1) a sample pad for sample deposition, (2) a conjugate pad to store the conjugated labels until the test begins, (3) a nitrocellulose membrane that contains test and control lines to indicate the test result and (4) absorbent pad at the end of the strip to wick the moisture from the membrane and aid in sample flow. Each component overlaps by at least 1–2 mm to enable the smooth capillary flow of the sample all over the strip in a horizontal orientation (Figure 7.8(a)).

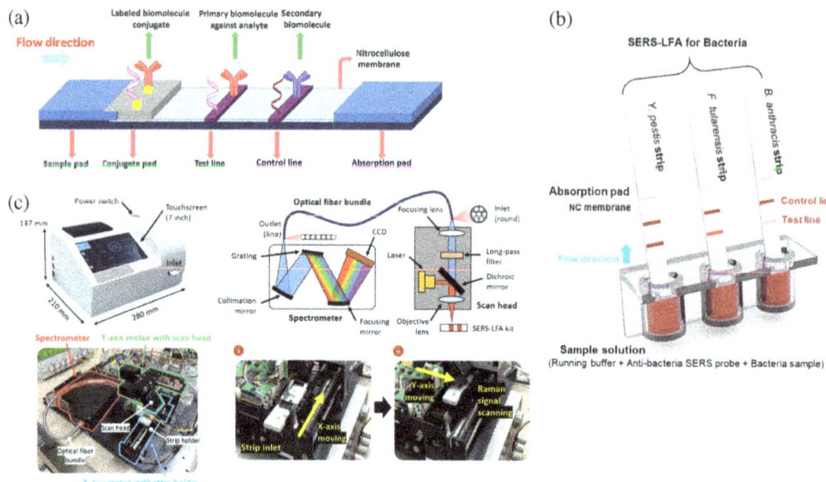

Figure 7.8. (a) Basic structure of the four components of a lateral flow strip showing horizontal flow direction. (b) Half-strip LFA design with a vertical flow direction. (c) Design of a portable SERS reader specified for lateral flow strips. Reproduced from Refs. [148], [154] and [158], respectively, with permission.

In some other designs, the strips are composed of only the nitrocellulose membrane and the absorbent pad in a format known as half-strip or dipstick test, where the strip is dipped into a mixture of the sample matrix and conjugated label to enable the vertical movement of the liquids in an upward orientation (Figure 7.8(b)) [145–147]. The lateral flow tests could be carried out via two methods, sandwich and competitive. These two methods work in a similar way, but they have different ways for displaying the results. In the sandwich assay, the target analyte binds to the conjugated label, then binds again to the binding reagents at the test line. Therefore, a test line coloration occurs and indicates a positive test, while the lack of line coloration indicates a negative test. In the less common competitive assay, the conjugated label and the binding reagents at the test line "compete" with each other for the binding with the target analyte. In the positive test, the target binds to the conjugated label and cannot bind to the binding reagents at the test line. Therefore, the test line will not be colored in positive tests, while a colored line indicates a negative result [148].

The most common conjugated labels that are used with lateral flow strips are composed of gold nanostructures conjugated passively or covalently with target-selective antibody or aptamer molecules for the specific detection of the target analyte in different matrices. To avoid any non-specific interference from the matrix components, the nanostructure's surface is usually backfilled with a protein such as bovine serum albumin. Gold nanostructures are chemically stable and have a strong optical property that makes them exceptionally strong absorbers and scatterers of light. Additionally, they offer strongly colored particles bound to the test lines on a white nitrocellulose strip, which simplify the test result interpretation by the naked eye [148].

There are many advantages of using lateral flow strips for rapid POC testing; however, they also possess major limitations in terms of poor sensitivity and quantification capability [145, 149]. Therefore, they might be inadequate for the early diagnosis and/or estimation of a specific level of a target [150]. To overcome these limitations, SERS detection was integrated with lateral flow strips in a single platform. As a powerful analytical technique, SERS improved the detection sensitivity and quantification capability of the conventional LFA. The approach of integrating SERS with lateral flow test in one platform has been extensively reported previously in many applications [151–154]. As a sensitive, stable, cost-effective, and user-friendly platform that is compatible with POC application, it showed a strong potential to be used as an alternative tool for traditional biomarker detection for on-site and facile diagnosis of different diseases [151, 155]. Additionally, this combination eliminated the need for expensive, highly patterned SERS substrates and for other separation technique instruments (such as high-performance liquid chromatography) in multiplexed analysis. For example, Zhang *et al.* demonstrated the use of a SERS lateral flow platform for the ultra-sensitive and high-throughput diagnosis of nucleic acids of respiratory tract infection pathogens in throat swab samples [156]. In this multiplexed assay, core-shell SERS tags encoded with two Raman reporters and selective single-stranded DNA (ssDNA) were chosen as signal labels and combined on a microarray immobilized onto a strip surface for the rapid quantification of the nucleic acids from eleven pathogens on a single strip. The reported detection limits were sub-picomolar for all the pathogens. The test benefitted from signal amplification of the encoded SERS tags and the 2×3 microarray embedded on the nitrocellulose membrane. In another application, selective novel antibodies were synthesized and used for the preparation of target-specific SERS tags. In this method, a duplex SERS-based LFA was demonstrated as a new test for the rapid detection of *Clostridium difficile (C. diff)* bacterial infection in synthetic stool matrix within 20 minutes. This was carried out via the quantification of new clinically relevant pathogenic biomarkers down to 0.01 pg/μL [150]. The reported test showed potential to be used in the future as an alternative diagnostic test for *C. diff* infection due to its high selectivity. Combined with simple manual operation, the proposed SERS lateral flow example demonstrated a strong potential for how SERS-based

LFA could be implemented for rapid clinical diagnosis application. However, it is still required to test this combination in a population wide-testing study before its implementation in real clinical applications.

One of the most required developments in SERS-based LFA is to move it from laboratory scale into field use. Since lateral flow strips could be easily integrated with portable readers, the POC diagnosis of different biomarkers could become more feasible. The use of the point-and-shoot feature of the portable Raman readers to scan the test line, instead of using the benchtop instruments, could make this platform easy to use without the need for special technical expertise [157]. Additionally, the readout time of the test lines would be much faster than the lengthy mapping scan of the benchtop Raman microscopes. Accordingly, this could enable the early and rapid clinical diagnosis of different biomarkers, as well as proper medical intervention in a timely manner [150]. The use of portable Raman readers with LFA was reported in multiple studies [150, 158–161]. For example, in a recent study Joung *et al.* reported the design of an on-site SERS-LFA reader with dimensions of 28 cm × 21 cm × 13.7 cm (Figure 7.8(c)) [158]. The system was designed to be operated by a battery to ensure its convenient movement. Additionally, it was provided with an embedded touch screen to eliminate the need for a separate computer connection. The device was equipped with a 638 nm diode laser as a light source, and the laser beam was focused on the strips through an objective lens to scan the beam at 10 μm intervals by moving the laser head. In order to improve the measurement reproducibility, a fast-mapping technique was used in the reader to measure the pixel-to-pixel Raman signal intensities for the test and control lines, which were then averaged to obtain a final value. The sample loading required 10 minutes and the time to read and process the data with the reader required an additional 5 minutes; thus, the total assay time was estimated to be 15 minutes. Another portable reader for SERS-LFA application was developed by Tran *et al.* for the fast scanning of the strips within a few seconds [159]. The developed instrument scans the test line via a line illumination along the entire width by a custom-designed fiber optical probe, with a line focus in combination with a compact diode laser source. By using a motorized stage, the instrument can collect different scans from 50 positions all over the strip within five seconds.

To sum up, the miniaturization ability of SERS-based LFA makes lateral flow test strips a promising biosensor for limited-resource surroundings and emergency divisions, and a better alternative to the conventional diagnostic methods. The use of SERS in combination with lateral flow strips could become the right combination for reliable and accurate testing, with the merits of a quick and large number of tests [151]. However, more improvement and optimization procedures are still required before this integration could be used for broader applications. For example, there is a continuous need for the synthesis of stable and reproducible SERS tags. Additionally, the use of advanced data treatment methods to aid the rapid and high-throughput reliable analysis of clinical data is also needed. Moreover, an accessible data library for clinical Raman spectral data needs to be extended to allow the use for multiple disease targets [152]. Furthermore, the principle itself should be cross-validated against other standard techniques like PCR before clinical use.

7.4.2 *Microfluidics Paper-Based Analytical Devices*

Microfluidics is a well-established technology that is used in several applications [162]. The use of microfluidic technology in analytical science enabled several advantages, such as miniaturization of analytical equipment with high analysis efficiency and reduced reagent consumption [163]. Usually the conventional microfluidic devices use glass and polydimethylsiloxane as substrates for their fabrication using photolithography, etching, electron beam lithography and printing methods [161]. Apart from the conventional microfluidic devices, paper-based microfluidics are characterized with many advantages, such as the capability of storing reagents. Additionally, the naturally occurring microchannels in paper combine the simple fabrication along with the advantages of microfluidics [164]. Moreover, the natural capillary-driven fluidic flow through cellulose fibers enables the samples and reagents to move freely through the porous paper network without the need for external pushing forces such as pressure pumps or additional liquid phase centrifugation [164, 165]. Like lateral flow test strips, microfluidic paper-based analytical devices (μPADs) have attracted increasing attention for POC application. They are miniaturized, disposable, user friendly and could be customizable in a range of analysis scenarios [165]. Compared to lateral flow strips, μPAD would be more straightforward, economical, easier to make using established patterning methods, and devoid of LFA assembling and antibody spraying.

The fabrication of μPAD can be carried out via many designs [166]; for example, they can be designed by dividing low-cost paper substrates (cellulose-based filter paper/membrane) into two regions, hydrophobic barriers and hydrophilic channels. The hydrophobic barriers could be fabricated using different methods such as wax printing and inkjet printing. They are placed to avoid the mixing of the reagents and enable the multiplexed assays [163, 167]. The hydrophilic channels contain sample-adding zones and a measurement zone. The channel dimensions are defined by the patterned hydrophobic barriers and the height of the channels depends on the thickness of the paper substrates (Figure 7.9(a)). In another example, Berry *et al.* described a cost-effective design of a paper-based microfluidic device ($0.03) for the measurement of hematocrit in a whole blood sample (Figure 7.9(b)) [168]. The device was designed using a chromatography paper and contained wax-printed hydrophobic and hydrophilic zones. The two zones were affixed with a patterned double-sided adhesive layer. The assay relied on metering the liquid volume (i.e., plasma) onto the device after applying the blood sample. The unimpeded transport of red blood cells through the device enabled a short assay time (30 minutes) and required only small amounts of EDTA and salt (NaCl) to perform the assay. Accordingly, we can see how the combination of microfluidic advantages with paper merits in one μPAD could result in a desirable biosensing platform for POC applications.

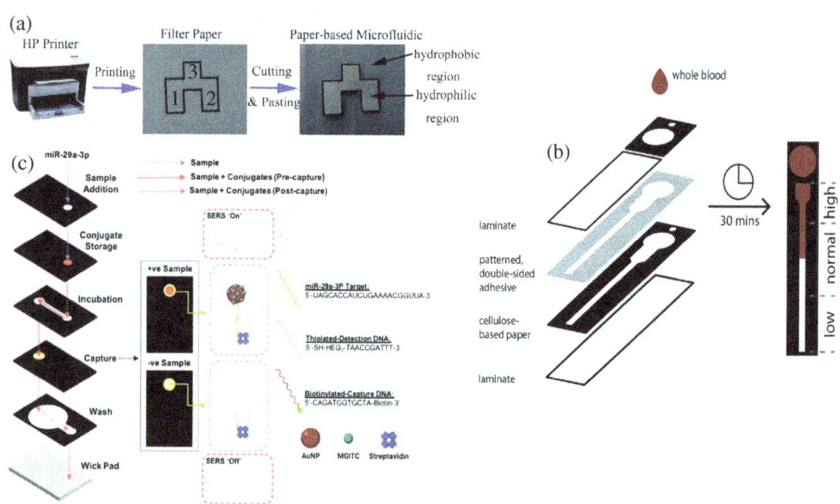

Figure 7.9. (a) The fabrication process of a μPAD via dividing the paper into hydrophobic and hydrophilic regions. Positions 1 and 2 denote sample addition zones, while position 3 is a measurement zone. (b) Schematic representation of a μPAD for hematocrit measurement in whole blood. The black and white regions represent the hydrophobic and hydrophilic zones of the paper, respectively. The grey layer denotes the double-sided adhesive used to affix the two layers. The guides indicate distances travelled by red blood cells over the device that correlate to different hematocrit levels. (c) Illustration of the 3D μPAD configuration. The dotted lines represent the sample pathway through the device, showing the mix with a conjugated label and forming an immunocomplex in the capture zone. Reproduced from Refs. [163], [168] and [175], respectively, with permission.

As in LFA, μPAD suffers from two major limitations: low detection sensitivity and limited quantitative detection capability [166]. The combined use of SERS with μPAD improved the sensitivity and the quantification ability of the system [169]. The SERS signals can be improved to further enhance the sensitivity via exploring a range of nanoparticle sizes, morphologies and associated Raman reporters. Additionally, the integration of portable Raman readers with SERS-μPAD platforms shows a huge potential for miniaturization and field deployment. Many studies reported the SERS-μPAD integration for environmental, pharmaceutical, and chemical analysis and for biomedical diagnostics [166, 170–174]. For example, Mabbott *et al.* reported a 3D μPAD for the SERS detection of miRNA biomarker (miR-29a), associated with cardiovascular disease, down to 47 pg/μL [175]. The device is composed of six wax-patterned layers, which define hydrophilic and hydrophobic zones on the paper and control solution flow throughout the device (Figure 7.9(c)). From top to bottom, the first layer is for sample addition, the conjugate layer to store the SERS tag, and the incubation layer to enable the binding between the SERS tag and the miRNA as the sample travels laterally. The capture layer contains immobilized ssDNA to enable the formation of a sandwich complex for the SERS readout. The excess reagents are washed away from the capture zone in the wash layer to the wick pad. In another application, a SERS-μPAD platform was used for the detection of *S. typhimurium* bacterial infection in real food samples [165]. The assay used a dumbbell-shaped μPAD for the deposition of the conjugated label in one side. After drying, the target DNA was added to the same side and allowed to be mixed with the labeled conjugate and left to diffuse to the test point. The SERS measurement was carried out within 1 minute after adding the sample and the reported limit of detection was 3–4 CFU/mL. Interestingly, the SEM scans indicated that positive samples could diffuse further to the test point.

Another important aspect for the efficient implementation of SERS-μPAD in POC testing is to control the fluid flow over the substrate surface. Increasing the fluid flow time and decreasing the flow rate could improve the assay sensitivity (i.e., gives enough time for the sample to interact efficiently with the conjugated label) [176, 177]. This could be done through manipulating the μPAD design, using different approaches such as changing the paper's channel geometries, altering the permeability of the paper by using dissolvable materials such as wax, agarose, sucrose, and trehalose (dissolvable delay), carving channels on the paper and varying the paper wettability [178]. However, these approaches could lead to loss of considerable amount of fluid or even change the assay chemistries, due to mixing with dissolvable materials.

Another design direction to overcome these limitations is to use folded paper actuators and compressed cellulose sponges. In this design, the connection/separation of fluid flow channels is controlled by the vertical movements of the folded paper actuator or sponge. However, it is essential to avoid any false connection between channels before actuation. A similar approach reported a μPAD design for an aptamer-based SERS assay depending on the horizontal motion of a mechanical valve (paper arm) and a compressed sponge [178]. The horizontal direction movement prevented the problems that are often encountered in the vertical direction valves and provided robust detection. Additionally, a mixture of fructose and sucrose was used to form an effective localized dissolvable delay region that improved the SERS detection sensitivity down to 0.02 ng/mL.

Similar to LFA, the SERS-μPAD platform has the potential to play a role in converting current multistep laboratory assays into simple high-performance POC devices for clinical diagnostics purposes. However, the same considerations before introducing the system to clinical use should be maintained.

7.4.3 *Plasmonic Nanostructured Paper SERS Substrates*

Plasmonic nanostructured paper substrates are simple and convenient substrates for the infield SERS detection of different targets. The SERS measurement could be done after collecting the samples via many flexible ways such as the direct deposition onto the paper surface, or by dipping/swabbing the paper substrate itself onto the sample. Different types of paper were used for the fabrication of the plasmonic paper SERS substrates, such as filter paper, chromatography paper, printing A4-sized paper, etc. [179]. The porous nature of the paper enables the easy deposition and retention of the metallic nanostructures onto their surface with high stability and capacity. Additionally, their flexibility affords the potential of high-throughput roll-to-roll manufacturing [179]. Mostly, gold and silver nanostructures (nanospheres, nanostars, nanowires) are used for the manufacturing of the paper SERS substrates due to their strong plasmon resonance. Many approaches have been reported for the deposition of the active nanostructures onto the paper surface [179, 180]. However, the most commonly used methods are (1) *in situ* synthesis, (2) dip coating and (3) inkjet printing.

In situ synthesis fabrication method involves the formation of metallic nanostructures onto the rigid paper substrate. Usually, the paper is submerged into a solution of silver nitrate ($AgNO_3$) or chloroauric acid ($HAuCl_4$) with a reducing agent and then heated, as per the typical procedures of generating silver or gold nanoparticles. The heat leads to nucleation of nanoparticles on the paper fibers. In another approach, cellulose paper could be oxidized to expose the aldehyde groups and then treated with Tollens' reagent for the *in situ* synthesis of silver nanoparticles [181]. In order to improve the uniformity of nanostructure deposition over the paper surface, it is required to functionalize/modify the paper surface before nanostructure growth, to form a patterned paper sheet. For example, Luo *et al.* reported the *in situ* synthesis of gold nanoparticles onto a pseudo paper film [182]. The film was fabricated by mixing a derivatized cellulose solution with monodispersed silica (SiO_2) nanoparticles and then being casted and dried. Hydrofluoric acid was used to etch the embedded SiO_2 nanoparticles to create hydrophilic channels. Subsequently, gold nanoparticles were synthesized *in situ* using an iterative seeding method and firmly anchored onto the film surface using polyethylenimine. Since the porous and tangled fibrous structure of microcrystalline cellulose was destroyed after derivatization, the surface uniformity of the substrate was significantly improved and enabled the even distribution of nanoparticles, thus demonstrating a highly reproducible SERS measurement (relative standard deviation = 6.03%).

In the dip-coating method, the paper substrate is soaked into an already synthesized nanostructure colloid for the even distribution of nanostructures onto the paper surface. The dip coating enables some possible advantages over *in situ* synthesis, in terms of the fabrication simplicity and the possibility of coating the paper surface with complex and strongly plasmonic nanostructures that are difficult to be synthesized directly on the paper surface, thus improving the sensitivity of the SERS detection [179]. Nevertheless, it might take a longer fabrication time than the *in situ* growth method, as the paper is required to be soaked long enough in the colloidal solution to enable its efficient coating. As in the *in situ* synthesis method, paper pre-treatment is essential to improve the nanostructure absorption onto the paper surface. For example, Hasi *et al.* dipped a paper into NaCl solution before soaking in silver colloid [183]. The NaCl pre-treatment increased the silver nanoparticle loading onto the paper, which improved the SERS signal.

The inkjet printing method involves loading nanostructured colloids into cost-effective, commercial inkjet printers and using them as a SERS ink to print paper SERS substrates. While this can still be adapted for roll-to-roll fabrication, there is a requirement for many printing cycles to generate a paper substrate with a high density of nanostructures, which is essential to provide a strong SERS enhancement for the substrate [179, 180]. For example, Wang *et al.* demonstrated an ultra-sensitive design of paper SERS substrate by printing 30 layers of silver nanoparticle colloidal ink on a hydrophilic cellulose paper in a layer-by-layer manner [184]. Another direction is to concentrate the prepared colloid to enable complete coverage of the paper and strong enhancement in a single print. For example, Yu and White used glycerol with a concentrated silver nanoparticle colloid to adjust the viscosity and surface tension of the ink for optimal printing onto a hydrophobic paper to form sensing arrays [185].

The ability of the plasmonic paper SERS substrates to detect biological samples in an ultra-sensitive way, combined with their portability, stability, handling, and low cost, makes them feasible detection tools for on-site and POC testing for clinical application [186]. For example, Pan *et al.* reported a graphene oxide-gold nanostar hybrid paper biosensor for the label-free SERS detection of serum bilirubin for diagnosis of jaundice (Figure 7.10(a)). The graphene oxide nanosheet enabled high bilirubin enrichment over the substrate via strong electrostatic and π-π interactions, while the plasmonic gold nanostar imparted high sensitivity for the SERS detection. The reported detection limit was 0.436 μM [187]. In another application, a functionalized cellulose fiber plasmonic membrane was reported for the sensing of wound protein biomarkers as a non-invasive measure of cutaneous wound healing [188]. APTES linker molecules were assembled onto the whole substrate surface and used to facilitate the adhesion of plasmonic silver nanoparticles onto the membrane via sputtering (Figure 7.10(b)). The protein biomarkers were then assembled onto the plasmonic substate via gold-thiol (Au–S) bond formation. The exposure to the corresponding biomarker's antibodies tagged with 4-ATP (Raman reporter) resulted in a specific binding to protein biomarkers, which were quantified via monitoring the SERS signal of 4-ATP. These prototype designs of the plasmonic paper SERS substrates could pave the way in future for more rapid, accurate and sensitive applications for clinical diagnostics. However, the same pre-clinical measures that were previously discussed should be optimized first. Finally, for the development of a new clinical diagnostic approach that could serve at POC to monitor human health, a closer collaboration between physicians and laboratory researchers is critical for the fast and efficient translation from basic sciences to clinical applications [152].

Paper-based platforms are now at the forefront of POC devices as they are the platform which best encompasses the WHO's ASSURED criteria. In particular, lateral flows have really catapulted to the top, due to the

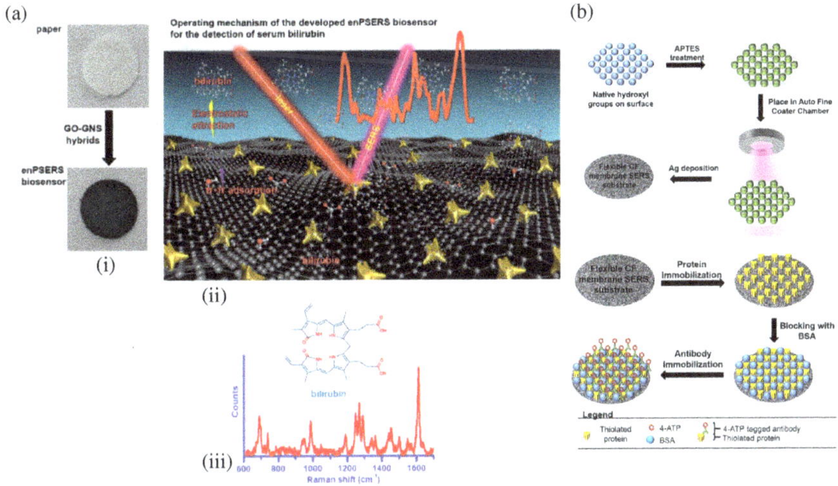

Figure 7.10. (a) i. Schematic illustrating the paper surface before and after graphene oxide-gold nanostar deposition onto the paper biosensor. ii. The operating principle of the developed biosensor for the label-free SERS detection of serum bilirubin. iii. Molecular structure and Raman spectrum of bilirubin detected by the paper biosensor. (b) Schematic illustration showing cellulose fiber SERS substrate fabrication and treatment for biomarker proteins sensing. Reproduced from Refs. [187] and [188], respectively, with permission.

COVID-19 pandemic as these tests have become a daily part of many people's lives. When combined with a SERS read-out instrument, a sensitive device is achieved. By creating an interface between the lateral flow strip and portable spectrometer, a powerful tool to detect clinically relevant biomarkers has been realized. However, further work needs to be done on reducing the associated costs of the spectrometer and being able to perform the analysis at safe laser powers without losing sensitivity for this technique to compete with other gold standard readers.

7.5 Conclusion

The global POC diagnostic market has exploded in recent years and is expected to reach USD 75.5 billion by 2027 from USD 45.4 billion in 2022 [189]. This can be attributed to the rising prevalence of infectious diseases such as COVID-19, shortage of technicians available to conduct lab-based tests, supportive government policies and the rising awareness about self-testing products. For SERS-POC to be included in this market as the go-to read-out instrument, further advancements in instrumentation, portability, interface between device and laser, usability and stability of nanoparticles themselves need to be addressed. Once a working prototype has been fixed upon, the clinical testing needs to be performed extensively on prospective samples and benchmarked against the current gold standard for that specific target. This takes significant time and investment but is the next necessary step in translating the potential of SERS into a clinically useful POC based assay format. The work reported here show the first steps in making SERS-POC a reality. Although still in its infancy, SERS-POC is possible when combined with portable read-out instrumentations and, thus, can provide rapid and quantitative assessment of clinical biomarkers to aid decision making, monitor diseases and assess treatment next to the patient.

References

1. Hocking, L., George, J., Broberg, E. K., Struelens, M. J., Leitmeyer, K. C., Deshpande, A., Parkinson, S., Francombe, J., Morley, K. I., and de Carvalho Gomes, H. (2021) Point of care testing for infectious disease in Europe: a scoping review and survey study. Front. Public Health **9**, 722943.
2. Rajendran, R. and Rayman, G. (2014) Point-of-care blood glucose testing for diabetes care in hospitalized patients: an evidence-based review. J. Diabetes Sci. Technol. **8**, 1081–1090.
3. Ebner, M., Birschmann, I., Peter, A., Spencer, C., Härtig, F., Kuhn, J., Blumenstock, G., Zuern, C. S., Ziemann, U., and Poli, S. (2017) Point-of-care testing for emergency assessment of coagulation in patients treated with direct oral anticoagulants. Crit. Care **21**, 32.
4. Joel, R. L. E. (2002) Home and point-of-care pregnancy tests: a review of the technology. Epidemiology **13**, S15–S18.
5. Hsiao, W. W. W., Le, T. N., Pham, D. M., Ko, H. H., Chang, H.-C., Lee, C. C., Sharma, N., Lee, C. K., and Chiang, W. H. (2021) Recent advances in novel lateral flow technologies for detection of COVID-19. Biosensors **11**, 295.
6. Nasseri, B., Soleimani, N., Rabiee, N., Kalbasi, A., Karimi, M., and Hamblin, M. R. (2018) Point-of-care microfluidic devices for pathogen detection. Biosensors Bioelectron. **117**, 112–128.
7. Naseri, M., Ziora, Z. M., Simon, G. P., and Batchelor, W. (2022) ASSURED-compliant point-of-care diagnostics for the detection of human viral infections, Rev. Med. Virol., **32**, e2263.
8. St John, A. and Price, C. P. (2014) Existing and emerging technologies for point-of-care testing. Clin. Biochem. Rev. **35**, 155–167.
9. Alonso, O., Franch, N., Canals, J., Arias-Alpízar, K., de la Serna, E., Baldrich, E., and Diéguez, A. (2020) An internet of things-based intensity and time-resolved fluorescence reader for point-of-care testing. Biosensors Bioelectron. **154**, 112074.

10. Ma, L., Abugalyon, Y., and Li, X. (2021) Multicolorimetric ELISA biosensors on a paper/polymer hybrid analytical device for visual point-of-care detection of infection diseases. Anal. Bioanal. Chem. **413**, 4655–4663.
11. Cruz, A. F., Norena, N., Kaushik, A., and Bhansali, S. (2014) A low-cost miniaturized potentiostat for point-of-care diagnosis. Biosens. Bioelectron. **62**, 249–254.
12. Abramczyk, H. and Brozek-Pluska, B. (2013) Raman imaging in biochemical and biomedical applications. Diagnosis and treatment of breast cancer. Chem. Rev. **113**, 5766–5781.
13. Langer, J., Jimenez de Aberasturi, D., Aizpurua, J., Alvarez-Puebla, R. A., Auguié, B., Baumberg, J. J., Bazan, G. C., Bell, S. E. J., Boisen, A., Brolo, A. G., *et al.* (2020) Present and future of surface-enhanced Raman scattering. ACS Nano **14**, 28–117.
14. Smith, W. (2008) Practical understanding and use of surface enhanced Raman scattering/surface enhanced resonance Raman scattering in chemical and biological analysis. Chem. Soc. Rev. **37**, 955–964.
15. Harper, M. M., McKeating, K. S., and Faulds, K. (2013) Recent developments and future directions in SERS for bioanalysis. *Phys. Chem. Chem. Phys.* **15**, 5312–5328.
16. Larmour, I. A., Faulds, K., and Graham, D. (2010) Improved versatility of silver nanoparticle dimers for surface-enhanced Raman spectroscopy. J. Phys. Chem. C **114**, 13249–13254.
17. Saha, K., Agasti, S. S., Kim, C., Li, X., and Rotello, V. M. (2012) Gold nanoparticles in chemical and biological sensing. Chem. Rev. **112**, 2739–2779.
18. Smith, E., Dent, G., and Wiley, J. (2005) *Modern Raman Spectroscopy: A Practical Approach*, John Wiley & Sons.
19. Bedics, M., Kearns, H., Cox, J., Mabbott, S., Ali, F., Shand, N., Faulds, K., Benedict, J., Graham, D., and Detty, M. (2015) Extreme red shifted SERS nanotags. Chem. Sci. **6**, 2302–2306.
20. Wang, L., Sun, Y. J., Li, Z., Wu, A. G., and Wei, G. (2016) Bottom-up synthesis and sensor applications of biomimetic nanostructures. Materials **9**, 53.
21. Kearns, H., Shand, N., Faulds, K., and Graham, D. (2015) Laser induced SERS switching using plasmonic heating of PNIPAM coated HGNs. Chem. Commun. **51**, 8138–8141.
22. Laing, S., Gracie, K., and Faulds, K. (2016) Multiplex in vitro detection using SERS. Chem. Soc. Rev. **45**, 1901–1918.
23. Sloan-Dennison, S., Laing, S., Graham, D., and Faulds, K. (2021) From Raman to SESORRS: moving deeper into cancer detection and treatment monitoring. Chem. Commun. **57**, 12436–12451.
24. Jamieson, L. E., Asiala, S. M., Gracie, K., Faulds, K., and Graham, D. (2017) Bioanalytical measurements enabled by surface-enhanced Raman scattering (SERS) probes. Annu. Rev. Anal. Chem. **10**, 415–437.

25. Berry, M. E., Kearns, H., Graham, D., and Faulds, K. (2021) Surface enhanced Raman scattering for the multiplexed detection of pathogenic microorganisms: towards point-of-use applications. Analyst **146**, 6084–6101.
26. Guerrini, L., Garcia-Rico, E., O'Loghlen, A., Giannini, V., and Alvarez-Puebla, R. A. (2021) Surface-enhanced Raman scattering (SERS) spectroscopy for sensing and characterization of exosomes in cancer diagnosis. Cancers **13**, 2179.
27. Dougan, J. A. and Faulds, K. (2012) Surface enhanced Raman scattering for multiplexed detection. Analyst **137**, 545–554.
28. Faulds, K., Littleford, R. E., Graham, D., Dent, G., and Smith, W. E. (2004) Comparison of surface-enhanced resonance Raman scattering from unaggregated and aggregated nanoparticles. Anal. Chem. **76**, 592–598.
29. McAnally, G., McLaughlin, C., Brown, R., Robson, D. C., Faulds, K., Tackley, D. R., Smith, W. E., and Graham, D. (2002) SERRS dyes. Part I. Synthesis of benzotriazole monoazo dyes as model analytes for surface enhanced resonance Raman scattering. Analyst **127**, 838–841.
30. McHugh, C., Docherty, F., Graham, D., and Smith, W. (2004) SERRS dyes Part 2. Syntheses and evaluation of dyes for multiple labeling for SERRS. Analyst **129**, 69–72.
31. Enright, A., Fruk, L., Grondin, A., McHugh, C. J., Smith, W. E., and Graham, D. (2004) SERRS dyes Part 3. Synthesis of reactive benzotriazole azo dyes for surface enhanced resonance Raman scattering. Analyst **129**, 975–978.
32. Lynn, K. A., McNay, G., Eustace, D. A., Shand, N. C., and Smith, W. E. (2010) Short-wave infrared excited SERS. Analyst **135**, 1904–1905.
33. Donahue, M., Huang, H., Brouillette, C., Smith, W., and Farquharson, S. (2011) Detecting explosives by portable Raman analyzers: a comparison of 785-, 976-, 1064-, and 1550-nm (retina-safe) laser excitation. https://www.spectroscopyonline.com/view/detecting-explosives-portable-raman-analyzers-comparison-785-976-1064-and-1550-nm-retina-safe-laser.
34. Asselin, K. J. and Chase, B. (1994) FT-Raman spectroscopy at 1.339 micrometers. Appl. Spectrosc. **48**, 699–701.
35. Anderson, R. R. and Parrish, J. A. (1981) The optics of human skin. J. Invest. Dermatol. **77**, 13–19.
36. Bashkatov, A., Genina, E., Kochubey, V., and Tuchin, V. (2005) Optical properties of human skin, subcutaneous and mucous tissues in the wavelength range from 400 to 2000 nm. J. Phys. D: Appl. Phys. **38**, 2543.
37. Culha, M., Cullum, B., Lavrik, N., and Klutse, C. K. (2012) Surface-enhanced Raman scattering as an emerging characterization and detection technique. J. Nanotechnol. **2012**, 971380.
38. Chen, I. H., Chu, S. W., Sun, C. K., Cheng, P. C., and Lin, B. L. (2002) Wavelength dependent damage in biological multi-photon confocal microscopy: A micro-spectroscopic comparison between femtosecond Ti: sapphire and Cr: forsterite laser sources. OQE **34**, 1251–1266.

39. Oldenburg, S. J., Westcott, S. L., Averitt, R. D., and Halas, N. J. (1999) Surface enhanced Raman scattering in the near infrared using metal nanoshell substrates. J. Chem. Phys. **111**, 4729–4735.
40. Wijesuriya, S., Burugapalli, K., Mackay, R., Ajaezi, G. C., and Balachandran, W. (2016) Chemically roughened solid silver: A simple, robust and broadband SERS substrate. Sensors **16**, 1742.
41. Gühlke, M., Heiner, Z., and Kneipp, J. (2015) Combined near-infrared excited SEHRS and SERS spectra of pH sensors using silver nanostructures. *Phys. Chem. Chem. Phys.* **17**, 26093–26100.
42. Kearns, H., Bedics, M. A., Shand, N. C., Faulds, K., Detty, M. R., and Graham, D. (2016) Sensitive SERS nanotags for use with 1550 nm (retina-safe) laser excitation. Analyst **141**, 5062–5065.
43. Milojevich, C. B., Mandrell, B. K., Turley, H. K., Iberi, V., Best, M. D., and Camden, J. P. (2013) Surface-enhanced hyper-Raman scattering from single molecules. J. Phys. Chem. Lett. **4**, 3420–3423.
44. Moreton, S., Faulds, K., Shand, N., Bedics, M., Detty, M., and Graham, D. (2015) Functionalisation of hollow gold nanospheres for use as stable, red-shifted SERS nanotags. Nanoscale **7**, 6075–6082.
45. Kearns, H., Shand, N., Smith, W., Faulds, K., and Graham, D. (2015) 1064 nm SERS of NIR active hollow gold nanotags. *Phys. Chem. Chem. Phys.* **17**, 1980–1986.
46. Kearns, H., Ali, F., Bedics, M. A., Shand, N. C., Faulds, K., Detty, M. R., and Graham, D. (2017) Sensitive SERS nanotags for use with a hand-held 1064 nm Raman spectrometer. Royal Soc. Open Sci. **4**, 170422.
47. Schmitt, J. M., Knuttel, A., Yadlowsky, M., and Eckhaus, M. (1994) Optical-coherence tomography of a dense tissue: statistics of attenuation and backscattering. Phys. Med. Biol. **39**, 1705.
48. Xie, H., Larmour, I. A., Chen, Y. C., Wark, A. W., Tileli, V., McComb, D. W., Faulds, K., and Graham, D. (2013) Synthesis and NIR optical properties of hollow gold nanospheres with LSPR greater than one micrometer. Nanoscale **5**, 765–771.
49. Izake, E. L. (2010) Forensic and homeland security applications of modern portable Raman spectroscopy. Forensic Sci. Int. **202**, 1–8.
50. Vítek, P., Ali, E. M., Edwards, H. G., Jehlička, J., Cox, R., and Page, K. (2012) Evaluation of portable Raman spectrometer with 1064nm excitation for geological and forensic applications. Spectrochim. Acta A **86**, 320–327.
51. Vítek, P., Jehlička, J., Edwards, H. G., Hutchinson, I., Ascaso, C., and Wierzchos, J. (2012) The miniaturized Raman system and detection of traces of life in halite from the Atacama Desert: some considerations for the search for life signatures on Mars. Astrobiology **12**, 1095–1099.
52. Roy, E., Wilcox, P. G., Hoffland, S., and Pardoe, I. (2015) Detection of munitions grade g-series nerve agents using Raman excitation at 1064 nm. https://doi.org/10.1117/12.2194027.

53. Jehlička, J., Edwards, H. G., and Oren, A. (2014) Raman spectroscopy of microbial pigments. Appl. Environ. Microbiol. **80**, 3286–3295.
54. Faulds, K., Jarvis, R., Smith, W. E., Graham, D., and Goodacre, R. (2008) Multiplexed detection of six labeled oligonucleotides using surface enhanced resonance Raman scattering (SERRS). Analyst **133**, 1505–1512.
55. Gracie, K., Correa, E., Mabbott, S., Dougan, J. A., Graham, D., Goodacre, R., and Faulds, K. (2014) Simultaneous detection and quantification of three bacterial meningitis pathogens by SERS. Chem. Sci. **5**, 1030–1040.
56. Kearns, H., Goodacre, R., Jamieson, L. E., Graham, D., and Faulds, K. (2017) SERS detection of multiple antimicrobial-resistant pathogens using nanosensors. Anal. Chem. **89**, 12666–12673.
57. Nicolson, F., Jamieson, L. E., Mabbott, S., Plakas, K., Shand, N. C., Detty, M. R., Graham, D., and Faulds, K. (2018) Multiplex imaging of live breast cancer tumour models through tissue using handheld surface enhanced spatially offset resonance Raman spectroscopy (SESORRS). Chem. Commun. **54**, 8530–8533.
58. Noonan, J., Asiala, S. M., Grassia, G., MacRitchie, N., Gracie, K., Carson, J., Moores, M., Girolami, M., Bradshaw, A. C., Guzik, T. J., *et al.* (2018) In vivo multiplex molecular imaging of vascular inflammation using surface-enhanced Raman spectroscopy. Theranostics **8**, 6195–6209.
59. Betz, J. F., Wei, W. Y., Cheng, Y., White, I. M., and Rubloff, G. W. (2014) Simple SERS substrates: powerful, portable, and full of potential. *Phys. Chem. Chem. Phys.* **16**, 2224–2239.
60. Cullum, B. M., Mobley, J., Chi, Z., Stokes, D. L., Miller, G. H., and Vo-Dinh, T. (2000) Development of a compact, handheld Raman instrument with no moving parts for use in field analysis. Rev. Sci. Instrum. **71**, 1602–1607.
61. Lieber, C. A. and Mahadevan-Jansen, A. (2007) Development of a handheld Raman microspectrometer for clinical dermatologic applications. Opt. Express **15**, 11874–11882.
62. Huang, H., Shende, C., Sengupta, A., Inscore, F., Brouillette, C., Smith, W., and Farquharson, S. (2012) Surface-enhanced Raman spectra of melamine and other chemicals using a 1550 nm (retina-safe) laser. J. Raman Spectrosc. **43**, 701–705.
63. Alvarez-Puebla, R. A. and Liz-Marzán, L. M. (2010) SERS-based diagnosis and biodetection. Small **6**, 604–610.
64. Jarvis, R. M. and Goodacre, R. (2004) Discrimination of bacteria using surface-enhanced Raman spectroscopy. Anal. Chem. **76**, 40–47.
65. Wu, X., Xu, C., Tripp, R. A., Huang, Y.-w., and Zhao, Y. (2013) Detection and differentiation of foodborne pathogenic bacteria in mung bean sprouts using field deployable label-free SERS devices. Analyst **138**, 3005–3012.
66. Chen, L., Mungroo, N., Daikuara, L., and Neethirajan, S. (2015) Label-free NIR-SERS discrimination and detection of foodborne bacteria by in situ synthesis of Ag colloids. J. Nanobiotechnology **13**, 45.

67. Kamińska, A., Witkowska, E., Kowalska, A., Skoczyńska, A., Ronkiewicz, P., Szymborski, T., and Waluk, J. (2016) Rapid detection and identification of bacterial meningitis pathogens in ex vivo clinical samples by SERS method and principal component analysis. Anal. Methods. **8**, 4521–4529.
68. Wang, H. N., Crawford, B. M., Fales, A. M., Bowie, M. L., Seewaldt, V. L., and Vo-Dinh, T. (2016) Multiplexed detection of microRNA biomarkers using SERS-based inverse molecular sentinel (iMS) nanoprobes. J. Phys. Chem. C **120**, 21047–21055.
69. Crawford, B. M., Wang, H. N., Stolarchuk, C., von Furstenberg, R. J., Strobbia, P., Zhang, D., Qin, X., Owzar, K., Garman, K. S., and Vo-Dinh, T. (2020) Plasmonic nanobiosensors for detection of MicroRNA cancer biomarkers in clinical samples. Analyst **145**, 4587–4594.
70. Papadopoulou, E. and Bell, S. E. (2012) Label-free detection of nanomolar unmodified single- and double-stranded DNA by using surface-enhanced Raman spectroscopy on Ag and Au colloids. Chem. Eur. J. **18**, 5394–5400.
71. Graham, D., Thompson, D. G., Smith, W. E., and Faulds, K. (2008) Control of enhanced Raman scattering using a DNA-based assembly process of dye-coded nanoparticles. Nat. Nanotechnol. **3**, 548–551.
72. Feng, E., Zheng, T., and Tian, Y. (2019) Dual-mode Au nanoprobe based on surface enhancement Raman scattering and colorimetry for sensitive determination of telomerase activity both in cell extracts and in the urine of patients. ACS Sensors **4**, 211–217.
73. Mabbott, S., Thompson, D., Sirimuthu, N., McNay, G., Faulds, K., and Graham, D. (2016) From synthetic DNA to PCR product: detection of fungal infections using SERS. Faraday Discuss. **187**, 461–472.
74. Gracie, K., Lindsay, D., Graham, D., and Faulds, K. (2015) Bacterial meningitis pathogens identified in clinical samples using a SERS DNA detection assay. Anal. Methods **7**, 1269–1272.
75. Marks, H., Huang, P. J., Mabbott, S., Graham, D., Kameoka, J., and Coté, G. (2016) Ferric plasmonic nanoparticles, aptamers, and magnetofluidic chips: toward the development of diagnostic surface-enhanced Raman spectroscopy assays. J. Biomed. Opt. **21**, 127005.
76. Zhang, H., Harpster, M. H., Wilson, W. C., and Johnson, P. A. (2012) Surface-enhanced Raman scattering detection of DNAs derived from virus genomes using Au-coated paramagnetic nanoparticles. Langmuir **28**, 4030–4037.
77. Donnelly, T., Smith, W. E., Faulds, K., and Graham, D. (2014) Silver and magnetic nanoparticles for sensitive DNA detection by SERS. Chem. Commun. **50**, 12907–12910.
78. Treerattrakoon, K., Roeksrungruang, P., Dharakul, T., Japrung, D., Faulds, K., Graham, D., and Bamrungsap, S. (2022) Detection of a miRNA biomarker for cancer diagnosis using SERS tags and magnetic separation. Anal. Methods **14**, 1938–1945.

79. Zhang, H., Ma, X., Liu, Y., Duan, N., Wu, S., Wang, Z., and Xu, B. (2015) Gold nanoparticles enhanced SERS aptasensor for the simultaneous detection of Salmonella typhimurium and Staphylococcus aureus. Biosensors Bioelectron. **74**, 872–877.
80. Diaz-Amaya, S., Lin, L.-K., Deering, A. J., and Stanciu, L. A. (2019) Aptamer-based SERS biosensor for whole cell analytical detection of E. coli O157:H7. Anal. Chim. Acta **1081**, 146–156.
81. Zhang, C., Wang, C., Xiao, R., Tang, L., Huang, J., Wu, D., Liu, S., Wang, Y., Zhang, D., Wang, S., *et al.* (2018) Sensitive and specific detection of clinical bacteria via vancomycin-modified Fe3O4@Au nanoparticles and aptamer-functionalized SERS tags. J. Mater. Chem. B **6**, 3751–3761.
82. Ni, J., Lipert, R. J., Dawson, G. B., and Porter, M. D. (1999) Immunoassay readout method using extrinsic Raman labels adsorbed on immunogold colloids. Anal. Chem. **71**, 4903–4908.
83. Neng, J., Harpster, M. H., Wilson, W. C., and Johnson, P. A. (2013) Surface-enhanced Raman scattering (SERS) detection of multiple viral antigens using magnetic capture of SERS-active nanoparticles. Biosens. Bioelectron. **41**, 316–321.
84. Neng, J., Li, Y., Driscoll, A. J., Wilson, W. C., and Johnson, P. A. (2018) Detection of multiple pathogens in serum using silica-encapsulated nanotags in a surface-enhanced Raman scattering-based immunoassay. J. Agric. Food Chem. **66**, 5707–5712.
85. Rathmell, C., Kearns, H., Graham, D., Jamieson, L. E., and Faulds, K. (2019) Rapid, portable pathogen detection with multiplexed SERS-based nanosensors. Spectroscopy **34**, 24–31.
86. Cheng, Z., Choi, N., Wang, R., Lee, S., Moon, K. C., Yoon, S.-Y., Chen, L., and Choo, J. (2017) Simultaneous detection of dual prostate specific antigens using surface-enhanced Raman scattering-based immunoassay for accurate diagnosis of prostate cancer. ACS Nano **11**, 4926–4933.
87. Zhang, W., Jiang, L., Diefenbach, R. J., Campbell, D. H., Walsh, B. J., Packer, N. H., and Wang, Y. (2020) Enabling sensitive phenotypic profiling of cancer-derived small extracellular vesicles using surface-enhanced Raman spectroscopy nanotags. ACS Sensors **5**, 764–771.
88. Tatar, A. S., Farcau, C., Vulpoi, A., Boca, S., and Astilean, S. (2022) Development and evaluation of a gold nanourchin (GNU)-based sandwich architecture for SERS immunosensing in liquid. Spectrochim. Acta A Mol. Biomol. Spectrosc. **273**, 121069.
89. Kozel, T. R. and Burnham-Marusich, A. R. (2017) Point-of-care testing for infectious diseases: past, present, and future. J. Clin. Microbiol. **55**, 2313–2320.
90. Mohammadi, M., Antoine, D., Vitt, M., Dickie, J. M., Jyoti, S. S., Wall, J. G., Johnson, P. A., and Wawrousek, K. E. (2022) A fast, ultrasensitive SERS immunoassay to detect SARS-CoV-2 in saliva. Anal. Chim. Acta **1229**, 340290.

91. Sharma, S., Zapatero-Rodríguez, J., Estrela, P., and O'Kennedy, R. (2015) Point-of-care diagnostics in low resource settings: present status and future role of microfluidics. Biosensors **5**, 577–601.
92. Schulte, T. H., Bardell, R. L., and Weigl, B. H. (2002) Microfluidic technologies in clinical diagnostics. Clin. Chim. Acta **321**, 1–10.
93. Olanrewaju, A., Beaugrand, M., Yafia, M., and Juncker, D. (2018) Capillary microfluidics in microchannels: from microfluidic networks to capillaric circuits. Lab Chip **18**, 2323–2347.
94. Park, S., Zhang, Y., Lin, S., Wang, T. H., and Yang, S. (2011) Advances in microfluidic PCR for point-of-care infectious disease diagnostics. Biotechnol. Adv. **29**, 830–839.
95. Zhang, H., Xu, Y., Fohlerova, Z., Chang, H., Iliescu, C., and Neuzil, P. (2019) LAMP-on-a-chip: Revising microfluidic platforms for loop-mediated DNA amplification. Trends Anal. Chem. **113**, 44–53.
96. Ng, A. H. C., Uddayasankar, U., and Wheeler, A. R. (2010) Immunoassays in microfluidic systems. Anal. Bioanal. Chem. **397**, 991–1007.
97. Nguyen, P. Q. M., Wang, M., Ann Maria, N., Li, A. Y., Tan, H. Y., Xiong, G. M., Tan, M.-K. M., Bhagat, A. A. S., Ong, C. W. M., and Lim, C. T. (2022) Modular micro-PCR system for the onsite rapid diagnosis of COVID-19. Microsyst. Nanoeng. **8**, 82.
98. Xu, D., Jiang, X., Zou, T., Miao, G., Fu, Q., Xiang, F., Feng, L., Ye, X., Zhang, L., and Qiu, X. (2022) A microfluidic system for rapid nucleic acid analysis based on real-time convective PCR at point-of-care testing. Microfluid. Nanofluid. **26**, 69.
99. Zhu, C., Hu, A., Cui, J., Yang, K., Zhu, X., Liu, Y., Deng, G., and Zhu, L. (2019) A lab-on-a-chip device integrated DNA extraction and solid phase PCR array for the genotyping of high-risk HPV in clinical samples. Micromachines **10**, 537.
100. Li, Z., Zhao, J., Wu, X., Zhu, C., Liu, Y., Wang, A., Deng, G., and Zhu, L. (2019) A rapid microfluidic platform with real-time fluorescence detection system for molecular diagnosis. Biotechnol. Biotechnol. Equip. **33**, 223–230.
101. Qiu, X., Ge, S., Gao, P., Li, K., Yang, S., Zhang, S., Ye, X., Xia, N., and Qian, S. (2017) A smartphone-based point-of-care diagnosis of H1N1 with microfluidic convection PCR. Microsyst. Technol. **23**, 2951–2956.
102. Farshidfar, N. and Hamedani, S. (2020) The potential role of smartphone-based microfluidic systems for rapid detection of COVID-19 using saliva specimen. Mol. Diagn. Ther. **24**, 371–373.
103. Gao, D., Liu, H., Jiang, Y., and Lin, J. M. (2013) Recent advances in microfluidics combined with mass spectrometry: technologies and applications. Lab Chip **13**, 3309–3322.
104. Zhao, Y., Tang, M., Liu, F., Li, H., Wang, H., and Xu, D. (2019) Highly integrated microfluidic chip coupled to mass spectrometry for online analysis of residual quinolones in milk. Anal. Chem. **91**, 13418–13426.

105. Chen, Q., Wu, J., Zhang, Y., and Lin, J. M. (2012) Qualitative and quantitative analysis of tumor cell metabolism via stable isotope labeling assisted microfluidic chip electrospray ionization mass spectrometry. Anal. Chem. **84**, 1695–1701.
106. Zhang, X., Bai, J., Wang, R., Wei, X., Chen, M., Yang, T., and Wang, J. (2022) Biological elemental analysis: A cute-meet of microfluidic device to inductively coupled plasma mass spectrometry. VIEW **4**, 20220035.
107. Lin, Q., Wen, D., Wu, J., Liu, L., Wu, W., Fang, X., and Kong, J. (2020) Microfluidic immunoassays for sensitive and simultaneous detection of IgG/IgM/Antigen of SARS-CoV-2 within 15 min. Anal. Chem. **92**, 9454–9458.
108. Man, Y., Li, A., Li, B., Liu, J., and Pan, L. (2019) A microfluidic colorimetric immunoassay for sensitive detection of altenariol monomethyl ether by UV spectroscopy and smart phone imaging. Anal. Chim. Acta **1092**, 75–84.
109. Antunes, P., Watterson, D., Parmvi, M., Burger, R., Boisen, A., Young, P., Cooper, M. A., Hansen, M. F., Ranzoni, A., and Donolato, M. (2015) Quantification of NS1 dengue biomarker in serum via optomagnetic nanocluster detection. Sci. Rep. **5**, 16145.
110. Panneerselvam, R., Sadat, H., Höhn, E. M., Das, A., Noothalapati, H., and Belder, D. (2022) Microfluidics and surface-enhanced Raman spectroscopy, a win–win combination?. Lab Chip **22**, 665–682.
111. Yue, S., Fang, J., and Xu, Z. (2022) Advances in droplet microfluidics for SERS and Raman analysis. Biosensors Bioelectron. **198**, 113822.
112. Lee, M., Lee, K., Kim, K. H., Oh, K. W., and Choo, J. (2012) SERS-based immunoassay using a gold array-embedded gradient microfluidic chip. Lab Chip **12**, 3720–3727.
113. Kamińska, A., Witkowska, E., Winkler, K., Dzięcielewski, I., Weyher, J. L., and Waluk, J. (2015) Detection of Hepatitis B virus antigen from human blood: SERS immunoassay in a microfluidic system. Biosens. Bioelectron. **66**, 461–467.
114. Wang, C., Madiyar, F., Yu, C., and Li, J. (2017) Detection of extremely low concentration waterborne pathogen using a multiplexing self-referencing SERS microfluidic biosensor. J. Biol. Eng. **11**, 9.
115. Wang, Y., Rauf, S., Grewal, Y. S., Spadafora, L. J., Shiddiky, M. J. A., Cangelosi, G. A., Schlücker, S., and Trau, M. (2014) Duplex microfluidic SERS detection of pathogen antigens with nanoyeast single-chain variable fragments. Anal. Chem. **86**, 9930–9938.
116. Li, J., Skeete, Z., Shan, S., Yan, S., Kurzatkowska, K., Zhao, W., Ngo, Q. M., Holubovska, P., Luo, J., Hepel, M., *et al.* (2015) Surface enhanced Raman scattering detection of cancer biomarkers with bifunctional nanocomposite probes. Anal. Chem. **87**, 10698–10702.
117. Gao, R., Ko, J., Cha, K., Jeon, J. H., Rhie, G. E., Choi, J., deMello, A. J., and Choo, J. (2015) Fast and sensitive detection of an anthrax biomarker using SERS-based solenoid microfluidic sensor. Biosens. Bioelectron. **72**, 230–236.

118. Yap, L. W., Chen, H., Gao, Y., Petkovic, K., Liang, Y., Si, K. J., Wang, H., Tang, Z., Zhu, Y., and Cheng, W. (2017) Bifunctional plasmonic-magnetic particles for an enhanced microfluidic SERS immunoassay. Nanoscale **9**, 7822–7829.
119. Wang, Y., Ruan, Q., Lei, Z. C., Lin, S. C., Zhu, Z., Zhou, L., and Yang, C. (2018) Highly sensitive and automated surface enhanced Raman scattering-based immunoassay for H5N1 detection with digital microfluidics. Anal. Chem. **90**, 5224–5231.
120. Syme, C. D., Martino, C., Yusvana, R., Sirimuthu, N. M. S., and Cooper, J. M. (2012) Quantitative characterization of individual microdroplets using surface-enhanced resonance Raman scattering spectroscopy. Anal. Chem. **84**, 1491–1495.
121. Gao, R., Choi, N., Chang, S. I., Lee, E. K., and Choo, J. (2014) Real-time analysis of diaquat dibromide monohydrate in water with a SERS-based integrated microdroplet sensor. Nanoscale **6**, 8781–8786.
122. Gao, R., Cheng, Z., deMello, A. J., and Choo, J. (2016) Wash-free magnetic immunoassay of the PSA cancer marker using SERS and droplet microfluidics. Lab Chip **16**, 1022–1029.
123. Gao, R., Cheng, Z., Wang, X., Yu, L., Guo, Z., Zhao, G., and Choo, J. (2018) Simultaneous immunoassays of dual prostate cancer markers using a SERS-based microdroplet channel. Biosensors Bioelectron. **119**, 126–133.
124. Dallari, C., Credi, C., Lenci, E., Trabocchi, A., Cicchi, R., and Pavone, F. S. (2020) Nanostars—decorated microfluidic sensors for surface enhanced Raman scattering targeting of biomolecules. J. Phys. Photonics **2**, 024008.
125. Dina, N. E., Colniță, A., Marconi, D., and Gherman, A. M. R. (2020) Microfluidic portable device for pathogens' rapid SERS detection. Proceedings **60**, 2.
126. Madiyar, F. R., Bhana, S., Swisher, L. Z., Culbertson, C. T., Huang, X., and Li, J. (2015) Integration of a nanostructured dielectrophoretic device and a surface-enhanced Raman probe for highly sensitive rapid bacteria detection. Nanoscale **7**, 3726–3736.
127. Liu, B., Wu, T., Yang, X., Wang, Z., and Du, Y. (2014) Portable microfluidic chip based surface-enhanced Raman spectroscopy sensor for crystal violet. Anal. Lett. **47**, 2682–2690.
128. Bardram, J. E. and Frost, M. (2016) The personal health technology design space. IEEE Pervasive Comput. **15**, 70–78.
129. He, X., Fan, C., Luo, Y., Xu, T., and Zhang, X. (2022) Flexible microfluidic nanoplasmonic sensors for refreshable and portable recognition of sweat biochemical fingerprint. npj Flex. Electron. **6**, 60.
130. Yuan, Y., Panwar, N., Yap, S. H. K., Wu, Q., Zeng, S., Xu, J., Tjin, S. C., Song, J., Qu, J., and Yong, K.-T. (2017) SERS-based ultrasensitive sensing platform: An insight into design and practical applications. Coord. Chem. Rev. **337**, 1–33.
131. Wang, Z., Zong, S., Wu, L., Zhu, D., and Cui, Y. (2017) SERS-activated platforms for immunoassay: probes, encoding methods, and applications. Chem. Rev. **117**, 7910–7963.

132. Marques, A. C., Águas, H., Martins, R., Costa-Silva, B., Sales, M. G., and Fortunato, E. (2022) Chapter 6 — Surface-Enhanced Raman Scattering Paper-Based Analytical Devices. In *Paper-based Analytical Devices for Chemical Analysis and Diagnostics* (de Araujo, W. R. and Paixão, T. R. L. C., Eds.), pp. 117–167, Elsevier.
133. Li, C., Liu, Y., Zhou, X., and Wang, Y. (2020) A paper-based SERS assay for sensitive duplex cytokine detection towards the atherosclerosis-associated disease diagnosis. J. Mater. Chem. B **8**, 3582–3589.
134. Gahlaut, S. K., Savargaonkar, D., Sharan, C., Yadav, S., Mishra, P., and Singh, J. P. (2020) SERS platform for dengue diagnosis from clinical samples employing a hand held raman spectrometer. Anal. Chem. **92**, 2527–2534.
135. Huang, C. C., Cheng, C. Y., and Lai, Y. S. (2020) Paper-based flexible surface enhanced Raman scattering platforms and their applications to food safety. Trends Food Sci. Technol. **100**, 349–358.
136. Alder, R., Hong, J., Chow, E., Fang, J., Isa, F., Ashford, B., Comte, C., Bendavid, A., Xiao, L., Ostrikov, K. K., *et al.* (2021) Application of plasma-printed paper-based SERS substrate for cocaine detection. Sensors **21**, 810.
137. Hassanain, W. A., Izake, E. L., Sivanesan, A., and Ayoko, G. A. (2017) Towards interference free HPLC-SERS for the trace analysis of drug metabolites in biological fluids. J. Pharm. Biomed. Anal. **136**, 38–43.
138. Hassanain, W. A., Izake, E. L., Schmidt, M. S., and Ayoko, G. A. (2017) Gold nanomaterials for the selective capturing and SERS diagnosis of toxins in aqueous and biological fluids. Biosensors Bioelectron. **91**, 664–672.
139. Ogundare, S. A. and van Zyl, W. E. (2019) A review of cellulose-based substrates for SERS: fundamentals, design principles, applications. Cellulose **26**, 6489–6528.
140. Vo-Dinh, T., Hiromoto, M. Y. K., Begun, G. M., and Moody, R. L. (1984) Surface-enhanced Raman spectrometry for trace organic analysis. Anal. Chem. **56**, 1667–1670.
141. Tran, C. D. (1984) Subnanogram detection of dyes on filter paper by surface-enhanced Raman scattering spectrometry. Anal. Chem. **56**, 824–826.
142. Boehringer, H. R. and O'Farrell, B. J. (2021) LFAs in infectious disease diagnosis. Clin. Chem. **68**, 52–58.
143. Guler, E., Yilmaz Sengel, T., Gumus, Z. P., Arslan, M., Coskunol, H., Timur, S., and Yagci, Y. (2017) Mobile phone sensing of cocaine in a LFA combined with a biomimetic material. Anal. Chem. **89**, 9629–9632.
144. Koczula, K. M. and Gallotta, A. (2016) LFAs. Essays Biochem. **60**, 111–120.
145. Choi, S., Hwang, J., Lee, S., Lim, D. W., Joo, H., and Choo, J. (2017) Quantitative analysis of thyroid-stimulating hormone (TSH) using SERS-based lateral flow immunoassay. Sensors Actuators B: Chem. **240**, 358–364.
146. Fu, X., Cheng, Z., Yu, J., Choo, P., Chen, L., and Choo, J. (2016) A SERS-based LFA biosensor for highly sensitive detection of HIV-1 DNA. Biosensors Bioelectron. **78**, 530–537.

147. Hwang, J., Lee, S., and Choo, J. (2016) Application of a SERS-based lateral flow immunoassay strip for the rapid and sensitive detection of staphylococcal enterotoxin B. Nanoscale **8**, 11418–11425.
148. Bahadır, E. B. and Sezgintürk, M. K. (2016) LFAs: Principles, designs and labels. Trends Anal. Chem. **82**, 286–306.
149. Blanco-Covián, L., Montes-García, V., Girard, A., Fernández-Abedul, M. T., Pérez-Juste, J., Pastoriza-Santos, I., Faulds, K., Graham, D., and Blanco-López, M. C. (2017) Au@Ag SERRS tags coupled to a lateral flow immunoassay for the sensitive detection of pneumolysin. Nanoscale **9**, 2051–2058.
150. Hassanain, W. A., Spoors, J., Johnson, C. L., Faulds, K., Keegan, N., and Graham, D. (2021) Rapid ultra-sensitive diagnosis of clostridium difficile infection using a SERS-based LFA. Analyst **146**, 4495–4505.
151. Yadav, S., Sadique, M. A., Ranjan, P., Kumar, N., Singhal, A., Srivastava, A. K., and Khan, R. (2021) SERS based lateral flow immunoassay for point-of-care detection of SARS-CoV-2 in clinical samples. ACS Appl. Bio. Mater. **4**, 2974–2995.
152. Kim, K., Kashefi-Kheyrabadi, L., Joung, Y., Kim, K., Dang, H., Chavan, S. G., Lee, M.-H., and Choo, J. (2021) Recent advances in sensitive surface-enhanced Raman scattering-based LFA platforms for point-of-care diagnostics of infectious diseases. Sensors Actuators B: Chem. **329**, 129214.
153. Saviñon-Flores, F., Méndez, E., López-Castaños, M., Carabarin-Lima, A., López-Castaños, K. A., González-Fuentes, M. A., and Méndez-Albores, A. (2021) A review on SERS-based detection of human virus infections: influenza and coronavirus. Biosensors **11**, 66.
154. Wang, R., Kim, K., Choi, N., Wang, X., Lee, J., Jeon, J. H., Rhie, G.-e., and Choo, J. (2018) Highly sensitive detection of high-risk bacterial pathogens using SERS-based LFA strips. Sensors Actuators B: Chem. **270**, 72–79.
155. Zhang, Y., Tran, V., Adanalic, M., and Schlücker, S. (2022) Chapter 9 — iSERS Microscopy: Point-of-Care Diagnosis and Tissue Imaging. In *Principles and Clinical Diagnostic Applications of Surface-Enhanced Raman Spectroscopy* (Wang, Y., Ed.), pp. 327–372, Elsevier.
156. Zhang, D., Huang, L., Liu, B., Ge, Q., Dong, J., and Zhao, X. (2019) Rapid and ultrasensitive quantification of multiplex respiratory tract infection pathogen via lateral flow microarray based on SERS nanotags. Theranostics **9**, 4849–4859.
157. Ellis, D. I., Muhamadali, H., Haughey, S. A., Elliott, C. T., and Goodacre, R. (2015) Point-and-shoot: rapid quantitative detection methods for on-site food fraud analysis — moving out of the laboratory and into the food supply chain. Anal. Methods **7**, 9401–9414.
158. Joung, Y., Kim, K., Lee, S., Chun, B. S., Lee, S., Hwang, J., Choi, S., Kang, T., Lee, M. K., Chen, L., *et al.* (2022) Rapid and accurate on-site immunodiagnostics of highly contagious severe acute respiratory syndrome coronavirus 2 using portable surface-enhanced Raman scattering-LFA reader. ACS Sensors **7**, 3470–3480.

159. Tran, V., Walkenfort, B., König, M., Salehi, M., and Schlücker, S. (2019) Rapid, quantitative, and ultrasensitive point-of-care testing: a portable SERS reader for LFAs in clinical chemistry. Angew. Chem. Int. Ed. **58**, 442–446.
160. Xiao, R., Lu, L., Rong, Z., Wang, C., Peng, Y., Wang, F., Wang, J., Sun, M., Dong, J., Wang, D., *et al.* (2020) Portable and multiplexed lateral flow immunoassay reader based on SERS for highly sensitive point-of-care testing. Biosensors Bioelectron. **168**, 112524.
161. Lee, S. H., Hwang, J., Kim, K., Jeon, J., Lee, S., Ko, J., Lee, J., Kang, M., Chung, D. R., and Choo, J. (2019) Quantitative serodiagnosis of scrub typhus using surface-enhanced Raman scattering-based LFA platforms. Anal. Chem. **91**, 12275–12282.
162. Carrell, C., Kava, A., Nguyen, M., Menger, R., Munshi, Z., Call, Z., Nussbaum, M., and Henry, C. (2019) Beyond the LFA: A review of paper-based microfluidics. Microelectron. Eng. **206**, 45–54.
163. Zhu, J., Chen, Q., Kutsanedzie, F. Y. H., Yang, M., Ouyang, Q., and Jiang, H. (2017) Highly sensitive and label-free determination of thiram residue using surface-enhanced Raman spectroscopy (SERS) coupled with paper-based microfluidics. Anal. Methods **9**, 6186–6193.
164. Saha, A. and Jana, N. R. (2015) Paper-based microfluidic approach for surface-enhanced Raman spectroscopy and highly reproducible detection of proteins beyond picomolar concentration. ACS Appl. Mater. Interfaces **7**, 996–1003.
165. Zhuang, J., Zhao, Z., Lian, K., Yin, L., Wang, J., Man, S., Liu, G., and Ma, L. (2022) SERS-based CRISPR/Cas assay on microfluidic paper analytical devices for supersensitive detection of pathogenic bacteria in foods. Biosensors Bioelectron. **207**, 114167.
166. Noviana, E., Ozer, T., Carrell, C. S., Link, J. S., McMahon, C., Jang, I., and Henry, C. S. (2021) Microfluidic paper-based analytical devices: from design to applications. Chem. Rev. **121**, 11835–11885.
167. Yetisen, A. K., Akram, M. S., and Lowe, C. R. (2013) Paper-based microfluidic point-of-care diagnostic devices. Lab Chip **13**, 2210–2251.
168. Berry, S. B., Fernandes, S. C., Rajaratnam, A., DeChiara, N. S., and Mace, C. R. (2016) Measurement of the hematocrit using paper-based microfluidic devices. Lab Chip **16**, 3689–3694.
169. Hariharan, A., Chelli, S. M., Muthukumar V, S., Belliraj, S. K., Ferrari, M., Krishna Narasimha, N., and Vishnubhatla, K. C. (2019) Paper-microfluidics based SERS substrate for PPB level detection of catechol. Opt. Mater. **94**, 305–310.
170. Chen, M., Yang, H., Rong, L., and Chen, X. (2016) A gas-diffusion microfluidic paper-based analytical device (μPAD) coupled with portable surface-enhanced Raman scattering (SERS): facile determination of sulphite in wines. Analyst **141**, 5511–5519.
171. Lee, J. C., Kim, W., and Choi, S. (2017) Fabrication of a SERS-encoded microfluidic paper-based analytical chip for the point-of-assay of wastewater. Int. J. Precis. Eng. **4**, 221–226.

172. Craig, D., Mazilu, M., and Dholakia, K. (2015) Quantitative detection of pharmaceuticals using a combination of paper microfluidics and wavelength modulated Raman spectroscopy. PLoS One **10**, e0123334.
173. Chen, J., Li, S., Yao, F., Bao, F., Ge, Y., Zou, M., Liang, P., and Chen, Q. (2022) Progress of microfluidics combined with SERS technology in the trace detection of harmful substances. Chemosensors **10**, 449.
174. Lim, W. Y., Goh, C. H., Thevarajah, T. M., Goh, B. T., and Khor, S. M. (2020) Using SERS-based microfluidic paper-based device (μPAD) for calibration-free quantitative measurement of AMI cardiac biomarkers. Biosens. Bioelectron. **147**, 111792.
175. Mabbott, S., Fernandes, S. C., Schechinger, M., Cote, G. L., Faulds, K., Mace, C. R., and Graham, D. (2020) Detection of cardiovascular disease associated miR-29a using paper-based microfluidics and surface enhanced Raman scattering. Analyst **145**, 983–991.
176. Rivas, L., Medina-Sánchez, M., de la Escosura-Muñiz, A., and Merkoçi, A. (2014) Improving sensitivity of gold nanoparticle-based LFAs by using wax-printed pillars as delay barriers of microfluidics. Lab Chip **14**, 4406–4414.
177. Fu, E., Lutz, B., Kauffman, P., and Yager, P. (2010) Controlled reagent transport in disposable 2D paper networks. Lab Chip **10**, 918–920.
178. Tu, D., Holderby, A., Dean, J., Mabbott, S., and Coté, G. L. (2021) Paper Microfluidic device with a horizontal motion valve and a localized delay for automatic control of a multistep assay. Anal. Chem. **93**, 4497–4505.
179. Restaino, S. M. and White, I. M. (2019) A critical review of flexible and porous SERS sensors for analytical chemistry at the point-of-sample. Anal. Chim. Acta **1060**, 17–29.
180. Romo-Herrera, J. M., Juarez-Moreno, K., Guerrini, L., Kang, Y., Feliu, N., Parak, W. J., and Alvarez-Puebla, R. A. (2021) Paper-based plasmonic substrates as surface-enhanced Raman scattering spectroscopy platforms for cell culture applications. Mater. Today Bio. **11**, 100125.
181. Li, Y., Zhang, K., Zhao, J., Ji, J., Ji, C., and Liu, B. (2016) A three-dimensional silver nanoparticles decorated plasmonic paper strip for SERS detection of low-abundance molecules. Talanta **147**, 493–500.
182. Luo, W., Chen, M., Hao, N., Huang, X., Zhao, X., Zhu, Y., Yang, H., and Chen, X. (2019) In situ synthesis of gold nanoparticles on pseudo-paper films as flexible SERS substrate for sensitive detection of surface organic residues. Talanta **197**, 225–233.
183. Hasi, W. L. J., Lin, X., Lou, X. T., Lin, S., Yang, F., Lin, D. Y., and Lu, Z. W. (2015) Chloride ion-assisted self-assembly of silver nanoparticles on filter paper as SERS substrate. Appl. Phys. A **118**, 799–807.
184. Wang, J., Yang, L., Liu, B., Jiang, H., Liu, R., Yang, J., Han, G., Mei, Q., and Zhang, Z. (2014) Inkjet-printed silver nanoparticle paper detects airborne species from crystalline explosives and their ultratrace residues in open environment. Anal. Chem. **86**, 3338–3345.

185. Yu, W. W. and White, I. M. (2010) Inkjet printed surface enhanced Raman spectroscopy array on cellulose paper. Anal. Chem. **82**, 9626–9630.
186. Cheng, H., Yi, L., Wu, J., Li, G., Zhao, G., Xiao, Z., Hu, B., Zhao, L., and Tian, J. (2021) Drug preconcentration and direct quantification in biofluids using 3D-printed paper cartridge. Biosensors Bioelectron. **189**, 113266.
187. Pan, X., Li, L., Lin, H., Tan, J., Wang, H., Liao, M., Chen, C., Shan, B., Chen, Y., and Li, M. (2019) A graphene oxide-gold nanostar hybrid based-paper biosensor for label-free SERS detection of serum bilirubin for diagnosis of jaundice. Biosensors Bioelectron. **145**, 111713.
188. Perumal, J., Lim, H. Q., Attia, A. B. E., Raziq, R., Leavesley, D. I., Upton, Z., Dinish, U. S., and Olivo, M. (2021) Novel cellulose fibre-based flexible plasmonic membrane for point-of-care SERS biomarker detection in chronic wound healing. Int. J. Nanomedicine **16**, 5869–5878.
189. https://www.marketsandmarkets.com/PressReleases/point-of-care-diagnostic.asp.

https://doi.org/10.1142/9789811264610_0008

Chapter 8

Raman Imaging and Screening of Bioactive Small Molecules

Hiroyuki Yamakoshi,[1] Jun Ando,[2] Syusuke Egoshi,[2,3] Kosuke Dodo,[2,3] Mikiko Sodeoka,[2,3] Katsumasa Fujita[4-6,*]

[1]*Graduate School of Pharmaceutical Sciences, Tohoku University, 6-3 Aoba, Aramaki, Aoba-ku, Sendai 980-8578, Japan*
[2]*RIKEN Cluster for Pioneering Research, 2-1 Hirosawa, Wako, Saitama 351-0198, Japan*
[3]*RIKEN Center for Sustainable Resource Science, 2-1 Hirosawa, Wako, Saitama 351-0198, Japan*
[4]*Department of Applied Physics, Osaka University, 2-1 Yamadaoka, Suita, Osaka 565-0871, Japan*
[5]*Advanced Photonics and Biosensing Open Innovation Laboratory, AIST-Osaka University, 2-1 Yamadaoka, Suita, Osaka 565-0871, Japan*
[6]*Transdimensional Life Imaging Division, Institute for Open and Transdisciplinary Research Initiatives, Osaka University, 2-1 Yamadaoka, Suita, Osaka 565-0871, Japan*
**Corresponding author: fujita@ap.eng.osaka-u.ac.jp*

8.1 Introduction

Pharmaceuticals and other bioactive compounds are used worldwide to maintain public health and cure various diseases and injuries. For example, more than US$10 billion are spent worldwide on anti-cancer drugs per year [1], and innovative drugs are being developed annually in fierce competition [2]. In drug development, it is necessary to study their distribution and metabolism in cells, organs, and the entire body and observe functional and morphological changes induced by drug administration. It is also important to study the interaction of bioactive compounds with their target molecules, such as enzymes and receptors, to elucidate their mechanisms of action at the molecular level. Various instruments and measurement methods have been used to analyze drug-body interactions, such as mass spectrometry [3], NMR [4], X-ray crystallography [5], fluorescence microscopy [6], liquid chromatography [7], absorption/emission spectroscopy [8], infrared spectroscopy [9], and Raman spectroscopy [10, 11]. Among these techniques, Raman spectroscopy is a unique and useful technology in pharmaceutical research and development because it provides label-free molecular structural information on drug molecules, even in aqueous environments, without sample destruction.

Raman spectroscopy is a vibrational spectroscopy technique that optically measures molecular vibrations. A laser beam comprising a single wavelength is irradiated onto a sample of interest, and the Raman scattered light generated by the molecules in the sample is measured as the signal light. In Raman scattering, the energy of the scattered light is lower (or higher), and the wavelength is longer (or shorter) than that of the incident light because of energy loss in the molecular vibration (or provided to the scattered light) during the scattering process. By acquiring the generated Raman scattered light with a spectrometer and determining the energy difference between the scattered and incident light, the vibrational energy of the molecule (type of chemical bonding) can be estimated, leading to the identification of the molecular species in the sample. The Raman shift (cm^{-1}) in the Raman scattering spectrum represents the difference between the wavenumber of the incident and scattered light, and larger values represent higher molecular vibration energies. Because Raman spectroscopy directly estimates the vibrations of molecules, and the Raman shift depends on the chemical structure, it can identify and analyze molecules in a sample without labeling and modification. Furthermore, Raman spectroscopy with a visible excitation light source can measure molecules in water in a non-contact and non-destructive manner. Therefore, it is useful for analyzing biomolecules and bioactive compounds, and various pharmaceutical studies have been conducted using Raman spectroscopy, such as studies on drug-protein interaction [12], pharmacokinetic profiling [13], including drug absorption, distribution, metabolism, and excretion, and the investigation of crystal polymorphism [14].

One of the challenges of Raman spectroscopy in life science and pharmaceutical research is its low sensitivity and long measurement times. The Raman scattering cross-section of the molecule is considerably lower than the absorption cross-section of the fluorescent dye (10^{-30} cm^2 vs. 10^{-16} cm^2). For this reason, in the past, measurements were often possible only when the concentration of the sample molecules was extremely high (e.g., molar or sub-molar range), or the time required for a single measurement was long (e.g., several minutes). In recent years, technological advances such as the development of laser light sources with high light intensity and narrow linewidth, improvement of optical filters that selectively transmit Raman scattered light, and development of photodetectors with high quantum yield and low noise have been achieved. These developments have addressed the issues associated with Raman spectroscopy, such as sensitivity and measurement time, and therefore, Raman spectroscopy is emerging as a powerful tool in biology and biomedicine. Additionally, the use of a parallel Raman spectral acquisition system [15] is a promising strategy for observing and analyzing large amounts of bioactive compounds or drug-treated cells with a relatively high yield. This review will discuss the analysis of pharmaceuticals and bioactive compounds using Raman spectroscopy, focusing on microscopic imaging systems and Raman tags for high-throughput imaging [15] and screening [16].

8.2 Imaging Small Molecules in Cells with Raman Tags

8.2.1 *Raman Microscopy and Small Molecules*

Confocal Raman microscopy has been widely used to perform two-dimensional Raman imaging and spectroscopy of biological samples [17, 18]. In this device, laser light is focused on a single point using an objective lens. The scattered light is collected by the same objective lens and then detected using a spectrophotometer through a pinhole. Raman spectra are sequentially acquired while scanning the sample or beam spot to obtain two-dimensional (2D) or three-dimensional (3D) Raman images of the sample. Because it produces high-resolution Raman images, it has been used to visualize intracellularly administered drugs [17]. However, the exposure time per point is often several seconds or longer. The total measurement time to obtain a high-resolution image with a field of view capturing the entire cell body is several tens of minutes to several hours or longer. To improve the imaging speed of Raman microscopy, parallel spectral acquisition systems have been developed, such as slit-scanning imaging systems with line-shaped laser illumination [19, 20] and multifocal imaging systems with 2D array illumination [21, 22]. In the slit-scanning Raman microscope, the laser beam was shaped into a line using a cylindrical lens and focused on the sample through an objective lens (Figure 8.1(a)). The Raman scattered light generated along the line-shaped illumination is collected by the same objective lens and imaged on the slit of

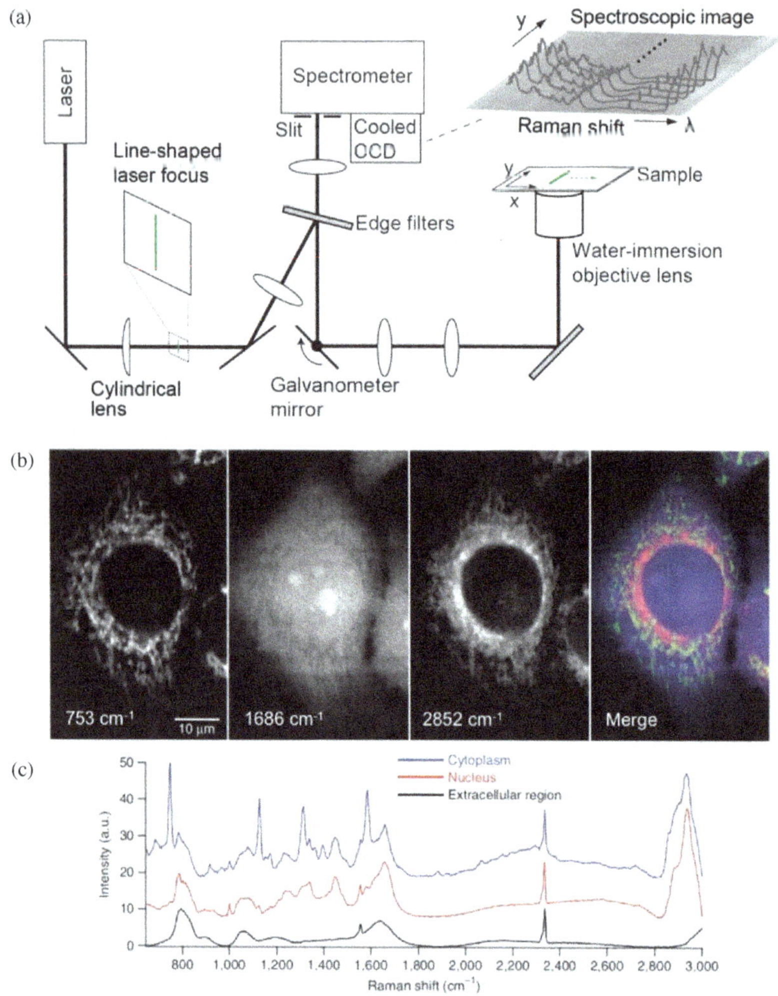

Figure 8.1. Raman image of live cells with parallel Raman acquisition system. (a) Schematic of a slit-scanning Raman microscope. (b) Reconstructed images from Raman signals at 753, 1686, and 2852 cm^{-1} and their superimposed images. (c) Average Raman spectra from cytoplasmic, nuclear, and extracellular regions. Adapted from Ref. [20] with permission.

an imaging spectrometer. The Raman spectra are recorded in parallel using a two-dimensional cooled CCD detector connected to the spectrometer. A hyperspectral Raman image of the sample is obtained by performing Raman spectrum measurements while scanning a line-shaped laser beam one-dimensionally using a galvanometer mirror. Compared with conventional Raman microscopes that acquire spectra from a sample one point at a time, this system can perform spectroscopic imaging more than 100 times faster. Figure 8.1(b) shows a Raman image of a HeLa cell obtained using the developed microscope. It was constructed based on the intensity of the Raman peaks at 753 cm^{-1} attributed to the respiratory vibration of the pyrrole ring, 1686 cm^{-1} attributed to the amide I vibration of the peptide bond, and 2852 cm^{-1} attributed to the stretching vibration of CH_2. The spatial distribution of cytochromes, proteins, and lipids in the cell can be visualized with a high spatial resolution that can identify cell organelles. The above Raman spectroscopic imaging can be completed within a few minutes to several tens of minutes. This imaging system has been used to analyze the distribution of small bioactive molecules in cells [23] and changes in cellular activities induced by bioactive compounds [24, 25] with high spatiotemporal resolution.

8.2.2 *Introduction to Raman-Tag Imaging*

Raman microscopy allows label-free visualization of biological molecules. However, it is unsuitable for specific molecular detection in cells because of the interference from endogenous molecular signals. Proteins are endogenous macromolecules composed of many amino acids linked together. Although the function of each protein varies, they all share the same structural element as a series of amide bonds. Therefore, current Raman microscopy techniques cannot distinguish between different proteins. In addition, Raman microscopy cannot distinguish between individuals for lipid detection. They are composed of similar C–H bonds. Externally added small bioactive molecules often consist of amides and C–H bonds. Hence, it is challenging to observe intracellularly administered drugs using Raman microscopy, and the narrow range of applicable molecules has limited the biological application of Raman microscopy. In such a situation, Sodeoka and co-workers introduced a concept of "Raman-tag imaging" that uses a functional group to provide a strong signal in a cellular silent region (1800–2800 cm^{-1}), where molecules in animal cells give no Raman signal [27]. The functional groups containing a triple bond (e.g., alkyne, nitrile) or C–D (carbon–deuterium) bonds show strong signals in the cellular silent region, thereby acting as Raman tags. In this section, we outline Raman-tag imaging using an example of Raman imaging of EdU (5-ethynyl-2'-deoxyuridine) by the Sodeoka group in 2011 [27].

EdU is an alkynylated analog of dT (thymidine) [28]. This compound is incorporated into replicating DNA and accumulates in the nucleus. The alkyne-tag moiety can be modified by copper-catalyzed alkyne-azide cycloaddition,

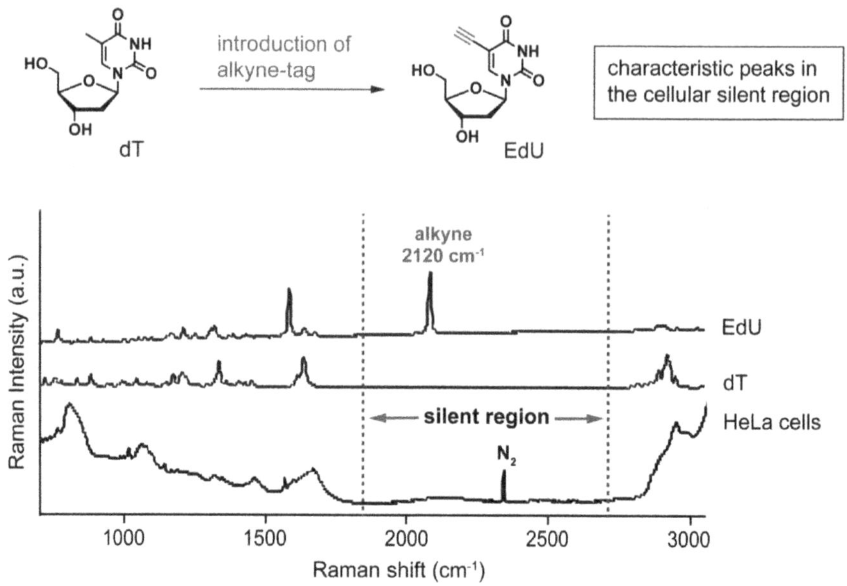

Figure 8.2. Raman spectra of thymidine analogs and a typical cellular spectrum of HeLa cells. Adapted from Ref. [26] with permission.

a representative reaction of "click chemistry" [26, 29–31], with an azide-modified fluorescent dye for the fluorescent detection of cell proliferation [32, 33]. However, fluorescence imaging is not applicable to live cell imaging of EdU due to toxicity and distribution issues of catalysts and dyes. In contrast, Raman microscopy allows live cell imaging of EdU. Figure 8.2 shows the Raman spectra of the dT, EdU, and HeLa cells. All peaks derived from dT overlapped with those from HeLa cells, indicating that dT is difficult to detect in these cells. In contrast, EdU showed a characteristic alkyne peak (2120 cm^{-1}) in the silent region, which allows live-cell Raman imaging.

Raman images of live HeLa cells treated with EdU are shown in Figure 8.3. An alkyne signal (2120 cm^{-1}) was detected in the nucleus of EdU-treated cells, whereas untreated control cells showed no signal (Figure 8.3(a)). These Raman images were reconstructed from the distribution of Raman signals at 749, 2120, and 2852 cm^{-1}. These peaks can be assigned to cytochromes, EdU, and lipid molecules, respectively (Figure 8.3(b)). The alkyne signal is recognized only in the nuclei of EdU-treated cells. Furthermore, Sodeoka *et al.* observed EdU uptake in HeLa cells using time-course Raman imaging. The results shows a good correlation between the doubling time of HeLa cells (~20 h) [34] and the ratio of cells that took up EdU. Through this, Raman-tag

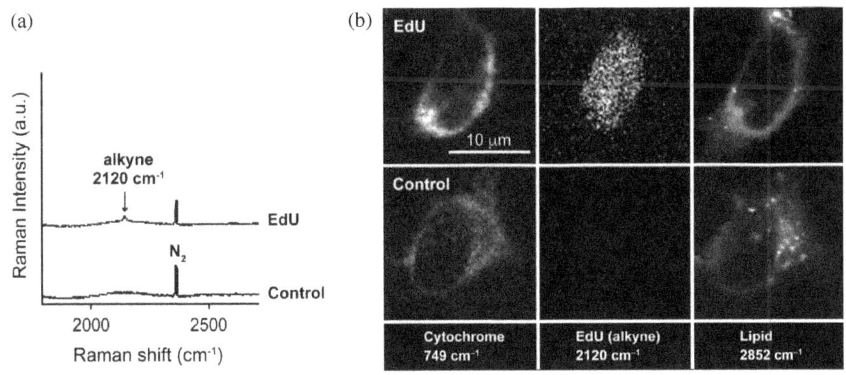

Figure 8.3. Raman imaging of EdU-treated and untreated (control) HeLa cells. (a) Average Raman spectra (silent region) obtained from nucleus. (b) Raman images at 749, 2150, and 2852 cm^{-1}. Adapted from Ref. [26] with permission.

imaging was proven effective in analyzing the distribution of Raman-tagged compounds in living cells.

Later, Sodeoka *et al.* investigated structure-Raman shift/intensity relationships (SIR) to design optimal Raman-tagged compounds [35]. For this purpose, they introduced the relative Raman scattering intensity (relative Raman intensity versus EdU), using EdU as the standard material. The signal intensity and wavenumbers of the Raman tags differ with the different functional groups of the tags and their substitution patterns. The details of SIR have been omitted due to limitations of space and scope of this review. Interested readers are referred to the original paper. Here, two-color alkyne-tag Raman imaging using two Raman-tagged compounds with different wavenumbers is presented (Figure 8.4). In the same report, AltQ2, an alkyne-labeled compound of mitochondrial lipid coenzyme Q (CoQ), was successfully imaged simultaneously with EdU.

Raman imaging of HeLa cells was performed using 40 μM EdU and 2 μM AltQ2. Two different alkyne peaks corresponding to EdU and AltQ2 were observed at 2122 and 2248 cm^{-1}, respectively. EdU (2122 cm^{-1}) accumulated in the nucleus, whereas AltQ2 (2248 cm^{-1}) co-localized with both mitochondria (747 cm^{-1}: cytochrome) and lipids (data not shown). These results demonstrate that the Raman tag is a promising tool for simultaneously studying the cellular accumulation of multiple compounds. Furthermore, the distribution of intracellular molecules, such as cytochromes and lipids, is a notable advantage of Raman microscopy.

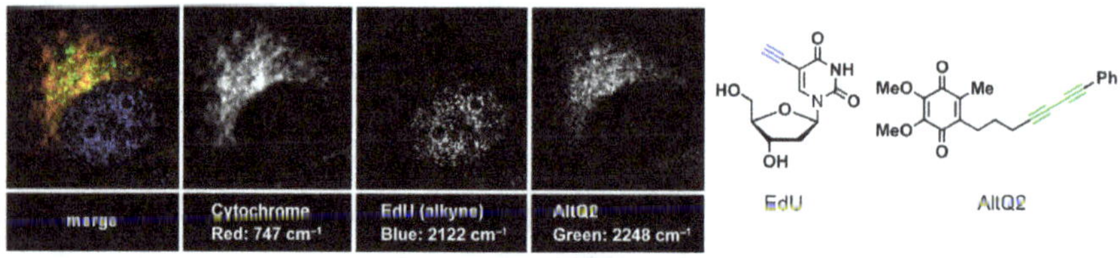

Figure 8.4. Two-color Raman-tag imaging. Images are overlays of the cytochrome (red), EdU (blue), and AltQ2 (green). Adapted from Ref. [35] with permission.

Table 8.1. Estimation of cellular concentration of AltQs. Adapted from Ref. [35] with permission.

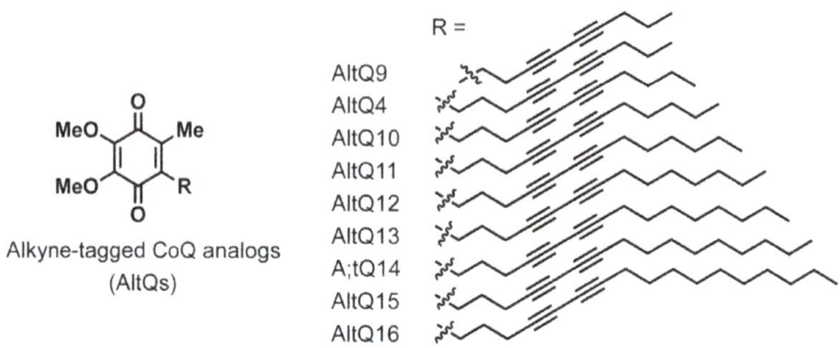

AltQs	AltQ9	AltQ4	AltQ10	AltQ11	AltQ12	AltQ13	AltQ14	AltQ15	AltQ16
Carbon length	C9	C10	C11	C12	C13	C14	C15	C16	C17
cLogP	3.1	3.6	4.1	4.7	5.2	5.7	6.2	6.8	7.3
Concentration (mM)	1.76	1.70	1.34	0.80	0.60	0.60	0.30	0.23	0.08

8.2.3 *Imaging Small Molecules in Cells with Raman Tags*

Raman-tag imaging enables estimating the concentration of small molecules in live cells. In contrast to fluorescent dyes used for fluorescent imaging, small Raman tags have a slight effect on labeled compounds. The first semi-quantitative Raman-tag analysis of small molecules was reported in 2012 by Sodeoka and co-workers [35]. They investigated the cellular accumulation of CoQ analogs (Table 8.1). CoQ_{10} is a lipid-soluble antioxidant and essential electron carrier in the respiratory chain. While CoQ_{10} supplements are commercially available, the bioavailability of exogenous CoQ_{10} is considered low owing to hydrophobicity. Analogs with shorter side chains have been developed, and their cellular accumulation correlates with hydrophobicity [36, 37]. However, studies on the cellular uptake of CoQ derivatives with different chain lengths are limited [38, 39]. Therefore, they designed and synthesized AltQ4 and AltQ9–16, with a 1,3-butadiyne structure as Raman tags, to investigate the relationship between the length of the alkyl side chain and cytosolic concentrations. AltQs have different side-chain carbon numbers (C9–16) and cover a wide range of overall lipophilicity with cLogP values of 3.1–7.3.

HeLa cells were incubated in Tyrode's solution containing 20 μM AltQs for 60 min, and the average Raman spectra of the cytoplasm were obtained at an excitation wavelength of 532 nm. Cellular concentrations were calculated based on a calibration curve prepared using the peak height and Raman spectra of AltQs measured separately in a DMSO solution. The shorter side-chain CoQ derivatives accumulated at higher concentrations. The concentration of AltQ9 with the shortest side chain was then estimated to be 1.8 mM. These results indicate that the CoQ derivatives accumulate at higher concentrations with lower lipophilicity. Differences in accumulation due to differences in only one carbon were detected, indicating that small Raman labeling (1,3-butadiyne tag: molecular weight 48) had negligible effects on the behavior of the compounds.

The C–D bonds are often used as Raman tags, although the signal intensities of C–D bonds are weaker than those of triple bonds, such as an alkyne and a nitrile [35, 40]. Because long-chain fatty acids can be labeled with a large amount of deuterium, several deuterated fatty acids are frequently employed to analyze cellular lipid metabolism [41]. Furthermore, in molecular reactions, such as chemical synthesis and metabolic pathways, the dissociation of C–D bonds is slower than that of C–H bonds. These kinetic isotope effects (KIEs) serve as inhibition against the enzymic oxidation of polyunsaturated fatty acids, such as the bis-allylic deuterated arachidonic acid [42, 43].

In 2021, Sodeoka and co-workers reported a mechanistic study of the tumor-selective cytotoxicity of γ-linolenic acids (GLA) using deuterium KIE and Raman imaging of C–D bonds (Figure 8.5) [44]. Several deuterated GLA derivatives were synthesized, and their resistance to enzymatic reactions was confirmed. Then, natural and deuterated GLA derivatives were evaluated for their cytotoxic effects on normal human fibroblast WI-38 cells and tumor VA-13 cells generated by the transformation of WI-38 with the SV40 virus (Figure 8.5(b)). Natural GLA was cytotoxic to both cell lines. In contrast, GLA with deuterium at all bis-allylic positions (partially D-GLA) was not cytotoxic to WI-38 cells but showed cytotoxicity toward VA-13 cells. All-deuterated GLA (all-D-GLA) was also synthesized for Raman imaging and showed similar

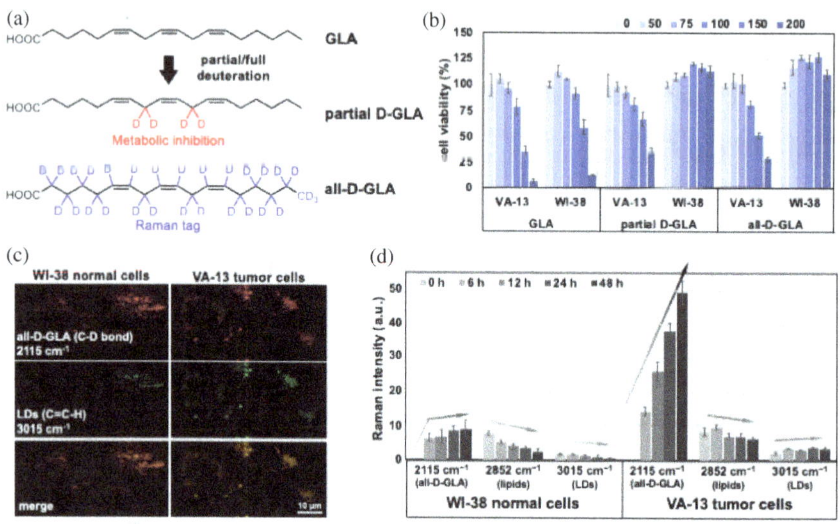

Figure 8.5. Mechanistic study of the tumor-selective cytotoxicity of GLA using deuterium-Raman imaging. (a) Partial/full deuteration of GLA for metabolic inhibition and Raman imaging. (b) Cytotoxicity test of natural GLA and partially/fully deuterated GLA. (c) Raman imaging in WI-38/VA-13 cells treated with 100 μM all-D-GLA for 48 h. (d) Semi-quantitative analysis for the lipid composition of LDs in WI-38/VA-13 cells. Adapted from Ref. [44] with permission.

selective cytotoxicity to those of partial D-GLA. These results indicate that GLA itself, not its oxidized metabolites, induced tumor-selective cytotoxicity.

Time-lapse Raman imaging was performed for WI-38 and VA-13 cells treated with 100 μM all-D-GLA. Figure 8.5(c) shows the intracellular distribution of all-D-GLA in both cell lines treated for 48 h. All-D-GLA was detected in lipid droplets (LDs) and the cytoplasm in WI-38 cells. In contrast, all-D-GLA was found in LDs but was negligibly detected in the non-LD region in VA-13. The lipid composition of LDs in both cell lines was determined via semi-quantitative analysis based on Raman signal intensities of all-D-GLA (2115 cm^{-1}, C–D bonds), endogenous lipids (2852 cm^{-1}, CH_2 bonds), and endogenous unsaturated fatty acids as indicators of LDs (3015 cm^{-1}, C–H bonds of *cis*-olefin) (Figure 8.5(d)). In WI-38 cells, the incorporation of all-D-GLA was limited. In contrast, all-D-GLA continuously accumulated in the VA-13 cells without restriction. These results imply that GLA itself shows tumor-selective cytotoxicity via accumulation in LDs.

The stable isotope labeling of molecules affects the Raman signals of several functional groups. For example, in addition to the C–D bonds, alkynes/nitriles labeled with stable isotopes exhibit blueshifts within the cellular silent region (e.g., the shift value is ~48 cm^{-1} for mono-^{13}C-alkyne, ~77 cm^{-1} for di-^{13}C-alkyne, ~28 cm^{-1} for ^{15}N-nitrile, ~54 cm^{-1} for ^{13}C-nitrile, and ~82 cm^{-1} for ^{13}C-^{15}N-nitrile) [45, 46]. These isotopically labeled alkynes and nitriles are often employed to perform multicolor Raman imaging with nonlinear Raman microscopy, such as stimulated Raman scattering (SRS) microscopy [45–49].

Deuteration affects the Raman signals of adjacent functional groups. For example, an approximately 30 cm^{-1} decrease in the Raman signal of the C=C bond is exhibited after the deuteration of vinylic positions [44, 50]. Therefore, the Raman signal of the deuterated C=C of all-D-GLA can be specifically observed and distinguished from the natural C=C bonds of endogenous biomolecules [44]. Furthermore, Sodeoka and co-workers demonstrated for the first time in 2021 [51] that the alkyne Raman signal shifts approximately 135 cm^{-1} upon deuteration. Deuterated alkynes (D-alkynes) are easily synthesized by the treatment of normal terminal alkynes (protonated alkynes, H-alkynes) in heavy water (D_2O)-containing bases. Furthermore, the H/D exchange of conjugated alkynes was faster than that of non-conjugated alkynes. Although D-alkynes were converted to H-alkynes in cells, approximately 90% of the non-conjugated D-alkynes were able to remain in cells for approximately six hours. Therefore, recent studies have shown that D-alkyne functions as a Raman tag for live cell Raman imaging and can be detected separately from the H-alkyne [51, 52]. Additionally, because D-alkyne and H-alkyne are compact Raman tags with almost identical chemical structures, similar small biomolecules can be distinguished and observed simultaneously by labeling them with D-/H-alkyne. For example, Figure 8.6 shows two-color Raman imaging in living

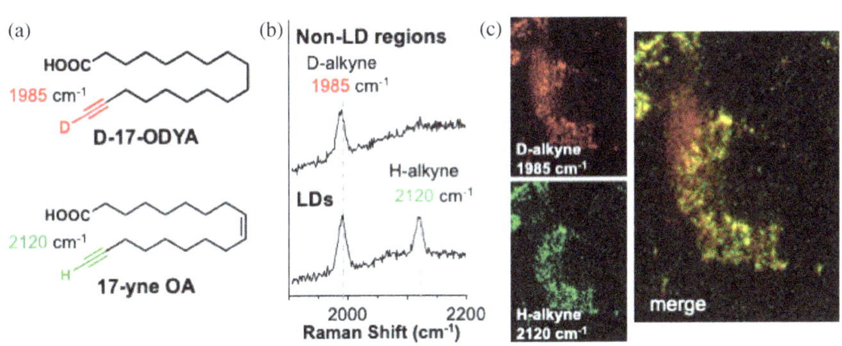

Figure 8.6. Two-color Raman imaging in living HeLa cells co-treated with 400 μM D-17-ODYA and 100 μM 17-yne OA for 6 h. (a) Structure of D-17-ODYA and 17-yne OA. (b) Raman spectra of non-LD regions and LDs. (c) Raman image of D-alkyne shown as red, H-alkyne shown as green, and their merged image. Adapted from Ref. [51] with permission.

HeLa cells co-treated with structurally similar D-alkyne-tagged C18 saturated fatty acids (D-17-ODYA) and H-alkyne-tagged unsaturated C18 unsaturated fatty acids (17-yne OA) (Figure 8.6(a)). Saturated fatty acids exhibit different intracellular metabolism/distributions compared to unsaturated fatty acids, even with chains of the same carbon number. D-17-ODYA with a Raman signal at 1985 cm^{-1} was localized to LDs and diffused through the cytoplasm, whereas 17-yne OA with a Raman signal at 2120 cm^{-1} was localized only at LDs (Figure 8.6(b, c)) [51].

Acidic compounds exist within the cell in an equilibrium mixture of molecular and ionic forms. Because Raman scattering provides structural information about molecules, two forms of acidic compounds can be distinguished via Raman microscopy. The first example of the structure-based imaging of a Raman-tagged compound in live cells was demonstrated with spontaneous Raman microscopy by Sodeoka and co-workers in 2014 [53]. FCCP is an uncoupler of mitochondrial oxidative phosphorylation, which was first reported by Heytler *et al.* [54]. It is a weak, lipid-soluble acid that can pass through the mitochondrial inner membrane in both its protonated molecular form and deprotonated ionic form, thereby acting as a proton ionophore. Because the pKa constant for FCCP is 6.0, the Raman spectra of deprotonated and protonated FCCP were measured using buffer solutions at pH 7.4 and 4.6 (Figure 8.7(a)). Significant differences in the Raman shifts of the nitrile peaks between the two states were observed at 2176 and 2195 cm^{-1} (deprotonated FCCP) and 2226 cm^{-1} (protonated FCCP).

Figure 8.7(b) shows Raman images of the FCCP-treated HeLa cells. The distribution of nitrile signals derived from deprotonated FCCP at 2176 and

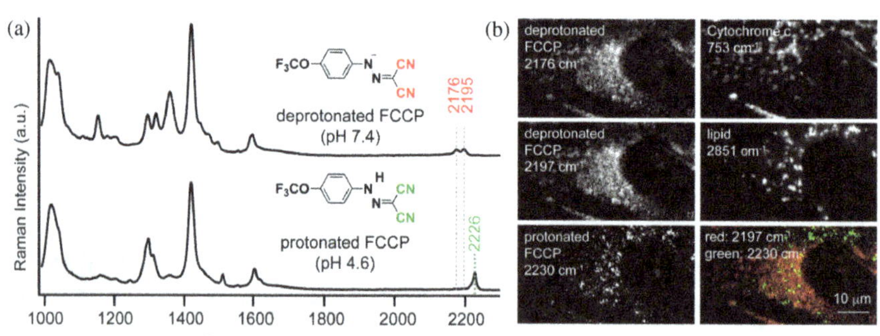

Figure 8.7. Structure-based imaging of protonated and deprotonated FCCP. (a) Raman spectra of protonated and deprotonated FCCP. (b) Raman imaging of protonated and deprotonated forms of FCCP. Adapted from Ref. [53] with permission.

2197 cm^{-1} was diffused throughout the cytoplasm, while the nitrile signal derived from protonated FCCP at 2230 cm^{-1} was co-localized with lipids (2851 cm^{-1}). Because FCCP is a weak acid, it is plausible that the deprotonated form is dominant in the cytoplasm. In contrast, deprotonated ionic FCCP tends to stay away from the hydrophobic environment, thereby protonated molecular FCCP is dominant in the LD.

In addition to Raman-tag imaging of bioactive molecules, several useful Raman sensors have been reported using spontaneous and SRS microscopy in recent years [55–59]. Notably, Raman-tag imaging itself reveals the localization of "labeled (tagged) molecules." In contrast, the Raman-tag sensor reveals the localization of "non-labeled endogenous molecules" using Raman probes (Raman-tagged molecules). Therefore, in the case of Raman sensors, the molecular size is not critical, and several Raman probes are based on dye structures. One might think that a fluorescent probe would be superior in terms of sensitivity if Raman probes were not very small. However, Raman probes have a superior wavelength resolution and are expected to provide more multicolor imaging than fluorescent dyes. As this chapter focuses on Raman-tag imaging, only representative Raman sensors are shown with their structures and detection mechanisms (Figure 8.8). The design of these sensors provides significant insights into Raman-tag imaging.

In 2016, Heo and co-workers developed a sensor H-Azo-3CN for biologically important hypochlorite anions (ClO^-), a reactive oxygen species [60]. The oxidation of hydrazobenzene to azobenzene by hypochlorite resulted in a shift of its electronic transition to longer wavelengths (H-Azo-3CN: 385 nm, Azo-3CN: 567 nm). This shift change allows the design of activatable Raman sensors. Under 532 nm laser excitation, the nitrile signal of non-resonant H-Azo-3CN was weak, whereas the resonant Azo-3CN gave a strong nitrile signal.

Raman sensor **1** for mitochondrial hydrogen sulfide (H_2S), with phenylazide as the reaction site and triphenylphosphine for mitochondrial targeting, was developed by Min and co-workers in 2018 [61]. When H_2S reduces phenylazide to phenylamine, the Raman signal peak of the conjugated diyne shifts from 2223 cm^{-1} to 2214 cm^{-1}. The ratio of each Raman signal peak intensity (2214 cm^{-1}/2223 cm^{-1}) provides a quantitative analysis of intracellular H_2S. H_2S is a gaseous signaling molecule that regulates many physiological effects; however, aberrant levels of H_2S cause many diseases, including Alzheimer's disease [62]

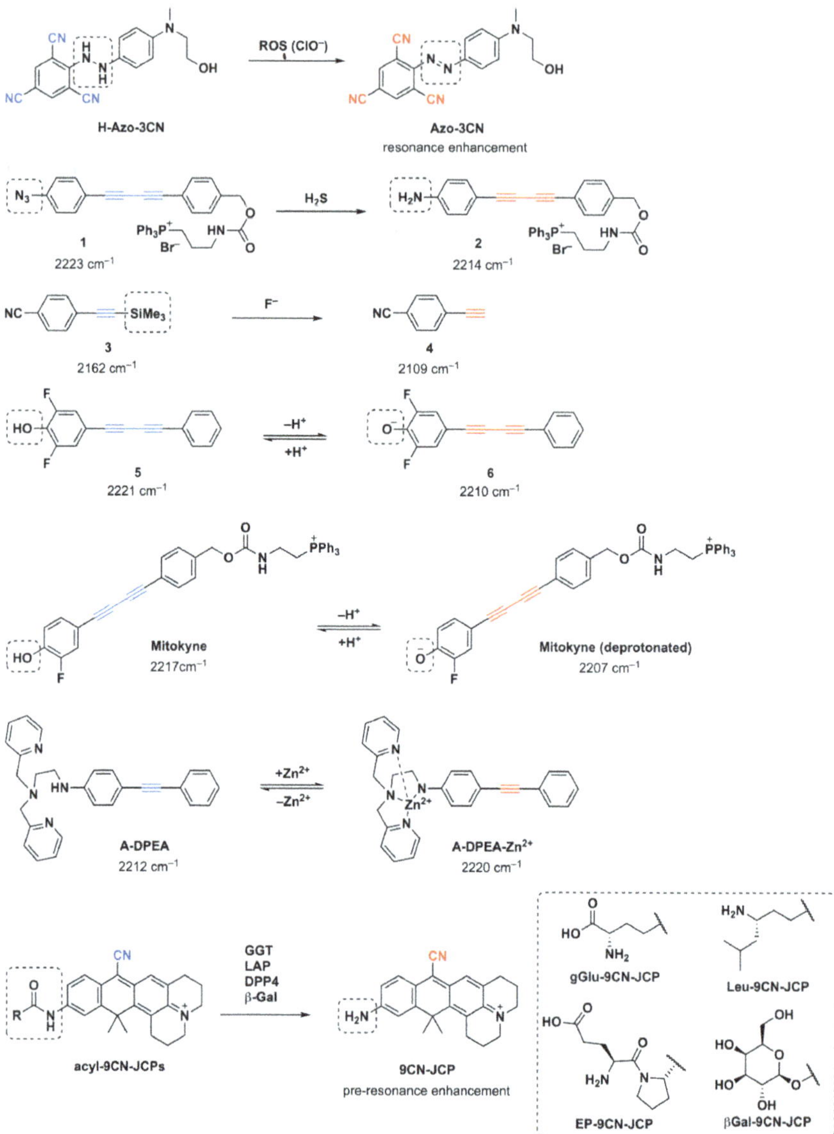

Figure 8.8. Structures of representative Raman sensors.

and liver cirrhosis [63]. Therefore, the selective sensor for H_2S in living cells is very important.

Tipping and co-workers reported a fluoride ion sensor **3** based on the desilylation of silylalkynes [64]. The Raman shift of the alkyne changes by 53 cm^{-1} with or without silyl groups (2162 and 2109 cm^{-1}). Sensor **3** has a nitrile group as the second Raman tag, which was used for ratiometric analysis. Using sensor **3**, fluoride concentrations as low as 125 μM were ratiometrically detected using a simple paper-based assay. The reported fluorescent dye-based fluoride sensors are used in organic solvents, whereas Raman sensor **3** functions in aqueous solvents, showing promising properties for groundwater analysis.

In 2020, alkyne-conjugated phenols **5** were developed by Wilson and co-workers [65]. Electron delocalization, associated with the presence or absence of phenolic protons, influences the alkyne stretching frequency. Because the pKa value of phenol **5** is close to the physiological pH range, it acts as an intracellular pH sensor. An alkyne signal of phenol **5** in buffer (pH 5.5) was observed at 2221 cm^{-1}, while that of phenoxide **6** in buffer at pH 7.5 was 2210 cm^{-1}. Using aniline, imidazole, pyridine, and phenol derivatives, they reported the development of a series of low-molecular-weight diyne compounds that exhibited pH sensitivity in different regions (pH range 2–10). Furthermore, they also found that the pKa value of alkyne-conjugated phenols could be finetuned by the fluorination of phenol. In 2021, Wilson and co-workers developed a Raman sensor for mitochondrial pH (mitokyne) by introducing triphenylphosphine to alkyne-conjugated phenols for mitochondria targeting [66]. The best Raman shifts of mitokynes for ratiometric imaging were determined to be 2230 cm^{-1} for mitokyne and 2216 cm^{-1} for ionized mitokyne from wavelength scans of mitokyne-treated HeLa cells at pH 6.0 and 8.5. The 2230 cm^{-1}/2216 cm^{-1} intensity ratio helps visualize mitochondrial pH changes.

Takemura and co-workers monitored zinc ion-ligand complexation using alkynylated (dipycolylamino)ethyl aniline (A-DPEA) as a Raman sensor [67]. A-DPEA exhibits a typical Raman signal from the alkyne at 2212 cm^{-1}. The addition of Zn^{2+} ions causes the complexation of A-DPEA, which decreases the π-electron density of the alkyne, and the Raman band shifts to 2220 cm^{-1}. A-DPEA was smoothly incorporated into the cells. A band shift from 2212 to 2220 cm^{-1} occurred with the administration of Zn^{2+} to the cells.

Kamiya and co-workers developed activatable Raman probes that show enhancement in the Raman signal via electronic pre-resonance (EPR) upon reaction with enzymes [68]. A series of xanthene derivatives with a nitrile group at position 9 was synthesized, as they showed a single, sharp, and strong Raman peak in the silent region under EPR conditions. Therefore, 9CN-JCP was identified as a scaffold dye. The blueshift absorption of Ac-9CN-JCP lies within the electronic non-resonant region (506 nm in phosphate-buffered saline), while that of 9CN-JCP lies within the EPR region (630 nm in phosphate-buffered saline) with the pump beam at 843 nm in the SRS imaging system. This difference in the absorption wavelengths causes a significant change in the Raman signal. Various probes were synthesized in which the substrate of the enzyme was linked to nitrogen instead of the acetyl group of Ac-9CN-JCP by acylation; these include gGlu-9CN-JCP, Leu-9CN-JCP, EP-9CN-JCP, and βGal-9CN-JCP. These probes released 9CN-JCP upon treatment with the corresponding enzyme for Raman detection. The four probes were analyzed simultaneously by combining isotopically labeled 9CN-JCP with ^{13}C and ^{15}N. Such multiple detections demonstrate the advantage of high-wavelength-resolution Raman microscopy and can be applied to the characterization of diseases and cells.

The enhancement of Raman intensities can be derived not only from the intracellular chemical/enzymatic environment but also from light manipulation. In 2021, Wei's group designed and developed photoactivatable Raman probes based on photocaged alkynes [69] and cyclopropenones, which are converted into alkynes by irradiation with UV light [70]. They synthesized three types of cyclopropenones: Me-Mito-^{13}C for mitochondria, Me-Lyso for endoplasmic reticulum, and Cyclo-LD for LDs (Fig 9a). After 405 nm illumination, these probes provided multiplexed live-cell imaging and tracking of the migration and interactions of subcellular organelles.

Raman peaks of photochromic molecules, such as diarylethene (DTE), can be reversibly changed by light manipulation [71, 72]. In 2021, Ji and co-workers developed a mitochondrial photoswitchable vibrational probe by introducing the alkyne and the mitochondria-targeting functional group into the photochromic DTE (DTE-Ph-Mito, Figure 8.9) [72]. UV irradiation induces photoisomerization of DTE from the open-ring state to the closed-ring state, while visible light irradiation induces reverse isomerization. In addition, during the ring closing of the DTE probes, the electronic absorption spectra show a redshift. Therefore, upon UV irradiation, the alkyne Raman signal of DTE-Ph-Mito was shifted from 2214 cm^{-1} to 2194 cm^{-1} and enhanced through the EPR effect in SRS imaging. Such properties are very useful for numerous biological investigations, such as tracking protein/organelle dynamics and monitoring intracellular environments.

Highly sensitive detection of biological molecules and drugs in cells has also been achieved using metal nanoparticles. Metal nanoparticles amplify the Raman scattering signals from molecules near the metal surface.

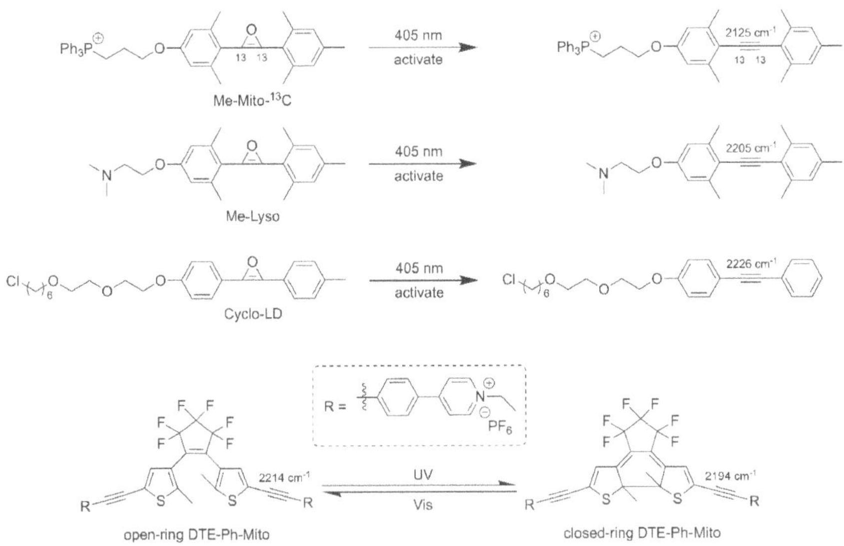

Figure 8.9. Structures of photoactivatable/photoswitchable Raman probes.

This phenomenon is known as surface-enhanced Raman scattering (SERS), which enables sensitive Raman measurements of biomolecules, including proteins, DNA, RNA, amino acids, and lipids [73]. When cells are cultured in a medium containing metal nanoparticles, they can take up the metal nanoparticles. This biological process is known as endocytosis and is often used to deliver metal nanoparticles into cells. Eventually, the nanoparticles accumulate in endosomes and lysosomes via the intracellular transport function, and they act as SERS probes that provide information on intracellular molecules in the vicinity of the metal surface [74]. Furthermore, SERS in cells with gold nanoparticles (AuNPs) is helpful for the detection of drugs introduced into cells from outside. In an early study, SERS detection of anti-cancer and anti-leukemic drugs in cells revealed the details of drug distribution and metabolism within the cell [75, 76]. Although SERS provides a strong Raman signal, it also has a strong background signal from endogenous molecules, as seen in the previous section, and often interferes with the specific detection of target drug molecules. In 2020, Fujita and co-workers developed a SERS measurement method for drug imaging with high molecular discrimination using an alkyne tag [77]. Similar to Raman spectroscopy with alkynes, the SERS signal of alkynes also exhibits a characteristic peak in the silent region (1800–2600 cm^{-1}), where biomolecules hardly show SERS signals. Therefore, molecules labeled with alkyne tags can be selectively detected without overlapping with endogenous biomolecules. In addition, the high affinity of alkynes for metal nanoparticles enhances the detection sensitivity of SERS for both electromagnetic and chemical enhancements. As a demonstration experiment, an alkyne tag was introduced into an inhibitor of cathepsin B, a drug target for tumor metastasis, and localized to lysosomes. AuNPs were used as probes accumulated by endocytosis into lysosomes inside macrophages. Alkyne-labeled inhibitors were added to the cell culture medium. Slit-scanning Raman microscopy of drug-treated cells revealed an increase in the bright spot originating from the alkyne SERS peak at 1980 cm^{-1} after drug administration (Figure 8.10(a)). The number of alkyne SERS signals was

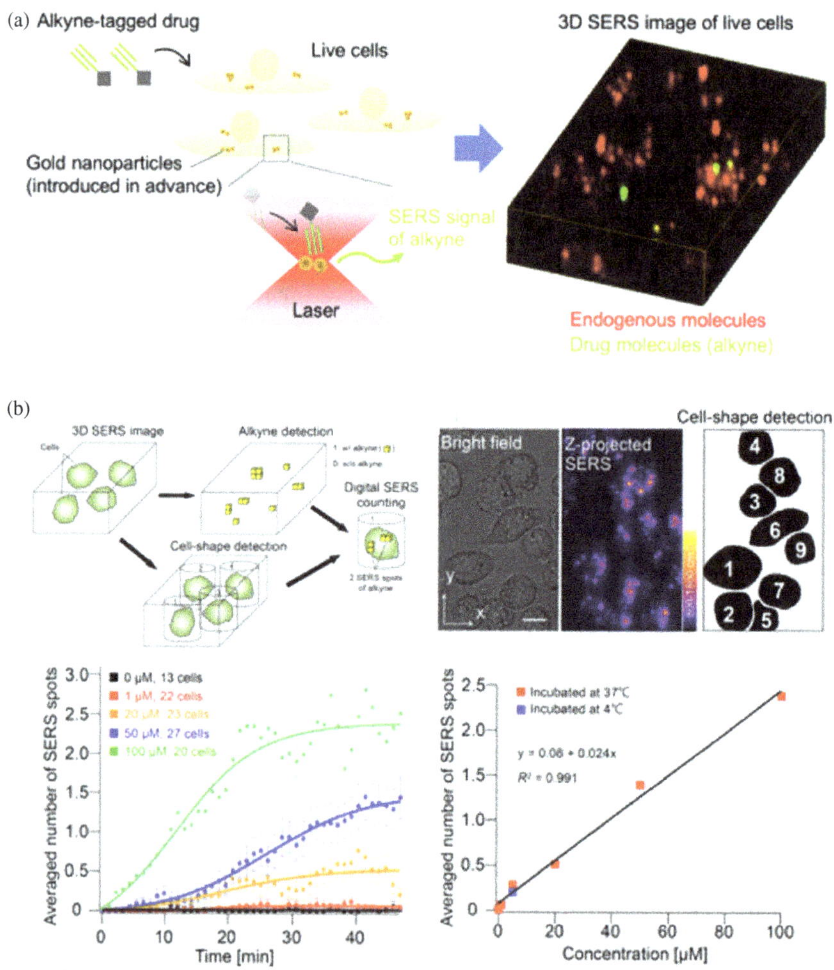

Figure 8.10. Monitoring cellular uptake of small molecule drugs by alkyne-tagged SERS imaging. (A) Schematic of the SERS detection of alkyne-labeled small molecule drugs in live cells. (B) Quantitative detection of SERS spots showing a peak of alkyne at ~1980 cm^{-1}. Adapted from Ref. [77] with permission.

counted to quantitatively evaluate the rate of inhibitor uptake (Figure 8.10(b)). SERS microscopy with alkyne tag offers a new method for analyzing the kinetics of drug uptake in living cells.

8.3 Raman Screening of Bioactive Small Molecules

Many drugs bind to specific cellular proteins to regulate their biological functions. Identification of the binding position of a drug in a protein will directly lead to the elucidation of the molecular mechanism of the drug. In the case of a drug that can form a covalent bond with a target protein [78], the binding site can be identified to the level of the amino acid side chain using a mass spectrometer based on the mass shift associated with the binding of the drug [3]. However, since the peptide-fragmented solution during the first stage of mass spectrometry is extremely complicated, it is not easy to search for a drug-binding peptide using only mass information.

In 2016, Fujita and co-workers developed a screening method using Raman spectroscopy to search for peptide fragments to which a drug has bound from a complex mixture and applied it to identify the drug binding site [16]. An alkyne was used as a label to specifically detect the Raman signals derived from a drug in a complex mixture of biomolecules. Because it has an extremely small molecular size, the possibility of inhibiting the binding between a drug and a protein by modification is significantly reduced. SERS with silver nanoparticles was used to increase the sensitivity of alkyne-Raman detection (Figure 8.11). The terminal alkyne was adsorbed on the surface of the transition metal. In addition to the chemical amplification mechanism due to the interaction between the metal and the alkyne, the electric field enhancement effect can be obtained with high efficiency by the localization of the sample molecule near the surface; thus, the SERS detection sensitivity of the alkyne is extremely high. In addition, trifluoroacetic acid (TFA) was found to promote the uniform aggregate formation of silver nanoparticles and alkyne-labeled molecules. Using TFA, aggregates exhibiting strong SERS signals can be uniformly formed on the surface of the substrate so that both the stability and sensitivity of alkyne SERS measurements can be improved. In fact, when measurements were taken using an alkyne-introduced peptide as a standard sample, a lower limit of detection of 100 fmol (3.3 nM upon conversion) was achieved (Figure 8.11(c)), with a dynamic range from 100 fmol to 100 pmol.

Drug-labeled proteins fragmented into peptides were fractionated by liquid chromatography and then sequentially subjected to mass spectrometry. In

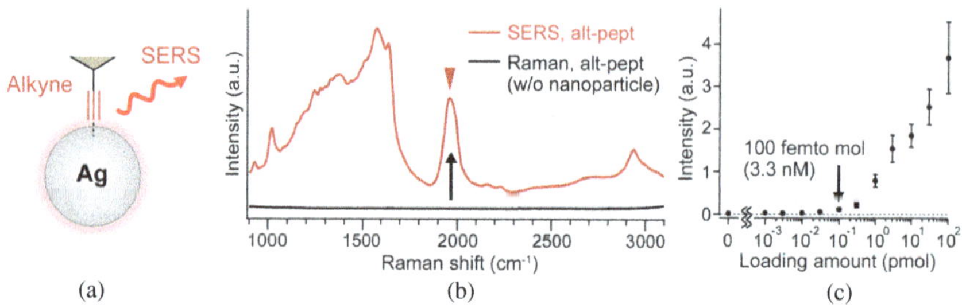

Figure 8.11. Alkyne SERS measurement with silver nanoparticles. (a) Schematics of alkyne SERS. (b) Comparison of Raman spectra of alkyne-labeled peptides with and without silver nanoparticles. When mixed with silver nanoparticles, a strong Raman peak of alkyne is observed at 1958 cm^{-1}. (c) Validation of detection sensitivity of alkyne SERS measurement. Vertical axis shows peak intensity at 1958 cm^{-1} and horizontal axis shows sample loading. Adapted from Ref. [80] with permission.

the method we developed, the sample, after fractionation, was sequentially dropped onto a multiwell plate. Alkyne SERS measurements were performed comprehensively on this multiwell plate to identify the peptide fragments to which the drug is bound (Figure 8.12). For the fraction narrowed down by alkyne SERS, intensive measurements were performed using a mass spectrometer to identify the binding site. Notably, this alkyne-SERS screening system was automated to measure multiple samples by synchronizing stage scanning and Raman measurements or using a multifocal Raman detection system designed for multiwell plates [79]. This is possible because the focal position suitable for SERS measurement can be fixed to the interface of the substrate without depending on the well, and SERS hot spots are uniformly formed on each well. This method was named Alkyne-Tag Raman Screening (ATRaS).

Based on the results of the studies described above, the binding position of Z-FG-AOMK, a covalent inhibitor of cathepsin B and a drug target for tumor metastasis, was investigated by ATRaS. Alt-AOMK, a drug containing an alkyne tag, was synthesized and acted on cathepsin B. Drug-bound cathepsin B was enzymatically fragmented and fractionated by liquid chromatography, and then the sample was dropped into a multiwell plate. Each well was mixed with AgNPs and TFA and screened for alkyne SERS. A heat map was created based on the Raman intensities of alkynes (Figure 8.13). The peptides contained in the alkyne-detected wells were subjected to mass spectrometry, and the peptide fragments modified with Alt-AOMK were observed. In addition, the binding residue of Alt-AOMK was identified as Cys29 of the peptide fragment (Figure 8.13(b)). Recently, this SERS screening system was combined with deep

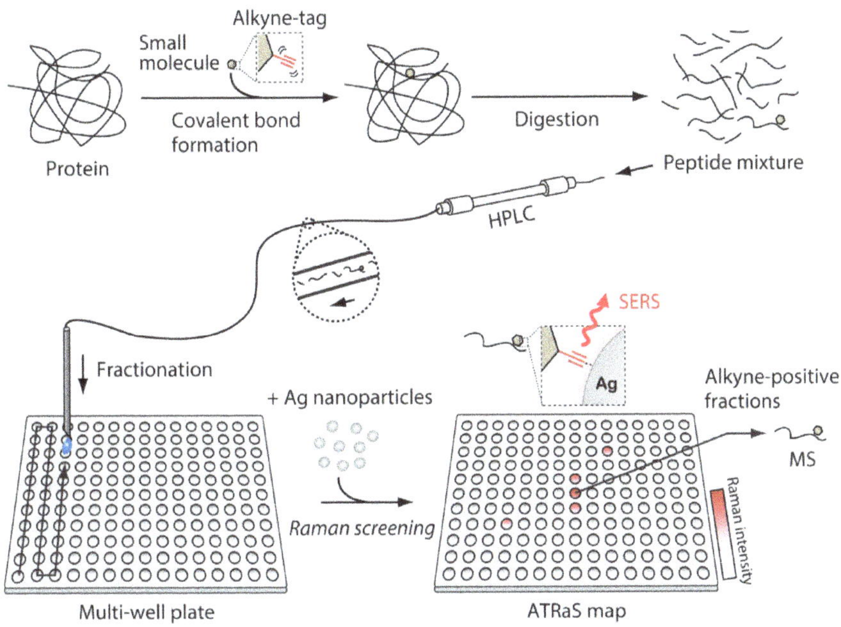

Figure 8.12. Schematic of the alkyne-tag Raman screening method. Alkyne-labeled small molecule-bound proteins are fragmented, fractionated by high-performance liquid chromatography, and arrayed in a multiwell plate. After mixing silver nanoparticles, each well is subjected to SERS measurement to search for fractions (containing peptides to which small molecules are bound) that yield an alkyne-derived Raman signal. Reproduced from Ref. [80] with permission.

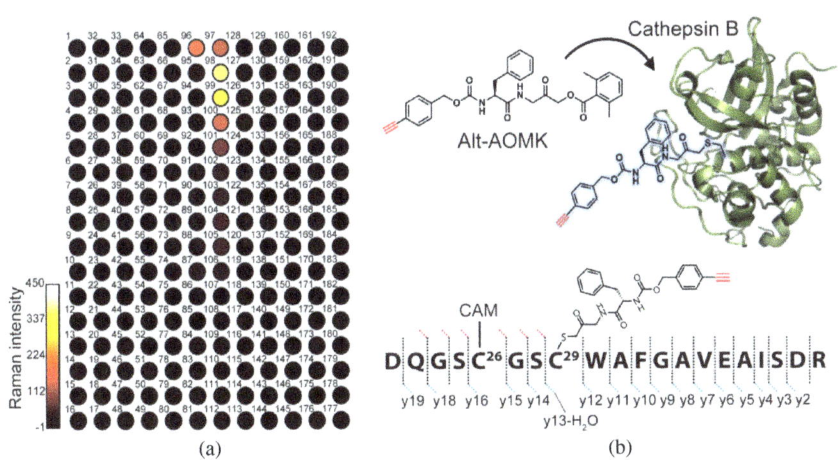

Figure 8.13. Binding site identification of cathepsin B to inhibitor (Alt-AOMK) by ATRaS. (a) Heat map of alkyne SERS per well. (b) Schematic and amino acid sequence of the binding site (C29) of Alt-AOMK identified via tandem mass spectrometry. Adapted from Ref. [80] with permission.

learning, which allows drug-modified peptide screening without an alkyne tag [80]. Various technological developments in Raman and SERS spectroscopy coupled with chromatographic techniques have allowed us to analyze complex mixtures with high sensitivity and molecular specificity.

8.4 Conclusions

In the 2000s, the selective detection of specific molecules was difficult in live cells using Raman microscopy. Researchers have attempted to develop technologically advanced laser sources, optical filters, and photodetectors. With the increased sensitivity resulting from these efforts and the advent of Raman tags, a wide variety of molecules has been visualized in the 2010s. Recent advances in Raman tag studies, including the development of Raman probes, have enabled the use of Raman-tagged molecules as tools in chemical biology and life sciences. In future, an increasing number of Raman probes based on Raman tags will be developed. In particular, simultaneous multimolecular detection and Raman screening methods will accelerate tailor-made medicine and drug development. Deuterium labeling will be increasingly necessary for the observation of various processes of endogenous molecules, such as absorption, distribution, metabolism, and excretion, each of which is expected to be observed both *in vitro* and *in vivo*. The development of deuteration chemical technologies is expected to accelerate the research advancements in this field. The key to success is the combination of fluorescent imaging and the accurate design of chemical modifications. Fluorescence and Raman imaging are complementary techniques, and their synergistic development will lead to the elucidation of biological phenomena. Chemical modifications of the nonlinear Raman-tag technique can address the issues associated with the low sensitivity of typical Raman imaging. Numerous avenues exist in which the Raman-tag technique can be explored and are expected to attract further attention from researchers in the coming decades.

References

1. Mullard, A. (2015) Cancer market hits $100 billion. Nat. Rev. Drug Discov. **14**, 373–373.
2. Brown, D. G., Wobst, H. J., Kapoor, A., Kenna, L. A. and Southall, N. (2022) Clinical development times for innovative drugs. Nat. Rev. Drug Discov. **21**, 793–794.

3. Meissner, F., Geddes-McAlister, J., Mann, M. and Bantscheff, M. (2022) The emerging role of mass spectrometry-based proteomics in drug discovery. Nat. Rev. Drug Discov. **21**, 637–654.
4. Pellecchia, M., Bertini, I., Cowburn, D., Dalvit, C., Giralt, E., Jahnke, W., James, T. L., Homans, S. W., Kessler, H., Luchinat, C., *et al.* (2008) Perspectives on NMR in drug discovery: a technique comes of age. Nat. Rev. Drug Discov. **7**, 738–745.
5. Blundell, T. L., Jhoti, H. and Abell, C. (2002) High-throughput crystallography for lead discovery in drug design. Nat. Rev. Drug Discov. **1**, 45–54.
6. Martinez, N. J., Titus, S. A., Wagner, A. K. and Simeonov, A. (2015) High-throughput fluorescence imaging approaches for drug discovery using in vitro and in vivo three-dimensional models. Expert Opin. Drug Discov. **10**, 1347–1361.
7. Masada, S., Tsuji, G., Arai, R., Uchiyama, N., Demizu, Y., Tsutsumi, T., Abe, Y., Akiyama, H., Hakamatsuka, T., Izutsu, K.-I., *et al.* (2019) Rapid and efficient high-performance liquid chromatography analysis of N-nitrosodimethylamine impurity in valsartan drug substance and its products. Sci. Rep. **9**, 1–6.
8. Benz, M., Asperger, A., Hamester, M., Welle, A., Heissler, S. and Levkin, P. A. (2020) A combined high-throughput and high-content platform for unified on-chip synthesis, characterization and biological screening. Nat. Commun. **11**, 5391.
9. Ruggeri, F. S., Habchi, J., Chia, S., Horne, R. I., Vendruscolo, M. and Knowles, T. P. J. (2021) Infrared nanospectroscopy reveals the molecular interaction fingerprint of an aggregation inhibitor with single Aβ42 oligomers. Nat. Commun. **12**, 688.
10. Paudel, A., Raijada, D. and Rantanen, J. (2015) Raman spectroscopy in pharmaceutical product design. Adv. Drug Deliv. Rev. **89**, 3–20.
11. Ling, J., Weitman, S. D., Miller, M. A., Moore, R. V. and Bovik, A. C. (2002) Direct Raman imaging techniques for study of the subcellular distribution of a drug. Appl. Opt. **41**, 6006–6017.
12. Mak, P. J., Denisov, I. G., Grinkova, Y. V., Sligar, S. G. and Kincaid, J. R. (2011) Defining CYP3A4 structural responses to substrate binding. Raman spectroscopic studies of a nanodisc-incorporated mammalian cytochrome P450. J. Am. Chem. Soc. **133**, 1357–1366.
13. Feizpour, A., Marstrand, T., Bastholm, L., Eirefelt, S. and Evans, C. L. (2021) Label-free quantification of pharmacokinetics in skin with stimulated Raman scattering microscopy and deep learning. J. Invest. Dermatol. **141**, 395–403.
14. Roy, S., Chamberlin, B. and Matzger, A. J. (2013) Polymorph discrimination using low wavenumber Raman spectroscopy. Org. Process Res. Dev. **17**, 976–980.
15. Ando, J., Palonpon, A. F., Sodeoka, M. and Fujita, K. (2016) High-speed Raman imaging of cellular processes. Curr. Opin. Chem. Biol. **33**, 16–24.
16. Ando, J., Asanuma, M., Dodo, K., Yamakoshi, H., Kawata, S., Fujita, K. and Sodeoka, M. (2016) Alkyne-tag SERS screening and identification of small-molecule-binding sites in protein. J. Am. Chem. Soc. **138**, 13901–13910.

17. Sijtsema, N. M., Wouters, S. D., De Grauw, C. J., Otto, C. and Greve, J. (1998) Confocal direct imaging Raman microscope: design and applications in biology. Appl. Spectrosc. **52**, 348–355.
18. Puppels, G. J., de Mul, F. F. M., Otto, C., Greve, J., Robert-Nicoud, M., Arndt-Jovin, D. J. and Jovin, T. M. (1990) Studying single living cells and chromosomes by confocal Raman microspectroscopy. Nature **347**, 301–303.
19. Hamada, K., Fujita, K., Smith, N. I., Kobayashi, M., Inouye, Y. and Kawata, S. (2008) Raman microscopy for dynamic molecular imaging of living cells. J. Biomed. Opt. **13**, 044027.
20. Palonpon, A. F., Ando, J., Yamakoshi, H., Dodo, K., Sodeoka, M., Kawata, S. and Fujita, K. (2013) Raman and SERS microscopy for molecular imaging of live cells. Nat. Protoc. **8**, 677–692.
21. Okuno, M. and Hamaguchi, H.-O. (2010) Multifocus confocal Raman microspectroscopy for fast multimode vibrational imaging of living cells. Opt. Lett. **35**, 4096–4098.
22. Samuel, A. Z., Yabumoto, S., Kawamura, K. and Iwata, K. (2015) Rapid microstructure characterization of polymer thin films with 2D-array multifocus Raman microspectroscopy. Analyst **140**, 1847–1851.
23. Harada, Y., Dai, P., Yamaoka, Y., Ogawa, M., Tanaka, H., Nosaka, K., Akaji, K. and Takamatsu, T. (2009) Intracellular dynamics of topoisomerase I inhibitor, CPT-11, by slit-scanning confocal Raman microscopy. Histochem. Cell Biol. **132**, 39–46.
24. Li, M., Liao, H.-X., Bando, K., Nawa, Y., Fujita, S. and Fujita, K. (2022) Label-free monitoring of drug-induced cytotoxicity and its molecular fingerprint by live-cell Raman and autofluorescence imaging. Anal. Chem. **94**, 10019–10026.
25. Okada, M., Smith, N. I., Palonpon, A. F., Endo, H., Kawata, S., Sodeoka, M. and Fujita, K. (2012) Label-free Raman observation of cytochrome c dynamics during apoptosis. Proc. Natl. Acad. Sci. **109**, 28–32.
26. Yamakoshi, H., Dodo, K., Okada, M., Ando, J., Palonpon, A., Fujita, K., Kawata, S. and Sodeoka, M. (2011) Imaging of EdU, an alkyne-tagged cell proliferation probe, by Raman microscopy. J. Am. Chem. Soc. **133**, 6102–6105.
27. Salic, A. and Mitchison, T. J. (2008) A chemical method for fast and sensitive detection of DNA synthesis in vivo. Proc. Natl. Acad. Sci. **105**, 2415–2420.
28. Kolb, H. C., Finn, M. G. and Sharpless, K. B. (2001) Click chemistry: Diverse chemical function from a few good reactions. Angew. Chem. Int. Ed. **40**, 2004–2021.
29. Tornøe, C. W., Christensen, C. and Meldal, M. (2002) Peptidotriazoles on solid phase: [1,2,3]-triazoles by regiospecific copper(i)-catalyzed 1,3-dipolar cycloadditions of terminal alkynes to azides. J. Org. Chem. **67**, 3057–3064.
30. Haldón, E., Nicasio, M. C. and Pérez, P. J. (2015) Copper-catalysed azide-alkyne cycloadditions (CuAAC): an update. Org. Biomol. Chem. **13**, 9528–9550.

31. Castelvecchi, D. and Ledford, H. (2022) Chemists who invented revolutionary "click" reactions win Nobel. Nature **610**, 242–243.
32. Beatty, K. E., Liu, J. C., Xie, F., Dieterich, D. C., Schuman, E. M., Wang, Q. and Tirrell, D. A. (2006) Fluorescence visualization of newly synthesized proteins in mammalian cells. Angew. Chem. Int. Ed. **45**, 7364–7367.
33. Hsu, T.-L., Hanson, S. R., Kishikawa, K., Wang, S.-K., Sawa, M. and Wong, C.-H. (2007) Alkynyl sugar analogs for the labeling and visualization of glycoconjugates in cells. Proc. Natl. Acad. Sci. **104**, 2614–2619.
34. Mu, Z. M., Le, X. F., Vallian, S., Glassman, A. B. and Chang, K. S. (1997) Stable overexpression of PML alters regulation of cell cycle progression in HeLa cells. Carcinogenesis **18**, 2063–2069.
35. Yamakoshi, H., Dodo, K., Palonpon, A., Ando, J., Fujita, K., Kawata, S. and Sodeoka, M. (2012) Alkyne-tag Raman imaging for visualization of mobile small molecules in live cells. J. Am. Chem. Soc. **134**, 20681–20689.
36. Telford, J. E., Kilbride, S. M. and Davey, G. P. (2010) Decylubiquinone increases mitochondrial function in synaptosomes. J. Biol. Chem. **285**, 8639–8645.
37. Lenaz, G. (1998) Quinone specificity of complex I. Biochim. Biophys. Acta Bioenerg. **1364**, 207–221.
38. Ross, M. F., Prime, T. A., Abakumova, I., James, A. M., Porteous, C. M., Smith, R. A. J. and Murphy, M. P. (2008) Rapid and extensive uptake and activation of hydrophobic triphenylphosphonium cations within cells. Biochem. J. **411**, 633–645.
39. Saito, Y., Fukuhara, A., Nishio, K., Hayakawa, M., Ogawa, Y., Sakamoto, H., Fujii, K., Yoshida, Y. and Niki, E. (2009) Characterization of cellular uptake and distribution of coenzyme Q10 and vitamin E in PC12 cells. J. Nutr. Biochem. **20**, 350–357.
40. Weeks, T., Schie, I., den Hartigh, L. J., Rutledge, J. C. and Huser, T. (2011) Lipid-cell interactions in human monocytes investigated by doubly-resonant coherent anti-Stokes Raman scattering microscopy. J. Biomed. Opt. **16**, 021117.
41. Egoshi, S., Dodo, K. and Sodeoka, M. (2022) Deuterium Raman imaging for lipid analysis. Curr. Opin. Chem. Biol. **70**, 102181.
42. Fomich, M. A., Bekish, A. V., Vidovic, D., Lamberson, C. R., Lysenko, I. L., Lawrence, P., Brenna, J. T., Sharko, O. L., Shmanai, V. V. and Shchepinov, M. S. (2016) Full library of (bis-allyl)-deuterated arachidonic acids: Synthesis and analytical verification. ChemistrySelect **1**, 4758–4764.
43. Navratil, A. R., Shchepinov, M. S. and Dennis, E. A. (2018) Lipidomics reveals dramatic physiological kinetic isotope effects during the enzymatic oxygenation of polyunsaturated fatty acids ex vivo. J. Am. Chem. Soc. **140**, 235–243.
44. Dodo, K., Sato, A., Tamura, Y., Egoshi, S., Fujiwara, K., Oonuma, K., Nakao, S., Terayama, N. and Sodeoka, M. (2021) Synthesis of deuterated γ-linolenic acid and application for biological studies: metabolic tuning and Raman imaging. Chem. Commun. **57**, 2180–2183.

45. Chen, Z., Paley, D. W., Wei, L., Weisman, A. L., Friesner, R. A., Nuckolls, C. and Min, W. (2014) Multicolor live-cell chemical imaging by isotopically edited alkyne vibrational palette. J. Am. Chem. Soc. **136**, 8027–8033.
46. Wei, L., Chen, Z., Shi, L., Long, R., Anzalone, A. V., Zhang, L., Hu, F., Yuste, R., Cornish, V. W. and Min, W. (2017) Super-multiplex vibrational imaging. Nature **544**, 465–470.
47. Woodbury, E. J. and Ng, W. K. (1962) Ruby laser operation in the near IR. Proc. Inst. Electr. Eng. **50**, 2367.
48. Bloembergen, N. (1967) The stimulated Raman effect. Am. J. Phys. **35**, 989–1023.
49. Freudiger, C. W., Min, W., Saar, B. G., Lu, S., Holtom, G. R., He, C., Tsai, J. C., Kang, J. X. and Xie, X. S. (2008) Label-free biomedical imaging with high sensitivity by stimulated Raman scattering microscopy. Science **322**, 1857–1861.
50. Schrötter, H. W. and Hoffmann, E. G. (1964) Raman- und Infrarot-Spektren einiger definiert an der Doppelbindung deuterierter Olefine. Justus Liebigs Ann. Chem. Ltd **672**, 44–54.
51. Egoshi, S., Dodo, K., Ohgane, K. and Sodeoka, M. (2021) Deuteration of terminal alkynes realizes simultaneous live cell Raman imaging of similar alkyne-tagged biomolecules. Org. Biomol. Chem. **19**, 8232–8236.
52. Bi, X., Miao, K. and Wei, L. (2022) Alkyne-tagged Raman probes for local environmental sensing by hydrogen-deuterium exchange. J. Am. Chem. Soc. **144**, 8504–8514.
53. Yamakoshi, H., Palonpon, A. F., Dodo, K., Ando, J., Kawata, S., Fujita, K. and Sodeoka, M. (2014) Simultaneous imaging of protonated and deprotonated carbonylcyanide p-trifluoromethoxyphenylhydrazone in live cells by Raman microscopy. Chem. Commun. **50**, 1341–1343.
54. Heytler, P. G. and Prichard, W. W. (1962) A new class of uncoupling agents — carbonyl cyanide phenylhydrazones. Biochem. Biophys. Res. Commun. **7**, 272–275.
55. Qian, N. and Min, W. (2022) Super-multiplexed vibrational probes: Being colorful makes a difference. Curr. Opin. Chem. Biol. **67**, 102115.
56. Bakthavatsalam, S., Dodo, K. and Sodeoka, M. (2021) A decade of alkyne-tag Raman imaging (ATRI): applications in biological systems. RSC Chem. Biol. **2**, 1415–1429.
57. Qiu, C., Cheng, Z., Lv, C., Wang, R. and Yu, F. (2021) Development of bioorthogonal SERS imaging probe in biological and biomedical applications. Chin. Chem. Lett. **32**, 2369–2379.
58. Xu, J., Yu, T., Zois, C. E., Cheng, J.-X., Tang, Y., Harris, A. L. and Huang, W. E. (2021) Unveiling cancer metabolism through spontaneous and coherent Raman spectroscopy and stable isotope probing. Cancers **13**, 1718.
59. Adamczyk, A., Matuszyk, E., Radwan, B., Rocchetti, S., Chlopicki, S. and Baranska, M. (2021) Toward Raman subcellular imaging of endothelial dysfunction. J. Med. Chem. **64**, 4396–4409.

60. Heo, J., Lim, C.-K., Baev, A., Kuzmin, A. N., Park, S. Y., Prasad, P. N. and Kim, S. (2016) Chromogenesis-based resonance Raman molecular sensor for reactive oxygen species. Dyes Pigm. **130**, 162–167.
61. Zeng, C., Hu, F., Long, R. and Min, W. (2018) A ratiometric Raman probe for live-cell imaging of hydrogen sulfide in mitochondria by stimulated Raman scattering. Analyst **143**, 4844–4848.
62. Eto, K., Asada, T., Arima, K., Makifuchi, T. and Kimura, H. (2002) Brain hydrogen sulfide is severely decreased in Alzheimer's disease. Biochem. Biophys. Res. Commun. **293**, 1485–1488.
63. Fiorucci, S., Antonelli, E., Mencarelli, A., Orlandi, S., Renga, B., Rizzo, G., Distrutti, E., Shah, V. and Morelli, A. (2005) The third gas: H2S regulates perfusion pressure in both the isolated and perfused normal rat liver and in cirrhosis. Hepatology **42**, 539–548.
64. Tipping, W. J., Wilson, L. T., Blaseio, S. K., Tomkinson, N. C. O., Faulds, K. and Graham, D. (2020) Ratiometric sensing of fluoride ions using Raman spectroscopy. Chem. Commun. **56**, 14463–14466.
65. Wilson, L. T., Tipping, W. J., Jamieson, L. E., Wetherill, C., Henley, Z., Faulds, K., Graham, D., Mackay, S. P. and Tomkinson, N. C. O. (2020) A new class of ratiometric small molecule intracellular pH sensors for Raman microscopy. Analyst **145**, 5289–5298.
66. Wilson, L. T., Tipping, W. J., Wetherill, C., Henley, Z., Faulds, K., Graham, D., Mackay, S. P. and Tomkinson, N. C. O. (2021) Mitokyne: A ratiometric Raman probe for mitochondrial pH. Anal. Chem. **93**, 12786–12792.
67. Takemura, S., Watanabe, H., Nishihara, T., Okamoto, A. and Tanabe, K. (2020) Monitoring intracellular metal ion complexation with an acetylene-tagged ligand by Raman spectroscopy. RSC Adv. **10**, 36119–36123.
68. Fujioka, H., Shou, J., Kojima, R., Urano, Y., Ozeki, Y. and Kamiya, M. (2020) Multicolor activatable Raman probes for simultaneous detection of plural enzyme activities. J. Am. Chem. Soc. **142**, 20701–20707.
69. Du, J. and Wei, L. (2022) Multicolor photoactivatable Raman probes for subcellular imaging and tracking by cyclopropenone caging. J. Am. Chem. Soc. **144**, 777–786.
70. Poloukhtine, A. and Popik, V. V. (2003) Highly efficient photochemical generation of a triple bond: synthesis, properties, and photodecarbonylation of cyclopropenones. J. Org. Chem. **68**, 7833–7840.
71. Shou, J. and Ozeki, Y. (2021) Photoswitchable stimulated Raman scattering spectroscopy and microscopy. Opt. Lett. **46**, 2176–2179.
72. Ao, J., Fang, X., Miao, X., Ling, J., Kang, H., Park, S., Wu, C. and Ji, M. (2021) Switchable stimulated Raman scattering microscopy with photochromic vibrational probes. Nat. Commun. **12**, 3089.
73. Ando, J., Yano, T.-A., Fujita, K. and Kawata, S. (2013) Metal nanoparticles for nano-imaging and nano-analysis. Phys. Chem. Chem. Phys. **15**, 13713–13722.

74. Ando, J., Fujita, K., Smith, N. I. and Kawata, S. (2011) Dynamic SERS imaging of cellular transport pathways with endocytosed gold nanoparticles. Nano Lett. **11**, 5344–5348.
75. Chourpa, I., Morjani, H., Riou, J. F. and Manfait, M. (1996) Intracellular molecular interactions of antitumor drug amsacrine (m-AMSA) as revealed by surface-enhanced Raman spectroscopy. FEBS Lett. **397**, 61–64.
76. Nabiev, I. R., Morjani, H. and Manfait, M. (1991) Selective analysis of antitumor drug interaction with living cancer cells as probed by surface-enhanced Raman spectroscopy. Eur. Biophys. J. **19**, 311–316.
77. Koike, K., Bando, K., Ando, J., Yamakoshi, H., Terayama, N., Dodo, K., Smith, N. I., Sodeoka, M. and Fujita, K. (2020) Quantitative drug dynamics visualized by alkyne-tagged plasmonic-enhanced Raman microscopy. ACS Nano **14**, 15032–15041.
78. Boike, L., Henning, N. J. and Nomura, D. K. (2022) Advances in covalent drug discovery. Nat. Rev. Drug Discov. **21**, 881–898.
79. Kawagoe, H., Ando, J., Asanuma, M., Dodo, K., Miyano, T., Ueda, H., Sodeoka, M. and Fujita, K. (2021) Multiwell Raman plate reader for high-throughput biochemical screening. Sci. Rep. **11**, 15742.
80. Peng, M., Wang, Z., Sun, X., Guo, X., Wang, H., Li, R., Liu, Q., Chen, M. and Chen, X. (2022) Deep learning-based label-free surface-enhanced Raman scattering screening and recognition of small-molecule binding sites in proteins. Anal. Chem. **94**, 11483–11491.

https://doi.org/10.1142/9789811264610_0009

Chapter 9

Coherent Anti-Stokes Raman Scattering (CARS) Microscopy and its Applications in Life Sciences

Shinichi Miyazaki,[1,2] Yusuke Murakami,[1,2] Sakiko Honjoh,[2] Yu Hayashi,[2,3,4] Hideaki Kano[5,6,*]

[1]*Ph.D. Program in Humanics, School of Integrative and Global Majors, University of Tsukuba, 1-1-1 Tennodai, Tsukuba, Ibaraki 305-8577, Japan*
[2]*International Institute for Integrative Sleep Medicine (WPI IIIS), 1-1-1 Tennodai, Tsukuba, Ibaraki 305-8575, Japan*
[3]*Department of Human Health Sciences, Graduate School of Medicine, Kyoto University, 53 Kawahara-cho, Shogoin, Sakyo-ku, Kyoto 606-8507, Japan*
[4]*Department of Biological Sciences, Graduate School of Science, University of Tokyo, Bunkyo-ku, Tokyo 113-0033, Japan*
[5]*Department of Chemistry, Faculty of Science, Kyushu University, 744, Motooka, Nishi-ku, Fukuoka, 819-0395, Japan*
[6]*Department of Applied Physics, Graduate School of Pure and Applied Sciences, University of Tsukuba, 1-1-1 Tennodai, Tsukuba, Ibaraki, 305-8573, Japan*
**Corresponding author: hkano@chem.kyushu-univ.jp*

9.1 Introduction

Spontaneous Raman scattering microscopy can provide spatial and temporal distributions of molecular information based on vibrational signatures. Since spontaneous Raman scattering microscopy does not require specific labels, such as fluorescent stains and genetically encoded fluorescent tags, it can be applied to a wide range of samples — from materials to biological specimens. Theoretically, any sample with Raman-active chemical bonds can be analyzed using spontaneous Raman scattering microscopy; however, it cannot be used practically for fast imaging or imaging of samples sensitive to light exposure because of its weak signal intensity.

Coherent Raman scattering (CRS) microscopy addresses the limitations of spontaneous Raman scattering microscopy through its higher intensity, which enables faster and more sensitive molecular vibrational imaging [1]. CRS is advantageous for imaging samples that produce weak signals or are sensitive to incident light, such as living cells and tissues, by boosting the weak Raman signal.

CRS microscopy is classified into several types, including coherent anti-Stokes Raman scattering (CARS) and stimulated Raman scattering (SRS) microscopy [1–3]. Recent developments in CRS microscopy instrumentation have significantly enhanced its performance in terms of chemical specificity and imaging speed [4]. In particular, CARS microscopy allows the acquisition of wide-range (up to 3000 cm^{-1}) broadband vibrational spectra, whereas SRS is useful for high-speed monochromatic and medium-range (~400 cm^{-1}) broadband vibrational imaging [5–7]. Recent advances in SRS microscopy have already been reviewed in a previous publication [8]. Here, we mainly focus on the recent progress in CARS microscopy.

This chapter focuses on the basic principles of CRS (Section 4.2), the brief history of CARS microscopy (Section 4.3), the practical implementation of CARS microscopy (Section 4.4), and the applications of CARS microscopy in life science (Section 4.5). Several important reviews [9–32] are included in the references.

9.2 Basic Principles

9.2.1 *Four Analogs in Coherent Raman Scattering*

First, we briefly review the four main CRS processes: CARS, stimulated Raman gain (SRG), stimulated Raman loss (SRL), and coherent Stokes Raman scattering (CSRS). The energy diagrams for each process are shown in Figure 9.1. In CRS processes, electric fields with angular frequencies of ω_P and ω_S interact with molecules with a vibrational resonance frequency of Ω. When $\omega_P - \omega_S = \Omega$ is satisfied, the CRS processes occur. As shown in Figure 9.1, the CRS processes result in the following spectral changes:

— Generation of electric field with a new angular frequency of $2\omega_P - \omega_S$: CARS;
— Increase in amplitude of electric field at ω_S: SRG;

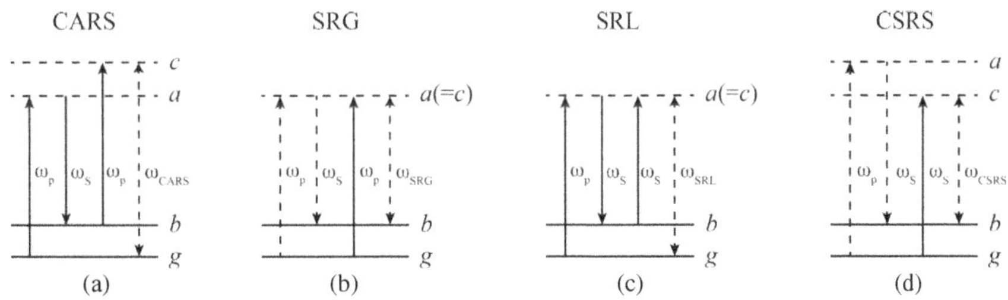

Figure 9.1. Energy-level diagrams of the four CRS processes: (a) CARS, (b) SRG, (c) SRL, (d) CSRS. The solid and broken arrows represent the interaction of the radiation field with molecules. Precisely, the solid up and dotted down arrows correspond to radiation at positive frequencies with phase factor of $e^{-i\omega t}$. Similarly, the solid down and dotted up arrows correspond to radiation at negative frequencies with a phase factor of $e^{i\omega t}$. The double-headed arrows represent the resulting third-order nonlinear polarization.

— Decrease in amplitude of electric field at ω_P: SRL;
— Generation of electric field with a new angular frequency of $2\omega_S - \omega_p$: CSRS.

Among them, SRL and SRG are classified into SRS.

The CRS processes provide a coherent sum of the signal electric fields, which can dramatically increase the signal intensity compared with spontaneous Raman scattering. The enhanced signal strength allows for fast signal acquisition, making it possible to perform real-time molecular vibrational imaging at video rates [33]. Among the four processes, this chapter is concerned with CARS. Surface-enhanced CARS has been reported as a useful technique for single-molecule vibrational spectroscopy [34–37]; however, it is beyond the scope of this chapter.

9.2.2 *Conditions for CARS Signal Acquisition and CARS Signal Features*

For the efficient generation of the CARS signal, the phase-matching condition is crucial. The phase-matching condition guarantees the constructive interference of the CARS signal generated from molecules within the focal volume. This condition is not always satisfied because the phase of the CARS electric field depends on the phases of the pump and Stokes electric fields, whose wavelengths differ from that of the CARS signal. Their phases are affected by the different refractive indices at the respective wavelengths, particularly when the interaction length is long (in microscopy, it corresponds to the length of the focus because the interaction length is typically longer than the focal length).

The first reported CARS microscope [38] considered the phase-matching condition in the two-beam configuration. Later, the collinear propagation of the pump and Stokes beams into the microscope objective was found to satisfy the phase-matching condition automatically [39, 40] because the large numerical aperture of the microscope objectives provides a large angular dispersion of the incident laser beam. Moreover, the short interaction length owing to tight focusing relaxes the phase-matching condition. Another consequence of phase matching is that intense CARS signal radiates in the forward direction [41] and not the other direction detected by the epi-detection setting. Epi-detection makes it possible to observe small particles or highly light-scattering samples, including biological tissues.

A theoretical study has shown that the CARS signal from an ensemble of N molecules is scaled by $N(N-1)$ using quantum electrodynamic treatment of the light fields [42]. Therefore, the CARS signal from a single molecule ($N = 1$) cannot be defined. The signal enhancement factor of the CARS process has been discussed by Scully's group, who theoretically and experimentally evaluated the signal amplitudes of CARS and spontaneous Raman scattering [43, 44]. The CARS signal is stronger by a factor of 100 than the spontaneous Raman signal for microscopy [43] and stronger by a factor of 10^5 for bulk materials because of the long coherence length [44].

CARS microscopy detects not only the vibrationally resonant signal but also the non-resonant background (NRB). Because NRB interferes with the vibrationally resonant CARS signal and distorts the CARS spectrum, several techniques have been reported to suppress NRB, including polarization control [45], time-resolved detection [46], and backscattering configuration [47]. NRB contamination can be partially avoided by using hyperspectral CARS microscopy to obtain the CARS spectrum; this issue is discussed in Section 9.4.4.

9.3 Early Development of CARS Microscopy

The first CARS microscope was reported in 1982 by Duncan *et al.* who used two synchronized dye laser sources [38]. They measured onion skin cells immersed in D_2O and reported CARS images in the OD stretching vibrational mode. Around 1999, tunable femtosecond solid-state laser sources came into wide use. Zumbusch *et al.* and Hashimoto *et al.* reported for the first time the application of CARS microscopy to live specimens, such as living cells. The light source was a combination of a Ti:sapphire laser amplifier system and an optical parametric amplifier system with repetition rates of 250 kHz [39] and 1 kHz [40]. Later, Cheng *et al.* [48] and Wurpel *et al.* [49] reported the development of a high-speed CARS microscope using two synchronized Ti:sapphire laser oscillators. Because two independent oscillators were used, matching the repetition frequencies of the two laser sources required sophisticated techniques to suppress jitter. The jitter was subsequently overcome in 2005 using an Nd:YVO_4 laser oscillator with an optical parametric oscillator (OPO), and a video-rate CARS microscope was reported [50]. The laser system comprising a picosecond mode-locked Nd:YVO_4 laser and OPO is widely used in CARS microscopy [51]. Although the laser source is tunable, the output wavelength is limited to a single color (or monochromatic). Therefore, most studies have focused on specific vibrational modes, such as the CH_2 symmetric stretching mode, to visualize lipids inside cells or tissues. The development of CARS/SRS microscopy up to the 2010s has been summarized in a previous publication [52].

In parallel with the development of ordinary CARS microscopy, various unique coherent Raman microscopy techniques were developed in the early 2000s. For instance, the pulse-shaping technique was applied to CARS microscopy [53], which uses multiple spectral components of femtosecond laser pulses simultaneously to accomplish the CARS process. Other examples include spatial resolution improvement using metal tips [54] and near-field optics [55].

9.4 Practical Implementation of CARS Microscopy

9.4.1 *Overview*

Here, we describe a typical implementation of the CARS microscope. Figure 9.2 shows a schematic of a CARS microscope. CARS microscopy employs two-color synchronized laser pulses called pump and Stokes pulses at angular frequencies of ω_P and ω_S (or ω_1 and ω_2), respectively. The parameters of the laser pulses are as follows: a temporal duration of 2–7 ps, repetition rate of ~100 MHz, wavelengths of ~800 nm and ~1000 nm for pump and Stokes, respectively, and an average power of 10–100 mW for each. The pump and Stokes pulses are combined in time and space by a sharp-edge dichroic mirror and then focused on a sample by an objective lens. When the frequency difference between them matches the vibrational frequency of the molecules,

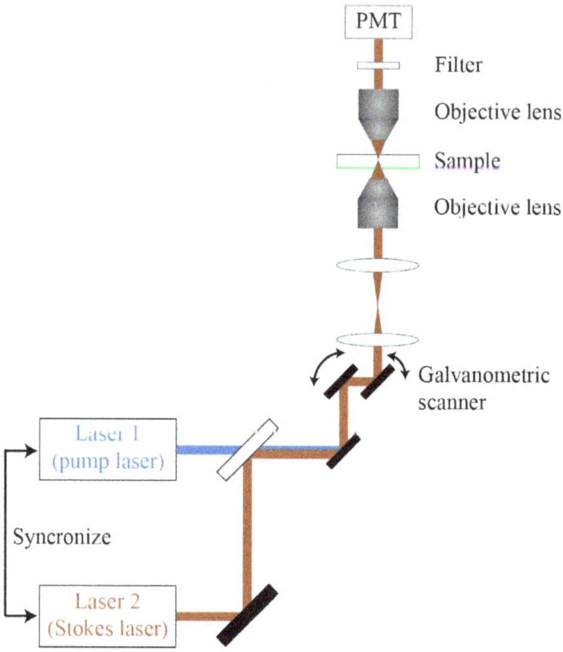

Figure 9.2. Schematic of a typical CARS microscope. Note that synchronization of the two lasers is achieved either passively or actively.

that is, $\omega_P - \omega_S = \Omega$, the CARS signal at $2\omega_P - \omega_2$ is generated in the focal volume. Finally, the CARS signal is detected either by another objective lens (transmission mode) or by the same objective lens (backscattering mode). After blocking the pump and Stokes pulses with an optical filter, the CARS signal is detected by an optical detector, such as a photomultiplier tube. For CARS imaging, the sample is scanned using laser scanning and/or stage scanning. In laser scanning, the propagation direction of the laser beam incident on the objective lens is controlled using a scanning mirror system, such as a galvanometric scanner, in the optical path. During stage scanning, the position of the stage is controlled using mechanical actuators. Finally, the CARS signal is obtained as a function of two- or three-dimensional spatial coordinates, from which we can reconstruct a CARS image at a particular angular frequency of $\omega_P - \omega_S = \Omega$.

Typical spatial resolution of CARS microscopy equipped with near-infrared laser is less than <0.5 μm in lateral and <1.5 μm in axial directions [48]. The spatial resolution depends on the wavelength of the laser and can be improved by using a shorter wavelength.

9.4.2 *Laser Sources for CARS Microscopy*

The laser sources for CARS microscopy are classified based on active and passive synchronization methods. In active synchronization, two independent lasers are synchronized using an external controller whereas, in passive synchronization, two-color laser pulses can be generated without external active control. Initial CARS microscopes [39, 40] used passively synchronized laser sources. An optical parametric amplifier is used to generate synchronized wavelength-tunable laser pulses. However, these laser systems typically have a low repetition rate of <1 MHz; therefore, they are incompatible with high-speed imaging. Further, actively synchronized Ti:sapphire lasers have been adapted to CARS microscopy, and extensive efforts have been made to synchronize two lasers with a low-timing jitter [56, 57]. Since Ti:sapphire oscillators can produce wavelength-tunable picosecond pulses with a narrow spectral width at a high repetition rate of ~80 MHz, they are suitable for CARS microscopy. Active synchronization also has a disadvantage in that it is typically sensitive to environmental perturbations, including physical shock and temperature changes.

To overcome these disadvantages, an OPO [58, 59] was proposed, which has become one of the most popular laser sources for CARS (and SRS) microscopy. OPO allows passive synchronization and is excited by a pulse train from a master laser, and the pulse train can yield optical parametric gain in a nonlinear optical crystal such as a KTP crystal only when the pulses pass through the crystal. Consequently, OPO can generate optical pulses synchronized with the master laser pulses. Various laser configurations have been adopted as master laser sources, including mode-locked solid-state laser oscillators using Nd:YVO_4 as a gain material [58]. Currently, mode-locked Yb fiber lasers, which can generate ~3 ps pulses at a wavelength of ~1032 nm and a repetition rate of ~80 MHz, are also used [59]. Although OPO has wide wavelength tunability, wavelength tuning requires temperature control of the OPO crystal and mechanical control of the birefringent filter inside the OPO cavity. Therefore, wavelength tuning can take several tens of seconds to several minutes.

Extensive efforts have been devoted to realizing compact and practical laser sources based on fiber lasers and wavelength conversion technologies [60–62] including fiber optical parametric oscillators [63], optical parametric amplifiers [64], time-lens sources [65], and high-speed wavelength-swept fiber lasers [66]. Recently, several compact laser sources have been reported for CARS and SRS microscopy [62, 67–71]. For instance, a compact, fast, and tunable fiber-based laser source has been applied to frequency modulation CARS microscopy with spectral coverage between 700 and 3200 cm^{-1} via wavelength tuning within 5 ms [72].

9.4.3 *Hyperspectral Imaging Using CARS Microscopy*

Conventional CARS microscopy (monochromatic or single-color CARS) drives only one vibrational mode; in other words, $2\omega_P - \omega_S$ is a single value. Hyperspectral CARS excites multiple vibrational modes to obtain the CARS spectrum. Figure 9.3 summarizes the various methods of hyperspectral CARS and SRS imaging: (a) wavelength scanning [72–74], (b) spectral focusing [75, 76], (c) Fourier transformation [77, 78], and (d) multiplex method [79–83]. These four techniques are described in the following subsections.

9.4.3.1 *Wavelength Scanning*

In the wavelength-scanning method, CARS images at different vibrational modes are successively acquired by changing the laser wavelength, as shown

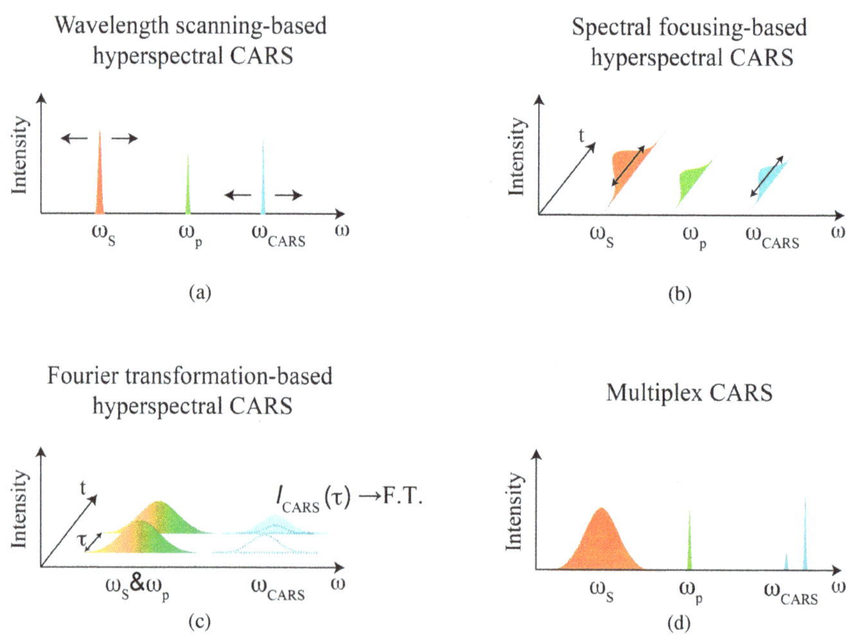

Figure 9.3. Hyperspectral CARS methods. (a) Wavelength scanning. (b) Spectral focusing. (c) Fourier-transform CARS. (d) Multiplex CARS.

in Figure 9.3(a). In the case of a laser system using OPO, this approach has a disadvantage in terms of the tuning speed of the OPO signal wavelength, which limits the imaging speed. Recently, fast wavelength-tunable lasers have been developed [84], making the wavelength scanning method practical.

9.4.3.2 *Spectral Focusing*

In the spectral focusing method, the pump and Stokes pulses are passed through dispersive elements such as glass rods such that they have the same frequency chirp (i.e., the time dependence of instantaneous optical frequency) and a long duration of time (typically several picoseconds). When the pump and Stokes pulses overlap in time, their frequency difference remains constant for picoseconds [76]. Furthermore, the frequency difference can be adjusted by tuning the delay between them, as shown in Figure 9.3(b). When the pulses are focused on a sample, a particular vibrational mode can be excited, which is chosen by the delay between the pump and Stokes pulses, leading to the generation of the CARS signal.

The typical spectral focusing method uses two-color femtosecond laser pulses as the pump and Stokes pulses for hyperspectral CARS imaging. This method does not require wavelength tuning and can achieve high spectral resolution [75]. Therefore, the requirements for laser sources are much more relaxed than those for the wavelength-scanning method. The spectral-focusing technique has been combined with a dual-comb laser source. All-fiber single-cavity dual-comb laser sources were used for CARS microscopy with a spectral focusing method [85].

9.4.3.3 *Fourier Transformation*

Similar to the Fourier-transform (FT) infrared spectrometer, the CARS spectrum can be obtained using the FT technique. FT-CARS techniques typically employ a single femtosecond laser source and an interferometer, such as a Michelson interferometer, to duplicate laser pulses that are introduced into a microscope [77, 86]. At the focus, the first pulse acts as the pump and Stokes pulses to impulsively excite vibrational coherence, while the second time-delayed pulse probes this coherence. Since the second pulse also generates the local oscillator to interfere with the CARS signal, the amplitude and phase information of the CARS signal is recorded as a delay function. The interferogram of the CARS signal is obtained by varying the delay time between the first and second pulses, as shown in Figure 9.3(c). The Fourier transform of the CARS interferogram provides the CARS spectrum. Because NRB appears only at the zero-delay time, it can be easily removed through FT analysis. The spectral bandwidth is determined using a laser source for impulsive Raman excitation. A combination of this method with a frequency comb has also been reported [87].

9.4.3.4 *Multiplex Method*

The multiplex or broadband CARS method [80–83, 88] enables simultaneous acquisition of the CARS spectrum in a broad spectral range using a set of broadband and narrowband laser pulses, as shown in Figure 9.3(d). The key component of the multiplex CARS method is a broadband laser source, such as a supercontinuum (SC) light source [4, 89] or a femtosecond laser source [90]. For SC generation, a portion of the master laser output is seeded into a tapered fiber [81] or a photonic crystal fiber (PCF) [82]. A cost-effective sub-nanosecond laser source can also be used as the master laser source for SC generation [91].

The CARS spectrum is measured using a spectrometer equipped with a multichannel detector, such as a charge-coupled device (CCD) or complementary metal oxide semiconductor (CMOS) camera. The spectral coverage of the multiplex CARS reaches more than 3500 cm^{-1}, which is sufficiently broad to detect all fundamental modes, including the fingerprint, C–H stretching, and O–H stretching regions.

For the multiplex method, the image acquisition speed depends mainly on the exposure and readout times of the multichannel photodetector, through which the pixel dwell time is restricted to be at least ~1 ms for broadband (>3500 cm^{-1}) spectral coverage [92, 93]. One of the advantages of multiplex CARS is its robustness against the motion of samples and the intensity fluctuation of the incident laser, owing to the short image acquisition time.

A typical experimental setup for multiplex CARS microscopy is shown in Figure 9.4(a). The wavelength, temporal duration, and repetition rate of the laser source are 1064 nm, 50 ps, and 1 MHz, respectively. The pulse energies of the ω_P and ω_S pulses are approximately 2 and 1 mJ, corresponding to peak powers of approximately 24 and 12 kW, respectively. The laser beam is divided into two parts: one is used as the pump beam (ω_P), while the other is used as the Stokes beam (ω_S) seeded into a PCF to generate SC. Because efficient CARS

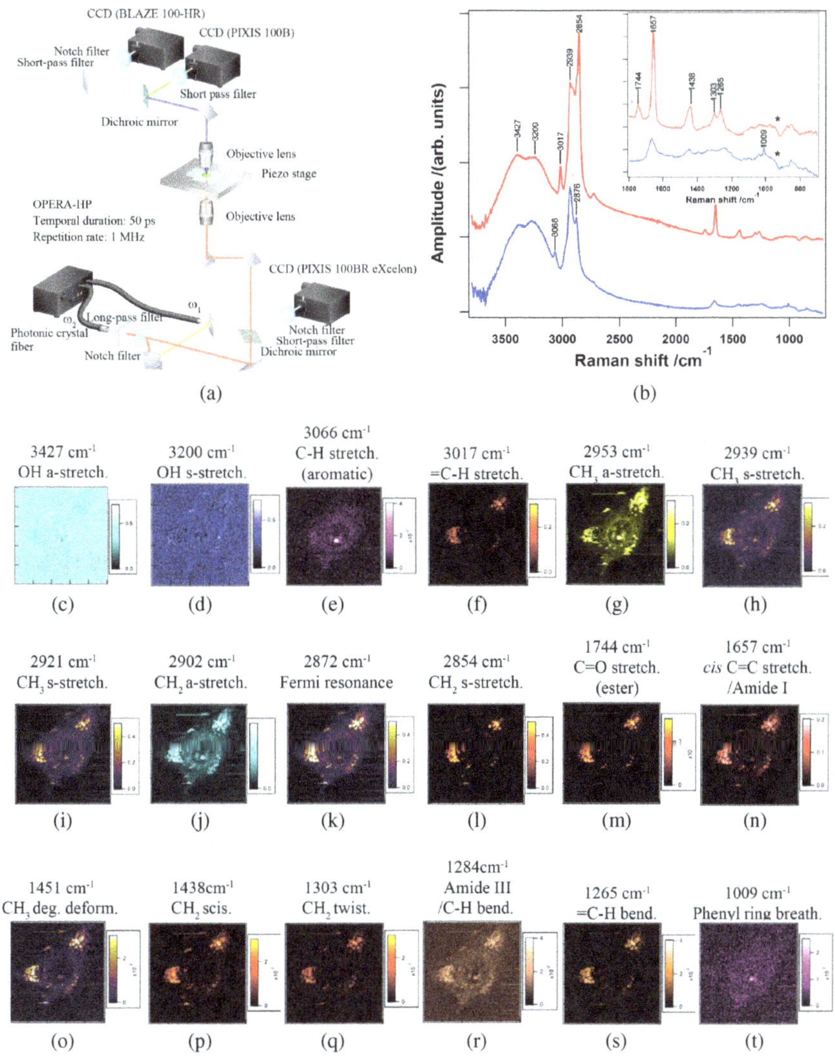

Figure 9.4. CARS spectroscopic imaging for living cells reveals various molecular distributions. (a) Schematic of multiplex CARS microscope. (b) Averaged Im[$\chi^{(3)}$] spectra of lipid droplet suspect regions (red) and nuclei (blue) of an A549 cell. (c–s) Ultra-multiplex CARS imaging of an A549 cell at (c) 3427, (d) 3200, (e) 3066, (f) 3017, (g) 2953, (h) 2939, (i) 2921, (j) 2902, (k) 2872, (l) 2854, (m) 1744, (n) 1657, (o) 1451, (p) 1438, (q) 1303, (r) 1284, (s) 1265, and (t) 1009 cm^{-1}, respectively. The exposure time per pixel was ~1.8 ms. Reproduced from Ref. [92] with permission.

signal generation requires a high spectral density around the near-infrared region, the PCF is fabricated to efficiently generate spectral components between 1100 and 1800 nm. SC contains a spectral component shorter than 1064 nm and will contaminate the CARS signal; therefore, a long-pass filter is utilized for blocking spectral components shorter than 1064 nm. The ω_P and ω_S laser pulses are superimposed using a sharp dichroic mirror and then introduced into a modified inverted microscope. The incident laser pulses are tightly focused onto the sample using the first objective lens. The sample is placed on a piezoelectric stage for microscopic imaging, and the CARS signal is collected using a second objective lens and dispersed using a spectrometer. Finally, the CARS signal is detected using a CCD camera.

9.4.4 *Retrieval of a Raman Spectrum from a CARS Spectrum*

Because the CARS signal has two contributions, NRB and vibrationally resonant CARS, the raw spectral profile can be obtained in a CARS interference of these two components. Because of this interference, the shape of the raw CARS spectrum is complex. It is especially challenging to calculate the signal and NRB using single-mode monochromatic CARS because the full spectral shape is not determined by monochromatic CARS. By contrast, hyperspectral CARS allows obtaining the full spectral shape of the raw CARS. We can then mathematically calculate the signal equivalent to spontaneous Raman signals if the NRB spectrum is obtained in the same experimental condition. Therefore, hyperspectral CARS is beneficial for accurately separating signals equivalent to the spontaneous Raman signals from NRB.

The spectral profile of the raw CARS signal is different from that of spontaneous Raman scattering; it should be converted into the spectrum equivalent of the spontaneous Raman spectrum using an adequate signal processing method. In particular, the spectral profile of the raw CARS signal is close to the real part of $\chi^{(3)}$ ($\mathrm{Re}[\chi^{(3)}]$); here, $\chi^{(3)}$ is a complex function of the vibrational frequency called third-order nonlinear susceptibility. The spontaneous Raman scattering signal is proportional to the absolute square of $\chi^{(3)}$. Assuming that the spectral profile is described by a complex Lorentzian function, the spontaneous Raman spectrum corresponds to the imaginary part of $\chi^{(3)}$ ($\mathrm{Im}[\chi^{(3)}]$) [94, 95].

Several techniques have been proposed to retrieve the $\mathrm{Im}[\chi^{(3)}]$ spectrum from the CARS spectrum (i.e., ~$\mathrm{Re}[\chi^{(3)}]$ spectrum), such as the maximum entropy method (MEM) [96], time-domain Kramers–Kronig formulation [97], and the phase-corrected Kramers–Kronig approach [98]. Recently, a deep learning technique was applied to remove NRB from the raw CARS spectra [99–101]. A fully automated model was able to process multiplex CARS spectra in real time.

Table 9.1. Vibrational bands and their assignments for intracellular Im[$\chi^{(3)}$] spectrum.

Typical Raman shift (cm^{-1})	Assignments	Main molecular components
3427	O–H a-stretch. with Fermi resonance	Water
3200	O–H s-stretch. with Fermi resonance	Water
3066	C–H stretch. (aromatic)	Proteins
3017	=C-H stretch.	Lipids
2953	CH_3 a-stretch.	DNAs and RNAs
~2930	CH_3 s-stretch.	Proteins/Lipids
2902	CH_2 a-stretch.	Lipids/Proteins
2872	Overtone of CH_3 deform. in Fermi resonance with CH_3 s-stretch.	Proteins/Lipids
2854	CH_2 s-stretch.	Lipids
1744	C=O stretch. (ester)	Lipids
1657	*cis* C=C stretch./Amide I	Lipids/Proteins
~1550	Purine ring (adenine and guanine)	DNAs and RNAs
1451	CH_3 deg. deform.	Proteins
1438	CH_2 scis.	Lipids
1303	CH_2 twist.	Lipids
~1284	Amide III/C–H bend.	Proteins
1265	=C–H bend.	Lipids
1004	Phenyl ring breath.	Proteins

Abbreviations: stretch.: stretching; deform.: deformation; rock.: rocking; twist.: twisting; scis.: scissors; bend.: bending; s-: symmetric; a-: antisymmetric; deg.: degenerate; breath.: breathing.

As an example, Figure 9.4(b) shows the intracellular averaged Raman-equivalent Im[$\chi^{(3)}$] spectrum of an A549 cell in the G1 phase. Using MEM, the Im[$\chi^{(3)}$] spectrum at each spatial position was calculated from the raw CARS spectra [89, 96]. MEM does not require *a priori* knowledge of the vibrational bands but can still retrieve the phase information of $\chi^{(3)}$ [96]. The CARS signal was observed between 600 and 3200 cm^{-1}. The assignments of the corresponding vibrational bands are listed in Table 9.1 [26, 102–109].

9.5 Applications of CARS Microscopy in Life Sciences

In the following sections, we review the applications of CARS microscopy in life sciences. First, monochromatic (single-color) CARS imaging is discussed, followed by hyperspectral (multicolor) CARS imaging. Some examples of applications in life sciences are then presented.

9.5.1 *Monochromatic (Single-Color) CARS Imaging*

Monochromatic CARS imaging uses a single molecular vibrational mode. Theoretically, any band is a target for monochromatic CARS imaging. However, most studies have focused on a band in the CH region (2800–3000 cm^{-1}) and not the fingerprint region (600–1800 cm^{-1}). The signal-to-noise ratio for a band in the CH region is sufficiently high owing to the large Raman scattering cross-section. Monochromatic CARS imaging using the fingerprint region (600–1800 cm^{-1}) is challenging due to the significant contribution from the NRB and low signal-to-noise ratio.

The primary target molecules of monochromatic CARS are lipids because of their large Raman scattering cross-sections. The vibrational mode at ~2850 cm^{-1} is frequently used to visualize lipids. The mode is assigned as a CH_2 symmetric stretching vibrational mode; because lipids contain long aliphatic chains, the signal at the band helps uncover the lipid distribution.

Monochromatic CARS microscopy allows the visualization of molecular distribution without labeling or fixation and with less phototoxicity than conventional fluorescence imaging. Several studies have shown that monochromatic CARS microscopy for lipids is comparable or superior to fluorescence imaging, although CARS microscopy does not require any labels [110–112]. Imaging without fixation is another advantage of CARS microscopy. Fixation stops the physiological changes of cells and affects the distribution of lipids and the structure of the cells. Imaging without fixation enables the assessment of lipid dynamics and physiological changes, such as differentiation, and is beneficial for rapid imaging and diagnosis for intraoperative pathological diagnosis [113]. The low phototoxicity of CARS lipid imaging is also an advantage. For lipid distribution imaging, 817-nm and 1064-nm laser sources are frequently used. These wavelengths are longer than those used for fluorescence microscopy; therefore, the phototoxicity is lower. The low phototoxicity allows long-lasting and repeated imaging for time-resolved analyses for up to several hours [114, 115].

Monochromatic CARS imaging of lipids is applicable to *in vivo* imaging. The most vital CARS signals propagate in the forwarding direction, and the most common detection method is the transmission mode. Signals in the CH region are strong enough to detect backscattering CARS signals.

In recent times, researchers have started preferring hyperspectral CARS over its monochromatic counterpart owing to the abundant molecular information it provides. However, monochromatic CARS is still useful for high-speed lipid imaging with accurate quantification.

9.5.2 *Hyperspectral (Multicolor) CARS Imaging*

Monochromatic CARS visualizes the lipid distribution without labels, as discussed previously. Hyperspectral (multicolor) CARS has the same advantages as monochromatic CARS; moreover, it enables the acquisition of not only lipids but also the distribution of other molecules, such as proteins, polysaccharides, and DNA/RNA. In addition to the distribution, hyperspectral CARS can reveal the saturation rate of lipids [115, 116] and the secondary structure of proteins [117, 118]. In particular, multiplex CARS (M-CARS) [119] or broadband CARS (B-CARS) [120] microspectroscopy with different spectral coverages enables multicolor CARS imaging to visualize molecular species in living cells and tissues [4, 21, 92, 93].

Cheng *et al.* [119] and Wurpel *et al.* [121] developed the initial M-CARS microscope using synchronized femtosecond and picosecond Ti:sapphire laser oscillators. The initial M-CARS microscope had two main limitations. The first was the difficulty in synchronizing the two independent lasers, requiring sophisticated techniques to ensure that the repetition rates of these two laser sources coincide. The second was the narrow spectral coverage. The spectral coverage was limited to ~300 cm^{-1} due to the spectral bandwidth of the femtosecond Stokes laser. This narrow coverage makes comprehensive molecular imaging difficult.

The initial M-CARS problems were later overcome using an ultra-broadband SC light source. The synchronization problem was solved because the M-CARS microscope used a single laser source; the SC was generated by seeding a portion of the pump laser pulses into a tapered fiber [81] or PCF [82]. The sources of the pump and Stokes (SC) laser pulses were identical; therefore, they were automatically synchronized. The second problem was solved because of the ultra-broadband spectral coverage of the SC (> 3000 cm^{-1}), which covers both the fingerprint and the C–H, N–H, and O–H stretching regions [120, 122]. CARS using SC is currently referred to as ultra-broadband multiplex CARS [82] (or ultra-multiplex CARS [93]) or B-CARS [4, 21, 120]. In the literature [21], spectroscopic techniques with bandwidths of hundreds of cm^{-1} are called M-CARS, while those with bandwidths on the scale of thousands of cm^{-1} are B-CARS. In this text, they are collectively referred to as hyperspectral CARS.

Here, we outline the applications of hyperspectral (multicolor) CARS in life sciences, such as imaging of cells, nematodes, tissue slices, and pathological samples, and in the environmental sciences, such as microplastic detection.

9.5.2.1 *Living Cells*

Living cells are frequently used in cell biology experiments. Visualizing the distribution of biomolecules helps characterize the physiological state of cells. Since CARS visualizes biomolecular information without any labels or invasion, it is an ideal method for assessing intact living cells.

One target of CARS imaging in living cells is lipids because the signal intensity of lipids is higher than that of other molecules. Nan *et al.* showed that lipid imaging using monochromatic CARS at 2845 cm^{-1} overlapped with Oil Red O and Nile Red staining in 3T3-L1 cells, a fibroblast cell strain derived from mice [110]. The authors also revealed that lipid dynamics can be assessed using CARS microscopy. They induced cell differentiation into adipocytes while conducting time-resolved CARS imaging for up to 96 h and showed that the initial lipid droplets decreased and later increased. These results demonstrate the utility of CARS in assessing intracellular lipid distribution and dynamics.

CARS allows selective imaging of saturated and unsaturated lipids [123], and quantitative imaging of lipid saturation and the order of lipids [116]. Heinrich *et al.* conducted lipid imaging of adipocytes using CARS signals at 2850 cm^{-1} and 3015 cm^{-1}, assigned to the –C–H and =C–H stretching modes, respectively [123]. Cells treated with stearic acid and arachidonic acid showed a difference in signal intensity at 3015 cm^{-1}; arachidonic acid-treated cells increased in signal intensity, indicating an increase in unsaturated lipids [123]. Rinia *et al.* evaluated the lipid unsaturation and acyl chain order using the CARS band ratios [116]. The authors used a ratio between ν_n(C=C) (1650 cm^{-1}) and $\delta(CH_2)$ (1450 cm^{-1}) vibrational modes to measure fatty acid unsaturation, as described in a spontaneous Raman scattering study [124], and they used a ratio between acyl chain-symmetric (2850 cm^{-1}) and -anti-symmetric (2880 cm^{-1}) vibrational modes to assess the acyl chain order. These indicators were used for adipocytes and revealed intracellular lipid heterogeneity.

Takei *et al.* conducted CARS lipid imaging of brown and white adipocytes (HB2 and 3T3-L1) using hyperspectral CARS (ultra-multiplex CARS) [115]. The authors utilized an onstage incubator and deuterium labeling technique to unveil the dynamics of fatty acid uptake for 9 h.

In addition to cultured mammalian cells, single-cell organisms are suitable for CARS microscopy. Oka *et al.* applied CARS microscopy to a living microalga, *Cyanidium caldarium* [125], to describe the characteristics of the organism. A broad and sharp Raman band at 505 cm^{-1} was observed at the periphery and inside the microalga. The band was assigned to polysulfides and glycogen and was confirmed by comparison with model samples. It was also confirmed by the second harmonic generation signal.

Here, we demonstrate that hyperspectral CARS is a powerful tool for comprehensive molecular imaging. Kano *et al.* reported the distribution of multiple molecules using ultra-broadband multiplex CARS spectroscopic imaging with a fast readout time (<1 ms) [93]. CARS images of 161 × 161 pixels were obtained for polymer beads with a total data acquisition time of approximately 28 s. Label-free and ultra-multiplex (18 colors) imaging of living cells was also performed with an effective exposure time of 1.8 ms based on the molecular fingerprint as well as the C–H and O–H stretching vibrational modes using a master oscillator fiber amplifier laser source (Figure 9.4(a)). The averaged spectrum contains multiple peaks (Figure 9.4(b)). CARS images were reconstructed for various Raman bands by analyzing the spectral profile at each cell position. Figure 9.4(c–t) summarizes the results of the ultra-broadband multiplex CARS imaging. It is apparent that the microscopic intracellular structures were successfully visualized based on their molecular fingerprint. Particle-like structures with diameters of a few micrometers were observed in the cytoplasm, as shown in Figures 9.4(f), (l), (j), (m), (p), (q), and (s). These bands were assigned to the C–H stretching vibrational mode of =C–H bonds (Figure 9.4(f)), CH_2 symmetric stretching vibrational mode (Figure 9.4(l)), C=O stretching mode of the ester (Figure 9.4(m)), CH_2 scissoring mode (Figure 9.4(p)), CH_2 twisting mode (Figure 9.4(q)), and =C–H bending mode (Figure 9.4(s)) — all of which are typically observed for lipids. Therefore, these organelles can be safely assigned as lipid droplets. As clearly shown in CARS images (Figures 9.4(f) and 9.4(s)), the lipid droplets contained rich unsaturated lipids. These results are consistent with the characteristics of the A549 cell, which is known to produce unsaturated lipids. By contrast, the CARS images at 2939 cm^{-1} (Figure 9.4(h)) and 2921 cm^{-1} (Figure 9.4(i)) indicate a dark round structure in the cell. This corresponds to the cell nucleus. The intranuclear bright spots can be assigned to the nucleolus, which introduces high vibrational contrast to CARS images in Figures 9.4(e), (g), (h), (i), (k), (o), and (t). These vibrational modes correspond to aromatic CH stretching (Figure 9.4(e)), CH_3 asymmetric stretching (Figure 9.4(g)), CH_3 symmetric stretching

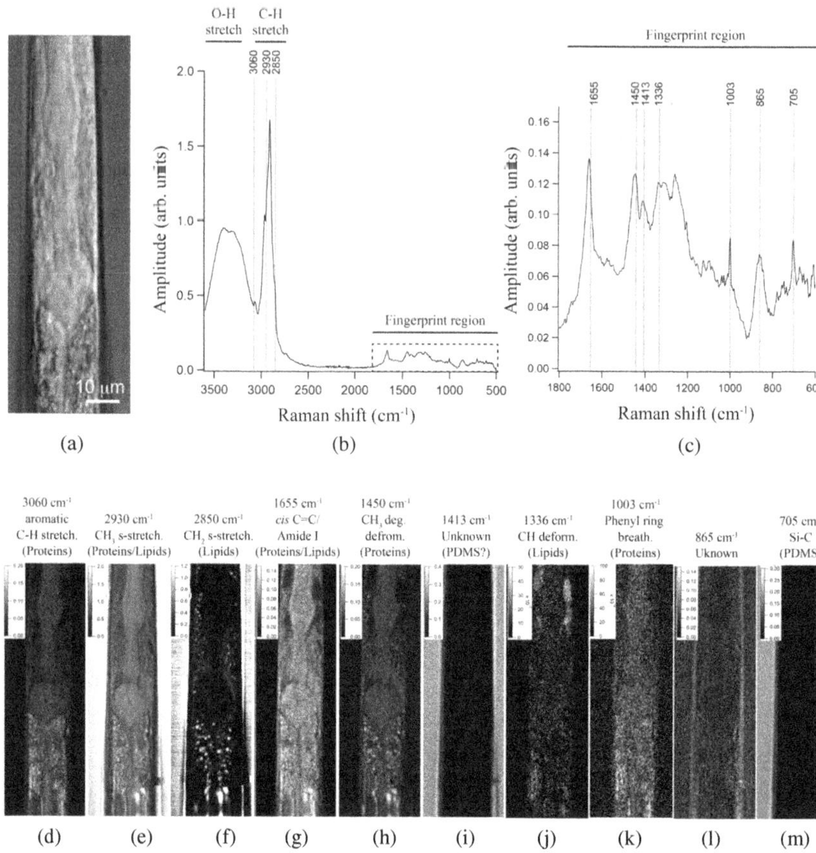

Figure 9.5. CARS spectroscopic imaging reveals molecular distributions in a nematode. (a) A raw CARS image of the head part of a nematode in the chamber. (b) The average CARS spectrum of a nematode shows multiple peaks assigned to vibrational modes. (c) An enlarged spectrum in the fingerprint region (600–1800 cm^{-1}). (d–m) CARS images at each Raman band (grey shaded areas in (b) and (c)). Reproduced from Ref. [127] with permission.

(Figures 9.4(h) and (i)), an overtone of CH_3 deformation in Fermi resonance with CH_3 symmetric stretching (Figure 9.4(k)), CH_3 degenerate deformation (Figure 9.4(o)), and phenyl ring breathing (Figure 9.4(t)) vibrational modes. On the contrary, the CARS images at 3427 cm^{-1} (Figure 9.4(c)) and 3200 cm^{-1} (Figure 9.4(d)), which correspond to the OH stretching vibrational modes, have low contrast in the field of view. These results suggest that hyperspectral (ultra-broadband) CARS reveals multiple molecular profiles of cells, such as lipid and protein distributions, without any label. Notably, multiple molecular profiles can be obtained by single imaging through hyperspectral CARS; thus, it provides a fast and detailed analysis of living cells.

9.5.2.2 *Nematodes*

Hyperspectral CARS is also useful for analyzing multicellular organisms. The tiny nematode *Caenorhabditis elegans* (*C. elegans*) is frequently studied for hyperspectral CARS imaging. *C. elegans* offers several advantages when performing CARS microscopy, chiefly because it has a small (approximately 1 mm) and transparent body. Moreover, genetic tools are available for nematodes; CARS microscopy and genetics can thus be combined in a synergistic approach to unravel unresolved biological problems.

The initial targets of CARS microscopy were lipids, similar to the other samples. There are two main reasons lipids are a target of these studies, which are discussed below. Hellerer *et al.* investigated lipid droplets in nematodes using a CARS microscope [111]. The authors measured the number of lipid droplets in wild-type nematodes and compared them with those obtained via conventional fluorescent staining. CARS microscopy can be used to visualize lipid droplets that cannot be visualized by staining. CARS microscopy also allows volume imaging of lipid droplets in wild-type and mutant nematodes that accumulate excessive lipids in the body. Yen *et al.* also revealed that CARS microspectroscopy is considerably more sensitive for detecting lipid droplets in nematodes than several fluorescent staining methods [112]. These studies showed that CARS microscopy could reveal more detailed lipid distribution than conventional fluorescent imaging.

Furthermore, recent studies have used hyperspectral CARS microscopy to measure the number of lipids and characterize lipid dynamics in detail. Using SC laser-based hyperspectral (broadband) CARS and machine learning, Chen *et al.* revealed the diversity of lipid droplets within the nematode body [126]. Because hyperspectral (broadband) CARS spectra contain information on many types of molecules, the authors calculated the protein concentration and degree of lipid saturation using hyperspectral (broadband) CARS bands at 2850 cm^{-1}, 1650 cm^{-1}, and 1450 cm^{-1} to reveal the diversity among lipid-rich particles. Lipid-rich particles containing a high amount of protein are distributed to the progeny, whereas low protein-lipid particles are used for energy storage. This study showed that hyperspectral CARS allows for a more detailed analysis of lipid particles in organisms, such as protein content, degree of lipid saturation, and lipid order, whereas conventional fluorescence imaging is only applicable for quantifying lipid particles.

Here, we show that hyperspectral CARS and other nonlinear optical processes reveal the detailed molecular distribution of nematodes. Miyazaki *et al.* used a multimodal nonlinear optical microscope for nematodes (Figure 9.5(a)) [127]. The microscope configuration is shown in Figure 9.4(a). The authors simultaneously obtained hyperspectral (ultra-broadband multiplex) CARS and second and third harmonic generations (SHG and THG).

The average CARS spectra from the nematode body revealed that the microscope can obtain ultra-broadband (over 3000 cm^{-1}) spectra with an acceptable signal-to-noise ratio in both the CH stretch (Figure 9.5(b)) and fingerprint signals (Figure 9.5(c)). Each peak was fitted with a Gaussian function, the spectrum was deconvoluted with many Gaussians, and the concentration maps of each chemical bond were visualized. Images of the Raman shifts of 3060 cm^{-1} (Figure 5(d)), 2930 cm^{-1} (Figure 9.5(e)), 2850 cm^{-1} (Figure 9.5(f)), 1655 cm^{-1} (Figure 9.5(g)), 1450 cm^{-1} (Figure 9.5(h)), 1413 cm^{-1} (Figure 9.5(i)), 1336 cm^{-1} (Figure 9.5(j)), 1003 cm^{-1} (Figure 9.5(k)), 865 cm^{-1} (Figure 9.5(l)), and 705 cm^{-1} (Figure 9.5(m)) are shown in Figure 9.5.

The CH_2 stretching vibrational mode (2850 cm^{-1}, Figure 9.5(f)) visualized the lipid distribution. Certain small particle-shaped structures were observed, which might be lipid droplets. These results suggest that the intestine is the most abundant in lipid droplets, while some exist around the pharynx as well. Lipid droplets in the pharynx are smaller than those in the intestine. In addition, this result suggests that the lipid content of the pharyngeal muscle is much lower than that of other tissues. As Hellerer *et al.* suggested and Yen *et al.* confirmed, the CH_2 stretching vibrational mode is more advantageous for visualizing lipid distribution than fluorescent microscopy [111, 112].

Specific vibrational modes contain information about proteins in nematodes. 3060 and 1006 cm^{-1} showed high contrast in the intestine of nematodes, and the pharynx exhibited lower contrast than the intestine. These bands imply that more proteins with aromatic amino acids exist in the intestine than in the pharynx. By contrast, 2930 cm^{-1} (Figure 9.5(e)), 1655 cm^{-1} (Figure 9.5(g)), and 1450 cm^{-1} (Figure 9.5(h)) visualized the intestine and pharynx equally, suggesting that the overall protein content did not differ between the intestine and pharynx. The other feature is that some small particles showed a high intensity compared to the surrounding region. Some of these small particles overlapped with particles at 2850 cm^{-1}, suggesting that some were lipid droplets. Some of the lipid droplets contained proteins, which demonstrates the diversity of the lipid droplets, as shown in more detail in a recent study [126]. Thus, hyperspectral CARS provides detailed information on localized proteins without the use of labeling.

Nematodes are suitable for hyperspectral CARS owing to their simple body structure. They are among the few multicellular organisms that can be observed under a microscope without dissection. As shown here, hyperspectral CARS provides detailed information about biomolecules without labels. Moreover, established genetic tools and hyperspectral CARS can synergistically promote each other in the near future.

9.5.2.3 *Mouse Brain Tissues*

Hyperspectral CARS has also been used in tissue samples for investigation and diagnosis. Because hyperspectral CARS provides detailed molecular information compared with conventional imaging techniques, it can help uncover the molecular changes in biological tissues. The brain is a complex organ with over 100 million heterogeneous mammalian cells. Understanding the heterogenic properties of cells in the brain and their interactions is the primary goal of neuroscience. Hyperspectral CARS may be helpful for elucidating the molecular properties of the brain.

Multiphoton microscopy, or two-photon excited fluorescence microscopy, is widely used in neuroscience because of its high invasion depth and spatial resolution. However, the following problems remain: (1) Creating transgenic animals that express fluorescent proteins is technical, time-consuming, and costly. (2) Administration of fluorescent dyes is invasive and may alter the structure and function of the brain. Hyperspectral CARS microscopy, another type of multiphoton microscopy, is not as widely used as two-photon microscopy; however, it can overcome problems in two-photon microscopy.

Hyperspectral CARS microscopy allows high-resolution imaging without labeling. Evans *et al.* performed the initial application of CARS to brain tissue [128] (Figure 9.6). The authors showed that the CARS microscope is applicable to whole-brain imaging using the tiling method. Whole-brain images were produced by tuning the 2845 cm^{-1} due to CH_2 symmetric stretching mode. Brain myelin coating the axonal bundles is rich in CH_2 bonds, and thus the lipid CARS contrast produces an intense CARS signal and image contrast on the white matter. In a microscale image, they showed that a single-color CARS image at 2845 cm^{-1} enables discrimination of the layer structure in the

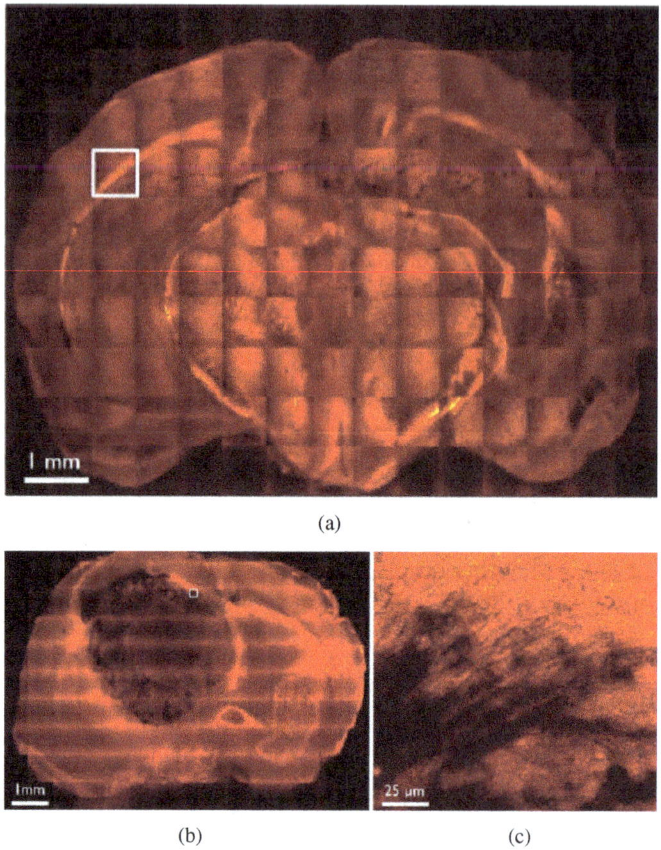

Figure 9.6. CARS imaging visualizes a healthy mouse brain and an astrocytoma. (a) Mosaic CARS image of a healthy mouse brain at 2846 cm^{-1}. Every single image is 700 × 700 μm in size. The brain slice was sectioned 2.8 mm posterior to the bregma. (b) Low-resolution, large-field-of-view mosaic CARS image of an astrocytoma at 2846 cm^{-1}. (c) Higher resolution CARS image corresponding to the area enclosed by the rectangle in (b). The image visualizes microscopic infiltration at the boundary between the tumor and normal tissue. Adapted from Ref. [128] with permission.

brain. In addition, the neuronal cell bodies were visualized with a combination of 2955 cm^{-1} and 2845 cm^{-1}; the multicolor CARS image contrasted the hematoxylin and eosin stain images. The authors applied CARS imaging to discriminate between healthy brain tissue and astrocytoma. The healthy tissue and astrocytoma tissue differed at 2845 cm^{-1}, indicating that astrocytoma could be distinguished from CARS without any label.

Fu *et al.* applied hyperspectral CARS microscopy to brain slices and showed that label-free imaging of myelin sheaths at a three-dimensional submicron resolution is possible [129]. In addition, they further tested the capability of CARS microscopy to image the *in vivo* brain of the parietal cortex and white matter. The authors have simultaneously shown that CARS microscopy helps provide sharper contrast and avoids photobleaching compared to lipophilic dye-labeled two-photon excitation fluorescence imaging.

The fingerprint region (600–1800 cm^{-1}), as well as the CH region (2800–3000 cm^{-1}), are applicable for CARS brain slice imaging; the laser source development increases the signal-to-noise ratio of bands in the fingerprint region to an acceptable level. Camp *et al.* applied hyperspectral (broadband) CARS to distinguish tumors from intact brain tissue [4, 130]. The authors found an overall reduction in the lipid-protein ratio (2850 cm^{-1}/1004 cm^{-1}) in tumor cells relative to that in healthy brain tissues, as shown by the spectra.

Murakami *et al.* conducted comprehensive hyperspectral CARS imaging of brain slices [131]. Hyperspectral CARS imaging was performed along the longitudinal axis of the brain (Figure 9.7). Images based on several Raman bands were reconstructed at different positions along the anterior-posterior axis. The hyperspectral CARS images at CH_2 symmetric stretching (Figure 9.7) and CH_2 scissoring vibrational bands (Figure 9.7) were assigned as lipids,

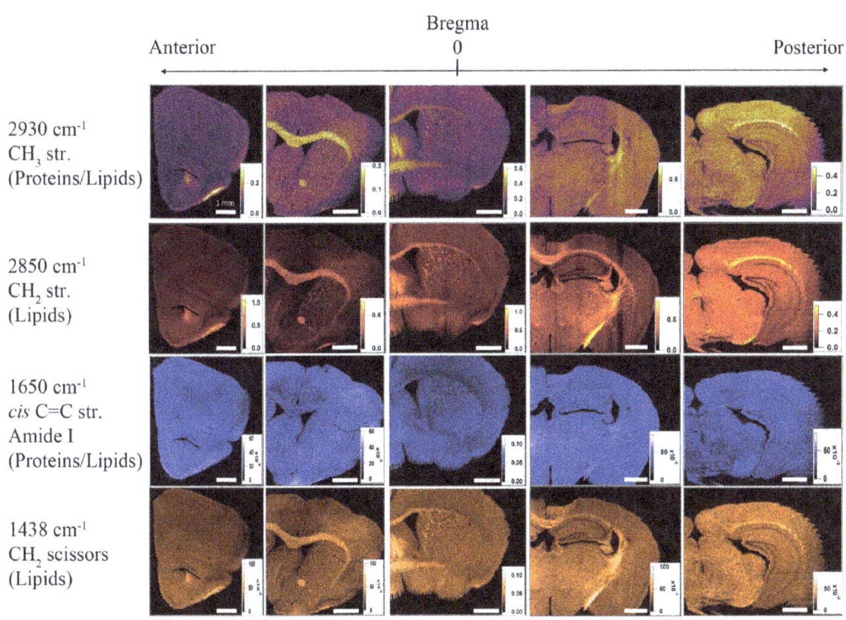

Figure 9.7. CARS microscopy for mouse brain showed molecular distribution throughout a brain. Each column represents each Raman band image from the anterior part of the brain (left) to the posterior (right). Scale bars are 1 mm. Reproduced from Ref. [131] with permission.

which allowed for visualization of the white matter due to the lipid-rich myelin sheath, similar to previous reports [128].

A recent study showed that CARS and another nonlinear optical process, THG, contrast differently in mice brain [132]. A combination of multiple nonlinear optical modalities, such as CARS, SHG, and THG, will complement each other for visualizing the brain structure and molecular profiles.

9.5.2.4 *CARS and Pathology*

Hyperspectral CARS is also used in pathological studies, particularly for malignant tumors. Because CARS imaging does not require fixation and staining, it is much faster than imaging with staining and is helpful for the rapid diagnosis of diseases. Here, we review the application of hyperspectral CARS in pathological samples.

Evans *et al.* demonstrated the brain structure and pathology imaging *ex vivo* [128] (Figure 9.6(a)). Since the brain myelin located in the oligodendrocyte sheaths coating the axonal bundles is lipid-rich, the CARS image at 2846 cm^{-1} provides excellent image contrast. Using fresh, unfixed *ex vivo* mouse brains, normal grey and white matter structures were identified on several scales to distinguish glioma from normal brain tissue and to clearly identify the tumor margin (Figure 9.6(b)). Camp *et al.* reported hyperspectral CARS images of healthy murine liver and pancreas tissues, as well as interfaces between xenograft brain tumors and the surrounding healthy brain matter [4]. Owing to the molecular fingerprint, a clear vibrational contrast is achieved for the nucleus, collagen, arterial wall, and lipid body.

Recently, hyperspectral CARS imaging has been combined with state-of-the-art deep/machine learning methods to determine the cancer boundary [133]. The authors used deep learning techniques to classify the data required for hyperspectral CARS. Another example is CARS imaging combined with generative adversarial networks (GAN). GAN was used to reconstruct conventional histopathological images, such as hematoxylin and eosin-stained images, using CARS images [134]. This decreases the pathologist's efforts because CARS images are complex, but GAN can reconstruct the CARS image into a pseudo-H&E image that is familiar to them.

Evidently, CARS imaging is advantageous in pathological studies; moreover, it is faster than conventional diagnostic imaging because it does not require fixation and staining.

9.5.2.5 *In Vivo CARS Imaging*

CARS is also applicable to *in vivo* imaging. In CARS microscopy, the signal photons are directly detected by photodetectors. This is a significant difference from SRS microscopy, which detects differences in the pump (or Stokes) light intensity modulated by the Stokes (or pump) light intensity. The photon detection scheme is advantageous for CARS microscopy in the backscattering configuration. To date, *in vivo* CARS imaging of skull cells [135], skin [136], adipose tissue [137], and zebrafish (*D. rerio*) [138] has been reported.

The endoscopic CARS apparatus has also been reported [139–143]. Lombardini *et al.* reported a flexible, compact CARS endoscope using a resonantly scanned hollow-core Kagome-lattice double-clad fiber [143]. Figure 9.8 shows an overview of the CARS endoscope and images of biological tissues. The femtosecond laser pulses can be delivered in a distortion-less manner. A combination of several lenses obtains a sub-micrometer spatial resolution over a large field of view of 320 mm. Endoscopic CARS as well as SHG and two-photon excitation fluorescence (TPEF) imaging of biological tissues, such as fresh fatty tissues, have been demonstrated at a rate of 0.8 frames per second. The endoscope visualizes lipids in the human colon (Figure 9.8(b)) and collagen fibers in rat tendons (Figure 9.8(c)). Moreover, the multimodal endoscope visualizes lipids and collagen simultaneously (Figure 9.8(d)). Yamato *et al.* developed a rigid CARS endoscope to visualize the peripheral nerves for nerve-sparing endoscopic surgery [113], wherein noise reduction was achieved using a deep learning method.

As shown here, *in vivo* CARS techniques benefit intraoperative diagnosis; for example, they can help determine the surgical margin for malignant tumors or spare intact nerves from the surrounding lesions.

9.5.2.6 *CARS and Environmental Science*

Finally, hyperspectral CARS can also be applied in environmental science, particularly for detecting microplastic pollution. The ingestion of marine microplastic debris by zooplankton in the ocean was visualized using CARS imaging [144]. Because microplastics provide a robust Raman band sufficiently quickly to distinguish the signal from a biological sample, hyperspectral CARS microscopy can help detect microplastic pollution. Figure 9.9 shows the CARS images of zooplankton. It can be observed that microplastics clumping in the posterior midgut were internalized

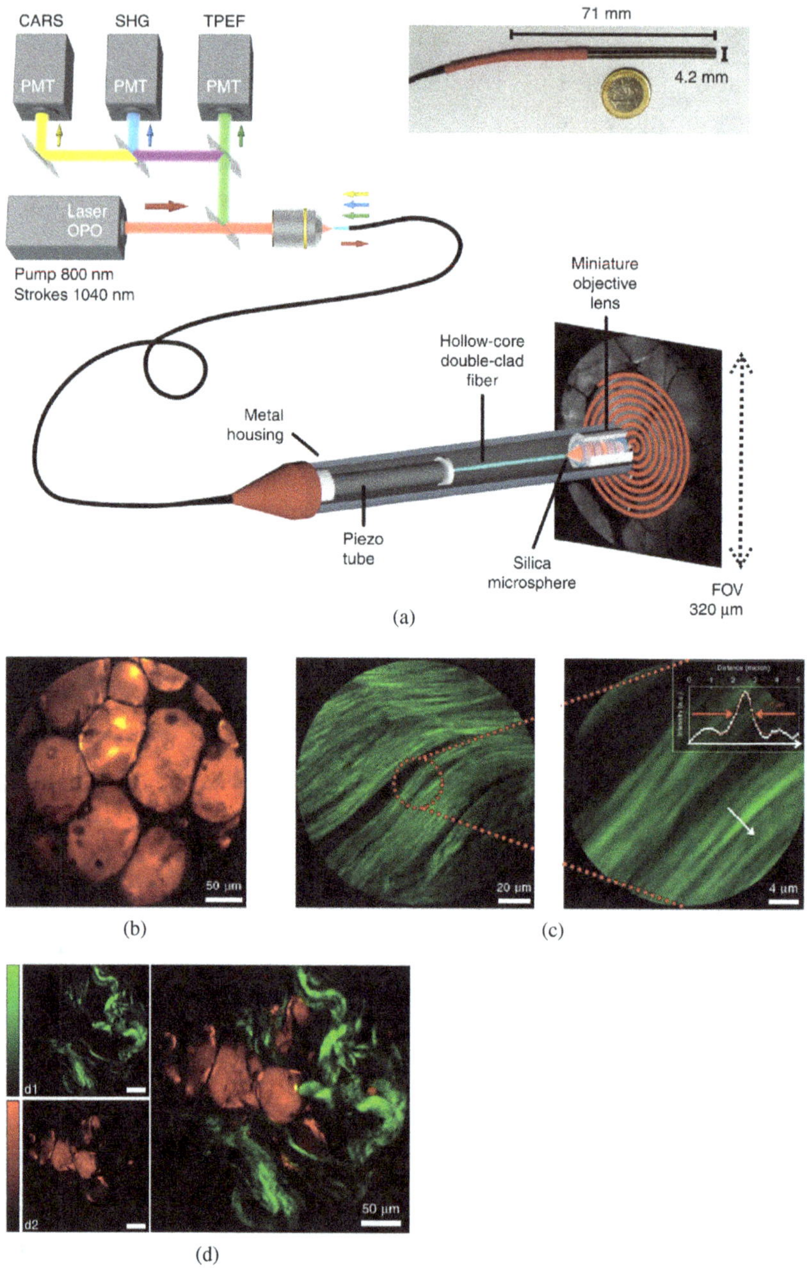

Figure 9.8. CARS, SHG, and TPEF endoscope visualize lipid content and collagen fibers. (a) Schematic of a multimodal endoscope. (b) CARS image of fresh fatty tissues in the human colon. (c) SHG image of collagen fibers in rat tendons. (d) Multimodal images of CARS and SHG in fresh human colon tissues below 50 mm from a sample surface. Reproduced from Ref. [143] with permission.

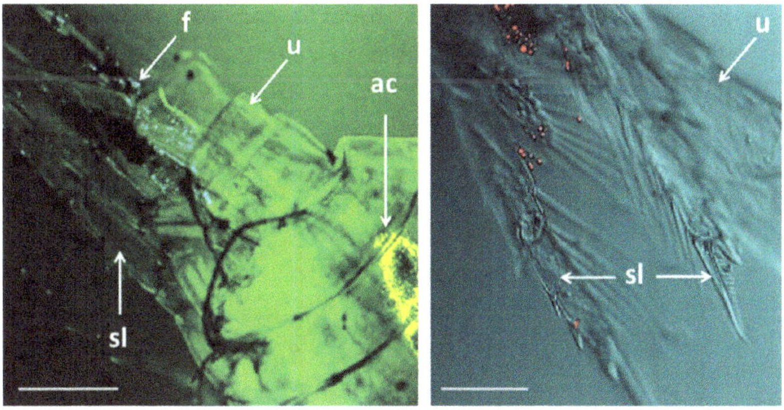

(a) (b)

Figure 9.9. CARS imaging revealed ingested microplastics in *Temora longicornis*. (a) Microplastics in the alimentary canal (ac, yellow particles) were visualized with CARS microscopy. Microplastics adhered to the urosome (u, blue particles), furca (f), and swimming legs (sl). (b) Microplastics were adhered to the swimming legs of *T. longicornis*. Scale bars are 50 mm. Adapted from Ref. [144] with permission.

(Figure 9.9(a); yellow dots). The images (Figures 9.9(a) and (b)) also showed microplastics adhering to the external appendages of the zooplankton. Polystyrene beads (0.4–3.8 μm) were found to be accumulated between the filamentous hairs on appendages, including the furca (Figure 9.9(a); blue dots), rear swimming legs (Figure 9.9(b); red dots), antennules, and between the segments of the carapace, particularly around the urosome and swimming legs. Using CARS microscopy, it may soon be possible to analyze and diagnose the function and health of living animals directly in the sea.

9.6 Summary

CARS microscopy is a versatile technique that can visualize various molecules by their vibrational modes. The CARS signal depends on vibrational modes, which in turn depend on the chemical bonds in a sample. Recent development of laser light sources allows high-speed and comprehensive spectral coverage of CARS microscopy. A higher imaging speed decreases the photodamage of the samples and further enables the live imaging of organisms. Increased spectral coverage enables obtaining Raman signals ranging from 600–3500 cm^{-1}. The state-of-the-art multiplex CARS can provide a detailed characterization of water, lipids, proteins, and DNA/RNA at high speed.

Recent CARS microscopy allows for the sensitive detection of molecular vibrational signatures of cells and tissues, thereby expanding its applications to label-free imaging, metabolic imaging, and ultra-multiplex imaging. Although challenges remain for imaging speed and apparatus miniaturization, CARS spectroscopic imaging has wide applications in cell biology, neuroscience, pathology, and environmental biology. We foresee promising outcomes that can be applied more effectively for a wider range of potential applications in these fields.

References

1. Freudiger, C. W., Min, W., Saar, B. G., Lu, S., Holtom, G. R., He, C. W., Tsai, J. C., Kang, J. X., Xie, X. S. (2008) Label-free biomedical imaging with high sensitivity by stimulated Raman scattering microscopy. Science **322**, 1857–1861.
2. Nandakumar, P., Kovalev, A., Volkmer, A. (2009) Vibrational imaging based on stimulated Raman scattering microscopy. New J. Phys. **11**, 033026.
3. Ozeki, Y., Dake, F., Kajiyama, S. i., Fukui, K., Itoh, K. (2009) Analysis and experimental assessment of the sensitivity of stimulated Raman scattering microscopy. Opt. Express **17**, 3651–3658.
4. Camp, C. H., Jr., Lee, Y. J., Heddleston, J. M., Hartshorn, C. M., Hight Walker, A. R., Rich, J. N., Lathia, J. D., Cicerone, M. T. (2014) High-speed coherent Raman fingerprint imaging of biological tissues. Nat. Photonics **8**, 627–634.
5. Ozeki, Y., Umemura, W., Otsuka, Y., Satoh, S., Hashimoto, H., Sumimura, K., Nishizawa, N., Fukui, K., Itoh, K. (2012) High-speed molecular spectral imaging of tissue with stimulated Raman scattering. Nat. Photonics **6**, 845–851.
6. Zhang, D. L., Wang, P., Slipchenko, M. N., Ben–Amotz, D., Weiner, A. M., Cheng, J. X. (2013) Quantitative vibrational imaging by hyperspectral stimulated Raman scattering microscopy and multivariate curve resolution analysis. Anal. Chem. **85**, 98–106.
7. Kong, L., Ji, M., Holtom, G. R., Fu, D., Freudiger, C. W., Xie, X. S. (2013) Multicolor stimulated Raman scattering microscopy with a rapidly tunable optical parametric oscillator. Opt. Lett. **38**, 145–147.
8. J.-X. Cheng, W. Min, Y. Ozeki, D. Polli (2022) *Stimulated Raman Scattering Microscopy: Techniques and Applications.* Elsevier.
9. Hashimoto, M. (2002) Coherent anti-Stokes Raman scattering microscopy. Acta Histochem. Cytoc. **35**, 83–86.
10. Cheng, J. X., Xie, X. S. (2004) Coherent anti-Stokes Raman scattering microscopy: Instrumentation, theory, and applications. J. Phys. Chem. B **108**, 827–840.

11. Volkmer, A. (2005) Vibrational imaging and microspectroscopies based on coherent anti-Stokes Raman scattering microscopy. J. Phys. D Appl. Phys. **38**, R59–R81.
12. Djaker, N., Lenne, P. F., Marguet, D., Colonna, A., Hadjur, C., Rigneault, H. (2007) Coherent anti-Stokes Raman scattering microscopy (CARS): Instrumentation and applications. Nucl. Instrum. Meth. A **571**, 177–181.
13. Muller, M., Zumbusch, A. (2007) Coherent anti-stokes Raman scattering microscopy. ChemPhysChem **8**, 2156–2170.
14. Volkmer, A., Radi, P. P., Zheltikov, A. M., Zumbusch, A. (2009) New trends and recent advances in coherent Raman microscopy and nonlinear optical spectroscopy: introduction to the special issue. J. Raman Spectrosc. **40**, 712–713.
15. Le, T. T., Yue, S. H., Cheng, J. X. (2010) Shedding new light on lipid biology with coherent anti-Stokes Raman scattering microscopy. J. Lipid Res. **51**, 3091–3102.
16. El-Diasty, F. (2011) Coherent anti-Stokes Raman scattering: Spectroscopy and microscopy. Vib. Spectrosc. **55**, 1–37.
17. Krafft, C., Dietzek, B., Schmitt, M., Popp, J. (2012) Raman and coherent anti-Stokes Raman scattering microspectroscopy for biomedical applications. J. Biomed. Opt. **17**, 040801.
18. Chung, C. Y., Boik, J., Potma, E. O. (2013) Biomolecular imaging with coherent nonlinear vibrational microscopy. Annu. Rev. Phys. Chem. **64**, 77–99.
19. Tu, H., Boppart, S. A. (2014) Coherent anti-Stokes Raman scattering microscopy: overcoming technical barriers for clinical translation. J. Biophotonics **7**, 9–22.
20. Zhang, D., Wang, P., Slipchenko, M. N., Cheng, J.-X. (2014) Fast vibrational imaging of single cells and tissues by stimulated Raman scattering microscopy. Acc. Chem. Res. **47**, 2282–2290.
21. Camp Jr, C. H., Cicerone, M. T. (2015) Chemically sensitive bioimaging with coherent Raman scattering. Nat. Photonics **9**, 295.
22. Cheng, J. X., Xie, X. S. (2015) Vibrational spectroscopic imaging of living systems: An emerging platform for biology and medicine. Science **350**, aaa8870.
23. Winterhalder, M. J., Zumbusch, A. (2015) Beyond the borders--Biomedical applications of non-linear Raman microscopy. Adv. Drug Deliv. Rev. **89**, 135–144.
24. Kano, H., Segawa, H., Okuno, M., Leproux, P., Couderc, V. (2016) Hyperspectral coherent Raman imaging — principle, theory, instrumentation, and applications to life sciences. J. Raman Spectrosc. **47**, 116–123.
25. Moura, C. C., Tare, R. S., Oreffo, R. O., Mahajan, S. (2016) Raman spectroscopy and coherent anti-Stokes Raman scattering imaging: prospective tools for monitoring skeletal cells and skeletal regeneration. J. Royal Soc. Interface **13**, 20160182.
26. Cicerone, M. T., Camp, C. H. (2017) Histological coherent Raman imaging: a prognostic review. Analyst **143**, 33–59.
27. Polli, D., Kumar, V., Valensise, C. M., Marangoni, M., Cerullo, G. (2018) Broadband coherent Raman scattering microscopy. Laser Photonics Rev. **12**, 1800020.

28. Hu, F., Shi, L., Min, W. (2019) Biological imaging of chemical bonds by stimulated Raman scattering microscopy. Nat. Methods **16**, 830–842.
29. Evans, C. L., Xie, X. S. (2008) Coherent anti-Stokes Raman scattering microscopy: chemical imaging for biology and medicine. Annu. Rev. Anal. Chem. **1**, 883–909
30. Min, W., Freudiger, C. W., Lu, S. J., Xie, X. S. (2011) Coherent nonlinear optical imaging: beyond fluorescence microscopy. Annu. Rev. Phys. Chem. **62**, 507–530.
31. Cicerone, M. (2016) Molecular imaging with CARS micro-spectroscopy. Curr. Opin. Chem. Biol. **33**, 179–185.
32. Rigneault, H., Berto, P. (2018) Tutorial: Coherent Raman light matter interaction processes. APL Photonics **3**, 091101.
33. Saar, B. G., Freudiger, C. W., Reichman, J., Stanley, C. M., Holtom, G. R., Xie, X. S. (2010) Video-rate molecular imaging in vivo with stimulated Raman scattering. Science **330**, 1368–1370.
34. Abedin, S., Roy, K., Jin, X., Xia, H., Brueck, S. R. J., Potma, E. O. (2022) Surface-enhanced coherent anti-Stokes Raman scattering of molecules near metal–dielectric nanojunctions. J. Phys. Chem. C **126**, 8760–8767.
35. Zhang, Y., Zhen, Y. R., Neumann, O., Day, J. K., Nordlander, P., Halas, N. J. (2014) Coherent anti-Stokes Raman scattering with single-molecule sensitivity using a plasmonic Fano resonance. Nat. Commun. **5**, 4424.
36. Liang, E. J., Weippert, A., Funk, J. M., Materny, A., Kiefer, W. (1994) Experimental observation of surface-enhanced coherent anti-Stokes Raman scattering. Chem. Phys. Lett. **227**, 115–120.
37. Koo, T.-W., Chan, S., Berlin, A. A. (2005) Single-molecule detection of biomolecules by surface-enhanced coherent anti-Stokes Raman scattering. Opt. Lett. **30**, 1024–1026.
38. Duncan, M. D., Reintjes, J., Manuccia, T. J. (1982) Scanning coherent anti-Stokes Raman microscope. Opt. Lett. **7**, 350–350.
39. Zumbusch, A., Holtom, G. R., Xie, X. S. (1999) Three-dimensional vibrational imaging by coherent anti-Stokes Raman scattering. Phys. Rev. Lett. **82**, 4142–4145
40. Hashimoto, M., Araki, T., Kawata, S. (2000) Molecular vibration imaging in the fingerprint region by use of coherent anti-Stokes Raman scattering microscopy with a collinear configuration. Opt. Lett. **25**, 1768–1770.
41. Cheng, J. X., Volkmer, A., Xie, X. S. (2002) Theoretical and experimental characterization of coherent anti-Stokes Raman scattering microscopy. J. Opt. Soc. Am. B **19**, 1363–1375.
42. Marx, C. A., Harbola, U., Mukamel, S. (2008) Nonlinear optical spectroscopy of single, few, and many molecules: Nonequilibrium Green's function QED approach. Phys. Rev. A **77**, 022110.
43. Petrov, G. I., Arora, R., Yakovlev, V. V., Wang, X., Sokolov, A. V., Scully, M. O. (2007) Comparison of coherent and spontaneous Raman microspectroscopies for noninvasive detection of single bacterial endospores. Proc. Natl. Acad. Sci. **104**, 7776–7779.

44. Pestov, D., Ariunbold, G. O., Wang, X., Murawski, R. K., Sautenkov, V. A., Sokolov, A. V., Scully, M. O. (2007) Coherent versus incoherent Raman scattering: molecular coherence excitation and measurement. Opt. Lett. **32**, 1725–1727.
45. Cheng, J. X., Book, L. D., Xie, X. S. (2001) Polarization coherent anti-Stokes Raman scattering microscopy. Opt. Lett. **26**, 1341–1343.
46. Volkmer, A., Book, L. D., Xie, X. S. (2002) Time-resolved coherent anti-Stokes Raman scattering microscopy: Imaging based on Raman free induction decay. Appl. Phys. Lett. **80**, 1505–1507.
47. Cheng, J. X., Volkmer, A., Book, L. D., Xie, X. S. (2001) An epi-detected coherent anti-Stokes Raman scattering (E-CARS) microscope with high spectral resolution and high sensitivity. J. Phys. Chem. B **105**, 1277–1280.
48. Cheng, J. X., Jia, Y. K., Zheng, G. F., Xie, X. S. (2002) Laser-scanning coherent anti-Stokes Raman scattering microscopy and applications to cell biology. Biophys. J. **83**, 502–509.
49. Wurpel, G. W. H., Schins, J. M., Muller, M. (2002) Chemical specificity in three-dimensional imaging with multiplex coherent anti-Stokes Raman scattering microscopy. Opt. Lett. **27**, 1093–1095.
50. Evans, C. L., Potma, E. O., Puoris'haag, M., Cote, D., Lin, C. P., Xie, X. S. (2005) Chemical imaging of tissue in vivo with video-rate coherent anti-Stokes Raman scattering microscopy. Proc. Natl. Acad. Sci. USA **102**, 16807–16812.
51. Ganikhanov, F., Carrasco, S., Xie, X. S., Katz, M., Seitz, W., Kopf, D. (2006) Broadly tunable dual-wavelength light source for coherent anti-Stokes Raman scattering microscopy. Opt. Lett. **31**, 1292–1294.
52. Cheng, J.-X. and Xie, S. X. (2012) *Coherent Raman Scattering Microscopy.* CRC Press.
53. Dudovich, N., Oron, D., Silberberg, Y. (2002) Single-pulse coherently controlled nonlinear Raman spectroscopy and microscopy. Nature **418**, 512–514.
54. Ichimura, T., Hayazawa, N., Hashimoto, M., Inouye, Y., Kawata, S. (2004) Tip-enhanced coherent anti-Stokes Raman scattering for vibrational nanoimaging. Phys. Rev. Lett. **92**, 220801.
55. Schaller, R. D., Ziegelbauer, J., Lee, L. F., Haber, L. H., Saykally, R. J. (2002) Chemically selective imaging of subcellular structure in human hepatocytes with coherent anti-Stokes Raman scattering (CARS) near-field scanning optical microscopy (NSOM). J. Phys. Chem. B **106**, 8489–8492.
56. Jones, D. J., Potma, E. O., Cheng, J. X., Burfeindt, B., Pang, Y., Ye, J., Xie, X. S. (2002) Synchronization of two passively mode-locked, picosecond lasers within 20 fs for coherent anti-Stokes Raman scattering microscopy. Rev. Sci. Instrum. **73**, 2843–2848.
57. Potma, E. O., Jones, D. J., Cheng, J. X., Xie, X. S., Ye, J. (2002) High-sensitivity coherent anti-Stokes Raman scattering microscopy with two tightly synchronized picosecond lasers. Opt. Lett. **27**, 1168–1170.
58. Jurna, M., Korterik, J. P., Offerhaus, H. L., Otto, C. (2006) Noncritical phase-matched lithium triborate optical parametric oscillator for high resolution

coherent anti-Stokes Raman scattering spectroscopy and microscopy. Appl. Phys. Lett. **89**, 251116.

59. Kieu, K., Saar, B. G., Holtom, G. R., Xie, X. S., Wise, F. W. (2009) High-power picosecond fiber source for coherent Raman microscopy. Opt. Lett. **34**, 2051–2053.
60. Lefrancois, S., Fu, D., Holtom, G. R., Kong, L. J., Wadsworth, W. J., Schneider, P., Herda, R., Zach, A., Xie, X. S., Wise, F. W. (2012) Fiber four-wave mixing source for coherent anti-Stokes Raman scattering microscopy. Opt. Lett. **37**, 1652–1654.
61. Coluccelli, N., Kumar, V., Cassinerio, M., Galzerano, G., Marangoni, M., Cerullo, G. (2014) Er/Tm:fiber laser system for coherent Raman microscopy. Opt. Lett. **39**, 3090–3093.
62. Freudiger, C. W., Yang, W. L., Holtom, G. R., Peyghambarian, N., Xie, X. S., Kieu, K. Q. (2014) Stimulated Raman scattering microscopy with a robust fibre laser source. Nat. Photonics **8**, 153–159.
63. Lamb, E. S., Lefrancois, S., Ji, M. B., Wadsworth, W. J., Xie, X. S., Wise, F. W. (2013) Fiber optical parametric oscillator for coherent anti-Stokes Raman scattering microscopy. Opt. Lett. **38**, 4154–4157.
64. Steinle, T., Kumar, V., Floess, M., Steinmann, A., Marangoni, M., Koch, C., Wege, C., Cerullo, G., Giessen, H. (2016) Synchronization-free all-solid-state laser system for stimulated Raman scattering microscopy. Light Sci. Appl. **5**, e16149-e16149.
65. Wang, K., Zhang, D., Charan, K., Slipchenko, M. N., Wang, P., Xu, C., Cheng, J.-X. (2013) Time-lens based hyperspectral stimulated Raman scattering imaging and quantitative spectral analysis. J. Biophotonics **6**, 815–820.
66. Karpf, S., Eibl, M., Wieser, W., Klein, T., Huber, R. (2015) A time-encoded technique for fibre-based hyperspectral broadband stimulated Raman microscopy. Nat. Commun. **6**, 6784.
67. Nose, K., Ozeki, Y., Kishi, T., Sumimura, K., Nishizawa, N., Fukui, K., Kanematsu, Y., Itoh, K. (2012) Sensitivity enhancement of fiber-laser-based stimulated Raman scattering microscopy by collinear balanced detection technique. Opt. Express **20**, 13958–13965.
68. Nose, K., Kishi, T., Ozeki, Y., Kanematsu, Y., Takata, H., Fukui, K., Takai, Y., Itoh, K. (2014) Stimulated Raman spectral microscope using synchronized Er- and Yb-fiber lasers. Jpn. J. Appl. Phys. **53**, 052401.
69. Seto, K., Tsukada, T., Okuda, Y., Tokunaga, E., Kobayashi, T. (2014) Development of a balanced detector with biased synchronous detection and application to near shot noise limited noise cancelling of supercontinuum pulse light. Rev. Sci. Instrum. **85**, 023702.
70. Crisafi, F., Kumar, V., Scopigno, T., Marangoni, M., Cerullo, G., Polli, D. (2017) In-line balanced detection stimulated Raman scattering microscopy. Sci. Rep. **7**, 10745

71. Kumar, V., Casella, M., Molotokaite, E., Gatti, D., Kukura, P., Manzoni, C., Polli, D., Marangoni, M., Cerullo, G. (2012) Balanced-detection Raman-induced Kerr-effect spectroscopy. Phys. Rev. A **86**, 053810.
72. Wuerthwein, T., Brinkmann, M., Hellwig, T., Wallmeier, K., Fallnich, C. (2021) High-sensitivity frequency modulation CARS with a compact and fast tunable fiber-based light source. Opt. Lett. **46**, 3544–3547.
73. Ozeki, Y., Umemura, W., Sumimura, K., Nishizawa, N., Fukui, K., Itoh, K. (2012) Stimulated Raman hyperspectral imaging based on spectral filtering of broadband fiber laser pulses. Opt. Lett. **37**, 431–433.
74. Fu, D., Lu, F. K., Zhang, X., Freudiger, C., Pernik, D. R., Holtom, G., Xie, X. S. (2012) Quantitative chemical imaging with multiplex stimulated Raman scattering microscopy. J. Am. Chem. Soc. **134**, 3623–3626.
75. Hellerer, T., Enejder, A. M. K., Zumbusch, A. (2004) Spectral focusing: High spectral resolution spectroscopy with broad-bandwidth laser pulses. Appl. Phys. Lett. **85**, 25–27.
76. Brückner, L., Buckup, T., Motzkus, M. (2016) Exploring the potential of tailored spectral focusing. J. Opt. Soc. Am. B **33**, 1482–1491.
77. Ogilvie, J. P., Beaurepaire, E., Alexandrou, A., Joffre, M. (2006) Fourier-transform coherent anti-Stokes Raman scattering microscopy. Opt. Lett. **31**, 480–482.
78. Hiramatsu, K., Luo, Y., Ideguchi, T., Goda, K. (2017) Rapid-scan Fourier-transform coherent anti-Stokes Raman scattering spectroscopy with heterodyne detection. Opt. Lett. **42**, 4335–4338.
79. Chen, J. X., Volkmer, A., Book, L. D., Xie, X. S. (2002) Multiplex coherent anti-stokes Raman scattering microspectroscopy and study of lipid vesicles. J. Phys. Chem. B **106**, 8493–8498.
80. Muller, M., Schins, J. M. (2002) Imaging the thermodynamic state of lipid membranes with multiplex CARS microscopy. J. Phys. Chem. B **106**, 3715–3723.
81. Kee, T. W., Cicerone, M. T. (2004) Simple approach to one-laser, broadband coherent anti-Stokes Raman scattering microscopy. Opt. Lett. **29**, 2701–2703.
82. Kano, H., Hamaguchi, H. (2005) Ultrabroadband (>2500 cm(−1)) multiplex coherent anti-Stokes Raman scattering microspectroscopy using a supercontinuum generated from a photonic crystal fiber. Appl. Phys. Lett. **86**, 121113.
83. Petrov, G. I., Yakovlev, V. V. (2005) Enhancing red-shifted white-light continuum generation in optical fibers for applications in nonlinear Raman microscopy. Opt. Express **13**, 1299–1306.
84. Bégin, S., Burgoyne, B., Mercier, V., Villeneuve, A., Vallée, R., Côté, D. (2011) Coherent anti-Stokes Raman scattering hyperspectral tissue imaging with a wavelength-swept system. Biomed. Opt. Express **2**, 1296–1306.
85. Qin, Y., Cromey, B., Batjargal, O., Kieu, K. (2021) All-fiber single-cavity dual-comb for coherent anti-Stokes Raman scattering spectroscopy based on spectral focusing. Opt. Lett. **46**, 146–149.

86. Hashimoto, K., Takahashi, M., Ideguchi, T., Goda, K. (2016) Broadband coherent Raman spectroscopy running at 24,000 spectra per second. Sci. Rep. **6**, 21036.
87. Ideguchi, T., Holzner, S., Bernhardt, B., Guelachvili, G., Picque, N., Hansch, T. W. (2013) Coherent Raman spectro-imaging with laser frequency combs. Nature **502**, 355–358.
88. Cheng, J. X., Volkmer, A., Book, L. D., Xie, X. S. (2002) Multiplex coherent anti-Stokes Raman scattering microspectroscopy and study of lipid vesicles. J. Phys. Chem. B **106**, 8493–8498.
89. Okuno, M., Kano, H., Leproux, P., Couderc, V., Day, J. P. R., Bonn, M., Hamaguchi, H. (2010) Quantitative CARS molecular fingerprinting of single living cells with the use of the maximum entropy method. Angew. Chem. Int. Ed. **49**, 6773–6777.
90. Isobe, K., Suda, A., Tanaka, M., Hashimoto, H., Kannari, F., Kawano, H., Mizuno, H., Miyawaki, A., Midorikawa, K. (2009) Single-pulse coherent anti-Stokes Raman scattering microscopy employing an octave spanning pulse. Opt. Express **17**, 11259–11266.
91. Okuno, M., Kano, H., Leproux, P., Couderc, V., Hamaguchi, H. (2007) Ultrabroadband (>2000 cm(−1)) multiplex coherent anti-Stokes Raman scattering spectroscopy using a subnanosecond supercontinuum light source. Opt. Lett. **32**, 3050–3052.
92. Yoneyama, H., Sudo, K., Leproux, P., Couderc, V., Inoko, A., Kano, H. (2018) CARS molecular fingerprinting using sub-100-ps microchip laser source with fiber amplifier. APL Photonics **3**, 092408.
93. Kano, H., Maruyama, T., Kano, J., Oka, Y., Kaneta, D., Guerenne, T., Leproux, P., Couderc, V., Noguchi, M. (2019) Ultra-multiplex CARS spectroscopic imaging with 1-millisecond pixel dwell time. OSA Continuum **2**, 1693–1705.
94. Evans, C. L., Potma, E. O., Xie, X. S. (2004) Coherent anti-Stokes Raman scattering spectral interferometry: determination of the real and imaginary components of nonlinear susceptibility $\chi(3)$ for vibrational microscopy. Opt. Lett. **29**, 2923–2925.
95. Hellwarth, R. W. (1977) Third-order optical susceptibilities of liquids and solids. Prog. Quantum. Electron. **5**, 1–68.
96. Vartiainen, E. M., Rinia, H. A., Müller, M., Bonn, M. (2006) Direct extraction of Raman line-shapes from congested CARS spectra. Opt. Express **14**, 3622–3630.
97. Liu, Y. X., Lee, Y. J., Cicerone, M. T. (2009) Broadband CARS spectral phase retrieval using a time-domain Kramers-Kronig transform. Opt. Lett. **34**, 1363–1365.
98. Karuna, A., Masia, F., Wiltshire, M., Errington, R., Borri, P., Langbein, W. (2019) Label-free volumetric quantitative imaging of the human somatic cell division by hyperspectral coherent anti-Stokes Raman scattering. Anal. Chem. **91**, 2813–2821.

99. Valensise, C. M., Giuseppi, A., Vernuccio, F., Cadena, A. D. l., Cerullo, G., Polli, D. (2020) Removing non-resonant background from CARS spectra via deep learning. APL Photonics **5**, 061305.
100. Houhou, R., Barman, P., Schmitt, M., Meyer, T., Popp, J., Bocklitz, T. W. (2020) Deep learning as phase retrieval tool for CARS spectra. Opt. Express **28**, 21002–21024.
101. Wang, Z., O'Dwyer, K., Muddiman, R., Ward, T., Camp, C. H., Hennelly, B. M. (2022) VECTOR: Very deep convolutional autoencoders for non-resonant background removal in broadband coherent anti-Stokes Raman scattering. J. Raman Spectrosc. **53**, 1081–1093.
102. Shimanouchi, T. (1977) Tables of molecular vibrational frequencies. Consolidated volume II. J. Phys. Chem. Ref. Data **6**, 993–1102.
103. Matthews, Q., Brolo, A., Lum, J., Duan, X., Jirasek, A. (2011) Raman spectroscopy of single human tumour cells exposed to ionizing radiation in vitro. Phys. Med. Biol. **56**, 19–38.
104. Krafft, C., Neudert, L., Simat, T., Salzer, R. (2005) Near infrared Raman spectra of human brain lipids. Spectrochim. Acta A **61**, 1529–1535.
105. Barry, B. W., Edwards, H. G. M., Williams, A. C. (1992) Fourier transform Raman and infrared vibrational study of human skin: Assignment of spectral bands. J. Raman Spectrosc. **23**, 641–645.
106. Deng, H., Bloomfield, V. A., Benevides, J. M., Thomas, G. J. (1999) Dependence of the Raman signature of genomic B-DNA on nucleotide base sequence. Biopolymers **50**, 656–666.
107. Snyder, R. G., Strauss, H. L., Elliger, C. A. (1982) Carbon-hydrogen stretching modes and the structure of n-alkyl chains. 1. Long, disordered chains. J. Phys. Chem. **86**, 5145–5150.
108. Snyder, R. G., Scherer, J. R. (1979) Band structure in the C–H stretching region of the Raman spectrum of the extended polymethylene chain: Influence of Fermi resonance. J. Chem. Phys. **71**, 3221–3228.
109. Brown, K. G., Bicknell-Brown, E., Ladjadj, M. (1987) Raman-active bands sensitive to motion and conformation at the chain termini and backbones of alkanes and lipids. J. Phys. Chem. **91**, 3436–3442.
110. Nan, X., Cheng, J. X., Xie, X. S. (2003) Vibrational imaging of lipid droplets in live fibroblast cells with coherent anti-Stokes Raman scattering microscopy. J. Lipid Res. **44**, 2202–2208.
111. Hellerer, T., Axäng, C., Brackmann, C., Hillertz, P., Pilon, M., Enejder, A. (2007) Monitoring of lipid storage in Caenorhabditis elegans using coherent anti-Stokes Raman scattering (CARS) microscopy. Proc. Natl. Acad. Sci. **104**, 14658–14663.
112. Yen, K., Le, T. T., Bansal, A., Narasimhan, S. D., Cheng, J.-X., Tissenbaum, H. A. (2010) A comparative study of fat storage quantitation in nematode Caenorhabditis elegans using label and label-free methods. PLOS One **5**, e12810.

113. Yamato, N., Niioka, H., Miyake, J., Hashimoto, M. (2020) Improvement of nerve imaging speed with coherent anti-Stokes Raman scattering rigid endoscope using deep-learning noise reduction. Sci. Rep. **10**, 15212.
114. Fu, Y., Sun, W., Shi, Y., Shi, R., Cheng, J.-X. (2009) Glutamate excitotoxicity inflicts paranodal myelin splitting and retraction. PLOS One **4**, e6705.
115. Takei, Y., Hirai, R., Fukuda, A., Miyazaki, S., Shimada, R., Okamatsu-Ogura, Y., Saito, M., Leproux, P., Hisatake, K., Kano, H. (2021) Visualization of intracellular lipid metabolism in brown adipocytes by time-lapse ultra-multiplex CARS microspectroscopy with an onstage incubator. J. Chem. Phys. **155**, 125102.
116. Rinia, H. A., Burger, K. N. J., Bonn, M., Müller, M. (2008) Quantitative label-free imaging of lipid composition and packing of individual cellular lipid droplets using multiplex CARS microscopy. Biophys. J. **95**, 4908–4914.
117. Bito, K., Okuno, M., Kano, H., Tokuhara, S., Naito, S., Masukawa, Y., Leproux, P., Couderc, V., Hamaguchi, H. (2012) Protein secondary structure imaging with ultrabroadband multiplex coherent anti-Stokes Raman scattering (CARS) microspectroscopy. J. Phys. Chem. B **116**, 1452–1457.
118. Chikishev, A. Y., Lucassen, G., Koroteev, N., Otto, C., Greve, J. (1992) Polarization sensitive coherent anti-Stokes Raman scattering spectroscopy of the amide I band of proteins in solutions. Biophys. J. **63**, 976–985.
119. Cheng, J.-X., Volkmer, A., Book, L. D., Xie, X. S. (2002) Multiplex coherent anti-Stokes Raman scattering microspectroscopy and study of lipid vesicles. J. Phys. Chem. B **106**, 8493–8498.
120. Parekh, S. H., Lee, Y. J., Aamer, K. A., Cicerone, M. T. (2010) Label-free cellular imaging by broadband coherent anti-Stokes Raman scattering microscopy. Biophys. J. **99**, 2695–2704.
121. Wurpel, G. W. H., Schins, J. M., Müller, M. (2002) Chemical specificity in three-dimensional imaging with multiplex coherent anti-Stokes Raman scattering microscopy. Opt. Lett. **27**, 1093–1095.
122. Okuno, M., Kano, H., Leproux, P., Couderc, V., Hamaguchi, H. (2008) Ultrabroadband multiplex CARS microspectroscopy and imaging using a subnanosecond supercontinuum light source in the deep near infrared. Opt. Lett. **33**, 923–925.
123. Heinrich, C., Hofer, A., Ritsch, A., Ciardi, C., Bernet, S., Ritsch-Marte, M. (2008) Selective imaging of saturated and unsaturated lipids by wide-field CARS-microscopy. Opt. Express **16**, 2699.
124. Davies, J. E. D., Hodge, P., Gunstone, F. D., Lie Ken Jie, M. S. F. (1975) Raman studies of some diunsaturated olefinic and acetylenic fatty acids and their derivatives. Chem. Phys. Lipids **15**, 48–52.
125. Oka, Y., Yoshida, M., Minoda, A., Leproux, P., Watanabe, M. M., Kano, H. (2021) Label-free detection of polysulfides and glycogen of Cyanidium caldarium using ultra-multiplex coherent anti-Stokes Raman scattering microspectroscopy. J. Raman Spectrosc. **52**, 2572–2580.

126. Chen, W.-W., Lemieux, G. A., Camp, C. H., Chang, T.-C., Ashrafi, K., Cicerone, M. T. (2020) Spectroscopic coherent Raman imaging of Caenorhabditis elegans reveals lipid particle diversity. Nat. Chem. Biol. **16**, 1087–1095.
127. Miyazaki, S., Leproux, P., Couderc, V., Hayashi, Y., Kano, H. (2020) Multimodal nonlinear optical imaging of Caenorhabditis elegans with multiplex coherent anti-Stokes Raman scattering, third-harmonic generation, second-harmonic generation, and two-photon excitation fluorescence. Appl. Phys. Express **13**, 072002.
128. Evans, C. L., Xu, X., Kesari, S., Xie, X. S., Wong, S. T. C., Young, G. S. (2007) Chemically-selective imaging of brain structures with CARS microscopy. Opt. Express **15**, 12076.
129. Fu, Y., Huff, T. B., Wang, H.-W., Cheng, J.-X., Wang, H. (2008) Ex vivo and in vivo imaging of myelin fibers in mouse brain by coherent anti-Stokes Raman scattering microscopy. Opt. Express **16**, 19396.
130. Camp Jr, C. H., Lee, Y. J., Heddleston, J. M., Hartshorn, C. M., Walker, A. R. H., Rich, J. N., Lathia, J. D., Cicerone, M. T. (2014) High-speed coherent Raman fingerprint imaging of biological tissues. Nat. Photonics **8**, 627–634.
131. Murakami, Y., Miyazaki, S., Boildieu, D., Rajaofara, Z., Helbert, D., Magnaudeix, A., Carré, P., Leproux, P., Honjoh, S., Kano, H. (2022) Toward whole brain label-free molecular imaging with single-cell resolution sing ultra-broadband multiplex CARS microspectroscopy. https://hal.science/hal-03531147/.
132. Abdeladim, L., Matho, K. S., Clavreul, S., Mahou, P., Sintes, J.-M., Solinas, X., Arganda-Carreras, I., Turney, S. G., Lichtman, J. W., Chessel, A., Bemelmans, A.-P., Loulier, K., Supatto, W., Livet, J., Beaurepaire, E. (2019) Multicolor multiscale brain imaging with chromatic multiphoton serial microscopy. Nat. Commun. **10**, 1662.
133. Li, J. S., Liu, J., Wang, Y., He, Y. J., Liu, K., Raghunathan, R., Shen, S. S., He, T. C., Yu, X. H., Danforth, R., Zheng, F. B., Zhao, H., Wong, S. T. C. (2021) Artificial intelligence-augmented, label-free molecular imaging method for tissue identification, cancer diagnosis, and cancer margin detection. Biomed. Opt. Express **12**, 5559–5582.
134. He, Y. J., Li, J. S., Shen, S., Liu, K., Wong, K. K., He, T. C., Wong, S. T. C. (2022) Image-to-image translation of label-free molecular vibrational images for a histopathological review using the UNet plus /seg-cGAN model. Biomed. Opt. Express **13**, 1924–1938.
135. Capitaine, E., Moussa, N. O., Louot, C., Bardet, S. M., Kano, H., Duponchel, L., Leveque, P., Couderc, V., Leproux, P. (2018) Fast epi-detected broadband multiplex CARS and SHG imaging of mouse skull cells. Biomed. Opt. Express **9**, 245–253.
136. Andreana, M., Le, T., Hansen, A., Verhoef, A., Jensen, O., Andersen, P., Slezak, P., Drexler, W., Fernández, A., Unterhuber, A. (2017) Epi-detecting label-free multimodal imaging platform using a compact diode-pumped femtosecond solid-state laser. J. Biomed. Opt. **22**, 091517.

137. Xu, D. Y., Liang, S. J., Xu, L., Bourdakos, K. N., Johnson, P., Read, J., Price, J. H. V., Mahajan, S., Richardson, D. J. (2021) Widely-tunable synchronisation-free picosecond laser source for multimodal CARS, SHG, and two-photon microscopy. Biomed. Opt. Express **12**, 1010–1019.
138. Andreana, M., Sturtzel, C., Spielvogel, C. P., Papp, L., Leitgeb, R., Drexler, W., Distel, M., Unterhuber, A. (2021) Toward quantitative in vivo label-free tracking of lipid distribution in a zebrafish cancer model. Front. Cell Dev. Biol. **9**, 675636.
139. Pshenay-Severin, E., Bae, H., Reichwald, K., Matz, G., Bierlich, J., Kobelke, J., Lorenz, A., Schwuchow, A., Meyer-Zedler, T., Schmitt, M., Messerschmidt, B., Popp, J. (2021) Multimodal nonlinear endomicroscopic imaging probe using a double-core double-clad fiber and focus-combining micro-optical concept. Light. Sci. Appl. **10**, 207.
140. Trägårdh, J., Pikálek, T., Šerý, M., Meyer, T., Popp, J., Čižmár, T. (2019) Label-free CARS microscopy through a multimode fiber endoscope. Opt. Express **27**, 30055–30066.
141. Legare, F., Evans, C. L., Ganikhanov, F., Xie, X. S. (2006) Towards CARS endoscopy. Opt. Express **14**, 4427–4432.
142. Belanger, E., Crepeau, J., Laffray, S., Vallee, R., De Koninck, Y., Cote, D. (2012) Live animal myelin histomorphometry of the spinal cord with video-rate multimodal nonlinear microendoscopy. J. Biomed. Opt. **17**, 021107.
143. Lombardini, A., Mytskaniuk, V., Sivankutty, S., Andresen, E. R., Chen, X., Wenger, J., Fabert, M., Joly, N., Louradour, F., Kudlinski, A., Rigneault, H. (2018) High-resolution multimodal flexible coherent Raman endoscope. Light Sci. Appl. **7**, 10.
144. Cole, M., Lindeque, P., Fileman, E., Halsband, C., Goodhead, R., Moger, J., Galloway, T. S. (2013) Microplastic ingestion by zooplankton. Environ. Sci. Technol. **47**, 6646–6655.

https://doi.org/10.1142/9789811264610_0010

Chapter 10

Raman Spectroscopy for Infection Diagnosis

Markus Salbreiter,[1,2] Aikaterini Pistiki,[2,3] Dana Cialla-May,[2,3] Petra Rösch,[1,2] Jürgen Popp[1-3,*]

[1]*Institute of Physical Chemistry and Abbe Center of Photonics, Friedrich Schiller University, Helmholtzweg 4, Jena, Germany*
[2]*InfectoGnostics Research Campus Jena, Center of Applied Research, Philosophenweg 7, 07743 Jena, Germany*
[3]*Leibniz Institute of Photonic Technology, Member of the Leibniz Research Alliance — Leibniz Health Technologies, Albert-Einstein-Str. 9, 07745 Jena, Germany*
Corresponding author: juergen.popp@ipht-jena.de

10.1 Introduction

Infectious diseases have always been a serious health issue and, despite the development of modern medicine, remain one of the leading causes of morbidity and mortality [1]. Infections can be caused by a wide range of organisms of gradable biological complexities, starting with viruses over to prokaryotes, eukaryotes up to complex eucoelomates (Figure 10.1). Every organism type is characterized by a different biology, life cycle as well as strategy in infecting the host and to survive and reproduce inside its body. All these parameters contribute to the development of infection-specific symptoms in the host, and depending on the pathogen type infections can be acute or chronic, mild or life threatening.

For the different types of pathogens, different detection methods are required to document the infection and treat the patient accordingly. In modern infectious disease laboratory diagnostics, these methods range from simple culture-based and staining techniques such as plating for bacterial

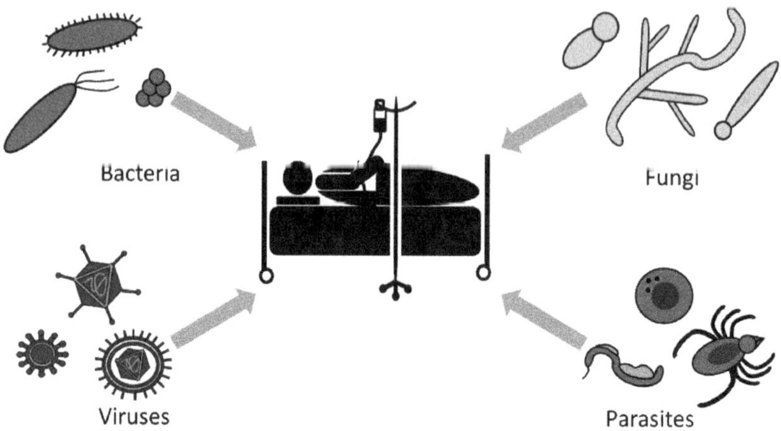

Figure 10.1. Major pathogen groups relevant in infectious diseases.

infections [2] and Giemsa stain for malaria [3] up to very complex techniques such as PCR-based methods [4] and mass spectrometry [5]. These methods provide a direct or indirect detection of the pathogen and come with several advantages and disadvantages in speed, precision, and costs. For bacterial and fungal infections, plating techniques combined with automatic devices for species differentiation and antibiotic susceptibility testing are broadly used and allow accurate identification of the pathogens in most cases [6]. However, these techniques are slow and require several days to provide results which is of obstacle especially in the case of acute, life-threatening infections [7]. This disadvantage in speed can be overcome by the use of PCR-based techniques that can provide accurate results within hours [8], but their high cost is prohibitive for many hospital units [9]. In the case of viruses, PCR-based techniques are the gold standard and the only option for their detection in many cases (e.g., HIV) [10]. Rapid antigen tests have been developed allowing fast detection of respiratory viruses; however, they require high virus load and this lack in sensitivity leaves many infections undiagnosed, allowing them to spread further [11]. Staining protocols followed by microscopy are commonly used for the detection of parasites such as malaria and *Trypanosoma* in blood or solid tissue samples [12]. Microscopy is also applied in the case of intestinal parasite such as *Ascaris* that allows the detection of the entire worms or their eggs [13]. However, these techniques are time consuming and require very experienced personnel that are able to (i) detect the pathogens in the sample and (ii) classify them from their morphology. Thus, these techniques are vulnerable to human error and cannot be standardized [14].

From the above it is clear that current infectious disease diagnostics can only partly cover the requirements for efficient patient care and many issues remain to be addressed towards this direction. Thus, new approaches for pathogen identification are gaining popularity. The task of developing quick procedures that are more simple, trustworthy, and specific remains a difficulty [15]. An attractive method capable of providing solutions to all these issues is Raman spectroscopy. It is a rapid, sensitive, and cost-effective analytical technique that can be applied onto a wide range of biological samples from single bacteria over single cells to complex tissues, providing biochemical information in a label-free way. It generates a spectroscopic fingerprint of the total biochemical composition within a sample deriving from its vibrational behavior [16, 17]. The direct pattern detection of characteristic "fingerprint" vibrations for specific chemical bonds is a key component of the Raman imaging approach. This invariably leads to the simultaneous observation of Raman signals from all biochemical components (e.g., nucleic acids, lipids, carbohydrates, proteins, and other low-molecular compounds), resulting in spectral features containing a large amount of data that could be valuable for diagnostic purposes. Because each pathogen has a unique biomolecular composition, these distinctions are captured in their Raman spectra ("optical fingerprint"), which may subsequently be examined and distinguished using chemometric methods [18, 19]. This distinctiveness allows for categorization, discrimination, and identification of pathogens on a species and even subspecies level [20].

Over the past decades, Raman spectroscopic techniques have been successfully applied to a wide range of pathogens and their development for routine infectious disease diagnostics could allow overcoming of the issues of the currently used standard techniques. In the following sections of this chapter, Raman-based techniques and their application in infectious disease diagnostics will be presented and analyzed.

10.2 Raman Spectroscopy

10.2.1 *Raman Spectroscopic Techniques*

The interacting of photons from a laser source with a vibrating molecule leads to inelastic scattering known as the Raman effect. In principle, Raman excitation wavelengths from the UV over the visible to the near-infrared (NIR) region can be used. Nevertheless, if the excitation wavelength is in resonance with an electronic absorption band, the resonance Raman spectra are enhanced by six orders of magnitudes allowing detection of molecules with low concentrations. For example, excitation with green wavelengths especially enhances chromophores like carotenoids, hem, or cytochromes [21–23].

Raman bands are very characteristic for the measured molecule. Since bacteria contain a large number of different molecules, the Raman spectrum of a cell is a spectral superposition of the complete molecular information in the measured volume. Microorganisms of different genera or species in principle contain the same type of molecules. However, due to changes in, e.g., the cell wall or the proteome, tiny variations in the Raman spectra occur which can then be used for differentiation (see Section 10.2.3) [24, 25]. Moreover, this also means that Raman spectroscopy is a phenotypic method. Therefore, various environmental influences and cultivation variations will alter the Raman spectroscopic signature of microorganisms (see Section 10.2.4) [26, 27].

Depending on the Raman setup, different measurement techniques are available. If there is sufficient time to generate biomass, bulk measurements are always the method of choice, since they allow averaging over a large number of bacteria making the analysis more stable [28]. In addition, bulk measurements normally require cultivation which can easily be standardized [29]. The disadvantage of bulk methods is the normally high amount of generated fluorescence, which partly or completely obscures the Raman spectrum. To overcome this, excitations in the NIR regions are used. Nevertheless, since the Raman intensity correlates to the excitation frequency with the power of four, NIR excitation normally results in Raman spectra of lower intensities but undamaged cells [23]. Raman bulk spectra are normally measured with a larger illumination field. One possibility is the application of a Raman fiber (Figure 10.2(a)). This enables collection of a Raman sum spectrum of the complete area and can also be used for averaging of heterogeneous samples [30, 31].

In contrast, Raman excitation in the ultraviolet range results in fluorescence-free spectra. UV resonance Raman spectroscopy (UVRR) with excitation wavelengths below 260 nm has the additional advantage that the Raman signals of DNA/RNA bases and aromatic amino acids are resonantly enhanced. However, due to photodegradation it is important to move the sample to avoid the measurement of burned cells (Figure 10.2(b)). Since mainly DNA information is included in the UVRR spectra, classifications using this method are expected to be particularly accurate [24, 32].

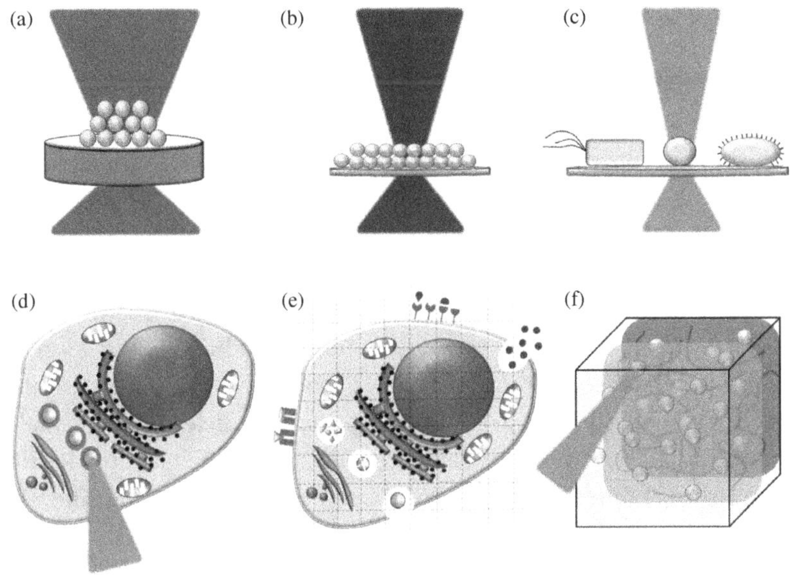

Figure 10.2. Different Raman spectroscopic techniques: (a) Raman fiber probe on colonies; (b) UVRR microscopy on bulk samples; (c) Raman microscopy on single bacterial cells; (d) Raman microscopy on intracellular bacteria; (e) 2D Raman mapping on host cells; (f) 3D Raman mappings on biofilms.

When a Raman setup is combined with a microscope, structures in the range of 1 μm are accessible. Therefore, single bacteria cells can be measured (Figure 10.2(c)) and directly used for identification [22, 33]. The advantages are clear: there is no need for cultivation, which speeds up the identification of a sample. Nevertheless, in this case isolation steps are required which can be performed <2 h (see Section 10.2.4). In addition, non-cultivatable microorganisms are also accessible for this type of investigation. A Raman microscope can also be used for analyzing small structures within eukaryotic cells (Figure 10.2(d)), which enables the investigation of intracellular bacteria (see Section 10.3.2) [24].

Apart from point measurements, Raman microscopes can also be used for larger areas. Here, two different techniques are available: Raman mapping scans the laser over the sample, generating one Raman spectrum for each position. This allows a 2D Raman map of, e.g., a eukaryotic cell (Figure 10.2(e) and Section 10.7) or a 3D approach when larger samples such as biofilms (see Section 10.3.3) are analyzed (Figure 10.2(f)). Raman imaging in contrary generates for each wavenumber a complete field of view. Normally, imaging techniques are faster than mapping approaches, but the spatial and spectral resolutions are quite different for both methods [34].

10.2.2 *Surface-Enhanced Raman Spectroscopy*

In order to augment the inherent weak Raman signal, signal-enhancing processes have garnered interest in the last decades within the framework of Raman spectroscopy. One amplification technique, which is widely used in bioanalytics, is surface-enhanced Raman spectroscopy (SERS), which is based on the usage of the exceptional optical properties of metallic nanostructures [35]. Here, due to the interaction with light, localized surface plasmon polariton modes are excited in mostly silver or gold nanostructures, which are associated with a strong electromagnetic field enhancement. Moreover, propagating surface plasmon polariton modes can be observed at the interface of a regularly nanostructured surface and a dielectric layer, making a nanosensing surface with a regular pattern doubly resonant as both localized and propagating modes contribute to the signal enhancement [36]. The strong electromagnetic field enhancement due to the plasmonic activity causes an enhancement of the Raman modes. The Raman scattered light can also interact with the electromagnetic field, resulting in an emission enhancement. The overall SERS enhancement is in most applications of 4–8 orders of magnitude [37, 38]. The second main SERS amplification contribution is the chemical enhancement, which summarizes signal enhancement due to charge transfer or the resonance Raman effect [39]. Under SERS conditions, Raman modes perpendicular to the metal surface are preferentially enhanced, allowing conclusions to be drawn about the orientation of the molecule of interest when investigating the band ratios of in-plane and out-of-plane vibrations [40]. Finally, the spectroscopic selection rules known in Raman spectroscopy are not valid in SERS as the strong electromagnetic field has an evanescent character and in the field gradient, Raman modes which are forbidden under normal Raman conditions are observable in SERS spectra [41].

The sensing schemes mainly used in biosensing by means of SERS are summarized in Figure 10.3. Label-free or direct SERS techniques are mostly applied [42, 43]. Here, the target analyte is required to have a high affinity towards the metallic surface and in the case of matrix molecules, they compete together for free binding sites at the sensing surface. The selectivity is achieved *via* a tailored affinity due to possible surface modifications. A further example of a SERS sensing detection scheme is the application of SERS labels or tags [44, 45]. Mostly gold nanoparticles are applied, which are equipped with a Raman reporter molecule providing unique fingerprint information as well as specific recognition elements such as antibodies or

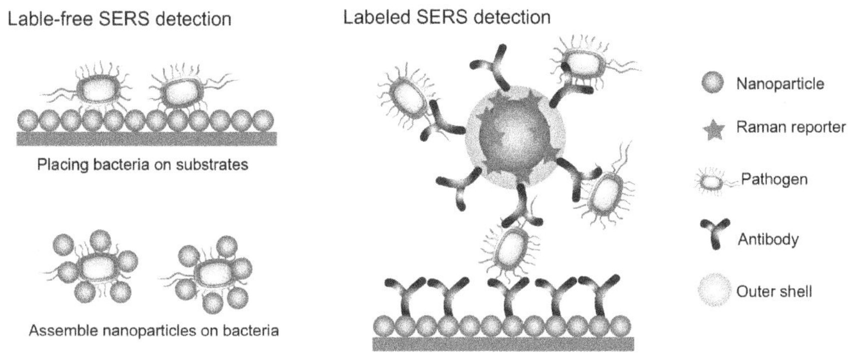

Figure 10.3. Illustration of the label-free as well as labeled SERS detection schemes for the detection of pathogens. Reproduced from Ref. [47] with permission.

aptamers. In immunosensing applications, their stability is surpassing that of fluorescent dye labels. Finally, a third main detection scheme in SERS is the usage of molecular sensors, which might be a powerful tool in infection diagnosis in future works [46]. Plasmonic-active nanoparticles are modified with a specific sensor molecule undergoing a chemical reaction with small molecules providing no or less Raman signals. Thus, the detection is achieved by following the changes within the SERS spectrum of the molecular sensor upon the interaction with the target. The same approach is available for the detection of ions or the pH value employing suitable ligand molecules.

SERS is a versatile tool for microbial diagnosis including the identification of the species, the assessment of the communication and response, the characterization of biofilms or resistance testing [35]. Here, SERS ensures the enhancement of the Raman signals by several orders of magnitude, allowing for the detection of fingerprint spectra in high throughput (e.g., by applying microfluidic devices) with less integration time as in normal Raman spectroscopy. However, by applying label-free SERS approaches, only molecules in close vicinity towards the metallic nanostructured sensing surface can contribute to the overall SERS spectrum, making SERS spectra of bacteria as well as biofilms unique in comparison to Raman spectra of the whole organism. Thus, SERS is selective for analyte molecules with high affinity towards the metallic surface and as a consequence, their appearance in the SERS spectrum is not necessarily reflecting their actual concentration in the whole organism. Mostly, SERS spectra of bacteria are dominated by low-molecular weight molecules such as adenosine monophosphate, adenine, guanine, hypoxanthine, xanthine and uric acid [48]. As the SERS-active structure is not incorporated in the bacterial cell in most of the application examples, the secretion of these small molecules, which are known to have a high affinity towards metallic sensor surfaces, are dominating the SERS spectrum. Moreover, as the secretion is a consequence of stress of the bacterial cell due to environmental conditions, their spectroscopic investigation and determination is performed for antibiotic susceptibility testing, showing the potential of SERS in clinical settings. However, for label-free SERS approaches, databases accompanied with chemometrics are required due to the complexity of the recorded SERS spectrum. To simplify the SERS spectral data analysis in the framework of the detection of pathogens, SERS labels equipped with antibodies and aptamers as recognition elements are available allowing for immunoassay or DNA-based detection schemes [49]. Here, the SERS spectrum is dominated by the contribution of the Raman reporter molecule and by thorough selection of a suitable label molecule, the Raman marker bands are not overlapping with possible background information; e.g., the vibrational modes of C≡N or C≡C triple bonds are in the Raman silent region making them perfectly suited moieties in Raman reporter molecules in SERS labels. Thus, a simplified data analysis alongside the application of handheld Raman instruments and cartridge solutions for an efficient sample preparation might level the path for these kind of SERS assays towards routine analytics in early and point-of-care detection of infectious diseases. Moreover, the application of SERS-based detection schemes of pathogens can be expanded to food matrices [47]. It is expected that food matrix components will interfere with the SERS spectral fingerprint information of the pathogens, showing the imminent importance of powerful sample preparation strategies. Magnetic plasmonic particles are composed of a magnetic core and a thin metallic layer equipped with biofunctionalization for the interaction with bacterial cells [50]. By applying external magnetic forces, the bacterial cells can be enriched even from complex matrices and finally, SERS spectra are recorded which are dominated by those molecules that are in close vicinity to the metallic SERS sensing surface. The capture efficiency and selectivity can be improved by tailoring the biofunctionalization towards the target bacteria.

10.2.3 *Statistical Evaluation of the Spectroscopic Data*

Since Raman spectra of different microorganisms are normally — independent of the applied method — very similar, the differentiation between genera, species, or strains is challenging and requires machine learning approaches [51, 52]. First of all, the Raman spectra need to be wavenumber and intensity calibrated to correct and eliminate potential setup-dependent differences and to be able to collect Raman databases over a longer time range [53–58]. Afterwards spectral pre-processing is applied to exclude, e.g., fluorescence or other artifacts [59, 60]. In particular, cosmic spikes need to be removed [61]. Also, fluorescence backgrounds or thermal fluctuation of the charged-coupled device are corrected with different baseline-removing algorithms like the Savitzky–Golay method or the SNIP algorithm [62, 63].

When designing a database for the identification of a pathogen, some important basic considerations must be made. One essential point is the reproducibility of the database. For this the variation within the classes (e.g., species) need to be sufficient, but also enough classes are required. A two-class problem is normally easy to solve und seldom reflects realistic scenarios. The size of a database is reflected by the amount of classes and within each class the number of biological and/or technical replicates [64]. This database should not be split in two dependent parts for classification and validation. Instead, the validation dataset should be independent at least with respect to different biological replicates, better when other previously not included strains are utilized [65]. In the end the identification step should be carried out with real patient or environmental samples [66]. Afterwards the appropriate selection of the discrimination algorithm should avoid over- or under-modeling the problem to allow a realistic scenario of the corresponding task to be generated [51, 67, 68]. If more than one device or one excitation wavelength is applied for the investigations, then model transfer algorithms are necessary to correct for device-to-device variations [69–78].

10.2.4 *Sample Preparation*

In principle, sample preparation for Raman spectroscopy is quite easy. Normally, the cells are deposited on a substrate and can then be directly measured, e.g., by means of a Raman microscope. For bulk measurements the Raman spectra can either be collected directly on the microcolonies on the agar plate [31] or bacterial films [79] are generated which can then be analyzed. These techniques require a huge amount of biomass and therefore a cultivation step. Here, it is important to keep in mind that as a phenotypic method, Raman spectroscopy is highly susceptible to changes during cultivation of bacteria [26]. This includes variations in media [80–85], temperature [83, 86], CO_2 content [29, 87] and the presence of antibiotics [88, 89] or heavy metals [90]. In addition, the sampling after different time points especially in the growth curve also alters the Raman spectra [84, 91, 92]. Apart from such biomass preparation parameters, preliminary factors like transport or sample storage can also influence the sample [29, 93].

For cultivation-free measurements the bacteria need to be isolated out of the samples of interest. The isolation step needs to be destruction-free and should not alter the cell chemistry of the bacteria since Raman spectroscopy as a phenotypic method is very sensitive towards such changes. For all isolation strategies the constitution of the sample, the initial bacteria concentration and the cell yield are the most important starting points for the decision on which isolation technique is appropriate. For isolation nearly every technique might be possible starting from pure washing steps, over filtration, (density) centrifugation, dielectrophoresis, optical trapping, immunocapture, to microfluidic setups (see Section 10.3.1) [79].

Especially when Raman microscopy is applied for the analysis of bacteria, the measured volume is quite small, being <4 μm^3. Nevertheless, apart from the cell information, nearly always spectral contribution of the used Raman substrate is found in the Raman spectrum. Therefore, Raman substrates should only exhibit one (or very few) Raman signals like CaF_2 or fused silica which do not alter with time. In addition, such substrate bands should not be in a spectral region where they superimpose important Raman bands from the microorganisms. Normal glass slides are most probably not useful, since the glass spectrum sometimes changes from lot to lot and in extreme cases even within one slide. An alternative approach is a metal surface. This can either be realized as a thin metal foil or as metal-coated glass substrates. For all these possible Raman substrates the applicability towards cell viability or attachment of the cells also needs to be considered. Therefore, the Raman substrates definitively depend on the planned experiment [94, 95].

In heterogenous samples it is sometimes helpful to mark microorganisms to locate them more easily. One possibility is fluorescence staining of the cells. Here, it is important to choose a stain which does not exhibit Raman signals and does not increase the already existing fluorescence background too much. This allows localization of the cells for the measurement [96, 97]. In addition, Raman tags can be applied. Here, either isotopes (see Section 10.3.6) or groups of chemically inert and small modifications like triple bonds are used. This approach makes it possible to localize microorganisms inside complex samples or to distinguish them from other non-targeted cells [98].

Another point concerns the use of samples that change during longer measurements or highly pathogenic samples that may not be analyzed everywhere. This requires suitable fixation or inactivation methods that do not change the cell chemistry too much and must not generate artifacts in the Raman spectra [99–101].

10.3 Bacteria Identification

10.3.1 *Single-Cell Analysis*

In order to prevent the spread of infection, rapid diagnosis and treatment of infectious diseases are required. When a patient with infection is admitted to the hospital, a sample is taken and cultured to identify the pathogen. The level of resistance of the pathogens must then be determined before an accurate treatment plan can be assessed. However, because of their high cost, maintenance and complexity, molecular approaches are not always available at laboratories, whereas traditional microbiological procedures require several days to produce data [9]. In contrast to culture-based techniques, Raman spectroscopy can offer this information in a few hours after pathogen isolation or even directly on the patient's bodily fluids. The analytical speed of this technology is important for patient care since it enables prompt treatment administration and the avoidance of a severe outcome [102].

The time allotted for the analysis will determine which Raman approach is most appropriate. If time is of the essence, single-cell analysis is the go-to method to use [23, 103]. The first stage in this process is always to isolate the causative pathogen without destroying it, which is followed by an identifying step. Since the majority of the isolation procedures can be completed in an hour, it usually takes two hours to identify the pathogen. With a validation accuracy of 95.1%, *Escherichia coli* and *Enterococcus faecalis* have been effectively detected in patient urine samples from 11 patients. Since urine samples often do not contain large cellular components or other interfering moieties, this was accomplished by using straightforward washing procedures. This shows that the identification of significant urinary tract infection bacteria within two hours without the requirement for a culture phase is possible when Raman microspectroscopy is used in conjunction with support vector machines (SVM) [104]. The same principle to separate and distinguish between different types of bacteria can be applied in ascitic fluid. As a result, a database was developed that contains more than 10,000 single-cell Raman spectra from 34 bacterial strains belonging to 13 distinct species. The model's accuracy was 83.6% at the species level and 96% at the genus level for Gram-negative and 97.7% for Gram-positive bacteria. All in all, the entire process of directly discriminating and identifying bacterial pathogens in ascitic fluid, which included sample pre-processing, measurement and data analysis, was achieved in just three hours [105].

Yet, the isolation method must be tailored to the matrix in which the sample is located or extracted. Bronchoalveolar lavage fluid, sputum, and blood are just some examples of more complex matrices. Density gradient centrifugation, for example, was used to isolate low concentrations of bacteria in bronchoalveolar lavage fluid and to see if this method affected the bacterial spectra. The isolation gradient had no discernible effect on the spectra and achieved yields of 63% and 78% [106]. The isolation of bacterial pathogens from a complex matrix, i.e., sputum, has proven to be a bit more complicated than "just washing steps". Sputum has a high degree of viscosity, so before isolation, a phase of liquefaction employing the proteolytic enzyme mixture Pronase E is necessary. To isolate the bacteria, further filtration and centrifugation procedures are used. Raman spectroscopy was used to identify the isolated pathogens with a 97.4% accuracy [107]. In a different study, Rusciano *et al.* were successful in identifying *Pseudomonas aeruginosa* and *Staphylococcus aureus* without the use of an isolation procedure in sputum samples from cystic fibrosis patients [108]. In the case of blood samples, the blood cells had to be lysed by Triton X-100 and the remnants of hemoglobin had to be removed by enzymatic digestion *via* Pronase E. Following sample preparation, the examined microorganisms could be accurately identified [109].

In a study by Stöckel *et al.*, mycobacteria were identified down to the species level using Raman microspectroscopy. The identification of *Mycobacterium tuberculosis* complex strains and the differentiation between pathogenic and commensal non-tuberculous mycobacteria were of particular interest. A spectral library containing more than 8,800 Raman spectra of individual bacterial cells was built using the suggested model, which takes into account 26 different mycobacteria species as well as antibiotic-susceptible and -resistant strains. Within 14 unknown samples, distinct mycobacterial strains, including *M. tuberculosis*, were correctly identified with an accuracy of 94.3% [110]. In addition, cerebrospinal fluid, which is transparent and colorless, can be used as a diagnostic tool for a number of neurological conditions, particularly meningitis brought on by bacteria or viruses. *M. tuberculosis*-positive cerebrospinal fluid samples provided Raman data that allowed for the precise and sensitive identification of tuberculous meningitis. Due to its high intrinsic specificity, minimal sample preparation, and lack of extended culture durations, it was recommended as an alternative to the conventional analytical approaches [111]. The spatial localization of cells, such as leukocytes, erythrocytes, and pathogens, in the crystal pattern of dried cerebrospinal fluid was also accomplished by Gonchukov *et al.* using confocal Raman microscopy [112].

The ubiquitous *Bacillus* genus contains symbiotic species as well as two parasitic harmful species, *B. cereus* and *B. anthracis*, which are responsible for food poisoning and anthrax, respectively. A two-stage classification model was created using Raman microscopy to distinguish between the endospores of 66 strains from 13 *Bacillus* and *Bacillus*-related species, including *B. anthracis*. 88–100% of a test set of 27 species, which comprised six *B. anthracis* strains and "unknown samples" in the database, were correctly identified [113]. A similar approach was employed to test for anthrax endospores in white powder samples (i.e., baking powder) which achieved typing accuracies of up to 99% [114]. Additionally, *Burkholderia mallei* and *B. pseudomallei* were quickly distinguished from broth cultures and pelleted animal feedstuff using Raman microspectroscopy. In addition to differentiating between *B. mallei* and *B. pseudomallei*, a two-stage classification model made up of two SVMs was also used to distinguish between five other *Burkholderia* species and four species of the closely related genus *Pseudomonas*. Accuracy rates for *B. mallei* and *B. pseudomallei* species identification ranged from 93.9–98.7% [115].

The most frequent cause of peritoneal dialysis (PD) is bacterial peritonitis, and prompt treatment with the appropriate medicines is crucial. Thus, Tien *et al.* use SERS to identify the bacteria present in the dialysate of patients with PD peritonitis, speeding up the process of identifying the bacteria and enabling timely treatment [116]. The most frequent infection in women (>60%) and the leading cause of nosocomial infections are urinary tract infections. Dielectrophoresis and Raman microspectroscopy were coupled by Schröder *et al.* to identify bacteria in urine samples. The only step in the preparation of the samples was filtration, which was done to remove bigger particles. In this study, a statistical classification model was used to distinguish between *E. faecalis* and *E. coli* in approximately 35 minutes [117]. Another study used multivariate statistical methods like principal component analysis (PCA), partial least square-discriminate analysis (PLS-DA), and SVM to assess five urinary tract infection-causing bacteria as pure and mixed cultures. The PLS-DA (73%) and the SVM (89%) were more effective in classifying the bacteria than the PCA [118].

Along with several beneficial symbionts, the family Enterobacteriaceae also contains many of the more well-known pathogens, including *Salmonella*, *E. coli*, *Klebsiella*, and *Shigella*. Raman spectroscopy was used to differentiate 24 clinical isolates of *E. coli*, *K. pneumoniae*, and *K. oxytoca* because it is difficult to distinguish pathogens from the Enterobacteriaceae family using the standard diagnostic tools. It was discovered that UVRR performed better than Raman microspectroscopy (532 nm), allowing 23 out of 24 isolates to be correctly classified at the genus level. Additionally, all three *K. oxytoca* isolates were correctly classified for the first time at the species level with 92% accuracy [119]. *Salmonella* species discrimination and identification have also been demonstrated utilizing either silver nanosphere SERS probes [120] or SERS characterization of the bacteria's O-antigen [121]. In addition, two multivariate chemometric approaches (PLS and PCA) were used to distinguish between four closely related *E. coli* strains: pathogenic enterohemorrhagic *E. coli* O157:H7, non-pathogenic *E. coli* C, *E. coli* Hfr K-12, and *E. coli* HF4714, with 95% accuracy [122]. In addition, SERS was used to detect and discriminate *E. coli* from the genetically closely related *Shigella spp*. In the presence of silver nanoparticles as opposed to absence, it was simple to distinguish between *E. coli* and *Shigella spp*. based on their distinctive Raman spectra [123].

Pseudomonas aeruginosa can cause serious infections in immunocompromised patients, and prompt and correct identification of the infectious agents is essential for effective antibiotic therapy of the infection. In order to identify *P. aeruginosa* infection, SERS was used to detect the presence of pyocyanin in 15 clinical sputum samples, achieving 95.6% sensitivity and 93.3% specificity [124]. Patients with cystic fibrosis have respiratory tract colonization by *P. aeruginosa* strains and *Burkholderia cepacia complex* (*Bcc*). Although it is challenging to distinguish between these strains phenotypically, species identification is important since they differ substantially in their capacity to cause disease. Three methods were applied to analyze a *Bcc* collection: Raman spectroscopy, AFLP and rep-PCR analysis. High resemblance was found using Raman spectroscopy for 40 strains; however, *Bcc* strains and *Pseudomonas* strains could be separated using Rep-PCR and AFLP for 96 and 112 strains, respectively. This study demonstrated that it was impossible to distinguish between *P. aeruginosa* and *Bcc* species using Raman spectroscopy [125].

10.3.2 *Intracellular Bacteria*

Given that the pathogens are concealed within the host cells, intracellular infections are frequently challenging to identify and manage. Pathogenic

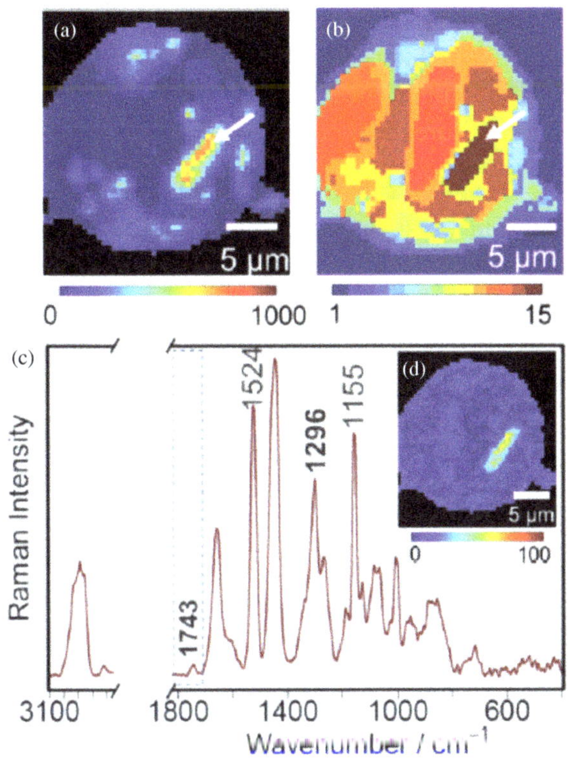

Figure 10.4. Raman map of an infected macrophage with noticeable compartmentalization. (a) Sum intensity of the bacterial Raman signal at 1524 and 1155 cm^{-1} within the cell matrix. (b) Corresponding plot of a hierarchical cluster analysis with 15 clusters. The cell compartment of interest is indicated by an arrow in both panels. (c) Mean spectrum of the indicated cluster. (d) Inset: Sum intensity of the Raman signal at 1743 cm^{-1} within the determined cell margins. Reproduced from Ref. [126] with permission.

mycobacteria are primarily found inside of macrophages during infections. Here, Raman microspectroscopy was used by Silge *et al.* to analyze *Mycobacterium gordonae* in macrophages (Figure 10.4). This study demonstrated not only the unique distribution of *M. gordonae* within macrophages, but also how bacteria outside or near the macrophages' outer membrane differed noticeably from their intracellular counterparts in terms of their spectral patterns. Furthermore, due to the chemical makeup of the macrophage milieu, the internal bacteria displayed different spectral and molecular information [126]. Raman microscopy, Fourier transform infrared absorption spectroscopy (FTIR), and atomic force microscopy were also used to investigate the biochemistry of mycobacteria and Gram-negative bacteria in both pure and mixed co-cultures. The outer membrane and cell walls of mycobacteria and Gram-negative bacteria have very different chemical compositions, which results in diversity in the spectral areas of each individual Raman spectrum. Raman and FTIR spectral pictures were used to determine the distribution of different cell types, and atomic force microscopy and Raman microspectroscopy were combined to measure the topography and cell surface [127].

Additionally, *Staphylococcus aureus* has the potential to function as an exceedingly challenging-to-treat facultative intracellular pathogen. In order to selectively identify internal *S. aureus* and localize it within endothelial cells, Große *et al.* used an innovative Raman-based imaging method that produced high-quality false-color images. The spectra showed that the internal bacteria are biochemically distinct from external bacteria and are in the exponential growth phase with a lower replication rate, demonstrating their adaptability to the host's internal environment [128]. The symbiotic and non-pathogenic *Protochlamydia amoebophila* and the human pathogen *Chlamydia trachomatis* were used to evaluate their intracellular and extracellular metabolic activity using Raman microscopy. Reticulate bodies and elementary bodies could be seen while isotope labeling was accomplished using ^{13}C-labeled phenylalanine. Both intracellular and long-term extracellular metabolic activity associated with the intake of the isotopically labeled amino acid were shown. The extracellular protein biosynthesis was then examined using mass spectrometry (MALDI-ToF) and two-dimensional gel electrophoresis [129]. The techniques described here are useful tools for illuminating the intricate internal workings of pathogens and for observing organisms that are otherwise challenging to culture.

10.3.3 *Bulk Analysis*

In contrast to single-cell analysis, bulk samples cannot be identified immediately because only pure cultures can be measured, necessitating a cultivation step. Normally, a thick bacteria suspension is dropped on a substrate and then the sample is dried to a homogenous film. Although this process takes longer than single-cell analysis, it is far more accurate in terms of discrimination and identification. De Siqueira e Oliveira *et al.* conducted a study to compare the Raman spectra of nine clinical species of bacteria isolated from infections, which included three Gram-positive and six Gram-negative species. A dispersive Raman spectrometer (830 nm) with an exposure time of 50 s was used to collect a total of 475 spectra from 115 distinct strains. The created classification model was capable of analyzing the entire spectrum as well as the peaks with the biggest discrepancies, and it did so with an overall accuracy of 89.5 and 90.1%, respectively [130].

Using confocal Raman microscopy (785 nm) and PCA, *Arcobacter* bacteria were detected and distinguished at the species level from the closely related genera *Campylobacter* and *Helicobacter*. All 18 *Arcobacter* species could be correctly identified down to the species level with an accuracy of 97.2%. The study also sought to establish the precise biomass proportion of a particular *Arcobacter* species in a mixture of bacteria that ranged from 5–100% [131].

Shen *et al.* were able to quickly receive Raman spectra from the microbial colonies in the petri dish by using a rapid fiber probe-based Raman approach with an excitation wavelength of 785 nm. With this procedure, eight species of bacteria and one yeast could be correctly classified and identified with an accuracy for validation and identification of above 99% [31]. In a different investigation, Rebrošová *et al.* used Raman spectroscopy to directly evaluate 254 strains of 20 species known to cause urinary tract infections in Petri dishes and were able to achieve an overall accuracy of above 97%. Additionally, they used optical tweezers along with Raman spectroscopy to study and distinguish single microbial cells directly in urine within a 10-minute time frame [132–134].

Maquelin *et al.* directly identified and distinguished bacterial species from microbial colonies using Raman spectroscopy and FTIR. Raman spectroscopy was used to evaluate 109 bacteria and 6 yeast strains, whereas FTIR spectroscopy was used to study 114 bacteria and 7 yeast strains. Both techniques produced excellent results on the species level, with an accurate identification rate of 98.3% for FTIR and 92.2% for Raman spectroscopy [135]. Almarashi *et al.* could demonstrate that by taking direct measurements of Raman spectra from 30 colonies and applying PCA, it is possible to distinguish between strains of *Staphylococcus epidermidis* and *E. coli* [136]. Samek *et al.* demonstrated that it was possible to discriminate between different clones of *S. epidermidis* by means of Raman spectroscopy directly from the petri dish. Additionally, differences in the Raman spectra of *S. epidermis*, *S. aureus* and *E. coli* were observed [137].

The investigation of microcolonies on petri dishes has also been conducted and analyzed by employing different vibrational spectroscopic techniques. For example, Choo-Smith *et al.* examined colony development for varied growth times (6, 12 and 24 h) using IR and Raman spectroscopy. Certain *S. aureus* strains' older colonies (12 and 24 h) displayed higher glycogen content in the surface layers, increasing levels of carotenoid pigmentation, and higher RNA content in the deeper layers. The 6 h microcolonies, in contrast, did not exhibit any observable spectrum distinctions, indicating that the molecular makeup may have been very homogeneous at this early stage of growth which would make them more suitable for inclusion in a spectral database [138]. Furthermore, Mathey *et al.* demonstrated that only a tiny percentage of bacteria in microcolonies are harmed or killed by laser exposure, whereas unaffected bacteria are still alive and continue to proliferate [139]. Finally, following 24-hour (macrocolonies) and 6-hour (microcolonies) incubation, Espagnon *et al.* examined colonies from 80 strains of nine bacterial and one yeast species directly on solid culture medium. Correct identification rates were 94.1% for macrocolonies and 91.5% for microcolonies, respectively [140]. This study was the first to truly compare macro- and microcolonies side by side without prior correction for water and medium variation.

The primary causes of urinary tract infections are *E. coli*, *K. pneumoniae*, and *Proteus mirabilis*; however, due to their similarities, accurate identification of *Enterobacteriaceae* is challenging and time consuming. Nakar *et al.* used an NIR Raman fiber probe to gather spectra from colonies on agar plates and from single cells using Raman microspectroscopy from 16 different Enterobacteriaceae strains from 8 genera (Figure 10.5). The results of single-cell analysis were insufficient, but the fiber probe spectra allowed for the accurate classification of all 16 isolates. In addition, the model was validated with an independent dataset and 15/16 strains were successfully identified with an overall accuracy of 94% [141].

10.3.4 *Biofilms*

A biofilm is a syntrophic consortium of microorganisms in which cells adhere to each other and frequently to a surface while embedded in an extracellular matrix made up of extracellular polymeric substances (EPSs). Typical EPS components produced by the bacteria consist of extracellular polysaccharides, proteins, lipids and DNA [142, 143]. Microbes form biofilms as a protective response to extracellular factors to survive hostile environments or to colonize new niches. Nutritional restrictions, UV light exposure, metal toxicity, acids, dehydration, salinity, phagocytosis, and several antibiotics and antimicrobial agents are just some examples of such factors [143]. In medicine, it is believed that about two-thirds of bacterial infections in humans are caused by biofilms, which prove difficult to combat [144]. This is primarily due to mature biofilms' antimicrobial tolerance and immune response evasion [145]. Infections

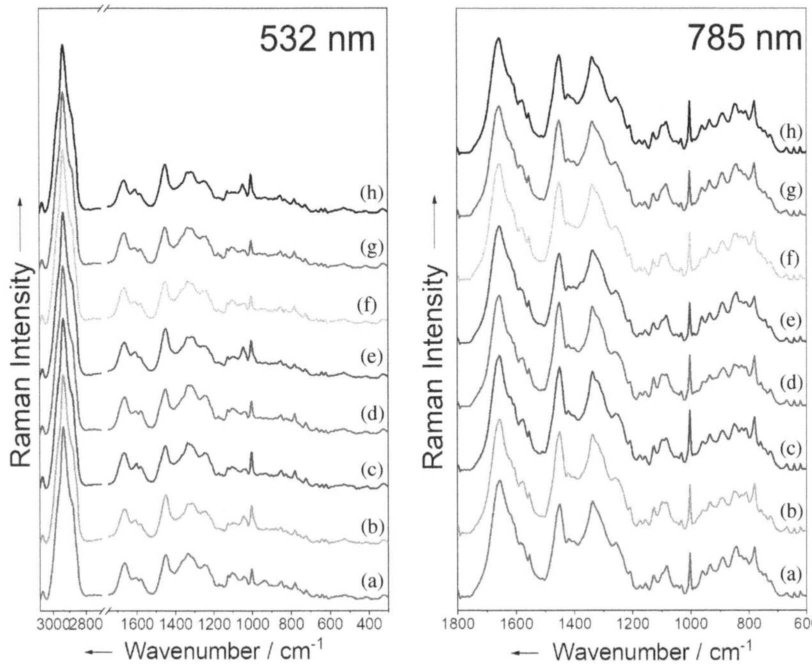

Figure 10.5. Mean spectra of different Enterobacteriaceae measured with single-cell Raman microspectroscopy (532 nm) and fiber-probe Raman spectroscopy (785 nm): (a) Citrobacter, (b) Enterobacter, (c) Escherichia, (d) Klebsiella, (e) Proteus, (f) Salmonella, (g) Serratia and (h) Shigella. Standard deviations are highlighted in gray. The spectra are normalized and vertically offset for visualization purposes. Reproduced from Ref. [141] with permission.

associated with the use of medical devices (e.g., catheters, prosthetic cardiac valves) are among the most difficult to treat [146].

There are two main categories of biofilms that can be discovered in the hospital environment: medical biofilms, which are found in patients with infections like on infected implants or joints, and environmental biofilms, which are found in places like the water supply system. Since pathogenic organisms like *P. aeruginosa* and *Legionella pneumophila* frequently generate environmental biofilms in the hospital setting, they can pose a health concern to patients. Raman spectroscopy is generally used to study biofilms with the primary goal of describing the composition of the biofilms [147, 148], the spatial distribution of bacteria, or the components of the EPS of bacterial [149–157] or yeast [158, 159] biofilms.

Bacterial biofilms are commonly responsible for endodontic persistent infections and are often characterized by an EPS matrix that protects the encased bacteria. Ramirez-Mora *et al.* used Raman spectroscopy and confocal scanning laser microscopy techniques to characterize the main components of *E. faecalis*, *Actinomyces naeslundii*, and dual-species biofilm matrices. The biomass of single-species biofilms was higher than that of two-species biofilms. Furthermore, Raman spectroscopy revealed that all samples contained carbohydrates, proteins, fatty acids, and nucleic acids. These biomolecules' varying expression allowed for spectroscopic differentiation using a PCA tool. These preliminary findings show differences in biomolecular components between mono-species and dual-species biofilms [148]. In order to investigate the hydrated *Pseudomonas spp.* biofilm matrix *in situ*, Liu *et al.* developed and used the confocal Raman mapping approach combined with non-negative matrix factorization (NMF) analysis (Figure 10.6). Within the various *Pseudomonas spp.* biofilm matrices, a variety of chemical elements, including proteins, bacteria, glycolipids, and polyhydroxyalkanoates were uncovered. Glycolipids and polyhydroxyalkanoates, however, were specific to the *P. aeruginosa* and *P. putida* biofilm matrices, respectively. Furthermore, it was shown that their large abundances in the lower part of the biofilm matrix were associated with particular physiological processes and local microenvironments [143].

Raman spectroscopy is also used to describe how biofilms age [160, 161], especially the transition from planktonic to sessile cells exhibits distinct Raman spectroscopic fingerprints [162, 163]. *E. faecalis* was studied as the bacterial model to examine the implications of the initial age of bacterial cells for biofilm production. Raman spectra were collected from bacterial cells in their exponential, stationary, and starvation phases. Bacterial cells in their starvation phase resulted in the formation of biofilms that contained more protein and less nucleic acid than those produced by cells in the exponential and stationary phases [164]. The transition between planktonic and biofilm states was observed in *Pseudomonas spp.* strain ADP using Raman microscopy and scanning electron microscopy. These spectra showed distinct differences between cells freely in suspension and in biofilm in the nucleic acid, carbohydrate, and protein regions of the Raman spectra. Scanning electron microscopy imaging visualized free and biofilm cells and attributed the majority of the differences to the presence of EPS in the matrix [162]. Furthermore, planktonic and sessile cells of *Cronobacter sakazakii*, which causes newborn meningitis, were described by Sharma *et al.* The intensity

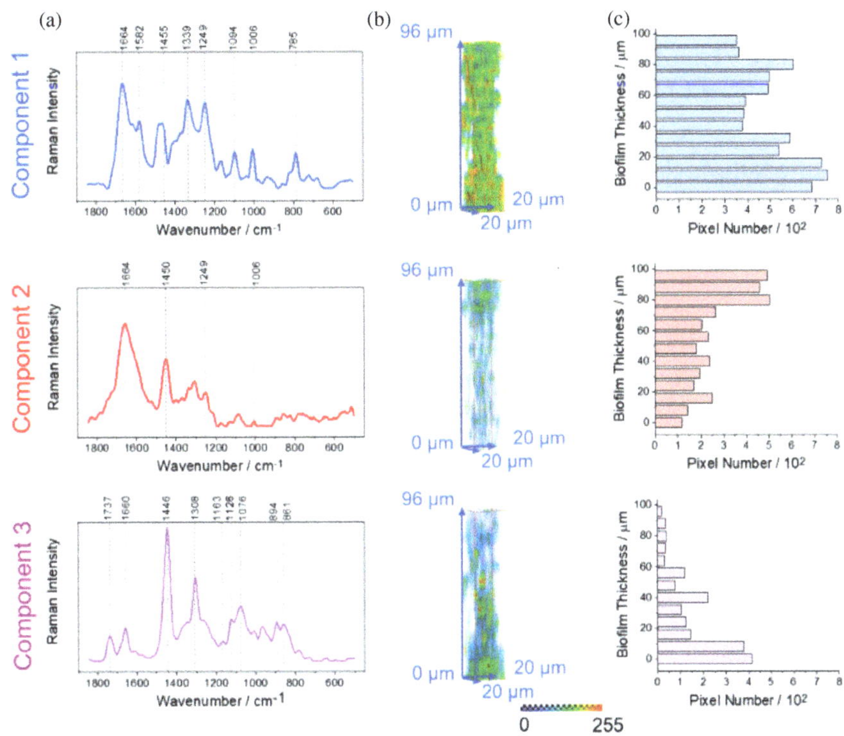

Figure 10.6. NMF analytical results of the *P. aeruginosa* biofilm matrix. (a) Calculated "pure" spectra of three major components in the biofilm: bacterial cells (Component 1), proteins (Component 2) and glycolipids (Component 3). (b) 3D distribution of the corresponding components in the biofilm matrix; the intensity was increased from blue to red. (c) Area coverage of each component in the biofilm with various depths. Zero marked the substrate surface. The scale on the z-axis represents the number of pixels whose Raman spectral abundance calculated by NMF analysis was above an automatically selected threshold. Reproduced from Ref. [152] with permission.

of the bands corresponding to carbohydrates, lipids, carotenoids, DNA, and tyrosine were more prominent in the sessile cell spectra compared to that of the planktonic cells [165].

In a different study, Kusić *et al.* examined biofilm formations and planktonic cells of diverse species of the *Legionella* genus, *P. aeruginosa*, *K. pneumoniae*, and *E. coli* by Raman microscopy. The Raman spectra of the sessile cells of six *Legionella* species revealed a higher lipid content opposed to their planktonic counterparts as well as the other investigated genera. In comparison to their planktonic cellular forms, *P. aeruginosa*, *K. pneumoniae*, and *E. coli* biofilms contained more polysaccharides [163]. In a related study, immunomagnetic separation was used to separate *Legionella* species' bacterial cells from their biofilms, and multivariate analysis was applied to identify the separated cells on a single-cell level. *P. aeruginosa*, *K. pneumoniae*, and *E. coli* cells were distinguished from isolated *Legionella* cells with an overall accuracy of 98.6%. Additionally, a classification accuracy of 86.3% for five separate *Legionella* strains was attained [166].

In a similar context, a biofilm model compiled of Raman spectra acquired from *Streptococcus sanguinis* and *Streptococcus mutans* was developed by Beier *et al.* [167]. PCA, in conjunction with a logistic regression technique, was used to examine the Raman spectra. Here, single-species biofilm spectra were used to validate the model, which had a 96% accuracy rate. Additionally, 97% of the Raman spectra of "pseudo-mixed" biofilms from various locations were accurately identified [167]. Raman spectra of the biofilm-forming *S. epidermidis* 1457 strain and its mutant *S. epidermidis* 1457-M10 strain were obtained by Samek *et al.* The PCA of the spectra clearly separated the two strains and showed the impact of the biofilm matrix components on the spectra, particularly that of polysaccharide intercellular adhesions [168].

Quorum sensing, a method of cell-to-cell communication used by the majority of bacterial biofilms, enables bacteria to track changes in the environment and cell density and to react accordingly. Both quorum sensing and biofilms are often involved in causing bacterial diseases. Here, Bodelón and colleagues applied special SERS tags to monitor the secretion of quorum sensing molecule pyocyanin over time in *P. aeruginosa* biofilms [169]. Guo *et al.* conducted a similar study in which they developed a method to monitor the gaseous metabolites of *P. aeruginosa*, *S. aureus*, and *E. coli* using specific SERS tags [170].

In stark contrast to the usual Raman methods, the use of a Raman fiber probe is an entirely different strategy. The data received from a fiber probe allowed Shen *et al.* to obtain Raman spectra from the embedded bacterial and yeast cells as well as the surrounding EPS matrix. The information from both the sessile cells and the EPS are examined thanks to the bigger detection area of ~50 μm. Based on the information received, a classification model was created, with a classification accuracy of 93.8%. Additionally, when clinical strains were employed for identification, the identification accuracy rose to 97.5%. The combination of Raman spectroscopy with chemometric analysis might serve recognition of medical biofilms or biofilm-related infections [30].

In conclusion, SERS and Raman spectroscopy are potential methods for determining the biofilm's amorphous and chaotic molecular makeup. These techniques have proven to be quite valuable with their quick processing times, non-destructiveness, cost-effectiveness, and straightforward applicability in comparison to the conventional methods. These strategies can be combined with several others to expand the use of these methods into new industries like the food, medical, and marine sectors.

10.3.5 *Antimicrobial Resistance*

After determining the infection-causing pathogen, it is necessary to assess any potential resistances. This is the most crucial information that doctors need in order to administer a successful treatment. Antimicrobial resistance is determined by two fundamental patterns, which are followed by Raman methods for antimicrobial susceptibility testing. The first, well-known method calls for treating the isolated pathogens with antimicrobial substances for a while before comparing their Raman spectra to those of untreated controls. Antibiotics drastically alter the biochemistry of cells of sensitive pathogens and produce considerable modifications from their control which can be detected using the RamanBioAssay™ technology. The alterations in resistant infections are minimal because the chemicals very marginally alter their biological makeup. In a recent study, clinical *E. coli* isolates were incubated for 90 min in the presence and absence of ciprofloxacin followed by Raman analysis for antimicrobial resistance determination. The results were equivalent to those of normal techniques used in clinical laboratory practice [171]. Furthermore, it was shown that high ciprofloxacin concentrations result in a simultaneous drop in the shoulder at 1485 cm^{-1} and an intensification of the Raman band at 1458 cm^{-1}. The ratio of the band intensities relates to growth and antibiotic-induced concentration-dependent growth inhibition. An on-chip Raman method provides sensitivity of 91% for differentiating between susceptible and resistant *E. coli* isolates after 2 h of incubation with the antibiotic [172]. Moreover, it was discovered that in samples that were resistant and untreated the relative intensity of the nucleic acid band at 1485 cm^{-1} was significantly decreased when compared to samples that were sensitive and treated. Using an *E. faecalis* strain that is vancomycin sensitive, it was possible to distinguish between treated and untreated samples with 94% accuracy after 30 minutes of vancomycin exposure [173]. Due to the considerable sample-to-sample variability, the cefoxitin treatment of methicillin-resistant (MRSA) and methicillin-susceptible (MSSA) isolates with concurrent Raman spectroscopy over a period of 4 h produced highly variable discrimination results of 33–100% [174].

Dekter *et al.* administered various antibiotics for 5 h to 133 Gram-positive and Gram-negative bacterial isolates. The susceptible strains received low amounts of the substance whereas the resistant strains received large concentrations. Comparing treated and untreated susceptible strains revealed distinct clustering, but resistant strains showed no clustering and an overall concordance of 89% when compared to the gold standard approach (Vitek-2). Susceptibility testing for ciprofloxacin was 100% consistent with Vitek-2 when the studies were repeated using *Enterobacter cloacae* that had already been cultured in blood culture flasks to imitate positive blood cultures [175]. Another study that used *E. coli* strains treated for 6 h with bacteriostatic and bactericidal antibiotics gave insight into how the drugs work by how they affected bacterial metabolism. The protein-to-lipid ratios I_{2936}/I_{2885} and I_{2936}/I_{2850} showed that both kinds of antibiotics supplied a shared stress signature, although the bactericidal chemicals caused reduced nucleic acid-to-protein (I_{812}/I_{830}) and nucleic acid-to-lipid (I_{1483}/I_{1452}) ratios in comparison to the bacteriostatic [176].

The second strategy is more challenging and is based on identifying the biochemical variations in genetic makeup and metabolic traits between resistant and susceptible cultures that have not previously been exposed to antibiotics. With the use of UVRR and Raman microspectroscopy the separation of extended-spectrum beta-lactamases and carbapenem-resistant Enterobacterales from susceptible clinical *E. coli* isolates was achieved with an accuracy of 75% and 70%, respectively [177]. Using deep learning to analyze data, it was possible to distinguish between MRSA and MSSA *S. aureus* with an accuracy of 89% [68]. Based on the MSSA strain's weaker staphyloxanthin bands, another study distinguished MRSA and MSSA strains [178]. By combining transcriptome analysis and Raman spectroscopy, Germond *et al.* were able to distinguish a parental isolate from 10 laboratory-evolved, resistant *E. coli* strains with an accuracy of 100%. When the strains were categorized in accordance with the antibiotic's mode of action, an accuracy of 99.4% was attained. The significant linear correlation between Raman spectral intensities and gene expression, along with the correlation between the wavenumber contribution to the classification model and the expression of particular genes linked to the resistance mode of action, were the most significant findings [179]. In a pilot study, Pistiki *et al.* evaluated the effectiveness and efficiency of three distinct label-free Raman spectroscopy techniques to distinguish

MRSA from MSSA. The most effective method was found to be single-cell analysis utilizing 532 nm excitation, which accurately predicted 87.5% of the strains and gathers data on the total biochemical makeup of the bacteria. UV resonance Raman microspectroscopy had a consistent accuracy of 62.5% but lacked the sensitivity to distinguish between MRSA and MSSA. With direct 785 nm excitation on the petri dish, a balanced accuracy of 87.5% was obtained, yet the distinction was based on staphyloxanthin bands, a cell component not connected to the presence of methicillin resistance [180].

These results demonstrate that particular information about a bacterium's antibiotic resistance may be extracted from its Raman spectrum, which was acquired in a label-free way.

10.3.6 *Isotope Labeling*

The application of stable isotope probing (SIP) to label microorganisms has recently gained in importance since this method can be used to introduce a harmless label into the cells [98]. Commonly used SIP labels are D, ^{13}C, ^{15}N, and ^{18}O. Here the most prominent shift can be observed from the C–H to the C–D stretching vibrations (Figure 10.7). In addition, the C–D signals are

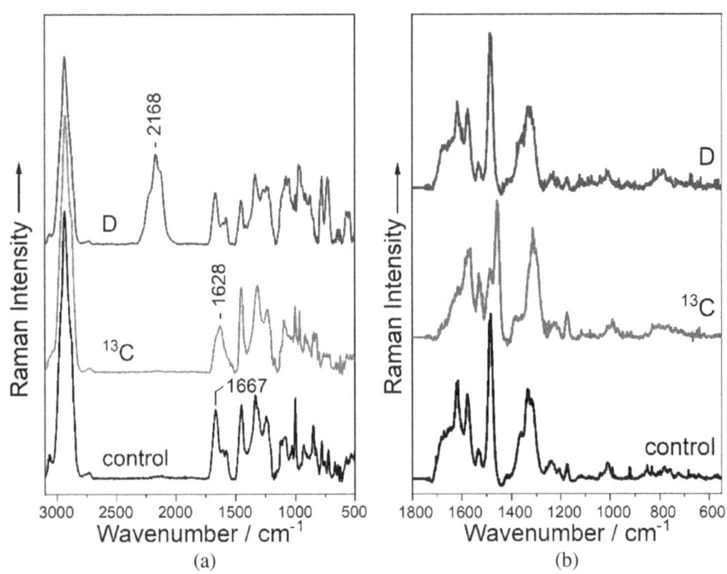

Figure 10.7. Isotope labeling of *E. coli* cultured with D-glucose or ^{13}C-glucose with an excitation wavelength of (a) 532 nm and (b) 244 nm. Reproduced from Ref. [181] with permission.

very easy to observe since they are in the so-called silent region of a Raman spectrum. Nevertheless, depending on the used excitation wavelengths and resonance enhancements, different labeling patterns can be monitored. In Figure 10.7 the UVRR spectra of isotopically labeled cells with an excitation wavelength of 244 nm are depicted. The application of heavier isotopes such as ^{13}C, ^{15}N, and ^{18}O are more complicated, since they lead to small variations in the fingerprint region where most of the signals are superimposed bands originating from different molecules [181, 182].

One of the most applied isotope labels is D_2O since here, the activity of microorganisms can be probed. The activity can be defined as the area of the C–D stretching vibrations in relation to the sum of the areas of the C–H and C–D stretching vibrations. Nevertheless, beside D_2O the applied carbon sources also influence the amount of deuterium which are incorporated from bacteria [183]. D_2O labeling can be used to track active groundwater microbes and understand their ecosystem function [184] or to study metabolic activities of single bacterial cells in human intestinal microbiota [185]. Other applications are the correlation of D incorporation with P-releasing activities of phosphate-solubilizing bacteria [186] or the detection of active cellulose degraders [187]. To better understand the mechanism of the deuterium uptake from D_2O in different bacterial species, two-dimensional Raman correlation spectroscopy is a suitable tool. Here, it is possible to highlight the different ways of, e.g., D incorporation into the cells [188]. Beside D_2O, D-labeled carbon sources can also be used. This approach not only leads to C–D stretching vibrations but also to different substituted phenylalanine rings [189]. Combining different carbon sources with D or ^{13}C labeling even allows revealing of which specific carbon source is preferentially utilized [190]. In addition, the labeling with different isotopes helps in assigning specific bands of unknown origin. In the study of Kubryk *et al.*, ^{13}C and ^{15}N was used to identify the band at ~730 cm^{-1} in the SERS spectra of bacteria as an adenine-related signal [191]. The correlation of Raman information with secondary-ion mass spectrometry makes it possible to quantify the spectral information. For this purpose, the bacteria were incubated in different $^{12}C/^{13}C$-glucose ratios and the position of the phenylalanine signals was used to estimate the amount of incorporated ^{13}C [192].

The use of ^{15}N allows a special look at nitrogen fixation. Here, diazotrophs were investigated by labeling with $^{15}N_2$. The study demonstrated that for quantification of N_2 fixation activity, the Raman spectroscopic approach is more sensitive than common methods [193]. This method can also be used to differentiate nitrogen-fixing bacteria in soil communities using cytochrome c as a marker molecule [194].

Combining isotope-labeling experiments with Raman-activated cell sorting allows not only the analysis of the differences due to isotope probing but also sorting according to such Raman spectroscopic changes. This will then enable sorting of the bacteria according to different properties and use them for further experiments [195].

These methods have been shown to find application in the hospital environment as wastewater surveillance, infection diagnostics and in determination of metabolically active bacteria in the hospital flora. Two studies coupled Raman spectroscopy with heavy water labeling and exposure to antibiotics to develop an activity-based antimicrobial susceptibility testing approach, directly applicable for clinical urine and blood samples within 2.5 h. In both studies the antimicrobial susceptibility detected with the Raman method was in line with standard methods [196, 197].

10.4 Viruses

SERS is known as a versatile tool in medical research for recording fingerprint information with molecular specificity as well as trace sensitivity due to the application of powerful SERS-active surfaces [198]. Thanks to the design and development of simplified Raman systems accompanied with elegant cartridge or microfluidic lab-on-a-chip devices, point-of-care applications of SERS in the detection of viruses have become more feasible [199]. To directly detect and identify the virus particles, the viruses are trapped in so-called hotspots of metallic nanostructures [200, 201]. Thus, the recorded SERS spectrum is originating from gene fragments or membrane proteins, i.e., those virus compartments being in close vicinity towards the metallic surface. Quantitative and multiplexed assays are achieved by SERS-based immunoassays, employing SERS labels equipped with specific antibodies to interact with the virus of interest. Within this paragraph, we aim to introduce the direct or label-free as well as indirect, i.e., by using SERS labels with specific recognition elements, detection of viruses to illustrate the potential of the SERS technique in this research field.

Gold nanocavities were applied to enhance the Raman scattered light of pseudo-virus particles located in the hotspot areas across the sensing surface [202]. The fingerprint information varies between different virus types which is associated with different surface proteins and virus components interacting with the metallic surface. However, in order to ensure a reproducible SERS signal from one virus type, the orientation of the biomacromolecules such as proteins needs to be constant as the SERS signal of Raman modes perpendicular to the metallic surface are preferentially enhanced. Inverted pyramidal sensing surfaces were applied to directly detect SERS fingerprint information from small volumes of hepatitis A virus particles down to a concentration of 13 pg/mL [203]. More examples of direct SERS sensing strategies in virus research involves the application of silicon nanowires equipped with silver nanoparticles [204] or Au nanopillars [205]. In order to allow for versatility in application scenarios such as wearable sensor surfaces, flexible SERS substrates were developed by means of lithographic processes and transfer printing [206]. SERS spectra of virus samples containing SARS-CoV-2 were recorded even in the complex matrix of saliva without sample preparation. By applying chemometrics, the authors illustrated that they could distinguish between different respiratory and non-respiratory viruses. SERS spectra were recorded from two different lentiviruses, which differ in the existence of a vector encoding a GFP gene, during their viral production in the media at varying concentrations using a 3D-printed SERS substrate [207]. By applying chemometrics, the viral titer of those virus particles containing the GFP gene were estimated, illustrating the potential of the technique in concentration-dependent measurements of viruses.

Instead of using solid SERS sensing surfaces for the direct detection of viruses, SERS-active nanoparticles have the advantage to form aggregations, i.e., hot spots allowing for a further signal enhancement due to the overlapping of electromagnetic fields. One example is the application of gold-copper nanostars for the detection of SERS spectra of SARS-CoV-2 virus particles, whose fingerprint information is dominated by the SERS signals of spike and nucleocapsid proteins [208]. Moreover, silver nanoparticles cleaned from citrate residues on the metallic surface are applied to detect reproducible SERS signals of SARS-CoV-2, Human Adenovirus 3 and H1N1 influenza virus particles [209]. In order to distinguish between the viruses, machine learning was applied allowing for a quantitative assessment. Here, the Raman marker mode of acetonitrile was applied as internal standard. For an efficient enrichment of SARS-CoV-2 from complex matrices such as wastewater or biofluids, the cellular receptor angiotensin-converting enzyme 2 (ACE2) was applied to functionalize the metallic, SERS-active sensing surface [210–212]. To identify the captured virus particles, machine learning needs to be implemented in the data analysis [211]. By using ACE2-modified magnetic

Fe_3O_4 gold nanocomposites to capture SARS-CoV-2 from nasal or throat swabs, the detection of SERS signals from those virus particles even from clinical samples became feasible [213]. A detection limit of 100 copies per mL was achieved while the analysis time was 15 min. The authors applied a SVM to identify contaminated swabs with an accuracy of 100%.

In the case of direct SERS investigations of viruses, sophisticated chemometric methods or machine learning procedures will be always needed for an identification of the target virus due to the complexity of the Raman fingerprint information, whereas the beauty of SERS immunoassays lies in the simplicity of the SERS spectrum being only dominated by the contribution of the Raman reporter molecule. Thus, the data analysis is simplified down to the identification of the marker mode of the Raman reporter and its integration, i.e., estimation of the signal intensity. To detect SARS-CoV-2, an immunoassay was created based on the usage of magnetic beads equipped with an antibody specific for the nucleocapsid protein as well as SERS tags being selective for the same target [214]. Thus, by using magnetic forces, the sensing platform is easily separated from the sample matrix. The assay was performed with SARS-CoV-2 lysates with virus concentrations between 0 and 10^4 PFU/mL and the authors found a detection limit of 5.1 PFU/mL, which reflects a higher level of sensitivity than commercially available rapid kits. Moreover, the same assay platform was applied to identify SARS-CoV-2 in human nasopharyngeal aspirates [215]. To illustrate the feasibility of the assay in clinical settings, a portable Raman spectrometer was applied, and the authors distinguished accurately between positive and negative clinical samples within 30 min. Thus, the assay showed excellent characteristics to be applied in point-of-care testing accompanied with an improved sensitivity in comparison to rapid tests. Using also magnetic nanoparticles as sensing platform as well as SERS tags, both equipped with antibodies specific for SARS-CoV-2 spike protein, an immunocomplex formation with a detection limit of 257 fg/mL within 30 min and in the matrix of viral transport medium was illustrated [216]. It was demonstrated that the assay is specific for B.1.1.7 (alpha), B.1.351 (beta), and B.1.617.2 (delta) spike proteins of SARS-CoV-2 and due to its high sensitivity, it has a high potential in point-of-care diagnosis and clinical settings when applying portable or handheld Raman devices for readout. Gold nanoparticles modified with a Raman reporter and SARS-CoV-2-specific anti-spike antibodies were applied to form nanoparticle aggregates in the presence of the target antigen, which is easily observed by the bare eye due to a color change from red to blue that is associated with the appearance of nanoparticle clusters [217]. Moreover, the formed hotspots were analyzed by means of SERS achieving a higher level of sensitivity in comparison to the colorimetric test. As the virus enters human cells *via* the expressed ACE2 moiety, the authors showed that viruses attached to the anti-spike antibody-modified SERS labels lost their capability to infect HEK293T cells. The application of a novel 6E3 monoclonal antibody as recognition element in a SERS-based immunoassay demonstrated the capability in detecting the H275Y neuraminidase mutation in influenza viruses [218]. Thus, the drug-resistant influenza virus was detected down to 10^2 PFU/mL and its application for the analysis of human nasopharyngeal aspirate samples showed its potential for diagnosis in clinical settings. Finally, a dual-mode SERS-based immunoassay being specific for the nucleoprotein of both influenza A and SARS-CoV-2 viruses was developed using the concept of a lateral flow assay [219]. The sensing strategy is illustrated in Figure 10.8, including the structure of the applied SERS tags as well as the test strip. Here, a single test strip is applied to detect both viruses simultaneously in virus lysates. Within a clinical test, the authors applied 39 patient samples, whereas 28 were SARS-CoV-2 positive, 6 were influenza A virus positives and 5 were the negative control, illustrating its efficacy in diagnosis.

As a further recognition element in SERS-based detection schemes employing SERS labels, aptamers were applied, being also specific towards virus particles. Silver nanoparticles were equipped with an aptamer containing

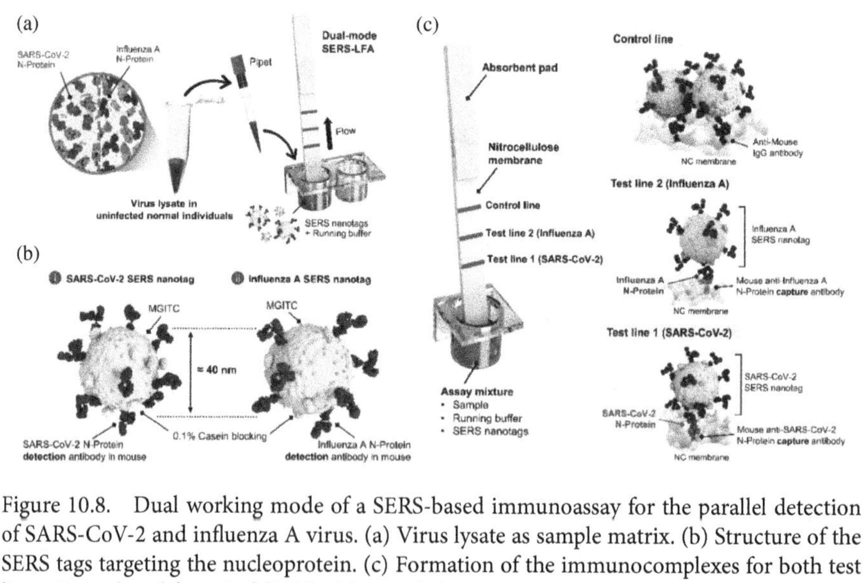

Figure 10.8. Dual working mode of a SERS-based immunoassay for the parallel detection of SARS-CoV-2 and influenza A virus. (a) Virus lysate as sample matrix. (b) Structure of the SERS tags targeting the nucleoprotein. (c) Formation of the immunocomplexes for both test lines. Reproduced from Ref. [219] with permission.

a G-quadruplex core to which the influenza A virus binds specifically [220]. In a competition assay, a dye molecule is realized from the sensor surface upon interaction with the virus particles, resulting in a decreased SERS signal of the Raman reporter as function of the virus concentration and a detection range of 10^3 to 5×10^{10} virus particles/mL is achieved. This concept of colloidal aptasensors was applied by the same group not only for influenza A viruses [220, 221] but also for the detection of SARS-CoV-2 [222]. By applying magnetic beads as a sensor platform to simplify the detection scheme applying magnetic forces, a SERS-based aptasensor was developed to detect SARS-CoV-2 *via* a locking amplifier strategy, which is only activated for the case of virus recognition by the aptamer [223]. For the detection of SARS-CoV-2, the authors found a detection limit of 260 TU/μL. The performance of the assay was validated by using tap water, river water and fish samples as complex matrices. Finally, a selective aptamer-based sensing scheme was developed for the parallel detection of SARS-CoV-2 and influenza A (H1N1) virus particles [224]. Here, a SERS-active sensing surface is decorated with dye-labeled DNA aptamers which are selective for the target viruses. A parallel detection is ensured due to the application of structurally different dye molecules as reporter with specific Raman maker modes, which are not overlapping. In the presence of the virus, the aptamer detaches from the surface, resulting in a decreased SERS intensity with increasing virus concentration. By applying an internal standard, quantitative assessments were made allowing for sensitive detection in a parallel fashion.

10.5 Fungi and Yeasts

Fungi are eukaryotic microorganisms which do not perform photosynthesis and are therefore more related to animals than to plants. These unicellular or multicellular organisms have chitin in their cell walls. Most of the fungi are dimorphic which means they can switch between hyphae and yeast cells. Such a morphology change is often associated with the change from commensals to pathogens. Fungi can be discriminated by means of Raman spectroscopy either directly according to their typical cell chemistry or by their special metabolites such as pigments or lipids.

10.5.1 *Pigments and Other Components*

Many fungi exhibit pigments depending on the environmental parameters. For *Basidiomycetes* (mushrooms) the pigment production is generated in close contact with other microbes. Such interaction zones can be analyzed by means of Raman microscopy which is non-invasive. This *in situ* application is able to analysis basidiomycete pigments in multi-partner cultures [225].

Apart from pigments, special components can also be localized in fungal hyphae. Raman mapping and coherent anti-Stokes Raman scattering microscopy can reveal the distribution of cytochrome, which can be used as marker for mitochondria in the hyphal tips of *Schizophyllum commune*. This study revealed that mitochondria are more active at the growing hyphal tips and at branching regions [226].

Oleaginous fungi of the *Mortierella spp.* are well known to produce high amounts of unsaturated lipids in vesicles inside the hyphae. The intensity ratio of the two Raman signals of =C–H and $-CH_2/-CH_3$ groups at 1270 and 1445 cm^{-1} can be used to determine the degree of unsaturation of the oil. It could be shown that the oil composition is homogeneous within one as well as between different individual hyphae of one fungal sample [227]. Nevertheless, the degree of unsaturation of the lipids vary between different species [228]. Also, the spores of macrofungi are rich in lipids, which can be used to discriminate them on the genus [229] and species level [230] by means of Raman microscopy.

Malassezia spp. belong to the skin flora of animals and are lipid dependent. The adaptation mechanism of *Malassezia* yeasts to their human and animal hosts is dependent on the lipid metabolism. A Raman fiber probe was used to monitor the differential ability of three *Malassezia spp.* to utilize lipid supplements [231].

The yeast cell wall of *Candida spp.* can be analyzed by SERS spectroscopy in combination with computational tools. The cell wall of yeasts contains mainly chitin and glucan apart from other polysaccharides. Three *Candida spp.* can then be differentiated *via* their SERS spectra [232].

10.5.2 *Identification of Fungi and Yeast Species*

Yeasts and fungi are eukaryotic cells with organelles exhibiting distinct Raman spectroscopic pattens. Nevertheless, the average Raman spectra can be used to differentiate between various species [233, 234].

From the yeasts *Dekkera bruxellensis*, *Saccharomyces cerevisiae*, and *Wickerhamomyces anomalus*, lysate and non-treated cells were analyzed by means of SERS spectroscopy. The SERS spectra of the lysate and non-treated cell samples reveal differences. In addition, yeast cells in spiked beer could also be analyzed [235].

Most studies to differentiate yeasts were performed on *Candida spp.* Here, several studies using Raman and/or FTIR spectroscopy achieved the classification of several different *Candida spp.* [236–238]. A Raman spectroscopic study of isolates from peritonitis patients from 93 reference strains belonging to 10 different *Candida spp.* achieved an accuracy of 90% [239]. The UVRR spectra of 22 clinically relevant *Candida* strains of 12 *Candida spp.* are illustrated in Figure 10.9 [240]. Using a SVM revealed that the differentiation accuracy differs strongly from species to species. Nevertheless, UVRR spectra of *Candida spp.* can be used as part of the decision criteria for microbiological documentation.

The Raman spectroscopic analysis of fungi is complicated since enhanced melanin concentrations exhibit a high level of fluorescence and in addition lead to photodamage of the cells. Therefore, mostly SERS spectroscopy is used to analyze fungal species. The application of silver nanoparticle synthesis directly on the fungal exoskeleton of the clinically relevant fungi *Aspergillus fumigatus* s.s., cryptic *A. fumigatus spp.*, and *Rhizomucor pusillus* resulted in very distinct SERS spectra which could easily be discriminated *via* chemometric models [241].

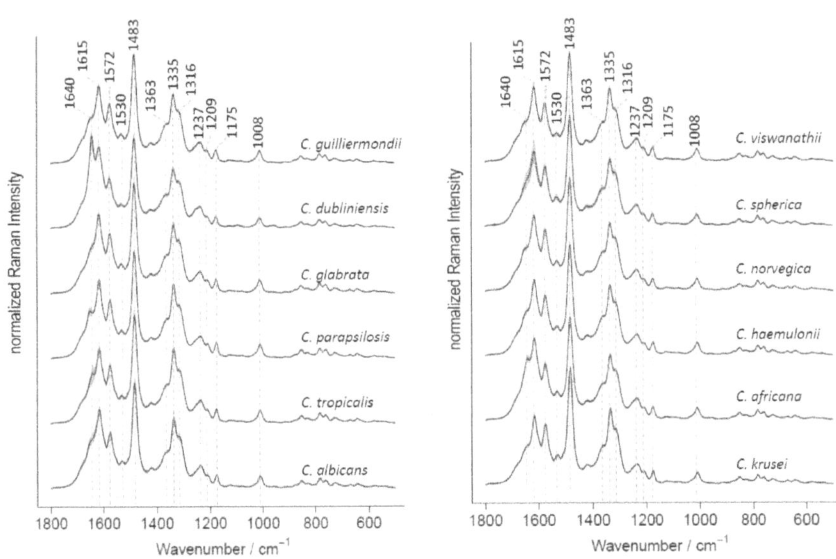

Figure 10.9. Mean UVRR spectra of the analyzed 12 *Candida* species. Reproduced from Ref. [240] with permission.

In addition, a SERS study was able to assign the main SERS signals of different fungi to the major constituents of the fungal cell wall chitin, galactomannan, and β-1,3-glucan. The SERS spectra were then used to differentiate the four fungal species *Aspergillus flavus, Trichophyton rubrum, Scopulariopsis brumptii,* and *Candida krusei*. In addition, skin samples infected with *T. rubrum* could also be discriminated from non-infected skin samples [242].

An *ex vivo* nail model of onychomycosis could discriminate between infection with the dermatophytes *T. rubrum*, *T. mentagrophytus* and *T. tonsurans* by means of Raman spectroscopy. In addition, infected nails from these species could be differentiated from that of non-dermatophytic species *Scopulariopsis brevicaulis* and *Candida albicans* [243, 244].

Individual fungal spores can be analyzed by Raman microscopy when the experimental parameters are set carefully to avoid laser damage. With this approach, it is possible to achieve different spectroscopic patterns for spores of fungal species encountered in indoor air or dust samples [245].

Another approach to differentiate between toxic mold species is the application of shifted-excitation Raman difference spectroscopy (SERDS) to separate the Raman spectrum from fluorescence. Conidial spores from *Aspergillus nidulans, A. flavus, A. oryzae, A. versicolor, A. fumigatus, A. niger, Stachybotrys chartarum*, and *Penicillium chrysogenum* reveal distinct SERDS spectra whereas the major features of the Raman spectra of each species can be correlated with the melanin biosynthesis pathway [246].

Highly pigmented spores from *A. fumigatus, A. niger, A. nidulans, A. calidoustus, Cladosporium herbarum, Alternaria alternata, Penicillium rubens,* and *Lichtheimia corymbifera* make it difficult to apply excitation wavelengths in the visible range. Therefore, UVRR spectroscopy was used to differentiate these spores associated with respiratory diseases [247].

10.6 Parasites

Parasites invading humans or animals can also be bacteria or fungi but here we will focus on animals belonging to the endoparasites such as protozoa and helminths as well as ectoparasites which either cause diseases or are vectors for other pathogens.

Ectoparasites such as mosquitos, sucking lice, ticks, or mites vector a large number of pathogens which are relevant for both human and animal diseases.

Especially for blood-feeding ticks the species information is important to estimate potential pathogens transmitted to the host. Despite finding the ticks on animals or humans and identifying them afterwards, one study analyses individual tick feces grains by means of Raman spectroscopy. Since tick feces is species specific, it can be used for typing. Applying Raman microscopy allows differentiation between feces of seven hard tick species from the family *Ixodidae* found on cattle. In addition, it is also possible to discriminate the tick developmental stage like nymphs, meta-nymphs, and adult ticks. In a proof-of-concept study, a hand-held Raman spectrometer was used to differentiate two *Amblyomma spp.* [248].

Endoparasites are either monocellular protozoa or multicellular hermits such as nematodes, trematodes, or cestodes. Nematodes do not only infect humans and animals but also plants. The burrowing nematode *Radopholus similis* for example invades banana plants (*Musa spp.*) and causes extensive root lesions. When treated with anigorufone, yellow droplets appear in the bodies of *R. similis*. With 2D Raman mapping it could be shown that lipids are localized within the droplets [249].

Other nematodes are common human parasites like *Ascaris*. Here, infection occurs orally through contaminated food, ingesting *Ascaris* eggs which adhere with their sticky surface on vegetables. The Raman spectra of different parts of unembryonated eggs from *Ascaris suum* revealed that inside the eggs a huge amount of lipids and proteins can be detected. In contrast, the Raman spectra of the shell indicates carbohydrates and few proteins [250].

Unicellular protozoa are eukaryotic parasites which exhibit a much broader diversity. *Leishmania* for example are transmitted by flies and occur in the human body in macrophages as amastigotes. Here, they replicate in an endolysosomal compartment called the parasitophorous vacuole (PV). SERS mapping reveal a high content of lipids and sterols inside the PV. In addition, proteophosphoglycans, ergosterol, and the phospholipid inositol could also be detected, which are specific for the parasite [251].

Trypanosoma spp. are unicellular flagellate protozoa which cause various diseases and are transmitted by insects. The chagas disease caused by *T. cruzi* is spread by infected feces of kissing bugs. The application of Raman spectroscopy could demonstrate that when treated with arachidonic acid, the lipid body in *T. cruzi* exhibits a higher content of this fatty acid [252]. Sleeping sickness is caused by *T. brucei rhodesiense* and *T. b. gambiense* transmitted by the tsetse fly. Since trypanosomes can be detected in skin biopsies, Raman spectroscopy was used to detect *T. brucei* in the skin of a murine model. Therefore, the information of 2D Raman mapping of a parasite was compared to these of *ex vivo* skin tissue. It could be shown that the Raman spectra of infected skin differ from those of non-infected skin [253].

The waterborne protozoan parasite *Cryptosporidium spp.* is considered the world's second most important causative agent of diarrheal diseases in children [254]. Applying SERS spectroscopy with silver nanoparticles on samples of *C. parvum* oocysts, *E. coli*, and *S. aureus* allows the discrimination of these three waterborne pathogens. This study discriminates the protozoa from the Gram-positive and Gram-negative bacteria by the chemistry of the cell surface [255]. Another study used Raman tweezers for the investigation of viable and neutralized oocysts. These sum spectra were then used to differentiate the *C. parvum* oocysts from other waterborne pathogens like *E. coli* and *V. cholerae* as well as the spores of *B. cereus* and *C. difficile* — common food pathogens [256].

Toxoplasma gondii is a protozoan parasite that infects up to 85% of the adults worldwide [254]. Infection is mainly acquired by the ingestion of oocysts shed by cats. Normally, primary infection is usually without symptoms but if the infection is acquired during pregnancy, it may cause severe damage to the fetus. Usually, the diagnosis of *T. gondii* requires a serological test to determine the immune condition of the patient. Here, Raman spectroscopy was used on colostrum samples to discriminate between infected and non-infected pregnant women [257]. Protozoa parasites cannot synthesize some amino acids and are therefore dependent on host-cell nutrients as carbon and energy sources. Labeled amino acids such as phenylalanine-D8 (Phe-D8) can be used to monitor the interaction between human retinal pigment epithelial cells (ARPE-19) infected by *T. gondii.* [258] Using an optical tweezer in combination with a Raman microscope can analyze human cerebrovascular endothelial cells infected by *T. gondii* at the very start of the infection process. Especially, the transfer of Phe-D8 from host cells to parasites can be measured in real time starting from the point of infection [259].

The protozoan parasite *Neospora caninum* is an important pathogen especially for cattle and is mainly transmitted vertically [254]. Using selective scanning Raman microscopy, *N. caninum* tachyzoites within individual live human brain microvascular endothelial cells (HBMEC) were analyzed. In Figure 10.10(a) the bright field image with the sampling points is shown in addition to the fluorescence image with the localization of the tachyzoite. The loading of PC2 and the corresponding map reveal the parasite with a

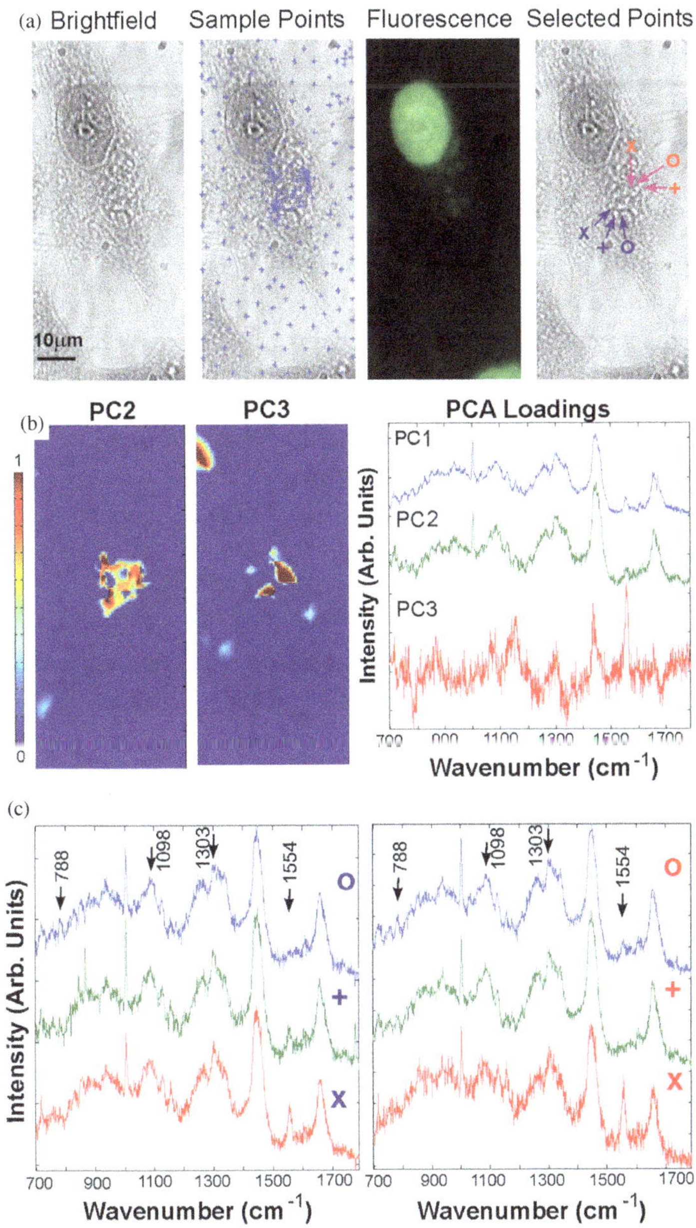

Figure 10.10. A typical example of spatially resolved Raman measurements obtained by selective scanning of a live HBMEC infected with *N. caninum*. (a) Bright field image, the distribution of the sampling point, acridine orange fluorescence image and positions of selected Raman spectra for (c). (b) The maps of the PC2 and PC3 scores and the corresponding loadings. (c) Spatially resolved Raman spectra at the positions indicated in (a). Reproduced from Ref. [260] with permission.

high content of phospholipids (Figure 10.10(b)). The Raman spectra from two infected regions of the cell are shown in Figure 10.10(c). The marks (o) indicate the parasite nuclei, (+) region rich in lipids and (x) high tryptophan concentrations most probably associated with parasite-host interactions [260].

Babsia bovis is transmitted by ticks and is the causative agent of the epidemic hemoglobinuria of cattle, thereby threatening livestock worldwide. The sporozoites of *Babesia spp.* exclusively infect erythrocytes [254]. The analysis of infected red blood cells (RBCs) by means of different vibrational spectroscopic methods shows a lower heme as well as a higher lipid content in the parasite as in the RBCs [261].

Malaria is caused by parasites of the genus *Plasmodium* and are transmitted by female *Anopheles* mosquitoes developing several blood-borne stages and finally infecting RBCs. The application of different Raman spectroscopic techniques can evaluate changes based on the molecular phenotype of the RBCs due to the presence of the parasite [262, 263]. Therefore, it is possible to monitor the effect of antimalarial drugs, on one hand, on the malaria parasite and, on the other hand, at the host RBC. In addition, it is possible to even diagnose subclinical levels of malaria infection. Especially the molecular changes that occur during the development of the parasite throughout the erythocytic cycle can be tracked. Here, the digestion of hemoglobin by the parasite and detoxification into the insoluble hemozoin form is especially suitable and therefore used as marker for most studies [264].

Hemozoin can be unambiguously identified by means of resonance Raman microscopy due to its extremely strong resonance enhancement of characteristic marker bands. Combining Raman mapping with partial dark-field microscopy achieves a fast localization of hemozoin deposits inside the RBCs and an unambiguous identification of the crystals *via* Raman spectroscopy [265]. Another approach is a fiber array-based hyperspectral Raman system. Here, Raman imaging of malaria-infected RBCs localizes the malaria pigment hemozoin in early ring stages of infected erythrocytes [266].

Also, various SERS substrates were used to differentiate between hemoglobin and hemozoin or between infected and non-infected RBCs. For this purpose silver particles [267], silver nanorods [268] also on magnetic substrates [269], nanostructured gold substrates [270], sandwich-based SERS probes [271], or even butterfly wings [272] were applied to detect the hemozoin marker signals. Combining SERS strategy with on-chip sample preparation and near-analyte silver nanoparticle synthesis can provide a quantitative hemozoin concentration in infected blood samples [273].

Nevertheless, malaria markers can also be detected in tissues other than RBCs. For a spleen study two female mice were infected with asynchronous *Plasmodium berghei* and Raman maps of their spleen sections were compared to those of non-infected mice. Here, an overall increase in heme-based Raman vibrations within the infected samples was observed due to an increase in hemozoin concentration [274].

A meta-analysis summarizes all vibrational spectroscopic studies on malaria research and their potential as a surveillance tool. For Raman spectroscopy the possibility to be used as a monitoring technique still need to be assessed. Nevertheless, it was recommended to evaluate the spectroscopic techniques in combination with multiple machine learning techniques in various epidemiological settings. For this, standardized protocols need to be established for both spectra collection and data analysis. Still, the development of rapid and cost-effective point-of-care Raman spectroscopic diagnostic tools may help to minimize further malaria outbreaks [275].

10.7 Host Response

Higher organisms are equipped with an immune system tasked to counter invading pathogens. In addition to chemical components such as the complement, the blood leukocytes are the main representatives of this system. These cells are very diverse, consisting of many different cell types with different abilities and characteristics. When a pathogen manages to overcome the natural barriers such as the skin or the mucosal, the immune system is activated and a cascade of action is triggered for its elimination [276]. These actions include the direct elimination of the pathogen performed by blood phagocytes, namely neutrophils and monocytes, that are the main representors of the innate immune system. It also includes the coordination of the immune response through cell signaling using cytokines and chemokines. The monocytes activate the T-lymphocytes through the presentation of the pathogen's antigen on their surface and this leads to the activation of B-lymphocytes that produce pathogen-specific antibodies [277]. The activation of all these mechanisms results in the alteration of the biochemical composition of all cell types involved. In the following chapter recent developments in label-free Raman spectroscopic techniques to extract, analyze, and translate this biochemical information is presented, providing inside on the cell's activation status but also about the invading pathogen itself. In addition, the translational potential of Raman data and the application of Raman approaches for diagnostic purposes in patients with infection will be also presented. For the Raman analysis of leukocytes two different strategies are applied. In the first strategy a highly focused laser spot is used, and the cells are scanned using a raster pattern, obtaining many spectra per cell which are afterwards averaged (Figure 10.2(e)). This provides a detailed analysis of the biochemical changes within the different areas of each measured cell, allowing the determination of activation at an intracell level. When the obtained spectra are averaged, the activation profile can be monitored at a cell level revealing the overall biochemical changes. The second strategy includes the acquisition of one spectrum per cell using a broader laser spot [278]. This significantly speeds up the process, allowing measurement of thousands of cells in limited time. This strategy is illustrated in Figure 10.11, where the cell mechanisms that are activated during the innate immune response are also shown. These mechanisms include phagocytosis, antigen degradation and presentation to T-lymphocytes, activation of pattern recognition receptors by pathogen-associated molecular patterns, as well as cytokine/chemokine secretion.

In vitro studies have shown that the determination of the cell's activation status is feasible *via* label-free Raman spectroscopy using the cell mapping mode. Toll-like receptor-4 stimulation with bacterial lipopolysaccharide (LPS) of THP-1 monocytes were compared to their unstimulated controls and could be differentiated with an accuracy of 87%. The first signs of cell activation were visible after 1 h through intense nucleic acid bands in the activated cells. After 3 and 8 h these bands were replaced by protein bands indicating ongoing transcriptional and translational activity. Correlation of these bands with data from cytokine gene expression and release confirmed this finding. In addition, spectral unmixing and Raman false-color images showed the distribution of several macromolecules as lipids, proteins and nucleic acids within the cell, allowing monitoring of the activation-derived biochemical changes overtime [279]. Another study used Raman spectroscopy to determinate the activation state of different immune cell types. THP-1 were activated with phorbol myristate acetate (PMA) and could be differentiated from their untreated controls with a sensitivity of 91%. The same results were provided from phytohemagglutinin (PHA)-stimulated Jurkat T-cells, whereas ionomycin- and PMA-stimulated Raji B cells provided a sensitivity of 95.2%. The activation of the lymphocytic cells was confirmed *via* the increase of

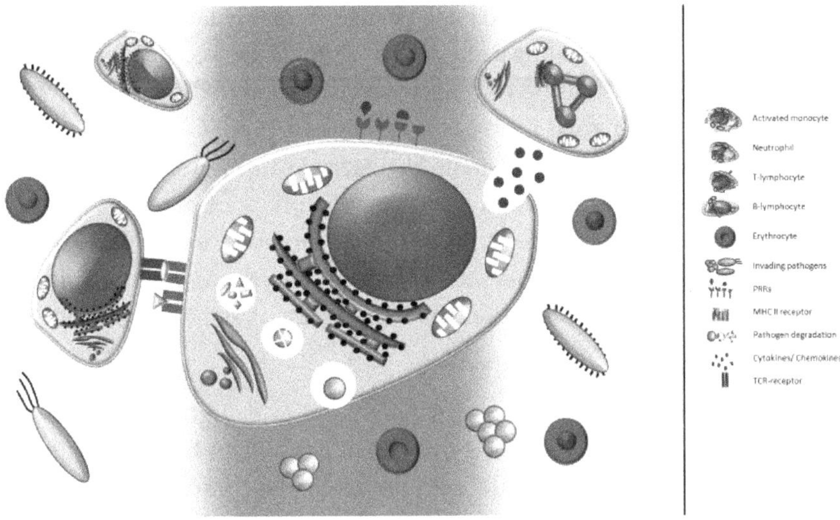

Figure 10.11. Schematic illustration of Raman spectroscopy performed on blood leukocytes to obtain information on the host response and host's immune status.

the activation marker CD69 on their cell surface and *via* increase of TNF-α expression in the monocyte cell line. Results were similar when the above cell population was isolated from the blood of healthy donors and activated *ex vivo* with the same stimulants where monocytes provided sensitivities of 95.2%, T-lymphocytes 90.9% and B-lymphocytes 89.9% when compared to their untreated controls. When peripheral blood mononuclear cells were treated with PHA and LPS an increase of sensitivity to 97.7% and 100%, respectively, was achieved, indicating ongoing cell signaling. Analysis of the Raman spectra revealed distinct protein and nucleic acid bands in all treated cells compared to their control, showing the activation-derived changes in biochemical composition [280]. In a mouse study it was shown that when challenging purified murine splenic $CD4^+$ T-lymphocyte with anti-CD3 and anti-CD28, application of Raman spectroscopy, using a mapping mode of 4×4 spots per cell, an overtime increase of biochemical differences could be evidenced compared to naïve controls. The increase of biochemical differences was parallel to the increase of CD69 expression on the cell's surface [281].

Similar findings were obtained from *in vivo* models in mice, providing first evidence for the translational potential of the host response determination through Raman spectroscopy. Raman analysis of splenic $CD4^+$ and $CD8^+$ lymphocytes from LPS-treated endotoxemic and saline-treated control mice revealed that the inflammation-related changes remained up to 10 days after LPS treatment. Raman imaging using scanning mode showed that in the CD4$^+$ lymphocytes of endotoxemic mice, transcriptional activity manifests after 4 days as nucleic acid signals increase in the nucleus. In the CD8$^+$ lymphocytes a shift of the observed amide I band is observed in the region of 1650 to 1610 cm^{-1} on the 4th and 10th day, indicating the presence of proteins with a different structural arrangement. When this approach was applied directly on the spleen tissue the accuracy for differentiation between individual mice spleen from LPS-treated and control mice 1 day after LPS injection was between 80–90% [282].

In the above-mentioned pre-clinical studies it is highlighted that the biochemical information obtained by Raman analysis of the host response allow the discrimination of different activation states *in vivo*. This ability could be a useful tool in clinical settings helping physicians to differentially diagnose and classify progressive inflammatory diseases. To test this, a pilot diagnostic clinical trial was designed to differentiate sterile inflammation from infection and sepsis. It was shown that application of Raman spectroscopy on blood leukocytes of hospitalized patients with infection and sepsis provided added diagnostic value compared to serum biomarkers alone (interleukin-6, C-reactive protein and procalcitonin). Raman spectra were obtained using a cell mapping mode and when considered in the model they allowed an 10% increase in the accuracy for differentiation of infection from sterile inflammation and an 18% increase in the differentiation of sepsis compared to biomarkers alone [283]. This indicates that the information on the host immune status hidden inside the Raman spectra has the potential to guide clinical decision making, when routinely applied in hospital settings.

Despite the determination of the cell's activation status, Raman analysis of leukocytes can also provide information on the infection-causing pathogen. Application of Raman mapping on *in vitro* infected EA.hy926 endothelial cells with *S. aureus* revealed the intracellular regions where the bacteria were present. The intracellular bacteria could be detected in the form of single bacteria as well as small colonies of 3–6 cells [284]. In another study the metabolic characteristics of an isolated *S. aureus* could be determined while the pathogen was inside EA.hy926 cells. It was shown that the intracellular pathogens did adapt to the host's conditions using strategies such as low replication rate while in exponential growth phase as well as by presenting different biochemical characteristics after 3–9 hours, compared to the extracellular lifestyle. In addition, 3D Raman mapping allowed precise localization of the bacteria inside the cells [128].

In other studies, and in order to investigate the diagnostic potential of Raman spectroscopy on infected cells, blood leukocytes were used. A recent *ex vivo* study revealed that Raman spectroscopy on blood leukocyte sub-population allows the identification of the pathogen type causing the infection. In this study a high-throughput Raman microscope was applied, capturing one spectrum per cell from thousands of cells per treatment. Multiple-step analysis of neutrophils from healthy donors that had phagocytosed *C. albicans*, *S. aureus* and *E. coli* isolates allowed design of a potential diagnostic algorithm for the determination of the causative pathogen. As a first step the discrimination of infection vs. non-infection was applied, using untreated controls, that yielded an accuracy of 90%. Afterwards discrimination of fungal vs. bacterial infection was applied that provided an accuracy of 92%, followed by the discrimination of neutrophils infected with Gram-positive vs. Gram-negative bacteria that provided an accuracy of 84%. Neutrophils infected with different pathogens revealed a distinct Raman profile in terms of lipid, protein, and nucleic acid bands, with specific features contributing to their differentiation. These differences in the spectral features have their origin in their different cell response to the pathogen. These data show that the pathogen information present inside the blood phagocytes can be extracted by Raman spectroscopy [285]. In another study the potential of extracting pathogen-related information from all major leukocyte sub-populations was investigated. In this study the cell mapping strategy was used. Neutrophils, monocytes, and lymphocytes from healthy donors were infected with *C. albicans*, *K. pneumoniae* and *S. aureus* clinical isolates. For the differentiation of fungal and bacterial pathogens, neutrophils provided an accuracy of 82%, lymphocytes 70% and monocytes 65%. The differentiation of Gram-positive and Gram-negative bacteria yielded an accuracy of 60% for monocytes. When the results from the *ex vivo* study were compared to Raman data from patients with infection of the same pathogens, common features could be detected (Figure 10.12), indicating the high translational potential of this method and its applicability in infectious disease diagnostics [286].

Determination of the cell response *via* Raman spectroscopy was also performed in the case of virus infections. Vero E6 cells were infected with SARS-CoV-2 and measles virus (MeV) and compared to naïve controls using Raman scans, aiming at the determination of virus-specific intracellular

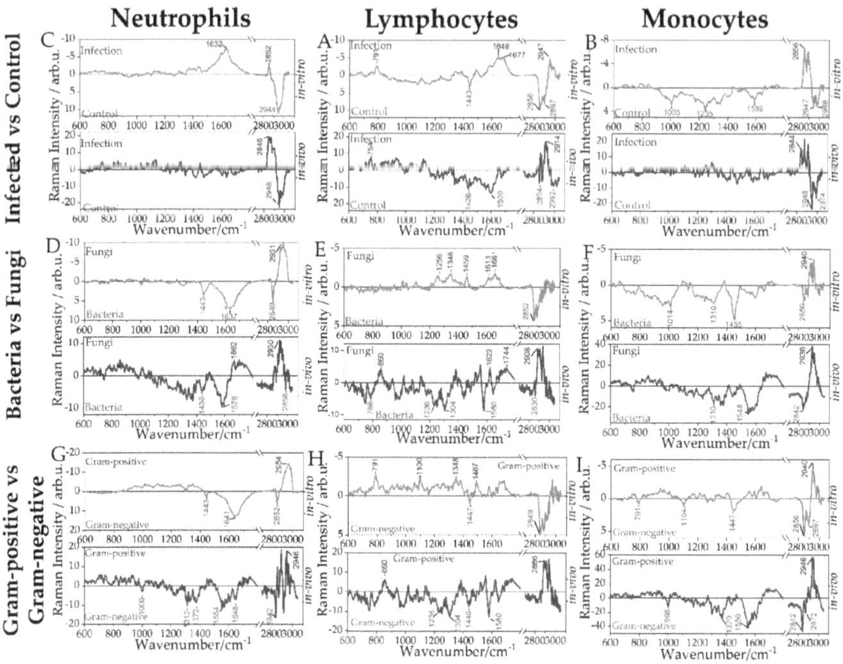

Figure 10.12. Raman difference spectra of the major leukocytes sub-populations infected *ex vivo* with different pathogen types compared to the same sub-populations derived from patients infected with the same pathogen. Reproduced from Ref. [286] with permission.

changes. Raman confocal images revealed a different distribution of the intercellular components, as well as lipids and proteins within the controls and the cells infected with SARS-CoV-2 and MeV. In addition, a different chemical composition of the intercellular components in each of the groups was revealed and higher intracellular tryptophan levels were found in SARS-CoV-2-infected cells. For the classification of SARS-CoV-2 and MeV infection compared to naïve controls, accuracies of 98.9 and 97.2% were yielded, respectively [287]. An identification success rate of 97% was yielded in the differentiation of Vero cells infected with the herpes family viruses HSV-1, HSV-2, and VZV from their uninfected controls [288]. Using Raman spectroscopy, the monitoring of replication kinetics of the Epstein–Barr Virus (EBV) in HMC-3 and U-87 microglial cells could be determined. The changes in band intensities post-EBV infection were monitored in the nucleus and cytosol in comparison to control cells at several time points to investigate the infection-related biochemical changes. During the course of infection, significant changes of the biochemical composition were monitored with the highest signals present in both cell types at the time spam of 24–36 h where the infection manifests.

Using Raman spectroscopy, a different cell-response profile was monitored by the two studied cell types, as reflected by the occurring biochemical changes in the different time points during the course of the EBV infection [289].

Another aspect of the host response approach is the application of Raman spectroscopy directly on the blood serum/plasma samples of infected individuals. The immune response to an infection is reflected through intense biochemical changes in the blood serum that can be analyzed using Raman spectroscopy [290]. In this approach, several Raman measurements are performed on a drop of a few μL of serum/plasma sample, a process that takes a few minutes, and the obtained spectra are then compared with those of healthy individuals or other infections. This method has found application especially in virus infections where a direct detection of their presence is challenging, and the advantages of Raman spectroscopy were used to design a fast screening test. These tests can be applied in the detection of specific viral infections as well as for differential diagnosis of infections causing similar clinical symptoms. Below, an overview of these methods is provided.

When applied on serum, Raman spectroscopy allowed the differentiation of healthy donors from patients with dengue fever. Distinct Raman features (750, 850, 1032, 1306, 1333, 1355, 1580, 1603 and 1660 cm^{-1}) could be observed in the patient sera, including Raman bands at 750 and 850 cm^{-1} deriving from ADT released into the serum by the rupturing of thrombocytes. In addition, the infected sera showed lower intensity in β-carotene bands at 1156 and 1516 cm^{-1} [291]. In another study, Raman spectroscopy was compared with quantification of Ns1, IgM and IgG using the ELISA method, the gold standard in dengue fever diagnosis. Results show that in the serum biomarker quantification, no correlation for the protein levels could be found since their level depended on several factors such as the day of infection. When Raman spectroscopy was applied on the sera, it provided 97.95% sensitivity and 95.40% specificity in detection of dengue fever when compared to healthy controls [292]. Dengue fever could also be differentiated from typhoid fever, two pathological conditions with similar symptomatology. Distinct spectral features were revealed in both conditions, allowing good differentiation using the PCA-LDA method. The results of this study show that Raman spectroscopy could also be a useful tool for differential diagnosis, allowing proper treatment of the patients [293]. Raman spectroscopy could also differentiate plasma from patients with fever, infected with malaria, infected with dengue virus and healthy individuals. The malaria-infected patients revealed distinct bands in their plasma, present only in this group showing a specific plasma biochemical composition of immunoglobulins, cortisone, amino acids and lipids. Multivariant regression analysis yielded a correlation coefficient R^2 of 0.981 between the predicted values and the accuracy for identification of unknown samples was 86% [294].

However, the most extensive research using this approach has been done for hepatitis. Several studies, using many different data analysis approaches, have shown that Raman spectroscopy allows the detection of hepatitis B and C (hepB and hepC) infection when applied in blood serum. With the use of several data analysis approaches, a recent study provided an accuracy of 98% for the differentiation of serum from hepB patients vs. healthy controls [295]. The use of neural networks provided an accuracy of 99.7% in the differentiation of Raman spectra for 600 blood plasma samples from hepB patients and 400 samples from healthy individuals [296]. Using an airPLS-PCA-PSO-SVM (PSO = particle swarm optimization) model, an accuracy of 93.1% was achieved in discriminating Raman spectra from serum samples of 500 hepB patients and 500 healthy controls. In addition, hepB patients showed lower intensity in numerous Raman bands compared to controls [297]. In another study, an radial basis function-based PCA-SVM model for the discrimination of Raman spectra from hepB and healthy blood plasma samples was developed and tested with an independent dataset to validate its diagnostic power. Similar results were obtained in the differentiation of plasma from hepC patients vs. healthy controls. In the PCA loadings, distinct Raman features could be identified in the hepC samples that allowed their differentiation from the healthy samples [298], and in another study an accuracy of 98.82% was yielded [299]. Using multiscale convolutional neural network a fast screening test was designed for the differentiation of the Raman spectra from the serum of healthy individuals and patients with infection from hepB and hepC. In a 3-class model the spectra from more than 1,300 cases were analyzed resulting in an accuracy for differentiation of 94.92%, and distinct Raman features, partly associated with liver disfunction, could be identified in both peak position and intensity that were characteristic for each group [300].

Similar Raman approaches have also been designed for the identification of SARS-CoV-2 infection. Raman analysis of the serum from 10 SARS-CoV-2 positive patients and 10 healthy controls revealed 87% sensitivity and 100% specificity for differentiation. In addition, data analysis of biochemical alterations related to SARS-CoV-2 infection in the serum could be revealed with patients presenting lower intensity in tryptophan bands and higher in bands of unsaturated lipids when compared to controls [301].

These data show that Raman analysis contains a large translational potential and could serve as a useful tool in everyday clinical practice. The development of this method for clinical applications could significantly contribute to overcoming the limitations of time-consuming, culture-based microbiology methods as well as cost-consuming molecular methods for microbiological documentation. In addition, information on the host immune status can provide added value in clinical decision making, improving patient care and mortality rates in the case of sepsis [294].

10.8 Conclusion and Outlook

The different techniques of Raman spectroscopy allow investigating and identifying all types of pathogenic microorganisms in food, environmental, and patient samples. Especially the capability of Raman spectroscopy to additionally obtain phenotypic information from pathogens is a useful add-on of this method. In addition, using single-cell analysis allows identification to be made within a few hours. Furthermore, bacteria normally inaccessible by culture-based detection methods, such as viable but not cultivable bacteria or persiters, can also be detected and identified.

Nevertheless, most of the studies describe a limited number of microorganisms or applications. Here, a more comprehensive approach would be necessary, including unlikely scenarios. For example, a study should include not only the (two) most common pathogens but all possible ones for the problem at hand. Likewise, possible contamination during the sampling with commensals or accompanying flora should be included in datasets. Care should also be taken to ensure that each genus or species has been included in the databases with sufficient variation in the amount and type of strains.

In case of single-cell measurements, the appropriate isolation techniques for each matrix need to be established. Here, the isolation procedure and respective sample preparation requires automatization, which will minimize the operator influence on the sample. In addition, a faster and parallelizable sample processing is also necessary. For cultivation-based approaches, the influences of media, temperature, pH, cultivation age, etc., must be standardized to obtain reliable, reproducible, and comparable Raman spectroscopic databases.

The machine learning algorithms to evaluate the different Raman databases need to establish approved and verifiable procedures, which allow a comprehensive approach. Here it would be necessary to enable identification of pathogens which are not included in the database as "new taxa". In addition, the possibility of identifying several pathogens simultaneously in one sample in rare cases must be taken into account. First steps towards comparable evaluations of databases are made with modern data analysis software (https://ramanmetrix.eu) [302].

To generalize the Raman spectroscopic approach for clinical settings, special devices need to be designed specifically for the identification of pathogens or the host response approach. Rigorous quality control is needed here to allow comparability of spectral information. Also, the database must be transferable from one device to another and verifiable. And in the end both the device and the cost per sample analysis must be in an economically reasonable range.

All in all, the potential of Raman spectroscopy for pathogen identification is high and has many advantages. Nevertheless, the above-mentioned issues need to be addressed in order to use this method as a full-fledged identification technique in a clinical environment.

In order to bring the advances of this research to the patient more quickly, translation structures are needed. What such translational research could look like in concrete terms is, e.g., demonstrated by the Leibniz Centre for Photonics in Infection Research (LPI) (see https://lpi-jena.de/en/). Within the framework of the LPI, diagnostic and targeted therapeutic light-based approaches will emerge through the combination of photonic methods with infection research, which, after appropriate approval, will be transferred directly to industrial production and clinical application. A central element within the framework of the LPI are technology scouts who, at the beginning of the value chain, work together with clinicians to identify precisely fitting photonic solution approaches that have already successfully proven their potential in proof-of-concept studies for specific medical issues.

Acknowledgement

Financial support of the Federal Ministry of Education and Research, Germany (Bundesministerium für Bildung und Forschung, Deutschland) in the project FastAlert (13GW0460B) as well as the Deutsche Forschungsgemeinschaft for the Collaborative Research Center AquaDiva (CRC 1076 AquaDiva) of the Friedrich Schiller University Jena are greatly acknowledged.

References

1. Murray, C. J. L., Ikuta, K. S., Sharara, F., Swetschinski, L., Robles Aguilar, G., Gray, A., Han, C., Bisignano, C., Rao, P., Wool, E., Johnson, S. C., Browne, A. J., Chipeta, M. G., Fell, F., Hackett, S., Haines-Woodhouse, G., Kashef Hamadani, B. H., Kumaran, E. A. P., McManigal, B., Agarwal, R., Akech, S., Albertson, S., Amuasi, J., Andrews, J., Aravkin, A., Ashley, E., Bailey, F., Baker, S., Basnyat, B., Bekker, A., Bender, R., Bethou, A., Bielicki, J., Boonkasidecha, S., Bukosia, J., Carvalheiro, C., Castañeda-Orjuela, C., Chansamouth, V., Chaurasia, S., Chiurchiù, S., Chowdhury, F., Cook, A. J., Cooper, B., Cressey, T. R., Criollo-Mora, E., Cunningham, M., Darboe, S., Day, N. P. J., De Luca, M., Dokova, K., Dramowski, A., Dunachie, S. J., Eckmanns, T., Eibach, D., Emami, A., Feasey, N., Fisher-Pearson, N., Forrest, K., Garrett, D., Gastmeier, P., Giref, A. Z., Greer, R. C., Gupta, V., Haller, S., Haselbeck, A., Hay, S. I., Holm, M., Hopkins, S., Iregbu, K. C., Jacobs, J., Jarovsky, D., Javanmardi, F., Khorana, M., Kissoon, N., Kobeissi, E., Kostyanev, T., Krapp, F., Krumkamp, R., Kumar, A., Kyu, H. H., Lim, C., Limmathurotsakul, D., Loftus, M. J., Lunn, M., Ma, J., Mturi, N., Munera-Huertas, T., Musicha, P., Mussi-Pinhata, M. M., Nakamura, T., Nanavati, R., Nangia, S., Newton, P., Ngoun, C., Novotney, A., Nwakanma, D., Obiero, C. W., Olivas-Martinez, A., Olliaro, P., Ooko, E., Ortiz-Brizuela, E., Peleg, A. Y., Perrone, C., Plakkal, N., Ponce-de-Leon, A., Raad, M., Ramdin, T., Riddell, A., Roberts, T., Robotham, J. V., Roca, A., Rudd, K. E., Russell, N., Schnall, J., Scott, J. A. G., Shivamallappa, M., Sifuentes-Osornio, J., Steenkeste, N., Stewardson, A. J., Stoeva, T., Tasak, N., Thaiprakong, A., Thwaites, G., Turner, C., Turner, P., van Doorn, H. R., Velaphi, S., Vongpradith, A., Vu, H., Walsh, T., Waner, S., Wangrangsimakul, T., Wozniak, T., Zheng, P., Sartorius, B., Lopez, A. D., Stergachis, A., Moore, C., Dolecek, C. and Naghavi, M. (2022) Global burden of bacterial antimicrobial resistance in 2019: a systematic analysis. Lancet **399**, 629–655.
2. Bauer, M., Kortgen, A. and Singer, M. (2015) Unmet medical needs in life-threatening infections — caring for the critically Ill. In *Modern Techniques for Pathogen Detection* (Popp, J. and Bauer, M., Eds.), pp. 1–18, John Wiley & Sons.
3. Jager, M. M., Murk, J. L., Pique, R. D., Hekker, T. A. and Vandenbroucke-Grauls, C. M. (2011) Five-minute Giemsa stain for rapid detection of malaria parasites in blood smears. Trop. Doct. **41**, 33–35.
4. Kai, S., Matsuo, Y., Nakagawa, S., Kryukov, K., Matsukawa, S., Tanaka, H., Iwai, T., Imanishi, T. and Hirota, K. (2019) Rapid bacterial identification by direct PCR amplification of 16S rRNA genes using the MinION nanopore sequencer. FEBS Open Bio. **9**, 548–557.
5. Jang, K. S. and Kim, Y. H. (2018) Rapid and robust MALDI-TOF MS techniques for microbial identification: a brief overview of their diverse applications. J. Microbiol. **56**, 209–216.

6. Ling, T. K., Tam, P. C., Liu, Z. K. and Cheng, A. F. (2001) Evaluation of VITEK 2 rapid identification and susceptibility testing system against gram-negative clinical isolates. J. Clin. Microbiol. **39**, 2964–2966.
7. Opota, O., Jaton, K. and Greub, G. (2015) Microbial diagnosis of bloodstream infection: towards molecular diagnosis directly from blood. Clin. Microbiol. Infect. **21**, 323–331.
8. Jung, J. Y., Yoon, H. K., An, S., Lee, J. W., Ahn, E. R., Kim, Y. J., Park, H. C., Lee, K., Hwang, J. H. and Lim, S. K. (2018) Rapid oral bacteria detection based on real-time PCR for the forensic identification of saliva. Sci. Rep. **8**, 10852.
9. https://www.who.int/publications/i/item/WHO-WSI-AMR-2019.1.
10. Rutsaert, S., Bosman, K., Trypsteen, W., Nijhuis, M. and Vandekerckhove, L. (2018) Digital PCR as a tool to measure HIV persistence. Retrovirology **15**, 16.
11. Peeling, R. W., Olliaro, P. L., Boeras, D. I. and Fongwen, N. (2021) Scaling up COVID-19 rapid antigen tests: promises and challenges. Lancet Infect. Dis. **21**, e290–e295.
12. Sivajothi, S. (2014) Detection of Trypanosoma evansi by different methods in bovines in Andhra Pradesh. J. Adv. Parasitology **1**, 35–38.
13. Karkashan, A., Khallaf, B., Morris, J., Thurbon, N., Rouch, D., Smith, S. R. and Deighton, M. (2015) Comparison of methodologies for enumerating and detecting the viability of Ascaris eggs in sewage sludge by standard incubation-microscopy, the BacLight Live/Dead viability assay and other vital dyes. Water Res. **68**, 533–544.
14. Makarewicz, O., Stein, C., Pfister, W., Loeffler, B. and Pletz, M. (2015) Identification Methods — An Overview. In *Modern Techniques for Pathogen Detection* (Popp, J. and Bauer, M., Eds.), pp. 1–18, John Wiley & Sons.
15. Hameed, S., Xie, L. and Ying, Y. (2018) Conventional and emerging detection techniques for pathogenic bacteria in food science: A review. Trends Food Sci. Technol. **81**, 61–73.
16. Niaura, G. (2000) Raman Spectroscopy in Analysis of Biomolecules. In *Encyclopedia of Analytical Chemistry* (Meyers, R. A., Ed.), pp. 645–676, John Wiley & Sons.
17. Arndt, M., Juffmann, T. and Vedral, V. (2009) Quantum physics meets biology. HFSP J. **3**, 386–400.
18. Li, Y.-S. and Church, J. S. (2014) Raman spectroscopy in the analysis of food and pharmaceutical nanomaterials. J. Food Drug Anal. **22**, 29–48.
19. Schmitt, M. and Popp, J. (2006) Raman spectroscopy at the beginning of the twenty-first century. J. Raman Spectrosc. **37**, 20–28.
20. Harz, M., Rösch, P. and Popp, J. (2009) Vibrational spectroscopy—A powerful tool for the rapid identification of microbial cells at the single-cell level. Cytometry A **75A**, 104–113.
21. AlMasoud, N., Muhamadali, H., Chisanga, M., AlRabiah, H., Lima, C. A. and Goodacre, R. (2021) Discrimination of bacteria using whole organism

fingerprinting: the utility of modern physicochemical techniques for bacterial typing. Analyst **146**, 770–788.

22. Cialla-May, D., Krafft, C., Rösch, P., Deckert-Gaudig, T., Frosch, T., Jahn, I. J., Pahlow, S., Stiebing, C., Meyer-Zedler, T., Bocklitz, T., Schie, I., Deckert, V. and Popp, J. (2022) Raman spectroscopy and imaging in bioanalytics. Anal. Chem. **94**, 86–119.
23. Lorenz, B., Wichmann, C., Stöckel, S., Rösch, P. and Popp, J. (2017) Cultivation-free Raman spectroscopic investigations on bacteria. Trends Microbiol. **25**, 413–424.
24. Stöckel, S., Kirchhoff, J., Neugebauer, U., Rösch, P. and Popp, J. (2016) The application of Raman spectroscopy for the detection and identification of microorganisms. J. Raman Spectrosc. **47**, 89–109.
25. Wang, L., Liu, W., Tang, J. W., Wang, J. J., Liu, Q. H., Wen, P. B., Wang, M. M., Pan, Y. C., Gu, B. and Zhang, X. (2021) Applications of Raman spectroscopy in bacterial infections: principles, advantages, and shortcomings. Front. Microbiol. **12**, 683580.
26. Hong, J. K., Kim, S. B., Lyou, E. S. and Lee, T. K. (2021) Microbial phenomics linking the phenotype to function: The potential of Raman spectroscopy. J. Microbiol. **59**, 249–258.
27. Senger, R. S. and Scherr, D. (2020) Resolving complex phenotypes with Raman spectroscopy and chemometrics. Curr. Opin. Biotechnol. **66**, 277–282.
28. Lee, K. S., Landry, Z., Pereira, F. C., Wagner, M., Berry, D., Huang, W. E., Taylor, G. T., Kneipp, J., Popp, J., Zhang, M., Cheng, J.-X. and Stocker, R. (2021) Raman microspectroscopy for microbiology. Nat. Rev. Meth. Primers **1**, 80.
29. Garcia-Timermans, C., Rubbens, P., Kerckhof, F. M., Buysschaert, B., Khalenkow, D., Waegeman, W., Skirtach, A. G. and Boon, N. (2018) Label-free Raman characterization of bacteria calls for standardized procedures. J. Microbiol. Meth. **151**, 69–75.
30. Shen, H., Rösch, P., Pletz, M. and Popp, J. (2022) Fiber probe based Raman spectroscopic identification on pathogenic biofilms. Anal. Chem. **94**, 5375–5381.
31. Shen, H., Rösch, P. and Popp, J. (2022) Fiber probe-based Raman spectroscopic identification of pathogenic infection microorganisms on agar plates. Anal. Chem. **94**, 4635–4642.
32. Maquelin, K., Kirschner, C., Choo-Smith, L. P., van den Braak, N., Endtz, H. P., Naumann, D. and Puppels, G. J. (2002) Identification of medically relevant microorganisms by vibrational spectroscopy. J. Microbiol. Meth. **51**, 255–271.
33. Rebrosova, K., Samek, O., Kizovsky, M., Bernatova, S., Hola, V. and Ruzicka, F. (2022) Raman spectroscopy-a novel method for identification and characterization of microbes on a single-cell level in clinical settings. Front. Cell. Infect. Microbiol. **12**, 866463.
34. Petersen, M., Yu, Z. L. and Lu, X. N. (2021) Application of Raman spectroscopic methods in food safety: a review. Biosensors **11**, 187.

35. Cialla, D., März, A., Böhme, R., Theil, F., Weber, K., Schmitt, M. and Popp, J. (2012) Surface-enhanced Raman spectroscopy (SERS): progress and trends. Anal. Bioanal. Chem. **403**, 27–54.
36. Cialla, D., Petschulat, J., Hübner, U., Schneidewind, H., Zeisberger, M., Mattheis, R., Pertsch, T., Schmitt, M., Möller, R. and Popp, J. (2010) Investigation on the second part of the electromagnetic SERS enhancement and resulting fabrication strategies of anisotropic plasmonic arrays. ChemPhysChem **11**, 1918–1924.
37. Tong, L., Zhu, T. and Liu, Z. (2011) Approaching the electromagnetic mechanism of surface-enhanced Raman scattering: from self-assembled arrays to individual gold nanoparticles. Chem. Soc. Rev. **40**, 1296–1304.
38. Yamamoto, Y. S., Ozaki, Y. and Itoh, T. (2014) Recent progress and frontiers in the electromagnetic mechanism of surface-enhanced Raman scattering. J. Photochem. Photobiol. C **21**, 81–104.
39. Jensen, L., Aikens, C. M. and Schatz, G. C. (2008) Electronic structure methods for studying surface-enhanced Raman scattering. Chem. Soc. Rev. **37**, 1061–1073.
40. Le Ru, E. C., Meyer, S. A., Artur, C., Etchegoin, P. G., Grand, J., Lang, P. and Maurel, F. (2011) Experimental demonstration of surface selection rules for SERS on flat metallic surfaces. Chem. Commun. **47**, 3903–3905.
41. Chulhai, D. V., Hu, Z., Moore, J. E., Chen, X. and Jensen, L. (2016) Theory of linear and nonlinear surface-enhanced vibrational spectroscopies. Annu. Rev. Phys. Chem. **67**, 541–564.
42. Lane, L. A., Qian, X. and Nie, S. (2015) SERS nanoparticles in medicine: from label-free detection to spectroscopic tagging. Chem. Rev. **115**, 10489–10529.
43. Zheng, X. S., Jahn, I. J., Weber, K., Cialla-May, D. and Popp, J. (2018) Label-free SERS in biological and biomedical applications: Recent progress, current challenges and opportunities. Spectrochim. Acta A **197**, 56–77.
44. Wang, Y. and Schlücker, S. (2013) Rational design and synthesis of SERS labels. Analyst **138**, 2224–2238.
45. Shan, B., Pu, Y., Chen, Y., Liao, M. and Li, M. (2018) Novel SERS labels: Rational design, functional integration and biomedical applications. Coord. Chem. Rev. **371**, 11–37.
46. Jahn, I. J., Mühlig, A. and Cialla-May, D. (2020) Application of molecular SERS nanosensors: where we stand and where we are headed towards? Anal. Bioanal. Chem. **412**, 5999–6007.
47. Qu, L. L., Ying, Y. L., Yu, R. J. and Long, Y. T. (2021) In situ food-borne pathogen sensors in a nanoconfined space by surface enhanced Raman scattering. Microchim. Acta **188**, 201.
48. Samek, O., Bernatova, S. and Dohnal, F. (2021) The potential of SERS as an AST methodology in clinical settings. Nanophotonics **10**, 2537–2561.

49. Berry, M. E., Kearns, H., Graham, D. and Faulds, K. (2021) Surface enhanced Raman scattering for the multiplexed detection of pathogenic microorganisms: towards point-of-use applications. Analyst **146**, 6084–6101.
50. Wang, C. G., Meloni, M. M., Wu, X. Z., Zhuo, M., He, T. G., Wang, J. F., Wang, C. W. and Dong, P. T. (2019) Magnetic plasmonic particles for SERS-based bacteria sensing: A review. AIP Adv. **9**, 010701.
51. Gautam, R., Vanga, S., Ariese, F. and Umapathy, S. (2015) Review of multidimensional data processing approaches for Raman and infrared spectroscopy. EPJ Techn. Instr. **2**, 8.
52. Guo, S. X., Popp, J. and Bocklitz, T. (2021) Chemometric analysis in Raman spectroscopy from experimental design to machine learning-based modeling. Nat. Protoc. **16**, 5426–5459.
53. Bocklitz, T. W., Dörfer, T., Heinke, R., Schmitt, M. and Popp, J. (2015) Spectrometer calibration protocol for Raman spectra recorded with different excitation wavelengths. Spectrochim. Acta A **149**, 544–549.
54. Dörfer, T., Bocklitz, T., Tarcea, N., Schmitt, M. and Popp, J. (2011) Checking and improving calibration of Raman spectra using chemometric approaches. Z. Physik. Chem. **225**, 753–764.
55. Gryniewicz-Ruzicka, C. M., Arzhantsev, S., Pelster, L. N., Westenberger, B. J., Buhse, L. F. and Kauffman, J. F. (2011) Multivariate calibration and instrument standardization for the rapid detection of diethylene glycol in glycerin by Raman spectroscopy. Appl. Spectrosc. **65**, 334–341.
56. Odake, S., Fukura, S. and Kagi, H. (2008) High precision in Raman frequency achieved using real-time calibration with a neon emission line: application to three-dimensional stress mapping observations. Appl. Spectrosc. **62**, 1084–1087.
57. Olsen, E. F., Baustad, C., Egelandsdal, B., Rukke, E. O. and Isaksson, T. (2010) Long-term stability of a Raman instrument determining iodine value in pork adipose tissue. Meat Sci. **85**, 1–6.
58. Swierenga, H., de Weijer, A. P., van Wijk, R. J. and Buydens, L. M. C. (1999) Strategy for constructing robust multivariate calibration models. Chemometr. Intell. Lab. **49**, 1–17.
59. Bocklitz, T., Walter, A., Hartmann, K., Rösch, P. and Popp, J. (2011) How to pre-process Raman spectra for reliable and stable models? Anal. Chim. Acta **704**, 47–56.
60. Simpson, J. V., Oshokoya, O., Wagner, N., Liu, J. and Jiji, R. D. (2011) Pre-processing of ultraviolet resonance Raman spectra. Analyst **136**, 1239–1247.
61. Ryabchykov, O., Bocklitz, T., Ramoji, A., Neugebauer, U., Foerster, M., Kroegel, C., Bauer, M., Kiehntopf, M. and Popp, J. (2016) Automatization of spike correction in Raman spectra of biological samples. Chemometr. Intell. Lab. **155**, 1–6.

62. Guo, S., Bocklitz, T. and Popp, J. (2016) Optimization of Raman-spectrum baseline correction in biological application. Analyst **141**, 2396–2404.
63. Liu, J. T., Sun, J. Y., Huang, X. Z., Li, G. J. and Liu, B. Q. (2015) Goldindec: a novel algorithm for Raman spectrum baseline correction. Appl. Spectrosc. **69**, 834–842.
64. Ali, N., Girnus, S., Rösch, P., Popp, J. and Bocklitz, T. (2018) Sample size planning for multivariate data: a Raman spectroscopy based example. Anal. Chem. **90**, 12485–12492.
65. Guo, S., Bocklitz, T., Neugebauer, U. and Popp, J. (2017) Common mistakes in cross-validating classification models. Anal. Meth. **9**, 4410–4417.
66. Ryabchykov, O., Schie, I., Popp, J. and Bocklitz, T. (2022) Errors and mistakes to avoid when analyzing Raman spectra. Spectroscopy **37**, 48–50.
67. Pradhan, P., Guo, S. X., Ryabchykov, O., Popp, J. and Bocklitz, T. W. (2020) Deep learning a boon for biophotonics? J. Biophotonics **13**, e201960186.
68. Ho, C.-S., Jean, N., Hogan, C. A., Blackmon, L., Jeffrey, S. S., Holodniy, M., Banaei, N., Saleh, A. A. E., Ermon, S. and Dionne, J. (2019) Rapid identification of pathogenic bacteria using Raman spectroscopy and deep learning. Nat. Commun. **10**, 4927.
69. Guo, S., Heinke, R., Stöckel, S., Rösch, P., Bocklitz, T. and Popp, J. (2017) Towards an improvement of model transferability for Raman spectroscopy in biological applications. Vib. Spectrosc. **91**, 111–118.
70. Guo, S., Heinke, R., Stöckel, S., Rösch, P., Popp, J. and Bocklitz, T. (2018) Model transfer methods for Raman spectroscopy based bacterial classification. J. Raman Spectrosc. **49**, 627–637.
71. Guo, S., Kohler, A., Zimmermann, B., Heinke, R., Stöckel, S., Rösch, P., Popp, J. and Bocklitz, T. W. (2018) Extended multiplicative signal correction based model transfer for Raman spectroscopy in biological applications. Anal. Chem. **90**, 9787–9795.
72. Guo, S. X., Beleites, C., Neugebauer, U., Abalde-Cela, S., Afseth, N. K., Alsamad, F., Anand, S., Araujo-Andrade, C., Askrabic, S., Avci, E., Baia, M., Baranska, M., Baria, E., de Carvalho, L., de Bettignies, P., Bonifacio, A., Bonnier, F., Brauchle, E. M., Byrne, H. J., Chourpa, I., Cicchi, R., Cuisinier, F., Culha, M., Dahms, M., David, C., Duponchel, L., Duraipandian, S., El-Mashtoly, S. F., Ellis, D. I., Eppe, G., Falgayrac, G., Gamulin, O., Gardner, B., Gardner, P., Gerwert, K., Giamarellos-Bourboulis, E. J., Gizurarson, S., Gnyba, M., Goodacre, R., Grysan, P., Guntinas-Lichius, O., Helgadottir, H., Grosev, V. M., Kendall, C., Kiselev, R., Kolbach, M., Krafft, C., Krishnamoorthy, S., Kubryck, P., Lendl, B., Loza-Alvarez, P., Lyng, F. M., Machill, S., Malherbe, C., Marro, M., Marques, M. P. M., Matuszyk, E., Morasso, C. F., Moreau, M., Muhamadali, H., Mussi, V., Notingher, I., Pacia, M. Z., Pavone, F. S., Penel, G., Petersen, D., Piot, O., Rau, J. V., Richter, M., Rybarczyk, M. K., Salehi, H., Schenke-Layland, K., Schlucker, S., Schosserer, M., Schutze, K., Sergo, V., Sinjab, F., Smulko, J., Sockalingum, G.

D., Stiebing, C., Stone, N., Untereiner, V., Vanna, R., Wieland, K., Popp, J. and Bocklitz, T. (2020) Comparability of Raman spectroscopic configurations: a large scale cross-laboratory study. Anal. Chem. **92**, 15745–15756.

73. Brouckaert, D., Uyttersprot, J. S., Broeckx, W. and De Beer, T. (2017) Calibration transfer of a Raman spectroscopic quantification method for the assessment of liquid detergent compositions between two at-line instruments installed at two liquid detergent production plants. Anal. Chim. Acta **984**, 1–18.
74. Brouckaert, D., Uyttersprot, J. S., Broeckx, W. and De Beer, T. (2017) Calibration transfer of a Raman spectroscopic quantification method from at-line to in-line assessment of liquid detergent compositions. Anal. Chim. Acta **971**, 14–25.
75. Brouckaert, D., Uyttersprot, J. S., Broeckx, W. and De Beer, T. (2018) Calibration transfer of a Raman spectroscopic quantification method for the assessment of liquid detergent compositions from at-line laboratory to in-line industrial scale. Talanta **179**, 386–392.
76. Chen, H., Zhang, Z. M., Miao, L., Zhan, D. J., Zheng, Y. B., Liu, Y., Lu, F. and Liang, Y. Z. (2015) Automatic standardization method for Raman spectrometers with applications to pharmaceuticals. J. Raman Spectrosc. **46**, 147–154.
77. Chen, H., Liu, Y., Lu, F., Cao, Y. B. and Zhang, Z. M. (2018) Eliminating non-linear Raman shift displacement between spectrometers via moving window fast Fourier transform cross-correlation. Front. Chem. **6**, 515.
78. Rodriguez, J. D., Westenberger, B. J., Buhse, L. F. and Kauffman, J. F. (2011) Standardization of Raman spectra for transfer of spectral libraries across different instruments. Analyst **136**, 4232–4240.
79. Pahlow, S., Meisel, S., Cialla-May, D., Weber, K., Rösch, P. and Popp, J. (2015) Isolation and identification of bacteria by means of Raman spectroscopy. Adv. Drug Del. Rev. **89**, 105–120.
80. Stöckel, S., Meisel, S., Böhme, R., Elschner, M., Rösch, P. and Popp, J. (2009) Effect of supplementary manganese on the sporulation of Bacillus endospores analysed by Raman spectroscopy. J. Raman Spectrosc. **40**, 1469–1477.
81. Silge, A., Schumacher, W., Rösch, P., da Costa Filho, P. A., Gérard, C. and Popp, J. (2014) Identification of water conditioned Pseudomonas aeruginosa by Raman microspectroscopy on a single cell level. Syst. Appl. Microbiol. **37**, 360–367.
82. Meisel, S., Stöckel, S., Rösch, P. and Popp, J. (2014) Identification of meat associated pathogens via Raman microspectroscopy. Food Microbiol. **38**, 36–43.
83. Harz, M., Rösch, P., Peschke, K. D., Ronneberger, O., Burkhardt, H. and Popp, J. (2005) Micro-Raman spectroscopic identification of bacterial cells of the genus Staphylococcus and dependence on their cultivation conditions. Analyst **130**, 1543–1550.
84. Hanson, C., Bishop, M. M., Barney, J. T. and Vargis, E. (2019) Effect of growth media and phase on Raman spectra and discrimination of mycobacteria. J. Biophotonics **12**, e201900150.

85. Mlynáriková, K., Samek, O., Bernatová, S., Růžička, F., Ježek, J., Háronikovа́, A., Šiler, M., Zemánek, P. and Holá, V. (2015) Influence of culture media on microbial fingerprints using Raman spectroscopy. Sensors **15**, 29635–29647.
86. Baritaux, J. C., Simon, A. C., Schultz, E., Emain, C., Laurent, P. and Dinten, J. M. (2016) A study on identification of bacteria in environmental samples using single-cell Raman spectroscopy: feasibility and reference libraries. Environ. Sci. Pollut. Res. Int. **23**, 8184–8191.
87. Wichmann, C., Bocklitz, T., Rösch, P. and Popp, J. (2021) Bacterial phenotype dependency from CO_2 measured by Raman spectroscopy. Spectrochim. Acta A **248**, 119170.
88. Münchberg, U., Rösch, P., Bauer, M. and Popp, J. (2014) Raman spectroscopic identification of single bacterial cells under antibiotic influence. Anal. Bioanal. Chem. **406**, 3041–3050.
89. Neugebauer, U., Schmid, U., Baumann, K., Holzgrabe, U., Ziebuhr, W., Kozitskaya, S., Kiefer, W., Schmitt, M. and Popp, J. (2006) Characterization of bacterial growth and the influence of antibiotics by means of UV resonance Raman spectroscopy. Biopolymers **82**, 306–311.
90. Walter, A., Kuhri, S., Reinicke, M., Bocklitz, T., Schumacher, W., Rösch, P., Merten, D., Büchel, G., Kothe, E. and Popp, J. (2012) Raman spectroscopic detection of Nickel impact on single Streptomyces cells — possible bioindicators for heavy metal contamination. J. Raman Spectrosc. **43**, 1058–1064.
91. Neugebauer, U., Schmid, U., Baumann, K., Ziebuhr, W., Kozitskaya, S., Deckert, V., Schmitt, M. and Popp, J. (2007) Towards a detailed understanding of bacterial metabolism: Spectroscopic characterization of Staphylococcus epidermidis. ChemPhysChem **8**, 124–137.
92. Hlaing, M. M., Dunn, M., Stoddart, P. R. and McArthur, S. L. (2016) Raman spectroscopic identification of single bacterial cells at different stages of their lifecycle. Vib. Spectrosc. **86**, 81–89.
93. Wichmann, C., Chhallani, M., Bocklitz, T., Rösch, P. and Popp, J. (2019) Simulation of transportation and storage and their influence on Raman spectra to bacteria. Anal. Chem. **91**, 13688–13694.
94. Mikoliunaite, L., Rodriguez, R. D., Sheremet, E., Kolchuzhin, V., Mehner, J., Ramanavicius, A. and Zahn, D. R. T. (2015) The substrate matters in the Raman spectroscopy analysis of cells. Sci. Rep. **5**, 13150.
95. Ramoji, A., Galler, K., Glaser, U., Henkel, T., Mayer, G., Dellith, J., Bauer, M., Popp, J. and Neugebauer, U. (2016) Characterization of different substrates for Raman spectroscopic imaging of eukaryotic cells. J. Raman Spectrosc. **47**, 773–786.
96. Krause, M., Radt, B., Rösch, P. and Popp, J. (2007) The investigation of single bacteria by means of fluorescence staining and Raman spectroscopy. J. Raman Spectrosc. **38**, 369–372.

97. Krause, M., Rösch, P., Radt, B. and Popp, J. (2008) Localizing and identifying living bacteria in an abiotic environment by a combination of Raman and fluorescence microscopy. Anal. Chem. **80**, 8568–8575.
98. Azemtsop Matanfack, G., Rüger, J., Stiebing, C., Schmitt, M. and Popp, J. (2020) Imaging the invisible — bioorthogonal Raman probes for imaging of cells and tissues. J. Biophotonics **13**, e202000129.
99. Kniggendorf, A.-K., Gaul, T. W. and Meinhardt-Wollweber, M. (2011) Effects of ethanol, formaldehyde, and gentle heat fixation in confocal resonance Raman microscopy of purple nonsulfur bacteria. Microsc. Res. Tech. **74**, 177–183.
100. Mariani, M. M., Lampen, P., Popp, J., Wood, B. R. and Deckert, V. (2009) Impact of fixation on in vitro cell culture lines monitored with Raman spectroscopy. Analyst **134**, 1154–1161.
101. Stöckel, S., Schumacher, W., Meisel, S., Elschner, M., Rösch, P. and Popp, J. (2010) Raman spectroscopy-compatible inactivation method for pathogenic endospores. Appl. Environ. Microbiol. **76**, 2895–2907.
102. Parvez, M. A. K., Ferdous, R. N., Rahman, M. S. and Islam, S. (2018) Healthcare-associated (HA) and community-associated (CA) methicillin resistant Staphylococcus aureus (MRSA) in Bangladesh — Source, diagnosis and treatment. J. Genet. Eng. Biotechnol. **16**, 473–478.
103. Pistiki, A., Salbreiter, M., Sultan, S., Rösch, P. and Popp, J. (2022) Application of Raman spectroscopy in the hospital environment. Transl. Biophotonics **4**, e202200011.
104. Kloß, S., Kampe, B., Sachse, S., Rösch, P., Straube, E., Pfister, W., Kiehntopf, M. and Popp, J. (2013) Culture independent Raman spectroscopic identification of urinary tract infection pathogens: a proof of principle study. Anal. Chem. **85**, 9610–9616.
105. Kloß, S., Rösch, P., Pfister, W., Kiehntopf, M. and Popp, J. (2015) Towards culture free Raman spectroscopic identification of pathogens in ascitic fluid. Anal. Chem. **87**, 937–943.
106. Wichmann, C., Rösch, P. and Popp, J. (2021) Isolation of bacteria from artificial bronchoalveolar lavage fluid using density gradient centrifugation and their accessibility by Raman spectroscopy. Anal. Bioanal. Chem. **413**.
107. Kloß, S., Lorenz, B., Dees, S., Labugger, I., Rösch, P. and Popp, J. (2015) Destruction-free procedure for the isolation of bacteria from sputum samples for Raman spectroscopic analysis. Anal. Bioanal. Chem. **407**, 8333–8341.
108. Rusciano, G., Capriglione, P., Pesce, G., Abete, P., Carnovale, V. and Sasso, A. (2013) Raman spectroscopy as a new tool for early detection of bacteria in patients with cystic fibrosis. Laser Phys. Lett. **10**, 075603.
109. Lorenz, B., Rösch, P. and Popp, J. (2019) Isolation matters — processing blood for Raman microspectroscopic identification of bacteria. Anal. Bioanal. Chem. **11**, 5445–5454.

110. Stöckel, S., Meisel, S., Lorenz, B., Kloß, S., Henk, S., Dees, S., Richter, E., Andres, S., Merker, M., Labugger, I., Rösch, P. and Popp, J. (2017) Raman spectroscopic identification of Mycobacterium tuberculosis. J. Biophotonics **10**, 727–734.
111. Sathyavathi, R., Dingari, N. C., Barman, I., Prasad, P., Prabhakar, S., Narayana Rao, D., Dasari, R. R. and Undamatla, J. (2013) Raman spectroscopy provides a powerful, rapid diagnostic tool for the detection of tuberculous meningitis in ex vivo cerebrospinal fluid samples. J. Biophotonics **6**, 567–572.
112. Gonchukov, S., Lonkina, T., Minaeva, S., Sundukov, A., Migmanov, T., Lademann, J., Darvin, M. and Bagratashvili, V. (2013) Confocal Raman microscopy of pathologic cells in cerebrospinal fluid. Laser Phys. Lett. **11**, 015602.
113. Stöckel, S., Meisel, S., Elschner, M., Rösch, P. and Popp, J. (2012) Identification of Bacillus anthracis via Raman spectroscopy and chemometric approaches. Anal. Chem. **84**, 9873–9880.
114. Stöckel, S., Meisel, S., Elschner, M., Rösch, P. and Popp, J. (2012) Raman spectroscopic detection of anthrax endospores in powder samples. Angew. Chem. Int. Ed. **51**, 5339–5342.
115. Stöckel, S., Meisel, S., Elschner, M., Melzer, F., Rösch, P. and Popp, J. (2015) Raman spectroscopic detection and identification of Burkholderia mallei and Burkholderia pseudomallei in feedstuff. Anal. Bioanal. Chem. **407**, 787–794.
116. Tien, N., Chen, H.-C., Gau, S.-L., Lin, T.-H., Lin, H.-S., You, B.-J., Tsai, P.-C., Chen, I.-R., Tsai, M.-F. and Wang, I.-K. (2016) Diagnosis of bacterial pathogens in the dialysate of peritoneal dialysis patients with peritonitis using surface-enhanced Raman spectroscopy. Clinica Chim. Acta **461**, 69–75.
117. Schröder, U.-C., Ramoji, A., Glaser, U., Sachse, S., Leiterer, C., Csaki, A., Hübner, U., Fritzsche, W., Pfister, W., Bauer, M., Popp, J. and Neugebauer, U. (2013) Combined dielectrophoresis–Raman setup for the classification of pathogens recovered from the urinary tract. Anal. Chem. **85**, 10717–10724.
118. Chawla, K., Bankapur, A., Acharya, M., D'Souza, J. S. and Chidangil, S. (2019) A micro-Raman and chemometric study of urinary tract infection-causing bacterial pathogens in mixed cultures. Anal. Bioanal. Chem. **411**, 3165–3177.
119. Nakar, A., Pistiki, A., Ryabchykov, O., Bocklitz, T., Rösch, P. and Popp, J. (2022) Label-free differentiation of clinical E. coli and Klebsiella isolates with Raman spectroscopy. J. Biophotonics **15**, e202200005.
120. Wang, Y., Lee, K. and Irudayaraj, J. (2010) Silver nanosphere SERS probes for sensitive identification of pathogens. J. Phys. Chem. C **114**, 16122–16128.
121. Osorio-Román, I., Aroca, R., Astudillo, J., Matsuhiro, B., Vásquez, C. and Pérez, J. (2010) Characterization of bacteria using its O-antigen with surface-enhanced Raman scattering. Analyst **135**, 1997–2001.
122. Hamasha, K., Mohaidat, Q. I., Putnam, R. A., Woodman, R. C., Palchaudhuri, S. and Rehse, S. J. (2013) Sensitive and specific discrimination of pathogenic and nonpathogenic Escherichia coli using Raman spectroscopy — a comparison of two multivariate analysis techniques. Biomed. Opt. Exp. **4**, 481–489.

123. Gong, J., Wang, X., Zeng, G., Cui, H. and Hu, J. (2011) Detection and discrimination of Escherichia coli and Shigella spp. using surface-enhanced Raman spectroscopy. China Environ. Sci. **31**, 1523–1527.
124. Wu, X., Chen, J., Li, X., Zhao, Y. and Zughaier, S. M. (2014) Culture-free diagnostics of Pseudomonas aeruginosa infection by silver nanorod array based SERS from clinical sputum samples. Nanomedicine **10**, 1863–1870.
125. Orelio, C., Beiboer, S., Morsink, M., Tektas, S., Dekter, H. and Van Leeuwen, W. (2014) Comparison of Raman spectroscopy and two molecular diagnostic methods for Burkholderia cepacia complex species identification. J. Microbiol. Meth. **107**, 126–132.
126. Silge, A., Abdou, E., Schneider, K., Meisel, S., Bocklitz, T., Lu-Walther, H. W., Heintzmann, R., Rösch, P. and Popp, J. (2015) Shedding light on host niches: label-free in situ detection of Mycobacterium gordonae via carotenoids in macrophages by Raman microspectroscopy. Cellular Microbiol. **17**, 832–842.
127. Tang, M., McEwen, G. D., Wu, Y., Miller, C. D. and Zhou, A. (2013) Characterization and analysis of mycobacteria and Gram-negative bacteria and co-culture mixtures by Raman microspectroscopy, FTIR, and atomic force microscopy. Anal. Bioanal. Chem. **405**, 1577–1591.
128. Große, C., Bergner, N., Dellith, J., Heller, R., Bauer, M., Mellmann, A., Popp, J. and Neugebauer, U. (2015) Label-free imaging and spectroscopic analysis of intracellular bacterial infections. Anal. Chem. **87**, 2137–2142.
129. Haider, S., Wagner, M., Schmid, M. C., Sixt, B. S., Christian, J. G., Häcker, G., Pichler, P., Mechtler, K., Müller, A. and Baranyi, C. (2010) Raman microspectroscopy reveals long-term extracellular activity of chlamydiae. Mol. Microbiol. **77**, 687–700.
130. de Siqueira e Oliveira, F. S., da Silva, A. M., Pacheco, M. T. T., Giana, H. E. and Silveira, L. (2021) Biochemical characterization of pathogenic bacterial species using Raman spectroscopy and discrimination model based on selected spectral features. Lasers Med. Sci. **36**, 289–302.
131. Wang, K., Chen, L., Ma, X., Ma, L., Chou Keng, C., Cao, Y., Khan Izhar, U. H., Gölz, G., Lu, X. and Master Emma, R. (2020) Arcobacter identification and species determination using Raman spectroscopy combined with neural networks. Appl. Environ. Microbiol. **86**, e00924–00920.
132. Rebrošová, K., Bernatová, S., Šiler, M., Uhlirova, M., Samek, O., Ježek, J., Holá, V., Růžička, F. and Zemanek, P. (2022) Raman spectroscopy — a tool for rapid differentiation among microbes causing urinary tract infections. Anal. Chim. Acta **1191**, 339292.
133. Rebrošová, K., Siler, M., Samek, O., Ruzicka, F., Bernatova, S., Hola, V., Jezek, J., Zemanek, P., Sokolova, J. and Petras, P. (2017) Rapid identification of staphylococci by Raman spectroscopy. Sci. Rep. **7**, 8.
134. Rebrošová, K., Šiler, M., Samek, O., Růžička, F., Bernatová, S., Ježek, J., Zemánek, P. and Holá, V. (2017) Differentiation between Staphylococcus aureus

and Staphylococcus epidermidis strains using Raman spectroscopy. Future Microbiol. **12**, 881–890.

135. Maquelin, K., Kirschner, C., Choo-Smith, L.-P., Ngo-Thi, N., Van Vreeswijk, T., Stammler, M., Endtz, H., Bruining, H., Naumann, D. and Puppels, G. (2003) Prospective study of the performance of vibrational spectroscopies for rapid identification of bacterial and fungal pathogens recovered from blood cultures. J. Clin. Microbiol. **41**, 324–329.
136. Almarashi, J. F., Kapel, N., Wilkinson, T. S. and Telle, H. H. (2012) Raman spectroscopy of bacterial species and strains cultivated under reproducible conditions. Spectroscopy Int. J. **27**, 361–365.
137. Samek, O., Telle, H., Harris, L., Bloomfield, M. and Mack, D. (2008) Raman spectroscopy for rapid discrimination of Staphylococcus epidermidis clones related to medical device-associated infections. Laser Phys. Lett. **5**, 465–470.
138. Choo-Smith, L.-P., Maquelin, K., Van Vreeswijk, T., Bruining, H., Puppels, G., Thi, N. N., Kirschner, C., Naumann, D., Ami, D. and Villa, A. (2001) Investigating microbial (micro) colony heterogeneity by vibrational spectroscopy. Appl. Environ. Microbiol. **67**, 1461–1469.
139. Mathey, R., Dupoy, M., Espagnon, I., Leroux, D., Mallard, F. and Novelli-Rousseau, A. (2015) Viability of 3 h grown bacterial micro-colonies after direct Raman identification. J. Microbiol. Meth. **109**, 67–73.
140. Espagnon, I., Ostrovskii, D., Mathey, R., Dupoy, M. G., Joly, P., Novelli-Rousseau, A., Pinston, F., Gal, O., Mallard, F. and Leroux, D. F. (2014) Direct identification of clinically relevant bacterial and yeast microcolonies and macrocolonies on solid culture media by Raman spectroscopy. J. Biomed. Opt. **19**, 027004.
141. Nakar, A., Wagenhaus, A., Rösch, P. and Popp, J. (2022) Raman spectroscopy for the differentiation of Enterobacteriaceae: a comparison of two methods. Analyst **147**, 3938–3946.
142. López, D., Vlamakis, H. and Kolter, R. (2010) Biofilms. Cold Spring Harb. Perspect. Biol. **2**, a000398.
143. Hall-Stoodley, L., Costerton, J. W. and Stoodley, P. (2004) Bacterial biofilms: from the natural environment to infectious diseases. Nat. Rev. Microbiol. **2**, 95–108.
144. Bjarnsholt, T., Jensen, P. Ø., Moser, C. and Høiby, N. (2011) *Biofilm Infections.* Springer.
145. Bryers, J. D. (2008) Medical biofilms. Biotechnol. Bioeng. **100**, 1–18.
146. Del Pozo, J., Rouse, M. and Patel, R. (2008) Bioelectric effect and bacterial biofilms. A systematic review. Int. J. Artif. Organs **31**, 786–795.
147. Habteyes, T. G. (2020) Anions as intermediates in plasmon enhanced photocatalytic reactions. J. Phys. Chem. C **124**, 26554–26564.
148. Ramirez-Mora, T., Davila-Perez, C., Torres-Mendez, F. and Valle-Bourrouet, G. (2019) Raman spectroscopic characterization of endodontic biofilm matrices. J. Spectrosc. **2019**, 1307397.

149. Kanematsu, H., Kudara, H., Kanesaki, S., Kogo, T., Ikegai, H., Ogawa, A. and Hirai, N. (2016) Application of a loop-type laboratory biofilm reactor to the evaluation of biofilm for some metallic materials and polymers such as urinary stents and catheters. Materials **9**, 824.
150. Kelestemur, S., Avci, E. and Culha, M. (2018) Raman and surface-enhanced Raman scattering for biofilm characterization. Chemosensors **6**, 5.
151. Kniggendorf, A. K., Nogueira, R., Kelb, C., Schadzek, P., Meinhardt-Wollweber, M., Ngezahayo, A. and Roth, B. (2016) Confocal Raman microscopy and fluorescent in situ hybridization — A complementary approach for biofilm analysis. Chemosphere **161**, 112–118.
152. Liu, X.-Y., Guo, S.-X., Bocklitz, T., Rösch, P., Popp, J. and Yu, H.-Q. (2022) Nondestructive 3D imaging and quantification of hydrated biofilm matrix by confocal Raman microscopy coupled with non-negative matrix factorization. Water Res. **210**, 117973.
153. Liu, X.-Y., Guo, S.-X., Ramoji, A., Bocklitz, T., Rösch, P., Popp, J. and Yu, H.-Q. (2020) Spatiotemporal organization of biofilm matrix revealed by confocal Raman imaging integrated with non-negative matrix factorization analysis. Anal. Chem. **92**, 707–715.
154. Meng, K.-L., Lv, X.-C., Che, H.-Y., Li, Y., Chen, X.-L., Hu, M.-X. and Yan, M. (2021) Joint protection strategies for Saccharomyces boulardii: exogenous encapsulation and endogenous biofilm structure. Appl. Microbiol. Biotechnol. **105**, 6469–6479.
155. Nguyen, C. Q., Thrift, W. J., Bhattacharjee, A., Ranjbar, S., Gallagher, T., Darvishzadeh-Varcheie, M., Sanderson, R. N., Capolino, F., Whiteson, K., Baldi, P., Hochbaum, A. I. and Ragan, R. (2018) Longitudinal monitoring of biofilm formation via robust surface enhanced Raman scattering quantification of Pseudomonas aeruginosa-produced metabolites. ACS Appl. Mater. Interf. **10**, 12364–12373.
156. Robuschi, L., Tomba, J. P. and Busalmen, J. P. (2017) Proving Geobacter biofilm connectivity with confocal Raman microscopy. J. Electroanal. Chem. **793**, 99–103.
157. Wickramasinghe, N. N., Hlaing, M. M., Ravensdale, J. T., Coorey, R., Chandry, P. S. and Dykes, G. A. (2020) Characterization of the biofilm matrix composition of psychrotrophic, meat spoilage pseudomonads. Sci. Rep. **10**, 16457.
158. Mattana, S., Cardinali, M. A., Caponi, S., Pierantoni, D. C., Corte, L., Roscini, L., Cardinali, G. and Fioretto, D. (2017) High-contrast Brillouin and Raman micro-spectroscopy for simultaneous mechanical and chemical investigation of microbial biofilms. Biophys. Chem. **229**, 123–129.
159. Roscini, L., Vassiliou, A., Corte, L., Pierantoni, D. C., Robert, V., Tascini, C., Mattana, S., Cardinali, M. A., Orfanos, S. E., Fioretto, D. and Cardinali, G. (2018) Yeast biofilm as a bridge between medical and environmental microbiology across different detection techniques. Infectious Dis. Ther. **7**, 27–34.

160. Chen, P., Wang, J. J., Hong, B., Tan, L., Yan, J., Zhang, Z., Liu, H., Pan, Y. and Zhao, Y. (2019) Characterization of mixed-species biofilm formed by Vibrio parahaemolyticus and Listeria monocytogenes. Front. Microbiol. **10**, 2543.
161. Yan, J. and Xie, J. (2020) Comparative proteome analysis of Shewanella putrefaciens WS13 mature biofilm under cold stress. Front. Microbiol. **11**, 1225.
162. Henry, V. A., Jessop, J. L. P. and Peeples, T. L. (2017) Differentiating Pseudomonas sp strain ADP cells in suspensions and biofilms using Raman spectroscopy and scanning electron microscopy. Anal. Bioanal. Chem. **409**, 1441–1449.
163. Kusić, D., Kampe, B., Ramoji, A., Neugebauer, U., Rösch, P. and Popp, J. (2015) Raman spectroscopic differention of planktonic bacteria and biofilms. Anal. Bioanal. Chem. **407**, 6803–6813.
164. Liu, H., Xu, Q., Huo, L., Wei, X. and Ling, J. (2014) Chemical composition of Enterococcus faecalis in biofilm cells initiated from different physiologic states. Folia Microbiol. **59**, 447–453.
165. Sharma, G. and Prakash, A. (2021) Combined use of Fourier transform infrared and Raman spectroscopy to study planktonic and biofilm cells of Cronobacter sakazakii. J. Microbiol. Biotechnol. Food Sci. **2021**, 310–314.
166. Kusić, D., Rösch, P. and Popp, J. (2016) Fast label-free detection of Legionella spp. in biofilms by applying immunomagnetic beads and Raman spectroscopy. Syst. Appl. Microbiol. **39**, 132–140.
167. Beier, B. D., Quivey Jr, R. G. and Berger, A. J. (2010) Identification of different bacterial species in biofilms using confocal Raman microscopy. J. Biomed. Opt. **15**, 066001–066005.
168. Samek, O., Al-Marashi, J. and Telle, H. (2010) The potential of Raman spectroscopy for the identification of biofilm formation by Staphylococcus epidermidis. Laser Phys. Lett. **7**, 378–383.
169. Bodelón, G., Montes-García, V., López-Puente, V., Hill, E. H., Hamon, C., Sanz-Ortiz, M. N., Rodal-Cedeira, S., Costas, C., Celiksoy, S. and Pérez-Juste, I. (2016) Detection and imaging of quorum sensing in Pseudomonas aeruginosa biofilm communities by surface-enhanced resonance Raman scattering. Nat. Mater. **15**, 1203–1211.
170. Guo, J., Liu, Y., Yang, Y., Li, Y., Wang, R. and Ju, H. (2020) A filter supported surface-enhanced Raman scattering "nose" for point-of-care monitoring of gaseous metabolites of bacteria. Anal. Chem. **92**, 5055–5063.
171. Kirchhoff, J., Glaser, U., Bohnert, J. A., Pletz, M. W., Popp, J. and Neugebauer, U. (2018) Simple Ciprofloxacin resistance test and determination of minimal inhibitory concentration within 2 h using Raman spectroscopy. Anal. Chem. **90**, 1811–1818.
172. Schröder, U. C., Kirchhoff, J., Hübner, U., Mayer, G., Glaser, U., Henkel, T., Pfister, W., Fritzsche, W., Popp, J. and Neugebauer, U. (2017) On-chip spectroscopic assessment of microbial susceptibility to antibiotics within 3.5 hours. J. Biophotonics **10**, 1547–1557.

173. Assmann, C., Kirchhoff, J., Beleites, C., Hey, J., Kostudis, S., Pfister, W., Schlattmann, P., Popp, J. and Neugebauer, U. (2015) Identification of vancomycin interaction with Enterococcus faecalis within 30 min of interaction time using Raman spectroscopy. Anal. Bioanal. Chem. **407**, 8343–8352.
174. Rousseau, A. N., Faure, N., Rol, F., Sedaghat, Z., Le Galudec, J., Mallard, F. and Josso, Q. (2021) Fast antibiotic susceptibility testing via Raman microspectrometry on single bacteria: an MRSA case study. ACS Omega **6**, 16273–16279.
175. Dekter, H. E., Orelio, C. C., Morsink, M. C., Tektas, S., Vis, B., te Witt, R. and van Leeuwen, W. B. (2017) Antimicrobial susceptibility testing of Gram-positive and -negative bacterial isolates directly from spiked blood culture media with Raman spectroscopy. Eur. J. Clin. Microbiol. Infect. Dis. **36**, 81–89.
176. Verma, T., Annappa, H., Singh, S., Umapathy, S. and Nandi, D. (2021) Profiling antibiotic resistance in Escherichia coli strains displaying differential antibiotic susceptibilities using Raman spectroscopy. J. Biophotonics **14**, e202000231.
177. Nakar, A., Pistiki, A., Ryabchykov, O., Bocklitz, T., Rösch, P. and Popp, J. (2022) Detection of multi-resistant clinical strains of E. coli with Raman spectroscopy. Anal. Bioanal. Chem. **414**, 1481–1492.
178. Ayala, O. D., Wakeman, C. A., Pence, I. J., Gaddy, J. A., Slaughter, J. C., Skaar, E. P. and Mahadevan-Jansen, A. (2018) Drug-resistant Staphylococcus aureus strains reveal distinct biochemical features with Raman microspectroscopy. ACS Infect. Dis. **4**, 1197–1210.
179. Germond, A., Ichimura, T., Horinouchi, T., Fujita, H., Furusawa, C. and Watanabe, T. M. (2018) Raman spectral signature reflects transcriptomic features of antibiotic resistance in Escherichia coli. Commun. Biol. **1**, 85.
180. Pistiki, A., Monecke, S., Shen, H., Ryabchykov, O., Bocklitz, T., Rösch, P., Ehricht, R. and Popp, J. (2022) Comparison of different label-free Raman spectroscopy approaches for the discrimination of isogenic MRSA and MSSA clinical isolates. Microbiol. Spectr. **10**, e0076322.
181. Azemtsop Matanfack, G., Pistiki, A., Rösch, P. and Popp, J. (2021) Raman stable isotope labeling of single bacteria in visible and deep UV-ranges. Life **11**, 1003.
182. Azemtsop Matanfack, G., Pistiki, A., Rösch, P. and Popp, J. (2021) Raman 18O-labeling of bacteria in visible and deep UV-ranges. J. Biophotonics **14**, e202100013.
183. Azemtsop Matanfack, G., Taubert, M., Guo, S., Houhou, R., Bocklitz, T., Küsel, K., Rösch, P. and Popp, J. (2020) Influence of carbon sources on quantification of deuterium incorporation in heterotrophic bacteria: a Raman-stable isotope labeling approach. Anal. Chem. **92**, 11429–11437.
184. Taubert, M., Stöckel, S., Geesink, P., Girnus, S., Jehmlich, N., von Bergen, M., Rösch, P., Popp, J. and Küsel, K. (2018) Tracking active groundwater microbes with D_2O labeling to understand their ecosystem function. Environ. Microbiol. **20**, 369–384.

185. Wang, Y., Xu, J. B., Kong, L. C., Liu, T., Yi, L. B., Wang, H. J., Huang, W. E. and Zheng, C. M. (2020) Raman-deuterium isotope probing to study metabolic activities of single bacterial cells in human intestinal microbiota. Microb. Biotechnol. **13**, 572–583.
186. Li, H. Z., Bi, Q. F., Yang, K., Zheng, B. X., Pu, Q. and Cui, L. (2019) D2O-Isotope-labeling approach to probing phosphate-solubilizing bacteria in complex soil communities by single-cell Raman spectroscopy. Anal. Chem. **91**, 2239–2246.
187. Olaniyi, O. O., Yang, K., Zhu, Y. G. and Cui, L. (2019) Heavy water-labeled Raman spectroscopy reveals carboxymethylcellulose-degrading bacteria and degradation activity at the single-cell level. Appl. Microbiol. Biotechnol. **103**, 1455–1464.
188. Azemtsop Matanfack, G., Taubert, M., Guo, S., Bocklitz, T., Küsel, K., Rösch, P. and Popp, J. (2021) Monitoring deuterium uptake in single bacterial cells via two-dimensional Raman correlation spectroscopy. Anal. Chem. **93**, 7714–7723.
189. Xu, J. B., Zhu, D., Ibrahim, A. D., Allen, C. C. R., Gibson, C. M., Fowler, P. W., Song, Y. Z. and Huang, W. E. (2017) Raman deuterium isotope probing reveals microbial metabolism at the single-cell level. Anal. Chem. **89**, 13305–13312.
190. Vinay Kumar, B. N., Guo, S., Bocklitz, T., Rösch, P. and Popp, J. (2016) Demonstration of carbon catabolite repression in naphthalene degrading soil bacteria via Raman spectroscopy based stable isotope probing. Anal. Chem. **88**, 7574–7582.
191. Kubryk, P., Niessner, R. and Ivleva, N. P. (2016) The origin of the band at around 730 cm(–1) in the SERS spectra of bacteria: a stable isotope approach. Analyst **141**, 2874–2878.
192. Chisanga, M., Muhamadali, H., McDougall, D., Xu, Y., Lockyer, N. and Goodacre, R. (2021) Metabolism in action: stable isotope probing using vibrational spectroscopy and SIMS reveals kinetic and metabolic flux of key substrates. Analyst **146**, 1734–1746.
193. Angel, R., Panholzl, C., Gabriel, R., Herbold, C., Wanek, W., Richter, A., Eichorst, S. A. and Woebken, D. (2018) Application of stable-isotope labelling techniques for the detection of active diazotrophs. Environ. Microbiol. **20**, 44–61.
194. Cui, L., Yang, K., Li, H. Z., Zhang, H., Su, J. Q., Paraskevaidi, M., Martin, F. L., Ren, B. and Zhu, Y. G. (2018) Functional single-cell approach to probing nitrogen-fixing bacteria in soil communities by resonance Raman spectroscopy with N-15(2) labeling. Anal. Chem. **90**, 5082–5089.
195. Lee, K. S., Pereira, F. C., Palatinszky, M., Behrendt, L., Alcolombri, U., Berry, D., Wagner, M. and Stocker, R. (2021) Optofluidic Raman-activated cell sorting for targeted genome retrieval or cultivation of microbial cells with specific functions. Nat. Protoc. **16**, 45.
196. Yang, K., Li, H.-Z., Zhu, X., Su, J.-Q., Ren, B., Zhu, Y.-G. and Cui, L. (2019) Rapid antibiotic susceptibility testing of pathogenic bacteria using heavy water labeled single-cell Raman spectroscopy in clinical samples. Anal. Chem. **91**, 6296–6303.

197. Zhang, M., Hong, W., Abutaleb, N. S., Li, J., Dong, P.-T., Zong, C., Wang, P., Seleem, M. N. and Cheng, J.-X. (2020) Rapid determination of antimicrobial susceptibility by stimulated Raman scattering imaging of D2O metabolic incorporation in a single bacterium. Adv. Sci. **7**, 2001452.

198. Ali, A., Nettey-Oppong, E. E., Effah, E., Yu, C. Y., Muhammad, R., Soomro, T. A., Byun, K. M. and Choi, S. H. (2022) Miniaturized Raman instruments for SERS-based point-of-care testing on respiratory viruses. Biosensors **12**, 590.

199. Mousavi, S. M., Hashemi, S. A., Rahmanian, V., Kalashgrani, M. Y., Gholami, A., Omidifar, N. and Chiang, W. H. (2022) Highly sensitive flexible SERS-based sensing platform for detection of COVID-19. Biosensors **12**, 466.

200. Huang, C.-C., Hsu, Z.-H. and Lai, Y.-S. (2021) Raman spectroscopy for virus detection and the implementation of unorthodox food safety. Trends Food Sci. Technol. **116**, 525–532.

201. Savinon-Flores, F., Mendez, E., Lopez-Castanos, M., Carabarin-Lima, A., Lopez-Castanos, K. A., Gonzalez-Fuentes, M. A. and Mendez-Albores, A. (2021) A review on SERS-based detection of human virus infections: influenza and coronavirus. Biosensors **11**, 66.

202. Sitjar, J., Xu, H. Z., Liu, C. Y., Wang, J. R., Liao, J. D., Tsai, H. P., Lee, H., Liu, B. H. and Chang, C. W. (2022) Synergistic surface-enhanced Raman scattering effect to distinguish live SARS-CoV-2 S pseudovirus. Anal. Chim. Acta **1193**, 339406.

203. Palermo, G., Rippa, M., Conti, Y., Vestri, A., Castagna, R., Fusco, G., Suffredini, E., Zhou, J., Zyss, J., De Luca, A. and Petti, L. (2021) Plasmonic metasurfaces based on pyramidal nanoholes for high-efficiency SERS biosensing. ACS Appl. Mater. Interf. **13**, 43715–43725.

204. Daoudi, K., Ramachandran, K., Alawadhi, H., Boukherroub, R., Dogheche, E., Khakani, M. A. E. and Gaidi, M. (2021) Ultra-sensitive and fast optical detection of the spike protein of the SARS-CoV-2 using AgNPs/SiNWs nanohybrid based sensors. Surf. Interfaces **27**, 101454.

205. Ansah, I. B., An, T., Yang, J. Y., Jung, H. S., Mun, C., Jung, S., Lee, S., Jang, Y., Kim, D. H., Kim, M. and Park, S. G. (2021) Electrochemical synthesis of 3D plasmonic — molecule nanocomposite materials for in situ label-free molecular detections. Adv. Mater. Interf. **8**, 2101201.

206. Paria, D., Kwok, K. S., Raj, P., Zheng, P., Gracias, D. H. and Barman, I. (2022) Label-free spectroscopic SARS-CoV-2 detection on versatile nanoimprinted substrates. Nano Lett. **22**, 3620–3627.

207. Morder, C. J., Scarpitti, B. T., Balss, K. M. and Schultz, Z. D. (2022) Determination of lentiviral titer by surface enhanced Raman scattering. Anal. Meth. **14**, 1387–1395.

208. Sanchez, J. E., Jaramillo, S. A., Settles, E., Velazquez Salazar, J. J., Lehr, A., Gonzalez, J., Rodriguez Aranda, C., Navarro-Contreras, H. R., Raniere, M. O., Harvey, M., Wagner, D. M., Koppisch, A., Kellar, R., Keim, P. and

Jose Yacaman, M. (2021) Detection of SARS-CoV-2 and its S and N proteins using surface enhanced Raman spectroscopy. RSC Adv. **11**, 25788–25794.

209. Zhang, Z., Li, D., Wang, X., Wang, Y., Lin, J., Jiang, S., Wu, Z., He, Y., Gao, X., Zhu, Z., Xiao, Y., Qu, Z. and Li, Y. (2022) Rapid detection of viruses: Based on silver nanoparticles modified with bromine ions and acetonitrile. Chem. Eng. J. **438**, 135589.
210. Zhang, D., Zhang, X., Ma, R., Deng, S., Wang, X., Wang, X., Zhang, X., Huang, X., Liu, Y., Li, G., Qu, J., Zhu, Y. and Li, J. (2021) Ultra-fast and onsite interrogation of Severe Acute Respiratory Syndrome Coronavirus 2 (SARS-CoV-2) in waters via surface enhanced Raman scattering (SERS) Water Res. **200**, 117243.
211. Yang, Y., Peng, Y., Lin, C., Long, L., Hu, J., He, J., Zeng, H., Huang, Z., Li, Z. Y., Tanemura, M., Shi, J., Lombardi, J. R. and Luo, X. (2021) Human ACE2-functionalized gold "virus-trap" nanostructures for accurate capture of SARS-CoV-2 and single-virus SERS detection. Nanomicro. Lett. **13**, 109.
212. Payne, T. D., Klawa, S. J., Jian, T., Kim, S. H., Papanikolas, M. J., Freeman, R. and Schultz, Z. D. (2021) Catching COVID: engineering peptide-modified surface-enhanced Raman spectroscopy sensors for SARS-CoV-2. ACS Sens. **6**, 3436–3444.
213. Li, Y., Lin, C., Peng, Y., He, J. and Yang, Y. (2022) High-sensitivity and point-of-care detection of SARS-CoV-2 from nasal and throat swabs by magnetic SERS biosensor. Sens. Actuat. B **365**, 131974.
214. Yu, Q., Wu, Y., Kang, T. and Choo, J. (2021) Development of surface-enhanced Raman scattering-based immunoassay platforms using hollow Au nanostars for reliable SARS-CoV-2 diagnosis. Bull. Korean Chem. Soc. **42**, 1699–1705.
215. Cha, H., Kim, H., Joung, Y., Kang, H., Moon, J., Jang, H., Park, S., Kwon, H. J., Lee, I. C., Kim, S., Yong, D., Yoon, S. W., Park, S. G., Guk, K., Lim, E. K., Park, H. G., Choo, J., Jung, J. and Kang, T. (2022) Surface-enhanced Raman scattering-based immunoassay for severe acute respiratory syndrome coronavirus 2. Biosens. Bioelectron. **202**, 114008.
216. Antoine, D., Mohammadi, M., Vitt, M., Dickie, J. M., Jyoti, S. S., Tilbury, M. A., Johnson, P. A., Wawrousek, K. E. and Wall, J. G. (2022) Rapid, point-of-care scFv-SERS assay for femtoGram-level detection of SARS-CoV-2. ACS Sens. **7**, 866–873.
217. Pramanik, A., Gao, Y., Patibandla, S., Mitra, D., McCandless, M. G., Fassero, L. A., Gates, K., Tandon, R. and Chandra Ray, P. (2021) The rapid diagnosis and effective inhibition of coronavirus using spike antibody attached gold nanoparticles. Nanoscale Adv. **3**, 1588–1596.
218. Kim, H., Kang, H., Kim, H. N., Kim, H., Moon, J., Guk, K., Park, H., Yong, D., Bae, P. K., Park, H. G., Lim, E. K., Kang, T. and Jung, J. (2021) Development of 6E3 antibody-mediated SERS immunoassay for drug-resistant influenza virus. Biosens. Bioelectron. **187**, 113324.

219. Lu, M., Joung, Y., Jeon, C. S., Kim, S., Yong, D., Jang, H., Pyun, S. H., Kang, T. and Choo, J. (2022) Dual-mode SERS-based lateral flow assay strips for simultaneous diagnosis of SARS-CoV-2 and influenza a virus. Nano Converg. **9**, 39.
220. Zhdanov, G., Nyhrikova, E., Meshcheryakova, N., Kristavchuk, O., Akhmetova, A., Andreev, E., Rudakova, E., Gambaryan, A., Yaminsky, I., Aralov, A., Kukushkin, V. and Zavyalova, E. (2022) A combination of membrane filtration and Raman-active DNA ligand greatly enhances sensitivity of SERS-based aptasensors for influenza A virus. Front. Chem. **10**, 937180.
221. Gribanyov, D., Zhdanov, G., Olenin, A., Lisichkin, G., Gambaryan, A., Kukushkin, V. and Zavyalova, E. (2021) SERS-based colloidal aptasensors for quantitative determination of influenza virus. Int. J. Mol. Sci. **22**, 1842.
222. Zavyalova, E., Ambartsumyan, O., Zhdanov, G., Gribanyov, D., Gushchin, V., Tkachuk, A., Rudakova, E., Nikiforova, M., Kuznetsova, N., Popova, L., Verdiev, B., Alatyrev, A., Burtseva, E., Ignatieva, A., Iliukhina, A., Dolzhikova, I., Arutyunyan, A., Gambaryan, A. and Kukushkin, V. (2021) SERS-based aptasensor for rapid quantitative detection of SARS-CoV-2. Nanomaterials (Basel) **11**, 1394.
223. Tian, C., Zhao, L., Qi, G., Zhu, J. and Zhang, S. (2022) One-pot and rapid detection of SARS-CoV-2 viral particles in environment using SERS aptasensor based on a locking amplifier. Sens. Actuat. B **371**, 132445.
224. Chen, H., Park, S. K., Joung, Y., Kang, T., Lee, M. K. and Choo, J. (2022) SERS-based dual-mode DNA aptasensors for rapid classification of SARS-CoV-2 and influenza A/H1N1 infection. Sens. Actuat. B **355**, 131324.
225. Tauber, J. P., Matthäus, C., Lenz, C., Hoffmeister, D. and Popp, J. (2018) Analysis of basidiomycete pigments in situ by Raman spectroscopy. J. Biophotonics **11**, e201700369.
226. Walter, A., Erdmann, S., Bocklitz, T., Jung, E.-M., Vogler, N., Akimov, D., Dietzek, B., Rösch, P., Kothe, E. and Popp, J. (2010) Analysis of the cytochrome distribution via linear and nonlinear Raman spectroscopy. Analyst **135**, 908–917.
227. Münchberg, U., Wagner, L., Spielberg, E. T., Voigt, K., Rösch, P. and Popp, J. (2013) Spatially resolved investigation of the oil composition in single intact hyphae of Mortierella spp. with micro-Raman spectroscopy. Biochim. Biophys. Acta **1831**, 341–349.
228. Münchberg, U., Wagner, L., Rohrer, C., Voigt, K., Rösch, P., Jahreis, G. and Popp, J. (2015) Quantitative assessment of the degree of lipid unsaturation in intact Mortierella fungi by Raman microspectroscopy. Anal. Bioanal. Chem. **407**, 3303–3311.
229. De Gussem, K., Vandenabeele, P., Verbeken, A. and Moens, L. (2007) Chemotaxonomical identification of spores of macrofungi: possibilities of Raman spectroscopy. Anal. Bioanal. Chem. **387**, 2823–2832.

230. De Gussem, K., Vandenabeele, P., Verbeken, A. and Moens, L. (2005) Raman spectroscopic study of Lactarius spores (Russulales, Fungi). Spectrochim. Acta A **61**, 2896–2908.
231. Petrokilidou, C., Pavlou, E., Gaitanis, G., Bassukas, I. D., Saridomichelakis, M. N., Velegraki, A. and Kourkoumelis, N. (2019) The lipid profile of three Malassezia species assessed by Raman spectroscopy and discriminant analysis. Mol. Cellul. Probes **46**, 101416.
232. Gherman, A. M. R., Dina, N. E., Chis, V., Wieser, A. and Haisch, C. (2019) Yeast cell wall — Silver nanoparticles interaction: A synergistic approach between surface-enhanced Raman scattering and computational spectroscopy tools. Spectrochim. Acta A **222**, 117223.
233. Rösch, P., Harz, M., Peschke, K. D., Ronneberger, O., Burkhardt, H. and Popp, J. (2006) Identification of single eukaryotic cells with micro-Raman spectroscopy. Biopolymers **82**, 312–316.
234. Rösch, P., Harz, M., Schmitt, M. and Popp, J. (2005) Raman spectroscopic identification of single yeast cells. J. Raman Spectrosc. **36**, 377–379.
235. Lemma, T., Wang, J., Arstila, K., Hytonen, V. P. and Toppari, J. J. (2019) Identifying yeasts using surface enhanced Raman spectroscopy. Spectrochim. Acta A **218**, 299–307.
236. Cardinali, M. A., Pierantoni, D. C., Caponi, S., Corte, L., Fioretto, D. and Cardinali, G. (2019) Meso-Raman approach for rapid yeast cells identification. Biophys. Chem. **254**, 106249.
237. Pezzotti, G., Kobara, M., Nakaya, T., Imamura, H., Miyamoto, N., Adachi, T., Yamamoto, T., Kanamura, N., Ohgitani, E., Marin, E., Zhu, W., Nishimura, I., Mazda, O., Nakata, T. and Makimura, K. (2022) Raman spectroscopy of oral Candida species: molecular-scale analyses, chemometrics, and barcode identification. Int. J. Mol. Sci. **23**, 5359.
238. Potocki, L., Depciuch, J., Kuna, E., Worek, M., Lewinska, A. and Wnuk, M. (2019) FTIR and Raman spectroscopy-based biochemical profiling reflects genomic diversity of clinical Candida isolates that may be useful for diagnosis and targeted therapy of Candidiasis. Int. J. Mol. Sci. **20**, 988.
239. Ibelings, M. S., Maquelin, K., Endtz, H. P., Bruining, H. A. and Puppels, G. J. (2005) Rapid identification of Candida spp. in peritonitis patients by Raman spectroscopy. Clin. Microbiol. Infect. **11**, 353–358.
240. Silge, A., Heinke, R., Bocklitz, T., Wiegand, C., Hipler, U.-C., Rösch, P. and Popp, J. (2018) The application of UV resonance Raman spectroscopy for the differentiation of clinically relevant Candida species. Anal. Bioanal. Chem. **410**, 5839–5847.
241. Dina, N. E., Gherman, A. M. R., Chis, V., Sarbu, C., Wieser, A., Bauer, D. and Haisch, C. (2018) Characterization of clinically relevant fungi via SERS fingerprinting assisted by novel chemometric models. Anal. Chem. **90**, 2484–2492.

242. Witkowska, E., Jagielski, T., Kaminska, A., Kowalska, A., Hryncewicz-Gwozdz, A. and Waluk, J. (2016) Detection and identification of human fungal pathogens using surface-enhanced Raman spectroscopy and principal component analysis. Anal. Meth. **8**, 8427–8434.
243. Smijs, T. G., Jachtenberg, J. W., Pavel, S., Bakker-Schut, T. C., Willemse-Erix, D., de Haas, E. R. M. and Sterenborg, H. (2014) Detection and differentiation of causative organisms of onychomycosis in an ex vivo nail model by means of Raman spectroscopy. J. Eur. Acad. Dermat. Venereol. **28**, 1492–1499.
244. Petrokilidou, C., Gaitanis, G., Bassukas, I. D., Velegraki, A., Guevara, E., Vardaki, M. Z. and Kourkoumelis, N. (2020) Emerging optical techniques for the diagnosis of Onychomycosis. Appl. Sci. **10**, 2340.
245. Ghosal, S., Macher, J. M. and Ahmed, K. (2012) Raman microspectroscopy-based identification of individual fungal spores as potential indicators of indoor contamination and moisture-related building damage. Environ. Sci. Technol. **46**, 6088–6095.
246. Strycker, B. D., Han, Z. H., Duan, Z., Commer, B., Wang, K., Shaw, B. D., Sokolov, A. V. and Scully, M. O. (2020) Identification of toxic mold species through Raman spectroscopy of fungal conidia. PLoS One **15**, e0242361.
247. Žukovskaja, O., Kloß, S., Blango, M. G., Ryabchykov, O., Kniemeyer, O., Brakhage, A. A., Bocklitz, T. W., Cialla-May, D., Weber, K. and Popp, J. (2018) UV-Raman spectroscopic identification of fungal spores important for respiratory diseases. Anal. Chem. **90**, 8912–8918.
248. Dou, T. Y., Ermolenkov, A., Hays, S. R., Rich, B. T., Donaldson, T. G., Thomas, D., Teel, P. D. and Kurouski, D. (2022) Raman-based identification of tick species (Ixodidae) by spectroscopic analysis of their feces. Spectrochim. Acta A **271**, 120966.
249. Holscher, D., Dhakshinamoorthy, S., Alexandrov, T., Becker, M., Bretschneider, T., Buerkert, A., Crecelius, A. C., De Waele, D., Elsen, A., Heckel, D. G., Heklau, H., Hertweck, C., Kai, M., Knop, K., Krafft, C., Maddula, R. K., Matthaus, C., Popp, J., Schneider, B., Schubert, U. S., Sikora, R. A., Svatos, A. and Swennen, R. L. (2014) Phenalenone-type phytoalexins mediate resistance of banana plants (Musa spp.) to the burrowing nematode Radopholus similis. Proc. Natl. Acad. Sci. **111**, 105–110.
250. Quiles, F., Balandier, J. Y. and Capizzi-Banas, S. (2006) In situ characterisation of a microorganism surface by Raman microspectroscopy: the shell of Ascaris eggs. Anal. Bioanal. Chem. **386**, 249–255.
251. Zivanovic, V., Semini, G., Laue, M., Drescher, D., Aebischer, T. and Kneipp, J. (2018) Chemical mapping of Leishmania infection in live cells by SERS microscopy. Anal. Chem. **90**, 8154–8161.
252. Toledo, D. A. M., Roque, N. R., Teixeira, L., Milan-Garces, E. A., Carneiro, A. B., Almeida, M. R., Andrade, G. F. S., Martins, J. S., Pinho, R. R., Freire-de-Lima, C. G., Bozza, P. T., D'Avila, H. and Melo, R. C. N. (2016) Lipid body organelles

within the parasite Trypanosoma cruzi: a role for intracellular arachidonic acid metabolism. PLoS One **11**, 0160433.

253. Girard, A., Cooper, A., Mabbott, S., Bradley, B., Asiala, S., Jamieson, L., Clucas, C., Capewell, P., Marchesi, F., Gibbins, M. P., Hentzschel, F., Marti, M., Quintana, J. F., Garside, P., Faulds, K., MacLeod, A. and Graham, D. (2021) Raman spectroscopic analysis of skin as a diagnostic tool for Human African Trypanosomiasis. PLoS Path. **17**, e1010060.
254. Lucius, R., Loos-Frank, B. and Lane, R. P. (2018) Biologie von Parasiten. Berlin: Springer.
255. Arslan, A. H., Ciloglu, F. U., Yilmaz, U., Simsek, E. and Aydin, O. (2022) Discrimination of waterborne pathogens, Cryptosporidium parvum oocysts and bacteria using surface-enhanced Raman spectroscopy coupled with principal component analysis and hierarchical clustering. Spectrochim. Acta A **267**, 120475.
256. Malyshev, D., Dahlberg, T., Oberg, R., Landstrom, L. and Andersson, M. (2022) Reference Raman spectrum and mapping of Cryptosporidium parvum oocysts. J. Raman Spectrosc. **53**, 1293–1301.
257. Araujo-Andrade, C., Pichardo-Molina, J. L., Barbosa-Sabanero, G., Frausto-Reyes, C. and Torres-Lopez, A. (2007) Detection of the presence of antibodies against Toxoplasma gondii in human colostrum by Raman spectroscopy and principal component analysis. J. Biomed. Opt. **12**, 034006.
258. Naemat, A., Elsheikha, H. M., Boitor, R. A. and Notingher, I. (2016) Tracing amino acid exchange during host-pathogen interaction by combined stable-isotope time-resolved Raman spectral imaging. Sci. Rep. **6**, 20811
259. Sinjab, F., Elsheikha, H. M., Dooley, M. and Notingher, I. (2020) Induction and measurement of the early stage of a host-parasite interaction using a combined optical trapping and Raman microspectroscopy system. J. Biophotonics **13**, e201960065.
260. Kong, K., Rowlands, C. J., Elsheikha, H. and Notingher, I. (2012) Label-free molecular analysis of live Neospora caninum tachyzoites in host cells by selective scanning Raman micro-spectroscopy. Analyst **137**, 4119–4122.
261. Ruther, A., Perez-Guaita, D., Poole, W. A., Cooke, B. M., Suarez, C. E., Heraud, P. and Wood, B. R. (2020) Vibrational spectroscopic based approach for diagnosing Babesia bovis infection. Anal. Chem. **92**, 8784–8792.
262. Christensen, D., Ruther, A., Kochan, K., Perez-Guaita, D. and Wood, B. (2019) Whole-organism analysis by vibrational spectroscopy. Annu. Rev. Anal. Chem. **12**, 89–108.
263. Wood, B. R. and McNaughton, D. (2006) Resonance Raman spectroscopy in malaria research. Exp. Rev. Proteomics **3**, 525–544.
264. Perez-Guaita, D., Marzec, K. M., Hudson, A., Evans, C., Chernenko, T., Matthaus, C., Miljkovic, M., Diem, M., Heraud, P., Richards, J. S., Andrew, D., Anderson, D. A., Doerig, C., Garcia-Bustos, J., McNaughton, D. and Wood, B. R. (2018)

Parasites under the spotlight: applications of vibrational spectroscopy to malaria research. Chem. Rev. **118**, 5330–5358.

265. Wood, B. R., Hermelink, A., Lasch, P., Bambery, K. R., Webster, G. T., Khiavi, M. A., Cooke, B. M., Deed, S., Naumann, D. and McNaughton, D. (2009) Resonance Raman microscopy in combination with partial dark-field microscopy lights up a new path in malaria diagnostics. Analyst **134**, 1119–1125.
266. Bruckner, M., Becker, K., Popp, J. and Frosch, T. (2015) Fiber array based hyperspectral Raman imaging for chemical selective analysis of malaria-infected red blood cells. Anal. Chim. Acta **894**, 76–84.
267. Chen, K. R., Yuen, C., Aniweh, Y., Preiser, P. and Liu, Q. (2016) Towards ultrasensitive malaria diagnosis using surface enhanced Raman spectroscopy. Sci. Rep. **6**, 20177
268. Chen, F. N., Flaherty, B. R., Cohen, C. E., Peterson, D. S. and Zhao, Y. P. (2016) Direct detection of malaria infected red blood cells by surface enhanced Raman spectroscopy. Nanomed. Nanotechnol. **12**, 1445–1451.
269. Yadav, S., Khanam, R. and Singh, J. P. (2022) A purview into highly sensitive magnetic SERS detection of hemozoin biomarker for rapid malaria diagnosis. Sens. Actuat. B **355**, 131303.
270. Wang, W., Dong, R. L., Gu, D. Y., He, J. A., Yi, P., Kong, S. K., Ho, H. P., Loo, J. F. C., Wang, W. and Wang, Q. (2020) Antibody-free rapid diagnosis of malaria in whole blood with surface-enhanced Raman spectroscopy using nanostructured gold substrate. Adv. Med. Sci. **65**, 86–92.
271. Mhlanga, N., Domfe, T., Skepu, A. and Ntho, T. A. (2020) Sandwich-based surface-enhanced Raman scattering probes for detection and quantification of malaria. J. Raman Spectrosc. **51**, 2416–2424.
272. Garrett, N. L., Sekine, R., Dixon, M. W. A., Tilley, L., Bambery, K. R. and Wood, B. R. (2015) Bio-sensing with butterfly wings: naturally occurring nano-structures for SERS-based malaria parasite detection. Phys. Chem. Chem. Phys. **17**, 21164–21168.
273. Yuen, C., Gao, X. H., Yong, J. J. M., Prakash, P., Shobana, C. R., Kaushalya, P. A. T., Luo, Y. M., Bai, Y. R., Yang, C., Preiser, P. R. and Liu, Q. (2021) Towards malaria field diagnosis based on surface-enhanced Raman scattering with on-chip sample preparation and near-analyte nanoparticle synthesis. Sens. Actuat. B **343**, 130162.
274. Frame, L., Brewer, J., Lee, R., Faulds, K. and Graham, D. (2018) Development of a label-free Raman imaging technique for differentiation of malaria parasite infected from non-infected tissue. Analyst **143**, 157–163.
275. Goh, B., Ching, K., Magalhaes, R. J. S., Ciocchetta, S., Edstein, M. D., Maciel-de-Freitas, R. and Sikulu-Lord, M. T. (2021) The application of spectroscopy techniques for diagnosis of malaria parasites and arboviruses and surveillance of mosquito vectors: A systematic review and critical appraisal of evidence. PLoS Neglect. Trop. Dis. **15**, e0009218.

276. Hato, T. and Dagher, P. C. (2015) How the innate immune system senses trouble and causes trouble. Clin. J. Am. Soc. Nephrol. **10**, 1459–1469.
277. Amarante-Mendes, G. P., Adjemian, S., Branco, L. M., Zanetti, L. C., Weinlich, R. and Bortoluci, K. R. (2018) Pattern recognition receptors and the host cell death molecular machinery. Front. Immunol. **9**, 2379.
278. Schie, I. W., Ruger, J., Mondol, A. S., Ramoji, A., Neugebauer, U., Krafft, C. and Popp, J. (2018) High-throughput screening Raman spectroscopy platform for label-free cellomics. Anal. Chem. **90**, 2023–2030.
279. Töpfer, N., Müller, M. M., Dahms, M., Ramoji, A., Popp, J., Slevogt, H. and Neugebauer, U. (2019) Raman spectroscopy reveals LPS-induced changes of biomolecular composition in monocytic THP-1 cells in a label-free manner. Integrative Biol. **11**, 87–98.
280. Chaudhary, N., Nguyen, T. N. Q., Cullen, D., Meade, A. D. and Wynne, C. (2021) Discrimination of immune cell activation using Raman micro-spectroscopy in an in-vitro & ex-vivo model. Spectrochim. Acta A **248**, 119118.
281. Ichimura, T., Chiu, L.-d., Fujita, K., Machiyama, H., Yamaguchi, T., Watanabe, T. M. and Fujita, H. (2016) Non-label immune cell state prediction using Raman spectroscopy. Sci. Rep. **6**, 37562.
282. Ramoji, A., Ryabchykov, O., Galler, K., Tannert, A., Markwart, R., Requardt, R. P., Rubio, I., Bauer, M., Bocklitz, T., Popp, J. and Neugebauer, U. (2019) Raman spectroscopy follows time-dependent changes in T lymphocytes isolated from spleen of endotoxemic mice. ImmunoHorizons **3**, 45.
283. Ramoji, A., Thomas-Rüddel, D., Ryabchykov, O., Bauer, M., Arend, N., Giamarellos-Bourboulis, E. J., Eugen-Olsen, J., Kiehntopf, M., Bocklitz, T., Popp, J., Bloos, F. and Neugebauer, U. (2021) Leukocyte activation profile assessed by Raman spectroscopy helps diagnosing infection and sepsis. Crit. Care Explor. **3**, e0394.
284. Neugebauer, U., Große, C., Bauer, M., Kemper, B., Barroso-Pena, A., Bauwens, A., Glueder, M., Woerdemann, M., Dewenter, L., Denz, C., Kloß, S., Rösch, P., Sabat, A., Schütze, K., Friedrich, A., Bally, G. v., Popp, J. and Mellmann, A. (2012) From infection to detection: imaging S. aureus — host interactions. Biomed. Techn. **57**, SI-1-Track-B.
285. Arend, N., Pittner, A., Ramoji, A., Mondol, A. S., Dahms, M., Rüger, J., Kurzai, O., Schie, I. W., Bauer, M., Popp, J. and Neugebauer, U. (2020) Detection and differentiation of bacterial and fungal infection of neutrophils from peripheral blood using Raman spectroscopy. Anal. Chem. **92**, 10560–10568.
286. Pistiki, A., Ramoji, A., Ryabchykov, O., Thomas-Rüddel, D., Press, A. T., Makarewicz, O., Giamarellos-Bourboulis, E. J., Bauer, M., Bocklitz, T., Popp, J. and Neugebauer, U. (2021) Biochemical analysis of leukocytes after in vitro and in vivo activation with bacterial and fungal pathogens using Raman spectroscopy. Int. J. Mol. Sci. **22**, 10481.

287. Salehi, H., Ramoji, A., Mougari, S., Merida, P., Neyret, A., Popp, J., Horvat, B., Muriaux, D. and Cuisinier, F. (2022) Specific intracellular signature of SARS-CoV-2 infection using confocal Raman microscopy. Commun. Chem. **5**, 85.
288. Huleihel, M., Shufan, E., Zeiri, L. and Salman, A. (2016) Detection of vero cells infected with herpes simplex types 1 and 2 and varicella zoster viruses using Raman spectroscopy and advanced statistical methods. PLoS One **11**, e0153599.
289. Tiwari, D., Jakhmola, S., Pathak, D. K., Kumar, R. and Jha, H. C. (2020) Temporal in vitro Raman spectroscopy for monitoring replication kinetics of Epstein-Barr virus infection in glial cells. ACS Omega **5**, 29547–29560.
290. Ramoji, A., Pahlow, S., Pistiki, A., Rueger, J., Shaik, T. A., Shen, H., Wichmann, C., Krafft, C. and Popp, J. (2022) Understanding viruses and viral infections by biophotonic methods. Transl. Biophotonics **4**, e202100008.
291. Khan, S., Ullah, R., Saleem, M., Bilal, M., Rashid, R., Khan, I., Mahmood, A. and Nawaz, M. (2016) Raman spectroscopic analysis of dengue virus infection in human blood sera. Optik **127**, 2086–2088.
292. Mahmood, T., Nawaz, H., Ditta, A., Majeed, M. I., Hanif, M. A., Rashid, N., Bhatti, H. N., Nargis, H. F., Saleem, M., Bonnier, F. and Byrne, H. J. (2018) Raman spectral analysis for rapid screening of dengue infection. Spectrochim. Acta A **200**, 136–142.
293. Naseer, K., Amin, A., Saleem, M. and Qazi, J. (2019) Raman spectroscopy based differentiation of typhoid and dengue fever in infected human sera. Spectrochim. Acta A **206**, 197–201.
294. Bilal, M., Saleem, M., Amanat, S. T., Shakoor, H. A., Rashid, R., Mahmood, A. and Ahmed, M. (2015) Optical diagnosis of malaria infection in human plasma using Raman spectroscopy. J. Biomed. Opt. **20**, 017002.
295. Khan, S., Ullah, R., Khan, A., Ashraf, R., Ali, H., Bilal, M. and Saleem, M. (2018) Analysis of hepatitis B virus infection in blood sera using Raman spectroscopy and machine learning. Photodiagnosis Photodyn. Ther. **23**, 89–93.
296. Ali, S., Hassan, M., Saleem, M. and Tahir, S. F. (2020) Deep transfer learning based hepatitis B virus diagnosis using spectroscopic images. Intern. J. Imag. Syst. Technol. **31**, 94–105.
297. Tong, D., Chen, C., Zhang, J., Lv, G., Zheng, X., Zhang, Z. and Lv, X. (2019) Application of Raman spectroscopy in the detection of hepatitis B virus infection. Photodiagnosis Photodyn. Ther. **28**, 248–252.
298. Ditta, A., Nawaz, H., Mahmood, T., Majeed, M. I., Tahir, M., Rashid, N., Muddassar, M., Al-Saadi, A. A. and Byrne, H. J. (2019) Principal components analysis of Raman spectral data for screening of Hepatitis C infection. Spectrochim. Acta A **221**, 117173.
299. Saleem, M., Ali, S., Khan, M. B., Amin, A., Bilal, M., Nawaz, H. and Hassan, M. (2020) Optical diagnosis of hepatitis B virus infection in blood plasma using Raman spectroscopy and chemometric techniques. J. Raman Spectrosc. **51**, 1067–1077.

300. Zhao, Y., Tian, S., Yu, L., Zhang, Z. and Zhang, W. (2021) Analysis and classification of hepatitis infections using Raman spectroscopy and multiscale convolutional neural networks. J. Appl. Spectrosc. **88**, 441–451.
301. Goulart, A. C. C., Silveira, L., Jr., Carvalho, H. C., Dorta, C. B., Pacheco, M. T. T. and Zangaro, R. A. (2022) Diagnosing COVID-19 in human serum using Raman spectroscopy. Lasers Med. Sci. **37**, 2217–2226.
302. Storozhuk, D., Ryabchykov, O., Popp, J. and Bocklitz, T. (2022) RAMANMETRIX: a delightful way to analyze Raman spectra. https://arxiv.org/abs/2201.07586.

https://doi.org/10.1142/9789811264610_0011

Chapter 11

Raman Spectroscopy Applied to Antimicrobial Resistance

Kamila Kochan,[1] Savithri Pebotuwa,[1,2] Thulya Chakkumpulakkal Puthan Veettil,[1] Anton Y. Peleg,[2] Xenia Kostoulias,[2] Bayden R. Wood[1,*]

[1]*Centre for Biospectroscopy, School of Chemistry, Monash University, 3800, Victoria, Australia*
[2]*Department of Infectious Diseases, The Alfred Hospital and Central Clinical School, 3800, Monash University*
**Corresponding author: bayden.wood@monash.edu*

11.1 Introduction

Antimicrobial resistance (AMR) is a phenomenon that arises when microorganisms, including bacteria, fungi and parasites, are no longer treatable with therapeutics to which they were once susceptible. It is a leading cause of morbidity and mortality globally, and has been declared as one of the top 10 global threats to public health by the World Health Organization (WHO) [1]. In fact, microorganisms that are resistant to all available antimicrobials are being increasingly reported [2, 3], raising concerns of a post-antimicrobial era. Unless urgent action is taken, it has been estimated that by the year 2050, AMR could kill as many as 10 million people per year [5]. In addition to the human cost, AMR has a significant economic impact with estimated costs of nine billion euros and 20 billion USD in Europe and the United States respectively, excluding the costs of lost productivity [6].

Infections with resistant microorganisms place a heavy burden on healthcare systems, leading to increased lengths of hospital stays, treatment failure and mortality [6]. Due to the escalating rates of AMR, empiric regimens in clinical practice are often inadequate and result in poor patient outcomes [7]. Early detection of resistance is therefore crucial to reduce the time to effective antimicrobial therapy, thereby improving patient outcomes and survival [8–10]. Indeed, an investigation into the impact of antibiotic therapy on the prognosis of adult patients with septic shock found that time to antibiotic administration was the strongest predictor of mortality [8]. Using traditional diagnostic tools, however, it can take up to 48 hours to determine the species and drug susceptibilities of bacteria from clinical specimens [11]. For slower growing microorganisms like fungi, this process can take much longer [12].

11.2 Bacteria

In 2019, there were an estimated 4.95 million deaths associated with bacterial AMR globally [7]. Within hospitals and other clinical settings, the emergence of highly drug-resistant bacteria is facilitated by the intensive and prolonged use of antibiotics [13]. The risk factors for developing a hospital-acquired infection include immunosuppression, indwelling medical devices, prolonged hospital stays and exposure to intensive care units [14]. A group of bacteria — *Enterococcus faecium*, *Staphylococcus aureus*, *Klebsiella pneumoniae*, *Acinetobacter baumannii*, *Pseudomonas aeruginosa* and *Enterobacter* species — aptly named the ESKAPE pathogens for their capacity to 'escape' the actions of antibiotics, make a significant contribution to the burden of disease in healthcare settings in both developed and developing nations [15]. ESKAPE pathogens are associated with severe, life-threatening hospital-acquired infections including bloodstream infections, meningitis and pneumonia [16]. This has led the WHO to include the ESKAPE pathogens in the list of bacteria for which new antibiotics are desperately required. Vancomycin-resistant *E. faecium* and vancomycin- and methicillin-resistant *S. aureus* (MRSA) have been listed as high-priority pathogens, while carbapenem-resistant *A. baumannii* and *P. aeruginosa* and extended spectrum β-lactamase producing and carbapenem-resistant *K. pneumoniae* and *Enterobacter* species have been listed as critical-priority pathogens [17].

Due to the overuse and misuse of antibiotics in human, industrial and agricultural activities and the environmental contamination of ESKAPE pathogens via hospital waste, community-acquired AMR infections also make a substantial contribution to global morbidity and mortality [18]. Perhaps the most significant community-acquired bacterial infection is tuberculosis

(TB), caused by *Mycobacterium tuberculosis*. TB was once the leading cause of death due to an infectious disease in humans, having been surpassed only recently by COVID-19 [19, 20]. In 2021, an estimated 10.6 million people contracted TB, resulting in 1.6 million deaths [20]. The growing incidence of drug resistance amongst *M. tuberculosis* isolates makes it a significant public health threat and is the target of an ambitious strategy by the WHO to end the TB epidemic by 2030 [20].

Bacteria have evolved a number of sophisticated mechanisms to avoid killing by antibiotics. One of the most successful AMR mechanisms employed by these bacteria is the production of enzymes that can destroy or inactivate the antibiotics used against them [16, 21]. Enzymes such as β-lactamases, for instance, destroy the β-lactam ring present in all β-lactam antibiotics (e.g., penicillin), thus rendering it ineffective [22]. Alternatively, aminoglycoside-modifying enzymes modify the structure of aminoglycoside antibiotics (e.g., gentamicin), thereby leading to their inactivation [23]. Another strategy employed by bacteria involves the modification of the binding site, which lowers the affinity of the antibiotic or prevents it from binding altogether [16, 21]. Additionally, bacteria can also reduce intracellular antibiotic accumulation via mechanisms that either reduce their entry or increase their removal from the cell [16, 21]. Perhaps the most important cause of AMR, however, is not due to these classical resistance mechanisms but rather due to the formation of bacterial biofilms. Biofilms can form on either biotic or abiotic surfaces and consist of complex microbial communities embedded in a matrix of extracellular polymeric substances. Biofilms impede the activity of antibiotics by providing both a physical and biochemical barrier that restricts drug penetration or attenuates its activity [16, 21].

11.2.1 *Raman Spectroscopy in Antimicrobial Resistance Studies*

The use of Raman spectroscopy (RS) in antibacterial resistance studies has been increasing rapidly over the past decade. RS is being utilized in AMR studies in a variety of contexts, including molecular characterization of the composition of various resistant strains [24], uncovering resistance mechanisms [25] or following the mechanisms of drug action [26]. However, by far the greatest and most explored application of RS in the AMR field lies in its potential use for rapid resistance detection. A vast array of studies emerged — in particular in the last decade — demonstrating the ability of RS to correctly identify resistance strains, with high sensitivity and specificity.

Indeed, RS has multiple advantages that position it as a strong candidate for a possible new, rapid antibiotic susceptibility test (AST). It provides detailed molecular characteristics of the interrogated sample, enabling the detection of differences in the chemical composition, including ones associated with resistant phenotypes [27]. Since water is a weak Raman scatterer and has minimal influence on the Raman spectra, the data can be collected from samples in the liquid state. Due to this, RS is perfectly suited to conduct measurements using body fluids, such as blood, urine and saliva [28]. The ability to use body fluids in diagnostics, in particular urine or saliva, is important from the clinical perspective, as their collection is relatively easy, fast and non-invasive. Furthermore, RS requires no or minimal sample preparation. The sample preparation stage is often long, laborious and requires specialized equipment. Eliminating the need for prolonged and complex sample preparation means that a potential RS-based AST could not only be faster, but also conducted on-site. Lastly, the recent rapid developments in RS instrumentation, with various hand-held or even spatially offset devices introduced to the market, means that Raman spectrometers are becoming portable and easy to use, without the need for specialized personnel or training.

Due to these attributes, RS is extensively explored in AMR research, with the focus on resistance detection. However, it should also be noted that RS is not free of challenges. Raman spectra are often of low intensity and suffer from overlapping fluorescence [29]. Spectral differences, even between various species, are too subtle to be observed with the naked eye. In the case of resistance profiling and detection, the spectral differences are even smaller due to high biomolecular similarities between resistant and susceptible strains of the same species [29]. Thus, coupling RS with advanced chemometric analysis is a necessity for achieving the desired discriminatory power.

One of the extensively explored approaches recently is a combination of RS and artificial intelligence through convolutional neural networks (CNN). In the first instance, this approach was demonstrated to be very powerful for species discrimination. For example, Lu *et al.* [30] used it for discrimination between 14 bacterial species and achieved an average accuracy of classification reaching 95.64% ± 5.46%. This work was conducted on a single-cell level, using Laser Tweezer RS.

The RS and CNN combination was recently used by Ho *et al.* [31] in an extensive study focused on discrimination between bacteria, including the aspect of drug resistance. Ho and colleagues collected an impressive database of 60,000 Raman spectra, originating from 30 isolates from Stanford Hospital. The isolates covered 94% of bacterial infections treated in Stanford Hospital in the years 2016–2017. They were selected to form a database (known as the Stanford Dataset) that is representative of the majority of bacterial infections in intensive care units worldwide [32]. The authors demonstrated the ability of RS to discriminate between the isolates with 82.2% ± 0.3% accuracy (for comparison, the standard normal variate-based discrimination achieved an accuracy of 74.9%). The work also showed the ability to discriminate between methicillin-sensitive *S. aureus* (MSSA) and MRSA (identified on the basis of 'gold standard' AST) with 89.0% ± 0.1% accuracy. The model was particularly tuned to achieve a higher sensitivity with a low false negative rate. This is due to the fact that a misdiagnosis of MRSA as MSSA is in practice more significant (and dangerous) than the opposite scenario, as it can have severe consequences for the patient's outcome. Interestingly, when the 30 different species used in this study were grouped based on the recommended empiric treatment, the RS-CNN classification models achieved 97.00% ± 0.3% accuracy. This shows the potential of RS not only to identify the resistant strains, but in fact to predict the most efficient treatment protocol.

The Sandford Dataset was further used by other research groups, with different chemometric approaches [29, 33]. Dang *et al.* [33] developed a multi-scale 1D CNN model, enabling the visualizing of the activated Raman wavenumber values and enhancing the discriminatory capabilities of this approach. Recently, Al-Shaebi *et al.* [29] demonstrated a deep learning U-Net approach that enabled them to further improve the discrimination based on the isolates, empiric treatment and resistance, and achieving accuracies of 86.3, 97.84 and 95% respectively. Figure 11.1 shows the confusion matrices for the U-Net model for isolates and empiric treatment.

The use of advanced chemometric methods can undoubtedly combat the complexity of spectral signatures and difficulties in isolating the subtle feature differences between resistant and susceptible profiles. However, they cannot influence the low-intensity RS signal, often combined with a relatively high level of noise. An improvement of the signal can be achieved using surface-enhanced Raman Spectroscopy (SERS). Numerous studies were published in the recent decade, showing the use of RS and SERS combined with deep learning to detect resistance in *S. aureus* [34–38], *A. baumanni* [35], *E. coli* [39–42] and *P. aeruginosa* [35].

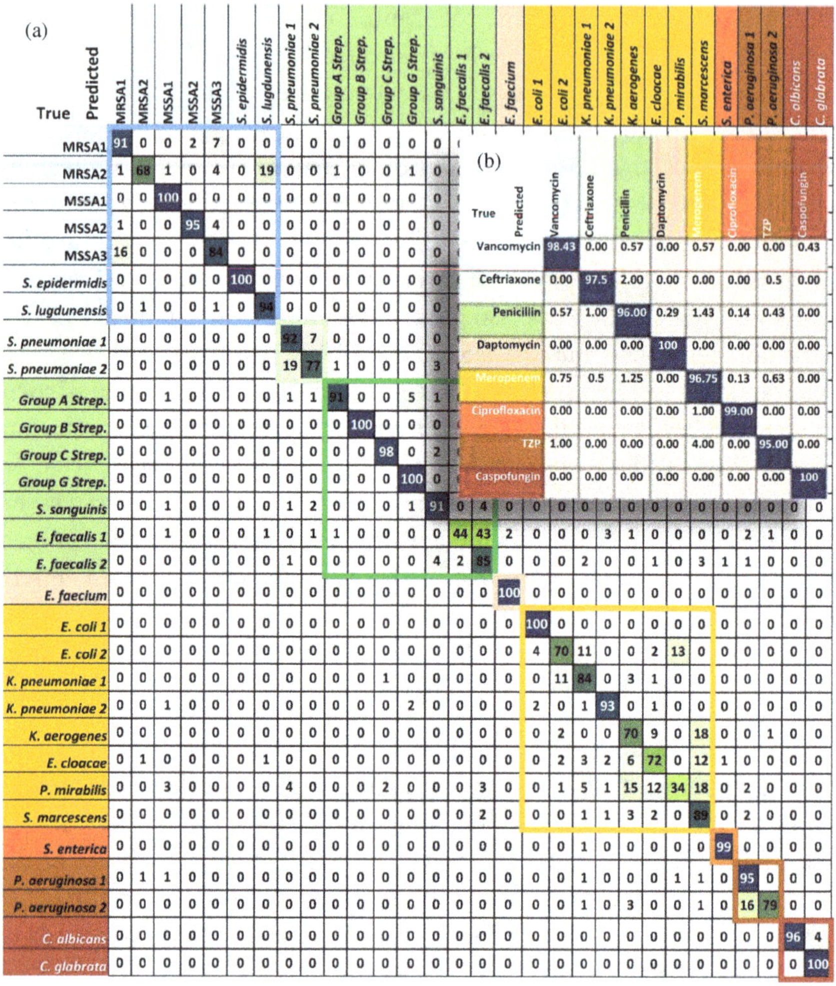

Figure 11.1. Confusion matrix for the U-Net model for (a) 30 isolates and (b) empiric treatment. The colored boxes are the treatment groups, containing one or multiple strains, treated with the antibiotics. Adapted from Ref. [29] with permission.

Ciloglu *et al.* [34] demonstrated that a combination of deep learning techniques with SERS provided additional improvement of signal, which allowed them to further improve the accuracy of discrimination between MSSA and MRSA up to 97.66%. The study nevertheless still required 24 h of culturing the bacteria and used spectra of pure isolates collected from the cultures. Chang *et al.* [39] developed a microfluidic device, combining membrane filtration and SERS-active substrate (MF-SERS), with the aim to perform an on-chip bacterial enrichment and *in situ* SERS measurements for susceptibility testing.

The authors first successfully demonstrated the utility of this device for efficient isolating and achieving a good signal-to-noise ratio, using *S. aureus* and *E. coli* samples (ATCC 25922 and HG 001). The lowest SERS detection limit for *E. coli* was established at the level of 10^3 CFU/mL, enabling significant reduction in the culture time. Furthermore, the authors demonstrated the possibility of using a microfluidic device for resistance detection by comparison of spectra of *E. coli* samples exposed to the antibiotic (kanamycin, 16 μg/mL).

Measuring the response to drug treatment is a common strategy in Raman-based AST approaches. In fact, the response to drug treatment is the underlying basis for the current 'gold star' AST method. In general, a positive response is indicative of a susceptible strain, whereas a negative response (or lack of one) characterizes a resistant strain. The current 'gold standard' AST test evaluates the drug response by monitoring the drugs' influence on growth, which requires at least 24 h (and often 48–72 h). The possibility of the use of RS to monitor drug-induced changes was previously reported by Kochan *et al.* [43]. In this study, two vibrational spectroscopy techniques, Raman and attenuated total reflection-infrared spectroscopy (ATR-IR), were coupled and analyzed in a multimodal, combined approach. The authors demonstrated that the drug-induced changes are prominent in the Raman spectra of MSSA, compared to the spectra of the same strain incubated in the same conditions but without the drug. The magnitude of these changes correlates directly to the antibiotic dose (<MIC (minimum inhibitory concentration), MIC, >MIC) and increases with incubation time. Interestingly, a 2 h incubation time with an antibiotic at MIC level is sufficient to observe drug-induced changes in MSSA. Principal Component Analysis (PCA) of MSSA strains after 2 h incubation with oxacillin showed a clear dose-dependent discrimination (Figure 11.2). For the MRSA strains on the other hand, introduction of antibiotic treatment had very little to no effect on the spectra.

In a similar manner, Li *et al.* [35] demonstrated the ability to discriminate between resistant and susceptible strains of *S. aureus*, *A. baumanni* and *P. aeruginosa* through varying spectral signatures between resistant and susceptible strains, grown on common and drug-sensitive plates. The study was conducted on 77 clinical isolates, enriched in blood culture bottles [35]. Lin *et al.* [44] presented a microfluidic device — a multiplex SERS-AST assay — that generates a continuous antibiotic concentration gradient, enabling the evaluation of the response to bacteria at different antibiotic concentrations. This system integrates all aspects of a SERS-AST test on a single chip, allowing one to perform the full procedure directly on the chip, using 20 μL of a

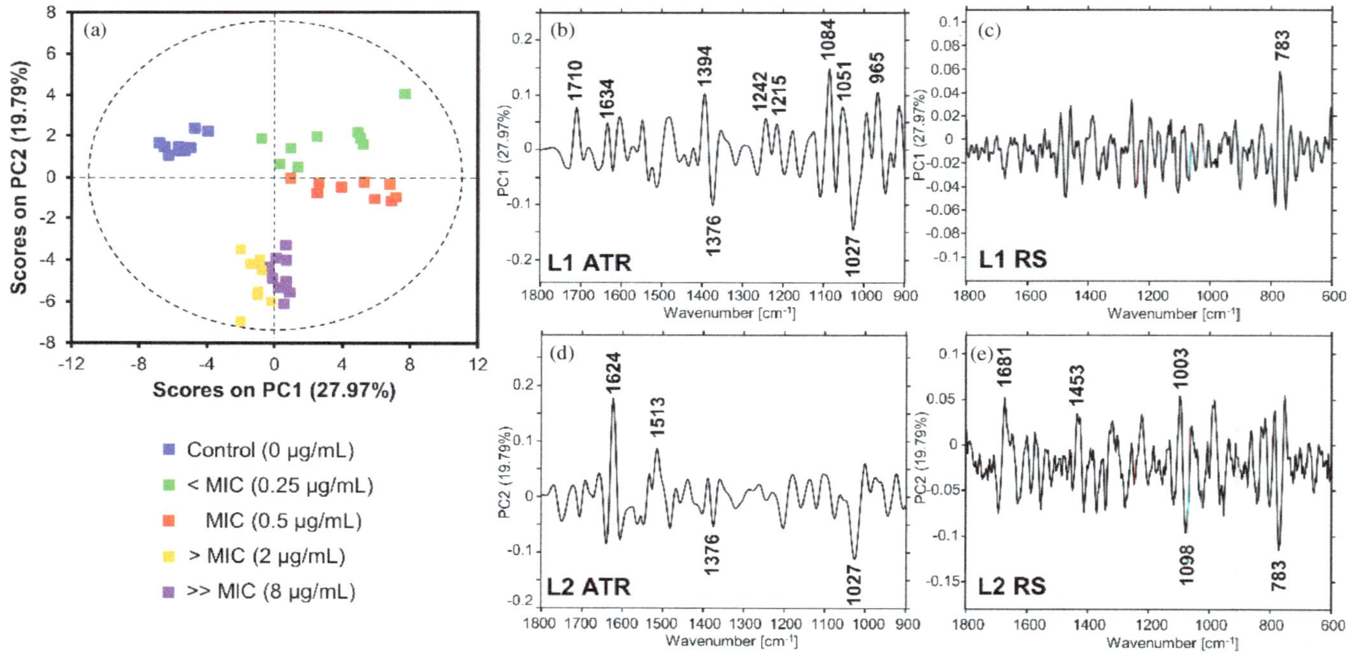

Figure 11.2. The results of PCA of multimodal dataset, containing ATR-IR and Raman data from the same samples in the spectral region of 1800–900 cm^{-1} (ATR-IR) and 1800–600 cm^{-1}: (a) scores plot and (b-e) corresponding loading plots. The dataset includes MSSA strains exposed for 2 h to oxacillin in the following concentrations: 0.25 μg/mL (<MIC), 0.5 μg/mL (MIC), 2 μg/mL (>MIC) and 8 μg/mL (>>MIC) in comparison to control (same strains incubated in the same medium without antibiotic addition). A clear dose-dependent discrimination is visible in the scores plot (a), reflecting the effects of oxacillin on MSSA strains. No such discrimination could be achieved for MRSA strains. Adapted from Ref. [43] with permission.

sample, with 5 h incubation. The performance of the system was shown using ampicillin-resistant and -susceptible strains [35]. Kirchoff *et al.* [45] demonstrated an elegant approach to determine ciprofloxacin resistance in *E. coli*, using a dielectrophoresis chip, enabling the automated collection of bacteria directly from the bacterial suspension. The authors were able to not only determine whether the investigated strains were susceptible or resistant, but in fact also establish the MIC of each strain, using an RS-based approach, in the timeframe of 2 h. The results of the RS- and SERS-based studies indicate that RS in general can capture the early response to drug treatment occurring on a molecular level and within a short period of time. Numerous examples of such studies can be found in the literature [46–54].

Recently, several studies demonstrated an interesting approach for studying bacterial activity and function *via* RS combined with stable isotope labeling [55–58]. In particular, the deuterium labeling results in the presence of a C–D peak located in the biologically silent region of the Raman spectra, which in turn can drastically increase the sensitivity of the technique [55, 56]. Stable D_2O labeling combined with RS gained particular interest in the context of AST [49, 58]. Yang *et al.* [49] developed an activity-based AST method, utilizing D_2O-RS performed at the single-cell level which is directly applicable to urine samples. This approach enabled the susceptibility vs. resistance determination within a 2.5 h timeframe from the moment of receiving patients' urine samples, drastically reducing the required time for diagnosis compared to the current gold standard. The authors showed that by using antibiotic treatment condition of 10 × Clinical Laboratory Standards Institute MIC they were able to overcome the effects of non-synchronous responses (activity vs. growth) on susceptibility testing. Furthermore, they were able to determine a simple cut-off value, based on relative C-D ratios, allowing them to determine susceptible and resistant strains. A similar approach was used by Yi *et al.* [58], who developed a fast Raman-assisted antibiotic susceptibility test (FRAST) based on single-cell RS and D_2O labeling, in combination with linear discriminant analysis. The study included six bacterial strains and response to 38 antibiotics, with 64,000 single-cell spectra in total. The FRAST approach was not only able to correctly classify between Gram-positive and Gram-negative bacteria and provide a susceptibility vs. resistance discrimination, but also enabled them to obtain MIC values, consistent with the ones obtained by broth microdilution methods (within a two-fold range) (Figure 11.3). The FRAST method was further validated using clinical samples: urine and blood. It allowed the AST readout to be obtained within 3 h for urine samples and 21 h for blood samples.

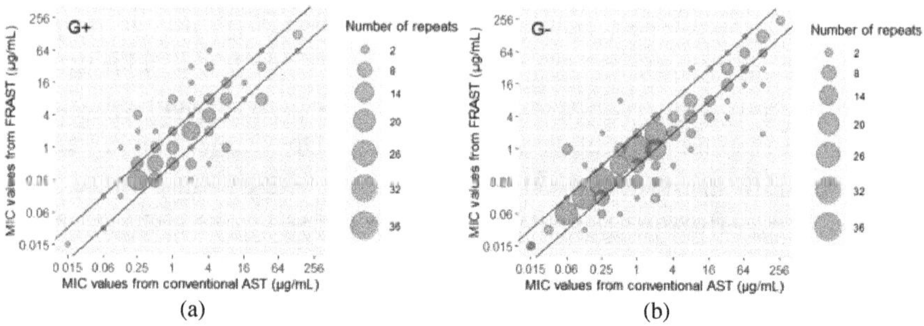

Figure 11.3. The MIC values obtained by broth microdilution method and FRAST approach for six ATCC quanlity control strains: (a) Gram-positive: ATCC 29212, ATCC 29213 and (b) Gram-negative: ATCC 27853, ATCC 35218, ATCC 25922, and ATCC 700603. The lines represent $y = 0.5x$ and $y = 2x$. The coordinates of the balloons represent the MIC values from one repetition and the sizes of the balloons correlate to the counts of their occurrence in all repetitions. Adapted from Ref. [58] with permission.

The plethora of AST-focused studies reflects the undoubtedly growing interest in RS as a potential alternative for susceptibility testing and determination of MICs or even as a potential tool for predicting the most efficient treatment protocol. For obvious reasons, research using the Raman-based AST alternative is the most explored avenue in the context of utilizing RS for AMR studies. However, aside from this, there are numerous interesting examples in the literature on the use of RS for basic research, such as following the mechanism of drug action [25, 59] or exploration of resistance development [24, 60].

Garmond *et al.* [24] demonstrated that RS can be used not only to determine resistance in bacteria, but also 'Raman resistance signatures' that reflect the transcriptomic features and can be linked to the genetic basis of acquired resistance. The authors used 11 *E. coli* strains, exhibiting resistance to various antibiotics, which differ in their mode of action. This included strains resistant to β-lactams (inhibition of cell wall synthesis), quinolones (action on DNA gyrase systems), trimethoprim (inhibition of DNA replication) and aminoglycosides and tetracyclines (inhibition of mRNA translation). To study the effects of resistance the authors used laboratory-evolved resistant strains (n = 16) and compared them to the parental strains (n = 48). Using this approach, the authors were able to determine the structural differences arising from resistance towards a specific class of antibiotics and thus the specific mode of action of the antibiotic. They identified multiple Raman bands contributing to the discrimination between resistances to different modes of action and were able to correlate them with gene expression (Figure 11.4).

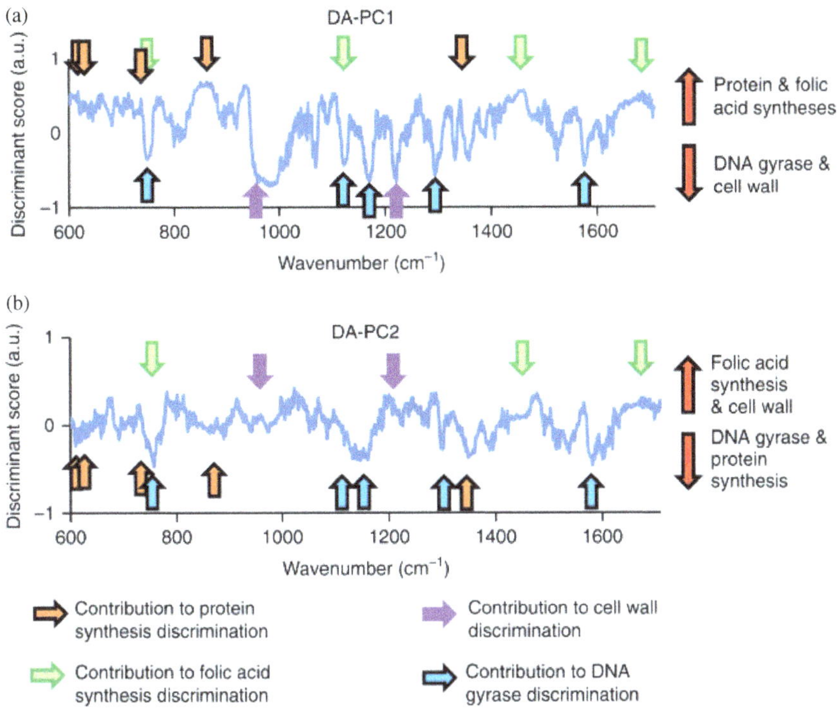

Figure 11.4. Results of PCA followed by discriminant analysis (DA-PC): vectors of the canonical discriminant analysis axes of the (a) first and (b) second dimensions. Arrows show the contribution of spectral peaks to the various modes of action of antibiotic resistance. The position of the arrows corresponds to the maximum value of some of the major spectral peaks. Adapted from Ref. [24] with permission.

This work truly showcased the ability of RS to provide an in-depth molecular characterization of bacteria, which not only allows the determination of resistance or susceptibility, but can in fact link specific changes in the chemical composition of a bacterium to the acquired resistance against a specific mode of action of antibiotics. It demonstrates that RS can significantly contribute to studies on new, emerging resistant strains and can help identify their acquired mechanism of resistance.

Further to that, Bernatova *et al.* [59] showed that RS can capture the differing biomolecular responses to various drugs. Using the example of *S. epidermidis*, the authors showed a prominent difference in biomolecular changes arising from bactericidal action of ciprofloxacin or penicillin and from bacteriostatic action of clindamycin and chloramphenicol [59]. Thus, RS can also be an invaluable tool for drug development studies, enabling determination (or confirmation) of the mode of action of the drug itself.

11.3 Fungi

Fungi are estimated to infect over a billion people annually, with severity ranging from mild skin and nail infections to life-threatening, invasive diseases [61, 62]. There are more than 150 million cases of severe fungal diseases, resulting in over 1.6 million deaths per year, similar to that reported for TB [61, 62]. Immunosuppression is one of the leading risks of invasive fungal disease and due to the increasing number of at-risk populations, the prevalence of fungal infections is also increasing globally [61, 63]. While over 600 different fungi have been reported to infect humans, the majority of deaths are due to a small number of species, including *Aspergillus*, *Candida*, *Cryptococcus* and *Pneumocystis* [64, 65]. However, in recent years the rise in at-risk populations has been accompanied by a re-emergence of fungal pathogens as well as infections by new fungal species that could pose a significant threat to human health [63]. For example, *Candida auris*, which was unknown prior to 2009, has since spread globally and is associated with therapeutic failure and high rates of mortality due to multidrug resistance [63, 66]. Due to the close evolutionary relationship between fungi and their human hosts, development of antifungal drugs that specifically target fungi without causing damage to human cellular function is uniquely challenging [64]. Therefore, there are a limited number of antifungal classes available for the treatment of invasive diseases, namely echinocandins, azoles, polyenes and flucytosine [67]. Their increased use in routine prophylaxis, empiric and directed therapy in critically ill patients and the widespread use of antifungal-based pesticides have led to an increase in the prevalence of drug resistance [68]. Given the limited number of available treatment options, the development of resistance to even one class of antifungals can pose significant therapeutic challenges.

Table 11.1 outlines four main antifungal drug classes and their molecular targets. Resistance to antifungals may be acquired through improper dosing and duration of antifungals or may intrinsically be present in the fungal species.

Resistance to azoles commonly occurs due to modifications to target enzymes whereby 14α-lanosterol demethylase is overexpressed or displays reduced binding affinity to the drug. The overexpression of efflux pumps which lower the intracellular concentration of the drug and ergosterol substitution

Table 11.1. Major classes of antifungals and their targets [69, 70–76].

Drug class	Drug	Target	Molecular target
Azoles	Miconazole Voriconazole Fluconazole Itraconazole	Fungal cell membrane synthesis	14α-lanosterol demethylase
Polyenes	Amphotericin B Nystatin Natamycin	Fungal cell membrane	Ergosterol
Echinocandins	Caspofungin Micafungin Anidulafungin	Fungal cell wall synthesis	1,3-β-D-glucan synthase
Pyrimidine analogs	Flucytosine	Fungal DNA, RNA and protein synthesis	Cytosine deaminase (encoded by the yeast gene *FCY1*)

by alteration of sterol biosynthesis have also been implicated with resistance [76]. Resistance to polyenes is reported to be relatively rare and have been attributed to mutations causing alteration of ergosterol biosynthesis [69, 77, 78]. Acquisition of resistance to echinocandins, although not as common as in azoles, is far from rare and have been correlated with prior exposure to other antifungals [76, 79]. Mutations in *FKS1*, the target protein, reduces the sensitivity to the drug. Reduced susceptibility to flucytosine have been attributed to inactivation of cytosine permeases and deaminases [80].

11.3.1 *Raman Spectroscopy for Antifungal Resistance*

There have been a handful of studies that have used RS with regard to AMR. A few studies examined the utility of RS for drug monitoring.

La Via *et al.* [81] investigated whether Resonant Raman Spectroscopy (RRS) could measure Amphotericin B (AmB) at therapeutic and sub-therapeutic concentrations in a system modeling the anterior chamber of the eye. The authors used a krypton-ion laser source (406.7 nm) for excitation and spectra were collected from a model anterior chamber. Results were used to develop a correlation curve for predicting AmB levels. The curve was then validated using a rabbit model and the predicted AmB concentrations measured by RRS were compared to those produced from high-performance liquid chromatography (HPLC). The authors reported that the predicted AmB closely approximated that measured by HPLC. Data from this study highlight the utility of RRS for non-invasive monitoring of intraocular drug concentrations and may pave the way for a novel method of drug monitoring.

Further to this, Berger *et al.* [82] developed and optimized a vertical-flow system with nitrocellulose membranes and a paper SERS sensor for therapeutic drug monitoring (Figure 11.5).

The authors used the vertical flow system to measure the level of flucytosine recovered from both water and serum using SERS. Five data points from the system were used to produce a linear regression model throughout the therapeutic range of flucytosine. The authors reported that they achieved detection of flucytosine down to 10 μg/mL in undiluted serum. This technique is reported to reduce the assay time to around 15 minutes, which is a significant improvement from current gold standard methods. The authors envision that the technique may enable near-patient drug monitoring, paving the way for rapid, safe and efficacious drug administration. They further highlight that future experiments would involve expanding the technique to filter cells from whole blood and application for detection of other drugs.

There have also been a few studies on investigating the capacity of RS for determining phenotypic variations of fungi, and their susceptibility and stress response due to antifungals.

Li *et al.* [83] investigated the utility of dynamic surface-enhanced Raman spectroscopy (D-SERS) combined with machine learning techniques to determine the phenotypic variations of fungal cells under antifungal influence. *Candida albicans* isolates were incubated with AmB, fluconazole and caspofungin at different time points and spectra were collected. A PCA model

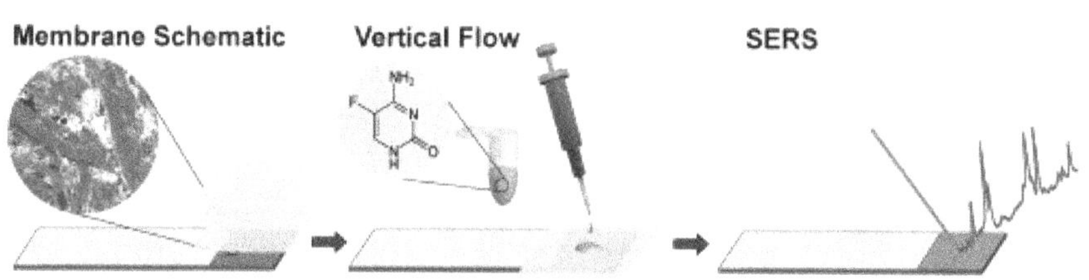

Figure 11.5. Schematic of the setup, vertical flow and detection. Flucytosine is separated from the serum via vertical flow using a microporous membrane. Scanning electron microscopy of silver nanoparticles on cellulose paper is shown. Paper SERS sensors are used to read the SERS signal. Adapted from Ref. [74] with permission.

was then established and the spectral profiles of the fungi in response to the antifungals were observed. The authors reported characteristic peaks that were specific to different antifungals and hypothesized that they correlated with the mechanisms of their action. Next, the authors also incorporated micafungin to examine the capability of the model to predict new antifungals using the model developed from the aforementioned antifungals. They reported that the PCA was able to accurately predict the mechanism of the antifungal owing to its score value clustering closer to those of caspofungin (Figure 11.6).

The authors envisioned that D-SERS combined with machine learning could open avenues for the rapid discovery and screening of new drugs in future.

Pezzotti *et al.* [84] utilized RS to monitor the susceptibility of two distinct clades of *C. auris* to antifungals AmB and flucytosine. The authors collected *in situ* Raman spectra of control and drug-exposed clades and used machine learning techniques to interpret the data. They reported major changes in cell-wall structures such as glucans and chitin, which were interpreted as results of regulatory mechanisms to compensate for the effect of the antifungals. In response to AmB, both clades formed structurally distinct biofilms while exposure to flucytosine resulted in distinct fungal morphogenesis in the two clades. The authors also reported that Raman analyses confirmed the main mechanisms of the drugs on the respective clades.

Although the literature on RS for fungal AMR is limited, these studies highlight the suitability of RS for drug monitoring, novel drug screening and

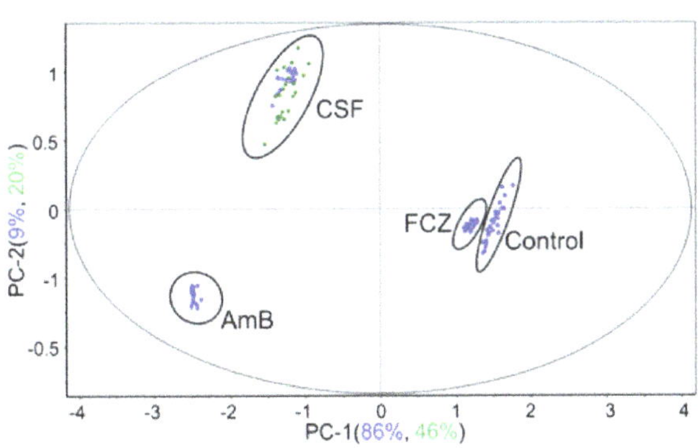

Figure 11.6. The PCA scores plot (PC1 versus PC2) of *C. albicans* treated with micafungin after 120 minutes of incubation. Blue points indicate the calibration set whilst the green scores indicate the predicted set. Adapted from Ref. [75] with permission.

for identifying novel cellular targets for fungal infection treatment. Thus, more studies in this area are required to further investigate the applications of this technique for AMR and for more species of fungi. Future studies may involve expanding to investigate more antifungals and detection from blood samples.

11.4 Raman Spectroscopy in Antimalarial Resistance Research

Malaria is considered to be one of the most catastrophic health issues in the world, caused by intraerythrocytic protozoa of the genus *Plasmodium*, with an estimated 300 million cases, resulting in 0.5–1 million deaths annually [85]. The greatest threat in regard to the alarming morbidity and mortality rates is antimalarial drug resistance, in particular resistance to *Plasmodium falciparum*, which challenges the treatment and control of malaria [86]. Several *Plasmodium* species have developed resistance to the common antimalarial drugs such as chloroquine (CQ), mefloquine, primaquine, and quinine. Hence, malaria, with a few exceptions, is now treated with combination therapy; in particular, artemisinin-based combination therapies are the current first-line agents for curative treatment [87]. However, resistance to artemisinin-based combination therapies, the standard treatments for malaria in Africa, has emerged in Southeast Asia which can be considered as a major threat in the upcoming years [86]. The conventional tools for surveillance of antimalarial drug resistance are the WHO micro test [88], isotopic approach [89, 90], ELISA [91] and flow cytometry. None of these methods have been able to fully explain the mechanism of antimalarial resistance at a molecular level and more importantly about the biochemical and phenotypic changes that accompany drug resistance. The human malaria parasite *P. falciparum* relies on the digestion of host red blood cell (RBC) hemoglobin in order to survive. This catabolic process occurs within a specialized acidic organelle known as the digestive vacuole. The by-product of this degradation is free heme, which is toxic to the parasite and is quickly sequestered into a crystalline lattice structure known as hemozoin [92]. Biochemically, the hemoglobin digestion has been shown to be downregulated in parasites that are resistant to artemisinin, whilst the antioxidant stress response mechanism of the parasite has been shown to be upregulated [93].

RS has been widely employed as a prominent vibrational spectroscopic tool in detecting and diagnosing a broad range of diseases. By providing simultaneous information on multiple biological molecules, such technologies generate a holistic biochemical "fingerprint", thus indicating the presence or absence of disease, and even the stage of disease progression [94]. Similarly, RS, especially RRS, has been widely applied to extract information related to drug-biomolecule interactions, especially antimalarial drugs with malaria biomarker, β-hematin molecule. A number of studies have reported the drug-hematin interactions in the literature using RS [95–97]. For example, mechanism of antimalarial action of cinchona alkaloids (a quinine derivative) is connected with their ability to create intermolecular H bonds which result in the protonation of quinine derivatives [98–100]. Oleksyn *et al.* reported that the cinchonine–nitrogen protonation resulted in a prominent band shift (a shift towards higher wavenumber values (up to 20 cm^{-1})) in the marker bands that appear in the wavenumber range 1350–1400 cm^{-1} [101]. Similarly, Solomonov *et al.* demonstrated that the quinoline-β-hematin binding has resulted in a modification of the surface and bulk propionic acid groups and an aggregation change in the crystal lattice [102].

In 2008, Webster *et al.* conducted an extensive research to monitor the effects of CQ treatment on cultures of *P. falciparum* trophozoites using the RRS approach [103]. Raman spectra were recorded by focusing the laser directly on the hemozoin pigment within the live infected RBCs with CQ-incubated cells and the non-treated cells (control). The intensity of characteristic hemozoin bands assigned to A_{1g} and B_{1g} modes have reduced in the CQ-treated cells. This indicates that CQ binds via π–π interactions between adjacent and orientated porphyrins thereby disrupting the hemozoin aggregate and reducing excitonic interactions between adjacent hemes. In another study by the same team, they reported that CQ acts as a molecular spacer and binds non-covalently through dispersion interactions, giving rise to π-π interactions between μ-oxo dimer units of Fe(III) PPIX as evinced by the decrease in intensity of ν_4 in the Raman spectrum as a function of increasing CQ mole ratio [104]. With the support of density functional theory calculations, RS elucidated the molecular mode of action of an antimalarial drug, halofantrine, through π-π interactions [105]. In detail, the strong bands at 1621 cm^{-1} and 1590 cm^{-1} in the UV/Raman spectrum are assigned to combined C=C stretching vibrations in the phenanthrene ring of halofantrine. These bands are considered as putative marker bands for interactions with the biological target molecules and these results were supported by the strong electron density distribution across the phenanthrene ring of halofantrine.

Khiavi *et al.* reported the first vibrational spectroscopic evidence of the formation of hydrogen bonding between a propionate group of heme and the tertiary amino nitrogen of CQ and quinacrine using ATR-IR and RS [106].

Although RS data does not provide any evidence to support the formation of a similar salt bridge in the complexes of ferriprotoporphyrin IX (FP) with quinine and mefloquine, it suggests that the interaction of these drugs with FP happens through coordination of the Fe(III) center of the porphyrin to the 9-hydroxy group of the drug.

A study by Kozicki *et al.* monitored the interactions between CQ and *P. falciparum*-infected RBCs using RS and FTIR-ATR spectroscopy [4]. A PCA analysis was carried out between CQ-treated and untreated malaria-infected RBCs and found that the cells treated with CQ showed higher levels of oxygenated hemoglobin compared to untreated controls (Figure 11.7). As can be

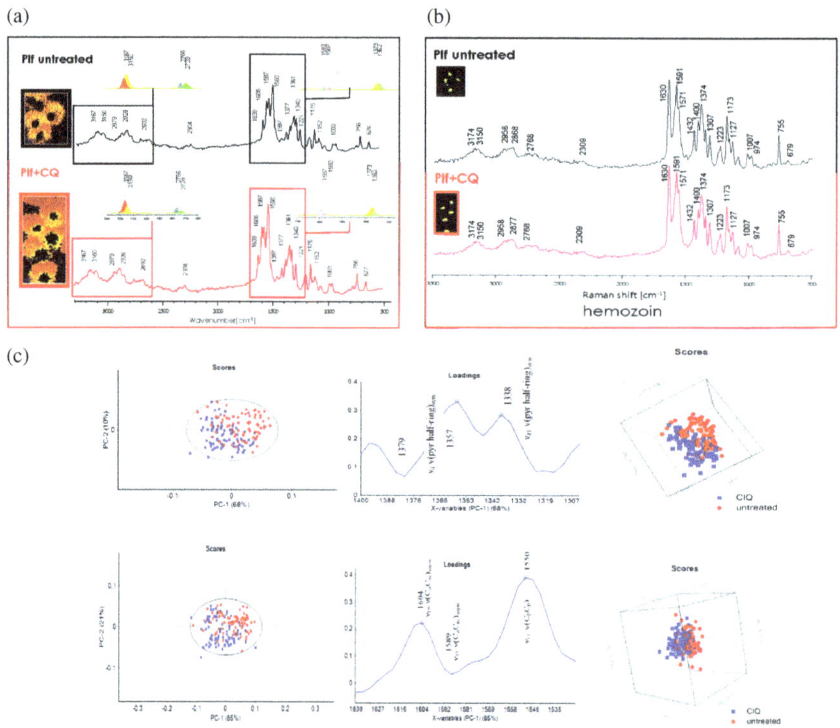

Figure 11.7. (a) Raman spectra of untreated (*P. falciparum* untreated) and CQ-treated (*P. falciparum* + CQ) from the hemoglobin region of *P. falciparum*-infected RBCs using 532 nm excitation. The insets show curve-fitted spectral ranges (left, 3300–2600 cm^{-1}; right, 1700–1300 cm^{-1}). (b) Raman spectra of untreated (*P. falciparum* untreated) and CQ-treated (*P. falciparum* + CQ) from the hemozoin region of *P. falciparum*-infected RBCs using 532 nm excitation. (c) PCA PC-1 vs. PC-2 applied to Raman spectra. The scores plot, corresponding loadings plot, PC-1 vs. PC-2 vs. PC-3, and 3D scores plot, showing a general separation between CQ-treated (blue dots) and -untreated (red dots) *P. falciparum*-infected RBCs for 1400–1300 cm^{-1} and 1640–1520 cm^{-1} regions using 532 nm excitation. Adapted from Ref. [4] with permission.

seen, a high oxygenated hemoglobin concentration in the CQ-treated infected RBCs is confirmed by the minima band at 1379 cm^{-1} which is assigned to ν_4, and this can be attributed to the presence of ferric heme, which is the oxidation state of the Fe ion when in the oxygenated state. Conversely, a higher concentration of deoxygenated hemoglobin is observed in the untreated infected RBCs as evidenced by the maxima band at 1357 cm^{-1}, which is typical for the oxidation state of a ferrous heme characteristic of deoxygenated hemoglobin.

In summary, although RS-based drug-hemozoin investigations show changes occurring within the cell metabolome, the direct detection of the drug in the cell is challenging because of its low concentration. However, RS has been an excellent tool in elucidating the drug-binding mechanisms for screening which will assist in structure-based design of new, effective antimalarials.

11.5 Conclusion

Raman spectroscopy offers tremendous potential as a new rapid AMR screening technique for bacteria, fungi and parasites. The underlying premise is that Raman spectroscopy can detect chemical changes associated with resistance, which precedes or accompanies any change in morphology or microbe death. For this reason, it has a number of advantages to offer over traditional diagnostic tools, which can take up to 48 hours to determine the species and drug susceptibilities from clinical specimens. Other advantages include: the technique requires little or minimal sample preparation, water does not interfere with the spectrum unlike infrared spectroscopy, a microscope can be used to target individual colonies, and it can be adapted to use in 96-well plates. The future will see the adaption of much cheaper Raman portable spectrometers with fiber optics that negate the need of a microscope facility. Recently, Raman and mid-infrared spectroscopy has been combined in one instrument known as optical photothermal infrared spectroscopy, which enables the simultaneous collection of an infrared and Raman spectrum at sub-micron spatial resolution. Unlike other infrared techniques which are based on detecting an evanescent beam using near-field optics, this system utilizes a pump-probe setup incorporating a tunable mid-IR quantum cascade laser which excites the sample by pumping photons into it, while a 532 nm continuous wave laser probes the sample. This technology has already been applied to study isotopically labeled bacteria [107, 108] and can obtain Raman and IR spectra at less than 500 nm spatial resolution. Combining infrared and Raman data into one matrix should improve the both the sensitivity and specificity of the technique, opening new avenues to explore AMR.

References

1. https://www.who.int/news-room/fact-sheets/detail/antimicrobial-resistance.
2. Jacobs, S. E., Jacobs, J. L., Dennis, E. K., Taimur, S., Rana, M., Patel, D., Gitman, M., Patel, G., Schaefer, S., Iyer, K., Moon, J., Adams, V., Lerner, P., Walsh, T. J., Zhu, Y., Anower, M. R., Vaidya, M. M., Chaturvedi, S. and Chaturvedi, V. (2022) Candida auris pan-drug-resistant to four classes of antifungal agents. Antimicrob. Agents Chemother. **66**, e0005322.
3. Karakonstantis, S., Kritsotakis, E. I. and Gikas, A. (2020) Pandrug-resistant Gram-negative bacteria: a systematic review of current epidemiology, prognosis and treatment options. J. Antimicrob. Chemother. **75**, 271–282.
4. Kozicki, M., Creek, D. J., Sexton, A., Morahan, B. J., Wesełucha-Birczyńska, A. and Wood, B. R. (2015) An attenuated total reflection (ATR) and Raman spectroscopic investigation into the effects of chloroquine on Plasmodium falciparum-infected red blood cells. Analyst **140**, 2236–2246.
5. O'Neill, J. (2016) Tackling Drug-Resistant Infections Globally: Final Report and Recommendations. The Review on Antimicrobial Resistance. https://amr-review.org/sites/default/files/160518_Final%20paper_with%20cover.pdf.
6. Dadgostar, P. (2019) Antimicrobial resistance: implications and costs. Infect. Drug Resist. **12**, 3903–3910.
7. Murray, C. J. L., *et al.* (2022) Global burden of bacterial antimicrobial resistance in 2019: a systematic analysis. Lancet **399**, 629–655.
8. Sherwin, R., Winters, M. E., Vilke, G. M. and Wardi, G. (2017) Does early and appropriate antibiotic administration improve mortality in emergency department patients with severe sepsis or septic shock? J. Emerg. Med. **53**, 588–595.
9. Bassetti, M., Carnelutti, A. and Peghin, M. (2017) Patient specific risk stratification for antimicrobial resistance and possible treatment strategies in gram-negative bacterial infections. Expert Rev. Anti. Infect. Ther. **15**, 55–65.
10. Morrell, M., Fraser, V. J. and Kollef, M. H. (2005) Delaying the empiric treatment of candida bloodstream infection until positive blood culture results are obtained: a potential risk factor for hospital mortality. Antimicrob. Agents Chemother. **49**, 3640–3645.
11. Maurer, F. P., Christner, M., Hentschke, M. and Rohde, H. (2017) Advances in rapid identification and susceptibility testing of bacteria in the clinical microbiology laboratory: implications for patient care and antimicrobial stewardship programs. Infect. Dis. Rep. **9**, 6839.

12. Wiederhold, N. P. (2021) Antifungal susceptibility testing: a primer for clinicians. Open Forum Infect. Dis. **8**, ofab444.
13. Prestinaci, F., Pezzotti, P. and Pantosti, A. (2015) Antimicrobial resistance: a global multifaceted phenomenon. Pathog. Glob. Health. **109**, 309–318.
14. Sydnor, E. R. and Perl, T. M. (2011) Hospital epidemiology and infection control in acute-care settings. Clin. Microbiol. Rev. **24**, 141–173.
15. Rice, L. B. (2008) Federal funding for the study of antimicrobial resistance in nosocomial pathogens: no ESKAPE. J. Infect. Dis. **197**, 1079–1081.
16. De Oliveira, D. M. P., Forde, B. M., Kidd, T. J., Harris, P. N. A., Schembri, M. A., Beatson, S. A., Paterson, D. L. and Walker, M. J. (2020) Antimicrobial resistance in ESKAPE pathogens. Clin. Microbiol. Rev. **33**, e00181–19.
17. Tacconelli, E., Carrara, E., Savoldi, A., Harbarth, S., Mendelson, M., Monnet, D. L., Pulcini, C., Kahlmeter, G., Kluytmans, J., Carmeli, Y., Ouellette, M., Outterson, K., Patel, J., Cavaleri, M., Cox, E. M., Houchens, C. R., Grayson, M. L., Hansen, P., Singh, N., Theuretzbacher, U., Magrini, N. and Group, W. H. O. P. P. L. W. (2018) Discovery, research, and development of new antibiotics: the WHO priority list of antibiotic-resistant bacteria and tuberculosis. Lancet Infect. Dis. **18**, 318–327.
18. Denissen, J., Reyneke, B., Waso-Reyneke, M., Havenga, B., Barnard, T., Khan, S. and Khan, W. (2022) Prevalence of ESKAPE pathogens in the environment: Antibiotic resistance status, community-acquired infection and risk to human health. Int. J. Hyg. Environ. Health. **244**, 114006.
19. Paulson, T. (2013) Epidemiology: A mortal foe. Nature **502**, S2–3.
20. https://www.who.int/publications/i/item/9789240061729.
21. Santajit, S. and Indrawattana, N. (2016) Mechanisms of antimicrobial resistance in ESKAPE pathogens. Biomed. Res. Int. **2016**, 2475067.
22. Munita, J. M. and Arias, C. A. (2016) Mechanisms of antibiotic resistance. Microbiol. Spectr. **4.**
23. Ramirez, M. S. and Tolmasky, M. E. (2010) Aminoglycoside modifying enzymes. Drug Resist. Updat. **13**, 151–171.
24. Germond, A., Ichimura, T., Horinouchi, T., Fujita, H., Furusawa, C. and Watanabe, T. M. (2018) Raman spectral signature reflects transcriptomic features of antibiotic resistance in Escherichia coli. Commun. Biol. **1**, 85.
25. Ma, L., Chen, L., Chou, K. C. and Lu, X. (2021) Campylobacter jejuni Antimicrobial resistance profiles and mechanisms determined using a Raman spectroscopy-based metabolomic approach. Appl. Environ. Microbiol. **87**, e0038821.
26. Bernatova, S., Samek, O., Pilat, Z., Sery, M., Jezek, J., Jakl, P., Siler, M., Krzyzanek, V., Zemanek, P., Hola, V., Dvorackova, M. and Ruzicka, F. (2013) Following the mechanisms of bacteriostatic versus bactericidal action using Raman spectroscopy. Molecules **18**, 13188–13199.

27. Pistiki, A., Salbreiter, M., Sultan, S., Rösch, P. and Popp, J. (2022) Application of Raman spectroscopy in the hospital environment. Transl. Biophotonics **4**, e202200011.
28. Choo-Smith, L. P., Edwards, H. G., Endtz, H. P., Kros, J. M., Heule, F., Barr, H., Robinson, J. S., Jr., Bruining, H. A. and Puppels, G. J. (2002) Medical applications of Raman spectroscopy: from proof of principle to clinical implementation. Biopolymers **67**, 1–9.
29. Al-Shaebi, Z., Uysal Ciloglu, F., Nasser, M. and Aydin, O. (2022) Highly accurate identification of bacteria's antibiotic resistance based on Raman spectroscopy and U-Net deep learning algorithms. ACS Omega **7**, 29443–29451.
30. Lu, W., Chen, X., Wang, L., Li, H. and Fu, Y. V. (2020) Combination of an artificial intelligence approach and laser tweezers Raman spectroscopy for microbial identification. Anal. Chem. **92**, 6288–6296.
31. Ho, C. S., Jean, N., Hogan, C. A., Blackmon, L., Jeffrey, S. S., Holodniy, M., Banaei, N., Saleh, A. A. E., Ermon, S. and Dionne, J. (2019) Rapid identification of pathogenic bacteria using Raman spectroscopy and deep learning. Nat. Commun. **10**, 4927.
32. Vincent, J. L., Rello, J., Marshall, J., Silva, E., Anzueto, A., Martin, C. D., Moreno, R., Lipman, J., Gomersall, C., Sakr, Y. and Reinhart, K. (2009) International study of the prevalence and outcomes of infection in intensive care units. JAMA **302**, 2323–2329.
33. Deng, L., Zhong, Y., Wang, M., Zheng, X. and Zhang, J. (2022) Scale-adaptive deep model for bacterial Raman spectra identification. IEEE J. Biomed. Health Inform. **26**, 369–378.
34. Ciloglu, F. U., Caliskan, A., Saridag, A. M., Kilic, I. H., Tokmakci, M., Kahraman, M. and Aydin, O. (2021) Drug-resistant Staphylococcus aureus bacteria detection by combining surface-enhanced Raman spectroscopy (SERS) and deep learning techniques. Sci. Rep. **11**, 18444.
35. Li, J., Wang, C., Shi, L., Shao, L., Fu, P., Wang, K., Xiao, R., Wang, S. and Gu, B. (2019) Rapid identification and antibiotic susceptibility test of pathogens in blood based on magnetic separation and surface-enhanced Raman scattering. Microchim. Acta **186**, 475.
36. Uysal Ciloglu, F., Saridag, A. M., Kilic, I. H., Tokmakci, M., Kahraman, M. and Aydin, O. (2020) Identification of methicillin-resistant Staphylococcus aureus bacteria using surface-enhanced Raman spectroscopy and machine learning techniques. Analyst **145**, 7559–7570.
37. Lorenz, B., Ali, N., Bocklitz, T., Rösch, P. and Popp, J. (2020) Discrimination between pathogenic and non-pathogenic E. coli strains by means of Raman microspectroscopy. Anal. Bioanal. Chem. **412**, 8241–8247.
38. Ho, C.-S., Jean, N., Hogan, C. A., Blackmon, L., Jeffrey, S. S., Holodniy, M., Banaei, N., Saleh, A. A. E., Ermon, S. and Dionne, J. (2019) Rapid identification

of pathogenic bacteria using Raman spectroscopy and deep learning. Nat. Commun. **10**, 4927.

39. Chang, K. W., Cheng, H. W., Shiue, J., Wang, J. K., Wang, Y. L. and Huang, N. T. (2019) Antibiotic susceptibility test with surface-enhanced Raman scattering in a microfluidic system. Anal. Chem. **91**, 10988–10995.
40. Nakar, A., Pistiki, A., Ryabchykov, O., Bocklitz, T., Rösch, P. and Popp, J. (2022) Label-free differentiation of clinical E. coli and Klebsiella isolates with Raman spectroscopy. J. Biophotonics **15**, e202200005.
41. Schröder, U.-C., Kirchhoff, J., Hübner, U., Mayer, G., Glaser, U., Henkel, T., Pfister, W., Fritzsche, W., Popp, J. and Neugebauer, U. (2017) On-chip spectroscopic assessment of microbial susceptibility to antibiotics within 3.5 hours. J. Biophotonics **10**, 1547–1557.
42. Zahn, J., Germond, A., Lundgren, A. Y. and Cicerone, M. T. (2022) Discriminating cell line specific features of antibiotic-resistant strains of Escherichia coli from Raman spectra via machine learning analysis. J. Biophotonics **15**, e202100274.
43. Kochan, K., Nethercott, C., Taghavimoghaddam, J., Richardson, Z., Lai, E., Crawford, S. A., Peleg, A. Y., Wood, B. R. and Heraud, P. (2020) Rapid approach for detection of antibiotic resistance in bacteria using vibrational spectroscopy. Anal. Chem. **92**, 8235–8243.
44. Lin, S.-J., Chao, P.-H., Cheng, H.-W., Wang, J.-K., Wang, Y.-L., Han, Y.-Y. and Huang, N.-T. (2022) An antibiotic concentration gradient microfluidic device integrating surface-enhanced Raman spectroscopy for multiplex antimicrobial susceptibility testing. Lab on a Chip **22**, 1805–1814.
45. Kirchhoff, J., Glaser, U., Bohnert, J. A., Pletz, M. W., Popp, J. and Neugebauer, U. (2018) Simple ciprofloxacin resistance test and determination of minimal inhibitory concentration within 2 h using Raman spectroscopy. Anal. Chem. **90**, 1811–1818.
46. Tao, Y., Wang, Y., Huang, S., Zhu, P., Huang, W. E., Ling, J. and Xu, J. (2017) Metabolic-activity-based assessment of antimicrobial effects by D2O-labeled single-cell Raman microspectroscopy. Anal. Chem. **89**, 4108–4115.
47. Moritz, T. J., Polage, C. R., Taylor, D. S., Krol, D. M., Lane, S. M. and Chan, J. W. (2010) Evaluation of Escherichia coli cell response to antibiotic treatment by use of Raman spectroscopy with laser tweezers. J. Clin. Microbiol. **48**, 4287–4290.
48. Teng, L., Wang, X., Wang, X., Gou, H., Ren, L., Wang, T., Wang, Y., Ji, Y., Huang, W. E. and Xu, J. (2016) Label-free, rapid and quantitative phenotyping of stress response in E. coli via ramanome. Sci. Rep. **6**, 34359.
49. Yang, K., Li, H.-Z., Zhu, X., Su, J.-Q., Ren, B., Zhu, Y.-G. and Cui, L. (2019) Rapid antibiotic susceptibility testing of pathogenic bacteria using heavy-water-labeled single-cell Raman spectroscopy in clinical samples. Anal. Chem. **91**, 6296–6303.
50. Han, Y.-Y., Lin, Y.-C., Cheng, W.-C., Lin, Y.-T., Teng, L.-J., Wang, J.-K. and Wang, Y.-L. (2020) Rapid antibiotic susceptibility testing of bacteria from patients'

blood via assaying bacterial metabolic response with surface-enhanced Raman spectroscopy. Sci. Rep. **10**, 12538.

51. Novelli-Rousseau, A., Espagnon, I., Filiputti, D., Gal, O., Douet, A., Mallard, F. and Josso, Q. (2018) Culture-free antibiotic-susceptibility determination from single-bacterium Raman spectra. Sci. Rep. **8**, 3957.
52. Fu, S., Wang, X., Wang, T., Li, Z., Han, D., Yu, C., Yang, C., Qu, H., Chi, H., Wang, Y., Li, S., Tian, B., Li, W. and Xia, Z. (2020) A sensitive and rapid bacterial antibiotic susceptibility test method by surface enhanced Raman spectroscopy. Braz. J. Microbiol. **51**, 875–881.
53. Thrift, W. J., Ronaghi, S., Samad, M., Wei, H., Nguyen, D. G., Cabuslay, A. S., Groome, C. E., Santiago, P. J., Baldi, P., Hochbaum, A. I. and Ragan, R. (2020) Deep learning analysis of vibrational spectra of bacterial lysate for rapid antimicrobial susceptibility testing. ACS Nano **14**, 15336–15348.
54. Thomsen, B. L., Christensen, J. B., Rodenko, O., Usenov, I., Grønnemose, R. B., Andersen, T. E. and Lassen, M. (2022) Accurate and fast identification of minimally prepared bacteria phenotypes using Raman spectroscopy assisted by machine learning. Sci. Rep. **12**, 16436.
55. Azemtsop Matanfack, G., Pistiki, A., Rösch, P. and Popp, J. (2021) Raman stable isotope probing of bacteria in visible and deep UV-ranges. Life **11**, 1003.
56. Wang, Y., Xu, J., Kong, L., Liu, T., Yi, L., Wang, H., Huang, W. E. and Zheng, C. (2020) Raman-deuterium isotope probing to study metabolic activities of single bacterial cells in human intestinal microbiota. Microb. Biotechnol. **13**, 572–583.
57. Azemtsop Matanfack, G., Taubert, M., Guo, S., Bocklitz, T., Küsel, K., Rösch, P. and Popp, J. (2021) Monitoring deuterium uptake in single bacterial cells via two-dimensional Raman correlation spectroscopy. Anal. Chem. **93**, 7714–7723.
58. Yi, X., Song, Y., Xu, X., Peng, D., Wang, J., Qie, X., Lin, K., Yu, M., Ge, M., Wang, Y., Zhang, D., Yang, Q., Wang, M. and Huang, W. E. (2021) Development of a fast Raman-assisted antibiotic susceptibility test (FRAST) for the antibiotic resistance analysis of clinical urine and blood samples. Anal. Chem. **93**, 5098–5106.
59. Bernatová, S., Samek, O., Pilát, Z., Serý, M., Ježek, J., Jákl, P., Siler, M., Krzyžánek, V., Zemánek, P., Holá, V., Dvořáčková, M. and Růžička, F. (2013) Following the mechanisms of bacteriostatic versus bactericidal action using Raman spectroscopy. Molecules **18**, 13188–13199.
60. Zhang, P., Fu, Y., Zhao, H., Liu, X., Wu, X., Lin, T., Wang, H., Song, L., Fang, Y., Lu, W., Liu, M., Liu, W. and Zheng, D. (2022) Dynamic insights into increasing antibiotic resistance in Staphylococcus aureus by label-free SERS using a portable Raman spectrometer. Spectrochim. Acta A **273**, 121070.
61. Bongomin, F., Gago, S., Oladele, R. O. and Denning, D. W. (2017) Global and multi-national prevalence of fungal diseases-estimate precision. J. Fungi (Basel). **3**, 57.

62. Kainz, K., Bauer, M. A., Madeo, F. and Carmona-Gutierrez, D. (2020) Fungal infections in humans: the silent crisis. Microb. Cell. **7**, 143–145.
63. Lockhart, S. R. and Guarner, J. (2019) Emerging and reemerging fungal infections. Semin. Diagn. Pathol. **36**, 177–181.
64. Geddes-McAlister, J. and Shapiro, R. S. (2019) New pathogens, new tricks: emerging, drug-resistant fungal pathogens and future prospects for antifungal therapeutics. Annu. N.Y. Acad. Sci. **1435**, 57–78.
65. Brown, G. D., Denning, D. W. and Levitz, S. M. (2012) Tackling human fungal infections. Science **336**, 647.
66. Satoh, K., Makimura, K., Hasumi, Y., Nishiyama, Y., Uchida, K. and Yamaguchi, H. (2009) Candida auris sp. nov., a novel ascomycetous yeast isolated from the external ear canal of an inpatient in a Japanese hospital. Microbiol. Immunol. **53**, 41–44.
67. Perlin, D. S., Rautemaa-Richardson, R. and Alastruey-Izquierdo, A. (2017) The global problem of antifungal resistance: prevalence, mechanisms, and management. Lancet Infect. Dis. **17**, e383–e392.
68. Schwartz, I. S. and Patterson, T. F. (2018) The emerging threat of antifungal resistance in transplant infectious diseases. Curr. Infect. Dis. Rep. **20**, 2.
69. Silva, S., Negri, M., Henriques, M., Oliveira, R., Williams, D. W. and Azeredo, J. (2012) Candida glabrata, Candida parapsilosis and Candida tropicalis: biology, epidemiology, pathogenicity and antifungal resistance. FEMS Microbiol. Rev. **36**, 288–305.
70. Campoy, S. and Adrio, J. L. (2017) Antifungals. Biochem. Pharmacol. **133**, 86–96.
71. Sheehan, D. J., Hitchcock, C. A. and Sibley, C. M. (1999) Current and emerging azole antifungal agents. Clin. Microbiol. Rev. **12**, 40–79.
72. Carrillo-Munoz, A., Giusiano, G., Ezkurra, P. and Quindós, G. (2006) Antifungal agents: mode of action in yeast cells. Rev. Esp. Quimioter. **19**, 130–139.
73. Prasad, R. and Kapoor, K. (2005) Multidrug resistance in yeast Candida. Int. Rev. Cyt. **242**, 215–248.
74. Chandra, J., Mohammad, S. and Ghannoum, M. A. (2009) Flucytosine: Site of Action, Mechanism of Resistance and Use in Combination Therapy. In *Antimicrobial Drug Resistance* (Mayers, D. L., Ed.), pp. 313–326, Springer.
75. Charlier, C., El Sissy, C., Bachelier-Bassi, S., Scemla, A., Quesne, G., Sitterlé, E., Legendre, C., Lortholary, O. and Bougnoux, M.-E. (2016) Acquired flucytosine resistance during combination therapy with caspofungin and flucytosine for Candida glabrata cystitis. Antimicrob. Agents Chemother. **60**, 662–665.
76. Ksiezopolska, E. and Gabaldón, T. (2018) Evolutionary emergence of drug resistance in Candida opportunistic pathogens. Genes. **9**, 461.
77. Vandeputte, P., Tronchin, G., Bergès, T., Hennequin, C., Chabasse, D. and Bouchara, J.-P. (2007) Reduced susceptibility to polyenes associated with a missense mutation in the ERG6 gene in a clinical isolate of Candida glabrata with pseudohyphal growth. Antimicrob. Agents Chemother. **51**, 982–990.

78. Sanglard, D. and Odds, F. C. (2002) Resistance of Candida species to antifungal agents: molecular mechanisms and clinical consequences. Lancet Infect. Dis. **2**, 73–85.
79. Vallabhaneni, S., Cleveland, A. A., Farley, M. M., Harrison, L. H., Schaffner, W., Beldavs, Z. G., Derado, G., Pham, C. D., Lockhart, S. R. and Smith, R. M. (2015) Epidemiology and risk factors for echinocandin nonsusceptible Candida glabrata bloodstream infections: data from a large multisite population-based candidemia surveillance program, 2008–2014. Open Forum Infect. Dis. **2**, ofv163.
80. Bassetti, M., Trecarichi, E. M., Righi, E., Sanguinetti, M., Bisio, F., Posteraro, B., Soro, O., Cauda, R., Viscoli, C. and Tumbarello, M. (2007) Incidence, risk factors, and predictors of outcome of candidemia. Survey in 2 Italian university hospitals. Diagn. Microbiol. Infect. Dis. **58**, 325–331.
81. La Via, W. V., Lambert, J. L., Pelletier, M. J., Michael Morookian, J., Sirk, S. J., Mickiene, D., Walsh, T. J. and Borchert, M. S. (2006) Measurement of Amphotericin B concentration by Resonant Raman Spectroscopy–a novel technique that may be useful for non-invasive monitoring. Med. Mycol. **44**, 169–174.
82. Berger, A. G., Restaino, S. M. and White, I. M. (2017) Vertical-flow paper SERS system for therapeutic drug monitoring of flucytosine in serum. Anal. Chim. Acta **949**, 59–66.
83. Li, H., Cao, Y. and Lu, F. (2021) Differentiation of different antifungals with various mechanisms using dynamic surface-enhanced Raman spectroscopy combined with machine learning. J. Innov. Opt. Health Sci. **14**, 2141002.
84. Pezzotti, G., Kobara, M., Nakaya, T., Imamura, H., Asai, T., Miyamoto, N., Adachi, T., Yamamoto, T., Kanamura, N. and Ohgitani, E. (2022) Raman study of pathogenic Candida auris: Imaging metabolic machineries in reaction to antifungal drugs. Front. Microbiol. **13**, 896359.
85. Veettil, T. C. P., Kochan, K., Karen, J. E., De Bank, P., Heraud, P. and Wood, B. R. (2022) Disposable coverslip for rapid throughput screening of malaria using attenuated total reflection spectroscopy. Appl. Spectrosc. **76**, 451–461.
86. Conrad, M. D. and Rosenthal, P. J. (2019) Antimalarial drug resistance in Africa: the calm before the storm? Lancet Infect. Dis. **19**, e338–e351.
87. Ippolito, M. M., Moser, K. A., Kabuya, J.-B. B., Cunningham, C. and Juliano, J. J. (2021) Antimalarial drug resistance and implications for the WHO global technical strategy. Curr. Epidemiol. Rep. **8**, 46–62.
88. Bloland, P. B. and World Health Organization (2001) *Drug Resistance in Malaria.* World Health Organization.
89. Chulay, J. D., Haynes, J. D. and Diggs, C. L. (1983) Plasmodium falciparum: assessment of in vitro growth by [3H] hypoxanthine incorporation. Exp. Parasitol. **55**, 138–146.

90. Desjardins, R. E., Canfield, C., Haynes, J. and Chulay, J. (1979) Quantitative assessment of antimalarial activity in vitro by a semiautomated microdilution technique. Antimicrob. Agents Chemother. **16**, 710–718.
91. Chaorattanakawee, S., Tyner, S. D., Lon, C., Yingyuen, K., Ruttvisutinunt, W., Sundrakes, S., Sai-gnam, P., Johnson, J. D., Walsh, D. S. and Saunders, D. L. (2013) Direct comparison of the histidine-rich protein-2 enzyme-linked immunosorbent assay (HRP-2 ELISA) and malaria SYBR green I fluorescence (MSF) drug sensitivity tests in Plasmodium falciparum reference clones and fresh ex vivo field isolates from Cambodia. Malar. J. **12**, 1–11.
92. Meshnick, S., Yang, Y., Lima, V., Kuypers, F., Kamchonwongpaisan, S. and Yuthavong, Y. (1993) Iron-dependent free radical generation from the antimalarial agent artemisinin (qinghaosu). Antimicrob. Agents Chemother. **37**, 1108–1114.
93. Siddiqui, G., Srivastava, A., Russell, A. S. and Creek, D. J. (2017) Multi-omics based identification of specific biochemical changes associated with PfKelch13-mutant artemisinin-resistant Plasmodium falciparum. J. Infect. Dis. **215**, 1435–1444.
94. Paraskevaidi, M., Matthew, B. J., Holly, B. J., Hugh, B. J., Thulya, C. P., Loren, C., StJohn, C., Peter, G., Callum, G. and Sergei, K. G. (2021) Clinical applications of infrared and Raman spectroscopy in the fields of cancer and infectious diseases. Appl. Spectrosc. Rev. **56**, 804–868.
95. Frosch, T., Küstner, B., Schlücker, S., Szeghalmi, A., Schmitt, M., Kiefer, W. and Popp, J. (2004) In vitro polarization-resolved resonance Raman studies of the interaction of hematin with the antimalarial drug chloroquine. J. Raman Spectrosc. **35**, 819–821.
96. Frosch, T., Schmitt, M., Schenzel, K., Faber, J. H., Bringmann, G., Kiefer, W. and Popp, J. (2006) In vivo localization and identification of the antiplasmodial alkaloid dioncophylline A in the tropical liana Triphyophyllum peltatum by a combination of fluorescence, near infrared Fourier transform Raman microscopy, and density functional theory calculations. Biopolymers **82**, 295–300.
97. Cîntă-Pînzaru, S., Peica, N., Küstner, B., Schlücker, S., Schmitt, M., Frosch, T., Faber, J., Bringmann, G. and Popp, J. (2006) FT-Raman and NIR-SERS characterization of the antimalarial drugs chloroquine and mefloquine and their interaction with hematin. J. Raman Spectrosc. **37**, 326–334.
98. Wesełucha-Birczyńska, A. and Nakamoto, K. (1993) UV resonance Raman studies on cinchonine-polynucleotide interactions. J. Mol. Struct. **294**, 127–129.
99. Karle, J. M. and Karle, I. L. (2002) Crystal structure of (−)-mefloquine hydrochloride reveals consistency of configuration with biological activity. Antimicrob. Agents Chemother. **46**, 1529–1534.

100. Wood, B. R. and McNaughton, D. (2006) Resonance Raman spectroscopy in malaria research. Expert Rev. Proteomics **3**, 525–544.
101. Oleksyn, B., Sliwinski, J., Kowalik, J. and Serda, P. (1991) *Organic Crystal Chemistry.* Oxford University Press.
102. Solomonov, I., Osipova, M., Feldman, Y., Baehtz, C., Kjaer, K., Robinson, I. K., Webster, G. T., McNaughton, D., Wood, B. R. and Weissbuch, I. (2007) Crystal nucleation, growth, and morphology of the synthetic malaria pigment β-hematin and the effect thereon by quinoline additives: the malaria pigment as a target of various antimalarial drugs. J. Am. Chem. Soc. **129**, 2615–2627.
103. Webster, G. T., Tilley, L., Deed, S., McNaughton, D. and Wood, B. R. (2008) Resonance Raman spectroscopy can detect structural changes in haemozoin (malaria pigment) following incubation with chloroquine in infected erythrocytes. FEBS Lett. **582**, 1087–1092.
104. Webster, G. T., McNaughton, D. and Wood, B. R. (2009) Aggregated enhanced Raman scattering in Fe (III) PPIX solutions: the effects of concentration and chloroquine on excitonic interactions. J. Phys. Chem. B **113**, 6910–6916.
105. Frosch, T. and Popp, J. (2010) Structural analysis of the antimalarial drug halofantrine by means of Raman spectroscopy and density functional theory calculations. J. Biomed. Opt. **15**, 041516.
106. Asghari-Khiavi, M., Vongsvivut, J., Perepichka, I., Mechler, A., Wood, B. R., McNaughton, D. and Bohle, D. S. (2011) Interaction of quinoline antimalarial drugs with ferriprotoporphyrin IX, a solid state spectroscopy study. J. Inorg. Biochem. **105**, 1662–1669.
107. Lima, C., Muhamadali, H. and Goodacre, R. (2022) Simultaneous Raman and infrared spectroscopy of stable isotope labelled Escherichia coli. Sensors **22**, 3928.
108. Lima, C., Muhamadali, H., Xu, Y., Kansiz, M. and Goodacre, R. (2021) Imaging isotopically labeled bacteria at the single-cell level using high-resolution optical infrared photothermal spectroscopy. Anal. Chem. **93**, 3082–3088.

https://doi.org/10.1142/9789811264610_0012

Chapter 12

Raman Spectral Cytopathology for Cancer Diagnostic Applications

Fiona M. Lyng,[1,2,3] Damien Traynor,[1,2] Isha Behl,[1,2]
Declan O'Dea,[1,4] Hugh J. Byrne[5,*]

[1]*Centre for Radiation and Environmental Science, FOCAS Research Institute, Technological University Dublin, City Campus, Dublin, Ireland*
[2]*School of Physics & Clinical & Optometric Sciences, Technological University Dublin, City Campus, Dublin, Ireland*
[3]*CERVIVA Research Consortium, Dublin, Ireland*
[4]*School of Biological and Health Sciences, Technological University Dublin, City Campus, Dublin, Ireland*
[5]*FOCAS Research Institute, Technological University Dublin, City Campus, Dublin, Ireland*
**Corresponding author: hugh.byrne@tudublin.ie*

12.1 Introduction

Histopathology is currently regarded as the "gold standard" patient sampling technique for cancer diagnostics. It involves extraction of a tissue sample, or biopsy, which is then sectioned and stained for evaluation by a pathologist [1]. Cytopathology, on the other hand, is the field of disease diagnosis at the cellular level [2], necessitating only the microscopic evaluation of samples of cells which can be harvested by less invasive methods such as exfoliative brushing, needle probes or from biofluids. Based on the identification of abnormalities in cellular appearance, cytopathology is currently widely used to aid in the screening of cancer, as well as for the diagnosis of some infectious diseases and other inflammatory conditions. Although highly specific, the methodology is notoriously low in sensitivity, however, which can potentially be addressed through emerging, more chemically sensitive analysis techniques [3–5].

The study of cells, generally termed cytology, emerged in the 17th century, with the development of optical microscopic techniques, during which time the term "cell" was coined by Robert Hooke [6]. Cytological analysis continued to evolve, particularly in the 19th century, with improved microscopic techniques and the development of specific cell stains, as well as the technique of exfoliative cytology [7]. Although there followed many demonstrations of the diagnostic potential of exfoliative cytology [7, 8], they were largely ignored until the 20th century, principally due to the work of Georgios Nikolaou Papanicolaou [9], who gives his name to the now widespread technique of stained cytological smear analysis, or Pap smear. Papanikolaou first reported that uterine cancer could be diagnosed by means of a vaginal smear in 1928 [10], although the work received little attention until it was published in 1941 [11] and 1943 [12]. On the basis of the technique, cervical cancer screening programs were trialed in the US and Canada throughout the 1950s, and, by the early 1960s, national screening programs began to emerge elsewhere [13]. This screening test for the early detection of cancer or lesions that may progress into cancer has dramatically reduced the morbidity rates of cervical cancer and is considered by some to be the singularly most significant advance in the control of cancer in the 20th century [10, 14].

The Pap smear test traditionally entails collecting exfoliated cellular material with a spatula or a cervical brush from the transformation zone of the uterine cervix. In the case of conventional smears, the cells are directly spread onto a glass slide, fixed in alcohol and ether and stained, using five stains in three solutions, the latter being a key element of the test [15, 16]. Using the prescribed protocol, the cells should remain fairly transparent, cell nuclei will stain dark blue, while the cytoplasm stains blue-green and keratin stains orange in color, such that squamous cells will stain green and keratinized cells will stain pink/orange. The staining technique has been adopted for analysis of a range of non-gynecological specimen preparations from exfoliated, needle probe and/or bodily fluid samples.

Liquid-based cytology (LBC) was introduced in the 1990s as a means of improving cytology test performance. Unlike in the conventional Pap test, the cells are not spread directly onto a slide, but the cervical brush is rinsed in a vial of preservative liquid which is then dispersed as a film on a glass slide, in which the cells are fixed and stained, after drying [17]. The LBC method improves sample quality by producing a more uniform layer of cells and helps remove unwanted cellular material such as red blood and inflammatory cells (leukocytes). Specimen cells can also be stored in the vials, allowing additional samples to be prepared for repeat or ancillary analysis. LBC samples are processed by either the Thinprep or Surepath™ methods. Thinprep uses a cell filtration system, while Surepath™ uses density gradient centrifugation to remove unwanted cells (red and white blood cells). Both result in a circular monolayer of cells on a glass slide. The introduction of automated image analysis has enabled identification of areas of interest on the slide that most likely contain abnormal cells, resulting in more rapid screening for each sample and a reduced detection error [18].

As an alternative to exfoliative cytology, fine needle aspiration (cytology/biopsy) is commonly used to sample cells from tissue lumps or masses. It is frequently used to investigate readily accessible palpable lesions in cases of thyroid cancer, breast cancer, and malignancy in the lymph nodes. A thin hollow needle (23–25 gauge (0.52 to 0.64 mm outer diameter)) is inserted into the tissue to extract cells which are then examined microscopically after fixing and staining, as for exfoliated cytological samples.

To use cytology for the identification of disease, one must first have an understanding of the regular function and growth patterns of the normal cells, and cytologists are trained to identify the type of cells that are normally present in different areas of the body, such that they can also detect either changes in the morphology of the cells or the presence of inappropriate cells that are associated with particular conditions. Microscopically observable changes in cell morphology, often accentuated by different staining techniques, have been recognized as indicators for cancer since the 19th century [19], and continue to be used in cytopathological screening to this day. Cell abnormalities indicative of cancer include changes in the cell size or shape, cell nuclear size, nuclear configuration, and changes in the number and size of nucleoli, in comparison to normal cells of the same origin. Specific nuclear aberrations may be used as prognostic indicators, and can be characteristic of certain tumor types [2, 20].

Cervical screening programs currently employ the Bethesda Classification system [21] for its terminology of squamous intraepithelial lesions (SIL). This is divided into three categories: 1) Low-grade SIL (LSIL) which includes HPV-associated cellular changes and mild dyskaryosis (Figure 12.1(left)); 2) High-grade SIL (HSIL) which includes moderate dyskaryosis and severe dyskaryosis (Figure 12.1(center)); 3) Squamous cell carcinoma (Figure 12.1(right)).

Cytological changes in squamous cells which are not normal and do not fit the criteria for SIL are classed as one of two subcategories of atypical squamous cells (ASC): 1) ASC-US — atypical squamous cells of

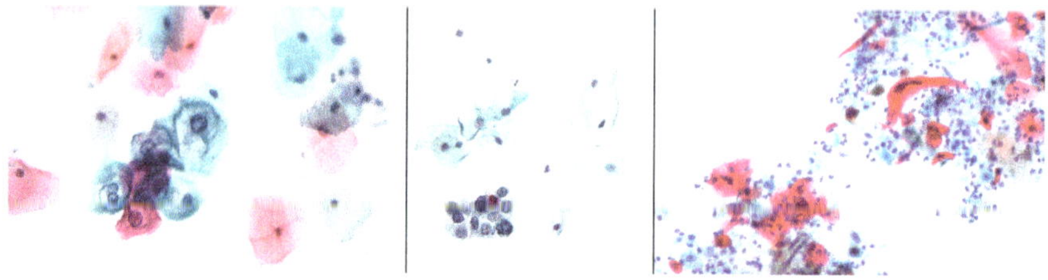

Figure 12.1. Cytological representation of LSIL (left) and HSIL (center) in a cervical Pap smear (Nephron, CC BY-SA 3.0, via Wikimedia Commons), squamous cell carcinoma (right) in a bronchial wash (Ed Uthman from Houston, TX, USA, CC BY 2.0, via Wikimedia Commons).

undetermined significance. 2) ASC-H — atypical squamous cells of undetermined significance but high-grade changes cannot be ruled out [22].

Cytopathology has proven itself to be an effective primary screening method for cervical cancer, with a specificity of 96.5% but a lower sensitivity of between 30–85% [23]. The low sensitivities are often associated with the subjectivity of the cytological assessment procedure, and in particular because the density of abnormal- compared to normal-looking cells in a cytological sample may be extremely low [24], resulting in a high proportion of classification as "no malignant cells seen" (NMCS), many of which can be false negatives (1.2–10.6% of breast cancer cases, 16% of squamous cervical cancers, 52% of glandular cervical cancers, and over 20% of thyroid cancer cases [25–28]), suggesting that morphological abnormality alone may not be the most sensitive diagnostic indicator for cytopathology.

Particularly in the case of the cervix, infection with human papilloma virus (HPV) has been identified as strongly associated with cancer [29]. There are over 100 different types of HPV, 12 of which have been identified as carcinogenic and associated with a higher risk of progression to malignancy, amongst which HPV 16 and 18 are associated with a higher risk of developing disease [30]. The virus/genome can be identified in exfoliated cells, which enables HPV testing to be performed on LBC samples. HPV DNA tests such as the Hybrid Capture 2 assay from Qiagen detect HPV DNA from 13 high-risk HPV types, including HPV 16 and 18 [31], while HPV DNA gentotyping tests such as the Roche Cobas 4800 assay identify HPV 16 and 18 individually together with a pool of 12 other high-risk HPV types [32]. HPV mRNA tests such as the APTIMA HPV assay detect mRNA for E6 and E7 viral oncoproteins of HPV high-risk types [33]. Because of a higher sensitivity than cytology, HPV testing has recently been implemented for primary cervical screening in many countries [34]. Due to the low specificity of HPV testing, cytology is performed as a triage test to avoid over-referral to colposcopy and over-treatment [35]. Molecular biomarkers, such as methylation markers and protein biomarkers, for instance p16INK4a, Ki67, minichromosome maintenance protein 2, and topoisomerases type IIa can also be utilized for the detection of transforming HPV infections for the management of women who test positive for HPV [36].

The presence of molecular biomarkers of disease, and even viral infection, suggests that biochemical changes at a cellular and subcellular level which can be diagnostic indicators at early stages of disease development should be identifiable, before morphological changes are apparent. Rather than being limited to individual molecular markers, these biochemical signatures of early-stage abnormalities are manifest in combinations of lipidic, proteinic, genomic content and across the cellular metabolism. Identifying and monitoring such changes therefore requires a more holistic, label-free approach. To this end, Raman microspectroscopic analysis of cytological samples has been extensively explored, leading to the concept of spectral cytopathology [37]. As an optical technique, in its confocal mode, Raman microspectrosccopy can investigate subcellular structures and organelles with a sub-micrometer resolution, depending on the wavelength of the source laser [38, 39], and has been employed, for example, to monitor uptake and subcellular distribution of chemotherapeutic agents [40] and nanoparticles [41], as well as the cellular responses [42]. In addition to biochemical perturbation induced by such toxic agents, as well as radiation [43, 44], it has been shown that Raman microspectroscopy can differentiate between cell lines with different HPV copy number [45]. In all cases, the analysis is based on the spectroscopic profiles of the cells, representing the biochemical content of the cell, or cellular region, and any changes to it because of exogenous insult or disease.

12.2 Review of Raman Cytology

12.2.1 *Cervical Spectral Cytology*

Cervical cancer ranks as the 7th highest of all cancers, at >600,000 new cases in 2020 [46]. While recognized as a hugely successful measure in limiting the occurrence of cervical cancer since its introduction in the 1960s, HPV testing has recently replaced cytology for primary cervical screening in many countries, although cytology triage is performed to minimize over-referral to colposcopy and over-treatment of women who are HPV positive. After an abnormal Pap screening test (HPV test with cytology triage), colposcopy is performed to visualize the cervix followed by a tissue biopsy and histopathology.

In the quest for improved screening methodologies, a number of Raman spectroscopic studies have been carried out to date using cervical exfoliated cells. High-risk HPV was identified in exfoliated cell pellets from 25 HPV-negative and 25 HPV-positive patients using Raman spectroscopy [47]. HPV-positive and HPV-negative cytology samples were discriminated based on spectral features of lipid, amino acid, protein and DNA, with an accuracy of 98.5% using a sparse multinomial logistic regression method.

Raman spectroscopy was also used to discriminate between exfoliated cell pellets from 45 patients with negative cytology and 49 patients with cervical cancer cytology [48]. Initially, principal component analysis-linear discriminant analysis (PCA-LDA) achieved classification of ~90%, although heme and fibrin bands from blood were the main discriminating features. Treatment of a further set of 28 negative and 29 cervical cancer exfoliated cell pellets with red blood cell lysis buffer resulted in successful blood removal, which was confirmed by the absence of heme and fibrin bands. PCA-LDA achieved classification of ~80% based on protein spectral features. This study was later extended to the analysis of 66 cervical (38 tumor and 28 normal) and 44 oral (29 tumor and 15 normal) exfoliated cell pellets [49]. Classification accuracies of 84% for cervical cancer and 86% for oral cancer were achieved based on DNA and protein spectral features.

A new method for recording Raman spectra from single exfoliated cells from ThinPrep samples was described by Bonnier *et al.* [50]. Pre-treatment of the slides with a hydrogen peroxide solution effectively removed blood contamination and significantly reduced variability in the spectral data. The hydrogen peroxide pre-treatment method was later adapted for Thinprep samples with excessive blood contamination [51]. Ramos *et al.* [52] applied this method for single exfoliated cells to routine Thinprep samples from a cervical screening program. Raman spectra were recorded from negative (n = 88), low grade (n = 35) and high-grade cytology samples (n = 43). Sensitivity and specificity >90% were achieved based on protein and nucleic acid spectral features.

Raman spectral signatures of the main cell types present in Pap test specimens, i.e., superficial, intermediate and parabasal cells, were defined by Kearney *et al.* [53]. In addition, Raman spectra from the cytoplasm were shown to exhibit significant variability due to different levels of glycogen present in samples taken during different phases of the menstrual cycle. Further work on hormone-associated variability, related to the menstrual cycle, menopause and the use of hormone-based contraceptives showed that although hormone-related spectral changes in glycogen and protein features were evident, biochemical changes due to pre-cancer were more pronounced than those due to the menstrual cycle or the use of hormone-based contraceptives [54].

Raman spectroscopy was also investigated as a potential triage test following HPV primary screening [55]. Discrimination between ThinPrep samples with transient and transforming HPV infection was based on increased nucleic acids, decreased glycogen and changes in protein features in the samples with a transforming HPV infection. Partial least squares discriminant analysis (PLS-DA) achieved classification accuracy of 93% following training on 60 ThinPrep samples and validation on a blinded independent test set of 14 ThinPrep samples.

The clinical utility of Raman spectroscopy for identifying cervical pre-cancer was recently shown [56]. PLS-DA achieved an accuracy of 91.3% following training on 662 ThinPrep samples and validation on a blinded independent test set of 69 ThinPrep samples. Raman imaging of liquid-based Pap smear samples from 30 patients prepared using a cytospin centrifuge together with deep convolutional neural networks achieved 100% accuracy for classification of negative, low-grade and high-grade cytology based on lipid, protein, polysaccharide, and nucleic acid spectral features [57].

Another Raman imaging study of single exfoliated cells from 96 patients showed accelerated glycogen metabolism in HPV-positive samples [58]. A further study on single exfoliated cells from 63 patients suggested a dual switch of lipid metabolism in cervical pre-cancer [59]. A decrease in lipid content in low-grade cytology samples and an increase in lipid content in high-grade cytology samples was observed compared to negative cytology samples.

Surface-enhanced Raman spectroscopy (SERS) using single exfoliated cells, cell pellets and extracted DNA on gold nanoparticle substrates was utilized to discriminate normal, high-grade pre-cancer and cervical squamous cell carcinoma [60]. Support vector machine analysis achieved classification accuracies of 94.46%, 71.6% and 97.72% for single exfoliated cells, cell pellets and extracted DNA, respectively, based on spectral features of nucleic acids and amino acids. Further work showed simultaneous detection of cervical cancer biomarkers in single exfoliated cells using a SERS tag functionalized with monoclonal antibodies against p16 and Ki67 [61].

12.2.2 *Oral Spectral Cytology*

There were >375,000 new cases of cancers of the lip and oral cavity worldwide in 2020 [46], the 16th highest of all cancers. Brush biopsy is generally a well-tolerated, minimally invasive and safe method for harvesting cells from the oral cavity, although oral cytology has not been widely adopted because of poor sensitivity for identification of dysplasia and cancer [62]. The sensitivity and specificity of oral cytology can be improved by augmentation with other techniques, such as analysis of DNA and other molecular markers, melanoma-associated antigen A, lamin-5, Tenascin-C and epidermal growth factor receptor [63]. However, a surgical biopsy coupled with histopathological assessment must be performed for definitive diagnosis of oral lesions. While cancerous cells can be collected from the surface, this does not currently qualify as a diagnosis, which requires histological proof of breach of basement membrane. Nevertheless, brush biopsy may be very useful for patients with multiple oral lesions or for monitoring oral potentially malignant disorders (OPMD).

Only a limited number of studies have explored Raman microspectroscopic analysis of oral exfoliated cells. Sahu *et al.* [64] demonstrated discrimination between samples from healthy volunteers and those from patients with oral cancer, using pelleted oral exfoliated cells. The discrimination was seen to be based on differences in protein secondary structure and increased DNA levels, and the work was extended to detection of OPMDs [65]. The same group also demonstrated the diagnostic potential of a combined, four-group model based on a dataset of exfoliated cell samples from oral and cervical sites, yielding high classification efficiencies of ~85% [49]. Behl *et al.* [66] sought to standardize the exfoliated cell sample preparation method, based on the LBC preparation on glass slides commonly employed for cervical samples. A complete methodology, incorporating sample collection, sample preparation, spectral acquisition and data pre-processing and analysis was described.

Using this sample preparation technique, further work by Behl *et al.* [67] analyzed brush biopsy cytological samples from healthy donors and from patients with OPMDs, leukoplakia, erythroplakia and erythroleukoplakia, showing mild, moderate or severe dysplasia on histological analysis. Sensitivities of 94% and 86% and specificity of 85% were achieved for discrimination between oral exfoliated cells from healthy donors and from patients with OPMDs, for spectra recorded from the cytoplasm and nucleus respectively.

The discrimination was seen to be mainly based on increased lipidic contributions from the OPMD samples. Through this explorative study, although there are many other contributing factors to the differentiating loading which were not fitted, it was successfully demonstrated that ceramides may play an important role in the discrimination of OPMD samples from healthy volunteer samples using Raman microspectroscopy and could therefore act as a spectral marker. Furthermore, this study also indicated that, in OPMDs, ceramide concentration increases in the cell, allowing differentiation of healthy volunteer samples from the OPMD patient samples.

The study also investigated the influence of a number of potential confounding factors on the classification model, amongst which, that of anatomical site was found to be significant. Raman spectra from buccal mucosa and the ventral surface of the tongue were found to be significantly different to the corresponding spectra from gingiva and alveolar mucosa. As both gingiva and alveolar mucosa are rich in lipids such as ceramides, saturated fatty acids and cholesterol, which act as an antibacterial barrier against infection, cells from these sites showed a similar lipidic spectral profile to cells from OPMDs. Thus, it was concluded that future studies should use separate classification models for buccal mucosa/tongue and for gingiva/alveolar mucosa, and notably, a discriminant model based only on buccal mucosa achieved sensitivities and specificities as high as 99% [67]. In contrast, neither age, gender, smoking nor alcohol consumption were seen to significantly influence the classification model.

Field cancerization, which can result in multiple OPMDs and in second primary tumors and recurrences, has also been investigated in oral cytology samples [68, 69]. In the studies of pellets of exfoliated cells, Sahu *et al.* observed an overlap of spectra of cells from contralateral normal sites and spectra from cells from tumor sites in oral cancer patients, indicative of field cancerization [68]. In the study of Behl *et al.*, oral exfoliated cells were collected from healthy volunteers and from patients with OPMDs, both from the lesion and from contralateral clinically normal mucosa. The study showed that the contralateral normal samples could be classified as spectrally different from the healthy volunteer samples and showed spectral features similar to the lesion samples, particularly in patients who had developed multiple lesions [69]. The effect of smoking, alcohol consumption, degree of dysplasia and gender were explored to understand the factors contributing to the spectral overlap between lesion samples and contralateral normal samples but none of these were found to be confounding factors. The ability of Raman microspectroscopic analysis of exfoliated cells to identify field cancerization is therefore potentially important for disease prognosis. Behl *et al.* also undertook a study of patients in a follow-up dysplasia clinic [70], indicating that classification according to Raman microspectroscopic analysis of exfoliated cells correlated well with histological analysis, if taken within the previous six months, indicating that such spectral cytopathological analysis can eliminate the need for multiple biopsies.

12.2.3 *Lung Spectral Cytology*

Lung cancer continues to be one of the most common cancer worldwide, with an estimated >2,200,000 cases in 2020 [46]. An estimated 13–14% of cases are categorized as small cell lung cancer, while the more common form of non-small cell lung cancer (NSCLC) accounts for approximately 85% of cases [71, 72], which in turn can be subdivided into histological subtypes of squamous cell carcinoma (SCC), adenocarcinoma (AC) and large cell carcinoma. Lung abnormalities are usually initially established using CT scanning or X-rays, after which bronchoscopy is employed as an investigatory technique to attain a cytological sample of the suspicious lesion for diagnostic analysis [73], by bronchial washing, brushing and bronchioalveolar lavage (BAL) [51–53].

O'Dea undertook a study of Raman microspectroscopic analysis of human bronchoscopy cytology samples, BALs and bronchial washes collected from 24 patients (9 females, 15 males), to evaluate the ability to characterize and diagnose NSCLC patients, for whom lung cancer was confirmed through final clinical diagnosis and final histology was recorded: 12 SCC, 5 AC, and 7 negative (no cancer diagnosed) [74]. Within each sample, the targeted cell types were identified as either bronchial epithelial cells, squamous cells, or lymphocytes. Based on analysis of the bronchial cellular nuclei, a three-way classification model to discriminate the negative, SCC, and AC cases yielded diagnostic sensitivities from 81–90% and specificities from 79–91%. Two-way models to discriminate the bronchial cell nuclei of negative cases vs. bronchial cells from SCC or AC cases yielded sensitivities of ≥91%, and specificities of ≥89%. The SCC cases were discriminated from the AC cases with a sensitivity and specificity of 90% and 86%, respectively. In the case of squamous cell nuclei, each two-way classification model yielded a sensitivity above 73% and a specificity above 78%, while for lymphocytes, the models yielded sensitivities and specificities above 82% for the discrimination of the SCC and AC subtypes. Combining all cell types, a two-way classifier of malignant and negative yielded a sensitivity of 89% and a specificity of 79%, while a classifier of SCC vs. AC yielded a sensitivity of 84% and a specificity of 69%.

O'Dea also compared the Raman microspectroscopic signatures of true negative, true positive (samples which had been classified as SCC on cytology and histology, and AC on cytology and histology), and false negative (NMCS on cytology and SCC on histology, and NMCS on cytology and AC on histology). The accuracy of the Raman microspectroscopic cytology analysis compared to the known histological result for true positives was 87–91% (SCC), 73–86% (AC) and for false negatives 73–84% (SCC), 91% (AC) [74]. The study demonstrates the particular advantage of Raman spectroscopic analysis of small samples in which obviously abnormal cells may be few and therefore unseen.

12.2.4 *Bladder Spectral Cytology*

Bladder cancer ranks 10th in the world for number of new cases worldwide in 2020, at >573,000 [46]. The current gold standard for detection of bladder cancer is cystoscopy, followed by biopsy, which are invasive and uncomfortable for patients. The majority of bladder tumors are urothelial carcinoma (UC), and, as there is a likelihood of recurrence, patients with a history of UC often undergo follow-up tests for years after initial treatment. As a result, bladder cancer is one of the costliest cancer diseases. Urine cytology is often used to aid in diagnosis, as it has relatively high specificity [75], although it has very low sensitivity, especially for low-grade tumors [76].

Shapiro *et al.* [77] undertook a study of 172 specimens of epithelial cells extracted from the urine of 50 patients without UC, 50 patients with low-grade tumor, and 72 patients with high-grade tumor (including 22 patients with carcinoma *in situ*). The Raman classification model achieved a sensitivity of 96% (100% of the high-grade tumors) and a specificity of 90% for prediction of bladder cancer, although all 50 patients without UC were classified as having low-grade UC. The algorithm was applied to a further 166 urine samples, and although 98% accuracy was achieved for high-grade UC, again all patients without UC were classified as having low grade. Note that the classification model is largely based on the strength of a single Raman band (1584 cm^{-1}), rather than multivariate analysis. The signature is similar to that of blood contamination in cervical samples, reported by [50], and Yousef *et al.* confirmed that the signal was from erythrocytes [78].

Yousef *et al.* used a combination of Raman, coherent anti-Stokes Raman scattering, and second harmonic generation imaging of urine samples from patients (n = 10) with pathologically confirmed high-grade UC and those without (n = 10) [78]. Based on the Raman spectral data, a multivariate classification model was constructed which could differentiate normal and cancer urothelial cells with 100% accuracy.

Hu *et al.* used SERS to examine the supernatant and sediment (including exfoliated cells) of the urine samples of 161 bladder cancer patients, further divided into high-grade (n = 80) and low-grade (n = 81), and of 87 healthy volunteers [79]. The sediment was processed to isolate the epithelial cells. Combining the SERS results for the urinary supernatant and sediment, the total diagnostic sensitivity and specificity were 100% and 98.85%, respectively, for high-grade tumors and 97.53% and 90.80%, respectively, for low-grade tumors.

12.3 Methods

Much of the proof-of-concept research in the field of spectral cytopathology has been undertaken at an academic level, and although some degree of consensus building around methodologies in the field in general was afforded by coordinated actions such as the EU FP6 "Diagnostic Applications of Synchrotron Infrared Microscopy (DASIM)" (2004–2008), the UK EPSRC Network CLIRSPEC (2013–2017) and the EU COST Network Raman4Clinics (2014–2018), there remains a significant diversity of approaches in the literature to aspects of sample preparation, measurement, instrumentation, data processing and analysis. To address this, Behl *et al.* attempted to standardize the protocol for oral spectral cytology of exfoliated oral cells [66], and Traynor *et al.* elaborated a more general protocol for Raman spectral cytopathology for use on LBC samples prepared on glass slides [80]. This protocol is described schematically in Figure 12.2 and details the specifics recommended for sample preparation, spectral acquisition, pre-processing and data analysis for spectral cytopathology for cervical, oral and lung cells.

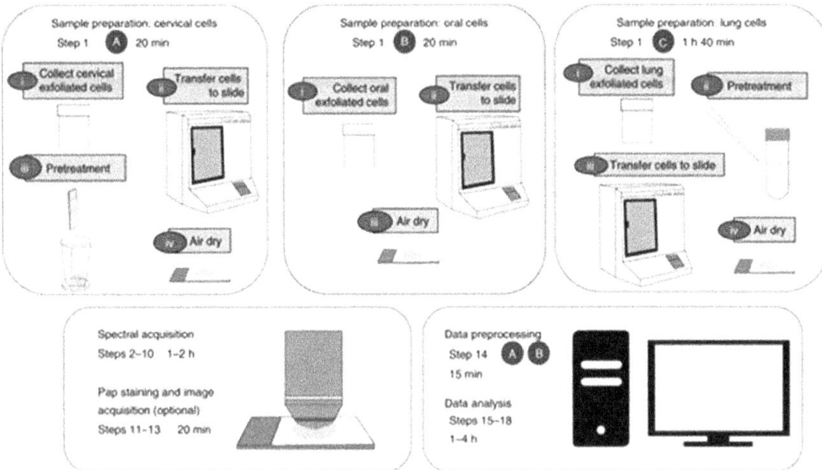

Figure 12.2. Schematic overview of the protocol for Raman spectral cytopathology for cervical, oral and lung cells. Reproduced from Ref. [80] with permission.

12.3.1 *Sample Preparation*

Methodologies of exfoliative cytology are well established for cervical, oral, lung, etc. However, as Raman spectroscopy can be very sensitive to chemical contaminants, additional steps may be required for sample preparation.

After collection in a cervical screening clinic, cell suspensions are annotated according to a blood scale index 0–3, 0 indicating a clear solution and 3 a very bloody one. Samples with a blood scale index of 2 or 3 are either rejected as unsuitable for analysis or treated with CytoLyt or alternatives to wash the cells before further sample processing. However, even in blood scale 0–1 samples, although not visible to the naked eye, residual blood can be detected in the Raman spectra of the samples, and even swamp the signatures of the cells [50]. This is particularly the case when using common green laser lines (e.g., 514.5 and 532 nm) as source, because the Raman signal of hemoglobin, with strong features between 1500 and 1650 cm^{-1}, is resonantly enhanced at these wavelengths. Bonnier *et al.* demonstrated a protocol to remove the residual blood using a hydrogen peroxide pretreatment, which effectively removed the spectral variability due to the contamination [50].

In the case of oral cytology, no sample pre-treatment is necessary and the protocol of Behl *et al.* advises minimal pressure on the cytobrush to avoid bleeding [66]. For bronchial washing or bronchial brushing/BAL samples, removal of mucus contamination is required, using a pre-treatment with dithiothreitol [74].

12.3.2 *Data Pre-Processing*

The general requirements for Raman spectral data pre-processing have been reviewed extensively [81–83]. In many cases, these requirements can be minimized by experimental design, and in this context, the most appropriate choice of substrate in Raman microspectroscopy has been long debated [84–86]. Most Raman microspectroscopy studies have been carried out using calcium fluoride substrates, as they have minimal spectral contributions, but they are very expensive, brittle, and it has been demonstrated that they may even perturb the cell cycle in *in vitro* cultures [87]. Critically, it has been argued that any new screening modality for diagnostic applications should be fully integrated into, and minimally disruptive of, the existing clinical workflow [88]. In the case of cytology, glass microscope slides are used to mount the samples for visualization and therefore it is desirable that the methodology of spectral cytopathology be adapted to suit. Metal oxide impurities in glass absorb in the near-infrared, giving commercial glass a characteristic green tint, and thus glass slides exhibit strong fluorescence on excitation with 785 nm but this can be avoided by using a blue or green source laser for Raman spectroscopy (e.g., 488, 514.5 and 532 nm).

Using 532 nm as source, two broad peaks at 550 cm^{-1} and 1100 cm^{-1} are evident in the Raman spectrum of glass (Figure 12.3). This glass spectral contribution can be minimized during recording by careful focusing into the cell and away from the substrate using a Raman microscope equipped with a confocal hole and a high numerical aperture objective lens (low focal depth). Residual glass contributions can then be removed, post-acquisition, using methods such as non-negatively constrained least squares (NNLS) [68] or extended multiplicative signal correction (EMSC) [69, 71, 92]. In both cases, after initially smoothing the spectra to reduce noise, a weighted sum of a glass spectrum, polynomial baseline, and cellular components are least squares fitted to the measured spectrum, and the weighted contribution of glass to the best fit is subtracted. In the NNLS method, the contributions of pure cell components, such as nucleic acids, proteins, and carbohydrates to the measured cellular spectrum are calculated according to a non-negatively constrained fitting routine. In the EMSC method, a

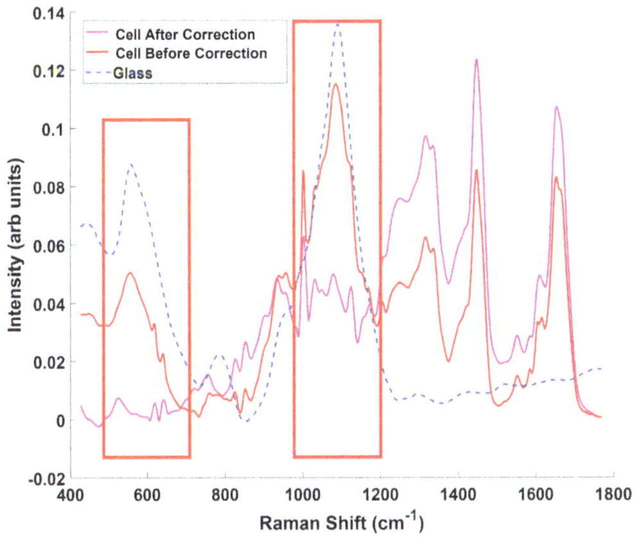

Figure 12.3. Raman spectrum of a cervical cell (red) on a glass microscope slide, the spectrum of which is shown in (blue). The main features of glass at ~550 cm^{-1} and ~1100 cm^{-1} are present in the cellular spectrum (indicated by red boxes), but can be removed by preprocessing to yield a corrected spectrum (magenta).

complete reference cellular spectrum, with no glass contribution (measured on a spectrally neutral substrate such as calcium fluoride or magnesium fluoride), is employed. For both NNLS and EMSC methods, a matrix of glass spectra should be recorded to cover the variability of the glass. After glass correction, vector normalization of the spectra of a group of cells is typically performed to minimize variance in the spectral dataset due to the measurement process. Both the NNLS and EMSC algorithms have been demonstrated to satisfactorily remove glass spectral contamination from spectral cytopathological datasets [89].

12.3.3 *Data Analysis*

Typically, a Raman spectrum contains ~1,000 points per spectral window and, depending on the spectral dispersion, 3–4 windows. The spectrum is multivariate, in that the spectral information which characterizes the pathological state of a sample can be contained in the relative strengths of multiple spectral features, each in turn comprised of multiple data points. Typically, a sample will be represented by multiple spectra taken from multiple cells, and these will be classified according to a database of spectra of known pathological states. The process relies on the use of multivariate statistical algorithms to, for example, reduce the dimensionality of the variance, and construct and validate a discriminant model to classify spectra of the dataset of reduced dimensionality according to the desired pathologies [81]. Although the choice of algorithms is ever increasing with the emergence of ever more sophisticated machine learning and artificial intelligence protocols, the basics of the processes can be described through the commonly employed methodologies of PCA and LDA [90].

PCA is an unsupervised method which is very commonly employed to reduce the dimensionality of the data based on the variation present in a dataset, whereby the first principal component (PC) identified describes the maximum variance of the dataset, the second PC describes the second highest variance, etc., such that the percentage contributions progressively decrease (PC1 > PC2 > PC3...). The scores of the PCs are described by the loading vector, which is a representation of this variance. In the context of spectroscopic analysis, the plot of the loadings vector provides an indication of the spectral features which differentiate two groups within a dataset [91]. PCA can thus be an extremely useful tool to verify that two sample sets are indeed differentiable (e.g., diseased and non-diseased) spectroscopically, and to provide an indication of the spectroscopic and therefore biochemical basis of that differentiation separating spectra into groups [92].

Having reduced the dimensionality of the dataset, a classification model can be established using, for example, LDA, a supervised algorithm which projects all the data points into a new space, normally of lower dimension, which maximizes the between-class separability while minimizing their within-class variability, based on calculation of the Mahalanobis distance between the sample data for each class, to identify the latent (spectral) variables which describe the discrimination, and therefore the features of highest diagnostic significance [93]. An LDA model is ideally constructed, or trained, and then tested using sets of data of well-characterized samples, which in reality are single datasets. Validation of the model is normally performed by a leave-k-out cross-validation routine, in which "k" samples are left out of the training dataset and used to test the model. Once trained, the model should be tested using unseen data. The performance of the model can be described by the (root mean squared) error of cross-validation and/or error of prediction. Note, it is important that spectra from the same sample/patient are not used to train and test the model, and therefore, in a dataset which has multiple spectra of the same sample/patient, a leave-one-patient-out protocol should be used.

12.4 Cervical Cancer

Cervical cancer begins in the basal layer of cells lining the cervix when the normal cells slowly change into pre-cancer cells that have the potential to turn into cancer. The gradual progression of cervical cancer can allow the detection of dysplastic changes before invasive cancer develops, through cervical cancer screening programs. These screening programs are common in developed countries, greatly reducing the mortality rates due to cervical cancer, but are not yet implemented in developing countries due to lack of infrastructure and funding [94]. Conventional cervical cytology is, however, notoriously low in sensitivity, largely because it relies on identification of morphological abnormalities [35]. Public health programs have therefore increasingly shifted towards screening for infection with high-risk HPV, increasing the complexity of the process. Cervical screening is therefore potentially an ideal and strategic target application for spectral cytopathology, and the progress to date will be described in detail.

Some of the challenges associated with cervical cytology samples have been mentioned in Sections 12.3.1 and 12.3.2. Contaminants such as blood can give rise to spectral features which can overwhelm those of the cells, unless they are removed during sample preparation (Section 12.3.1). Spectral contributions from the glass slide can also be an issue, unless removed effectively by methods such as EMSC or NNLS during data pre-processing (Section 12.3.2).

The most abundant cell types in a Pap test sample are the superficial, intermediate and parabasal epithelial cells. White blood cells, endocervical cells and squamous metaplastic cells are also commonly observed. Figure 12.4 shows typical superficial, intermediate and parabasal cells on a Pap-stained ThinPrep slide. Superficial cells stain pink due to their metabolic inactivity

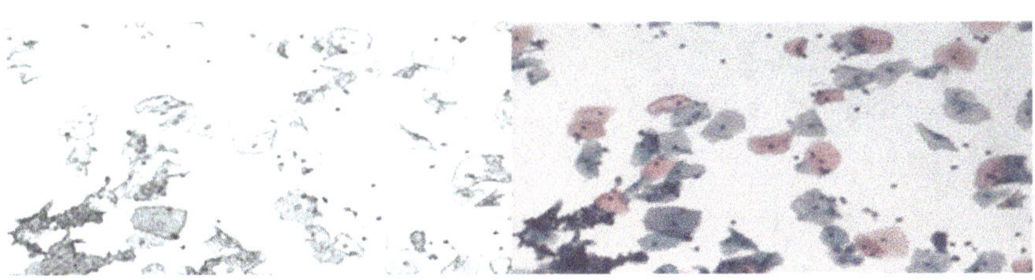

Figure 12.4. Unstained (left) and Pap-stained (right) images of negative cytology ThinPrep specimen, X10. After staining, superficial cells are pink and intermediate cells are blue. Reproduced from Ref. [95] with permission.

while intermediate and parabasal cells stain blue due to their metabolic activity. Unstained superficial and intermediate cell types can be difficult to distinguish from each other (Figure 12.4).

Raman spectra from superficial cells show strong spectral features of glycogen and nucleic acids at 480 cm^{-1}, 1380 cm^{-1} and 1490 cm^{-1}, while Raman spectra from intermediate cells show strong protein bands at 1450 cm^{-1} and 1670 cm^{-1} (Figure 12.5). Raman spectra from parabasal cells can be discriminated from superficial and intermediate cells on the basis of weaker signals from glycogen, nucleic acids and proteins due to a larger nuclear size for the parabasal cells (Figure 12.5).

The hormonal status of the woman at the time of sample collection can govern the ratio of superficial to intermediate cells in the Pap sample. The number of superficial cells can increase as the cervix matures, while the number of intermediate cells can increase in women taking the oral contraceptive pill [96].

Confounding factors related to hormonal changes in the woman at the time of sample collection (phase of the menstrual cycle and use of hormone-based contraceptives) can affect the reproducibility of the Raman spectra [53, 54]. Raman spectra from the cytoplasm already show significant variability due to the variable glycogen content and distribution within individual cells. As

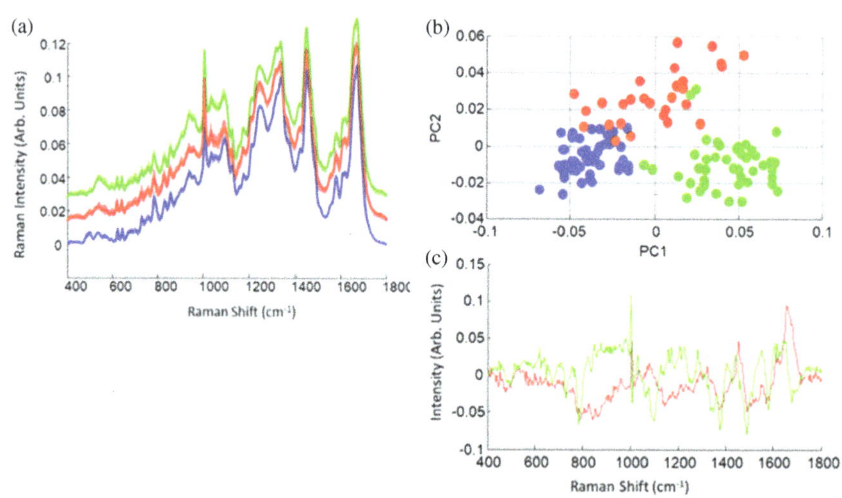

Figure 12.5. (a) Mean Raman spectra of superficial (blue), intermediate (green), and parabasal (red) cell nuclei. Shading denotes the standard deviation. Spectra have been offset for clarity. (b) PCA scatter plot and (c) PC1 (red) and PC2 (green) loadings. Reproduced from Ref. [53] with permission.

glycogen is present in pools in the cytoplasm, the glycogen contribution to the cellular spectrum can vary considerably depending on from where the spectrum is recorded. Glycogen levels in the cytoplasm can also vary due to the phase of the menstrual cycle and more prominent glycogen-related peaks (480, 850, 938, 1125, 1339 and 1380 cm^{-1}) are observed during days 14–28 (secretory phase) compared to days 5–13 (proliferative phase) (Figure 12.6) [53]. Hormone-related spectral changes are also observed to a lower extent in the Raman spectra from the nuclei, but biochemical changes due to cervical pre-cancer are more pronounced than the biochemical changes due to the menstrual cycle (Figure 12.7) or the use of hormone-based contraceptives [54].

A further challenge when working with cervical cytology samples is finding the rare abnormal cells on the unstained slide. Interestingly, Raman spectra from morphologically normal-appearing superficial and intermediate epithelial cells in pre-cancer cytology samples can be discriminated from superficial and intermediate epithelial cells in negative cytology samples (Figure 12.8). The latent variable (LV) scores scatter plot shows discrimination between the

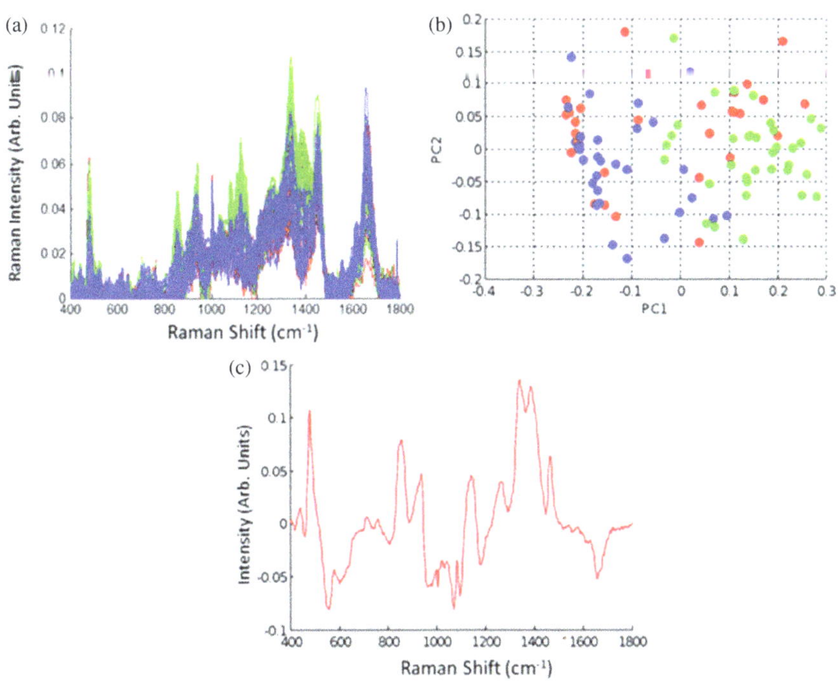

Figure 12.6. (a) Raman spectra of the cytoplasm of superficial cells from samples taken at different days of the menstrual cycle, days 5 to 13 (blue), days 13 to 14 (red), and days 14 to 28 (green). (b) PCA scatter plot. (c) PC1 loadings. Reproduced from Ref. [53] with permission.

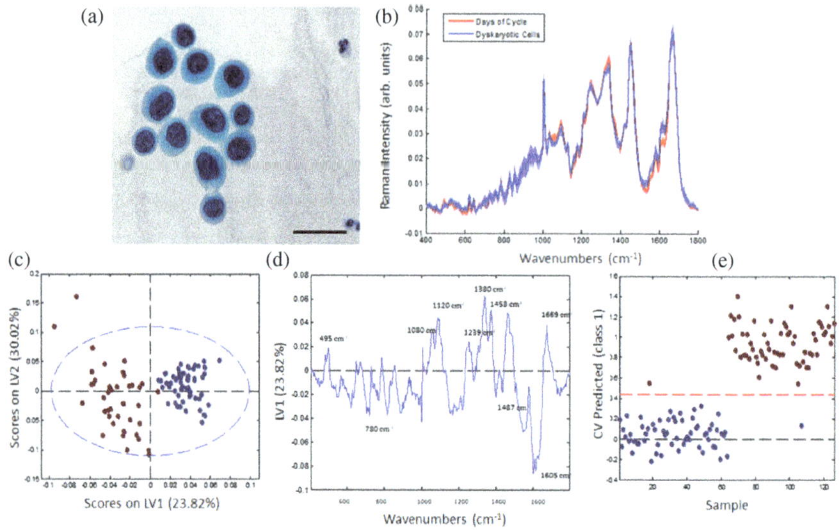

Figure 12.7. (a) Pap-stained cells with high-grade cytology. Bar = 35 μm. (b) Mean Raman spectra from negative samples from days 7 to 21 of the menstrual cycle (red) and spectra from high-grade cytology samples (blue). Shading denotes the standard deviation. (c) LV scores scatter plot of high-grade samples (red) and negative samples (blue). (d) LV1 loadings. (e) PLS-DA prediction plot. Reproduced from Ref. [54] with permission.

negative and pre-cancer cytology specimens, but overlap of the superficial and intermediate cells from each sample type. This indicates that morphologically normal cells near a pre-cancer lesion display biochemical features of pre-cancer [95].

With a full understanding of the challenges and confounding factors involved in working with cervical cytology samples, it is possible to obtain high-quality reproducible spectral datasets from the nuclei of cervical cells present on unstained ThinPrep specimens. Cervical exfoliated cells with negative cytology can then be discriminated from cervical exfoliated cells with pre-cancer cytology based on spectral features from glycogen (480, 850, 1381 cm^{-1}), nucleic acids (724, 780, 1578 cm^{-1}), proteins (1669 cm^{-1}) and lipids (1450 cm^{-1}) (Figure 12.9).

It has also been demonstrated that Raman spectroscopy can be utilized to detect HPV infection and its cellular consequences, such as increased proliferation and altered protein expression [45, 55]. Cervical cell lines with different HPV copy number (C33A (HPV negative), SiHa (1–2 integrated copies of HPV16), HeLa (20–50 integrated copies of HPV18) and CaSki

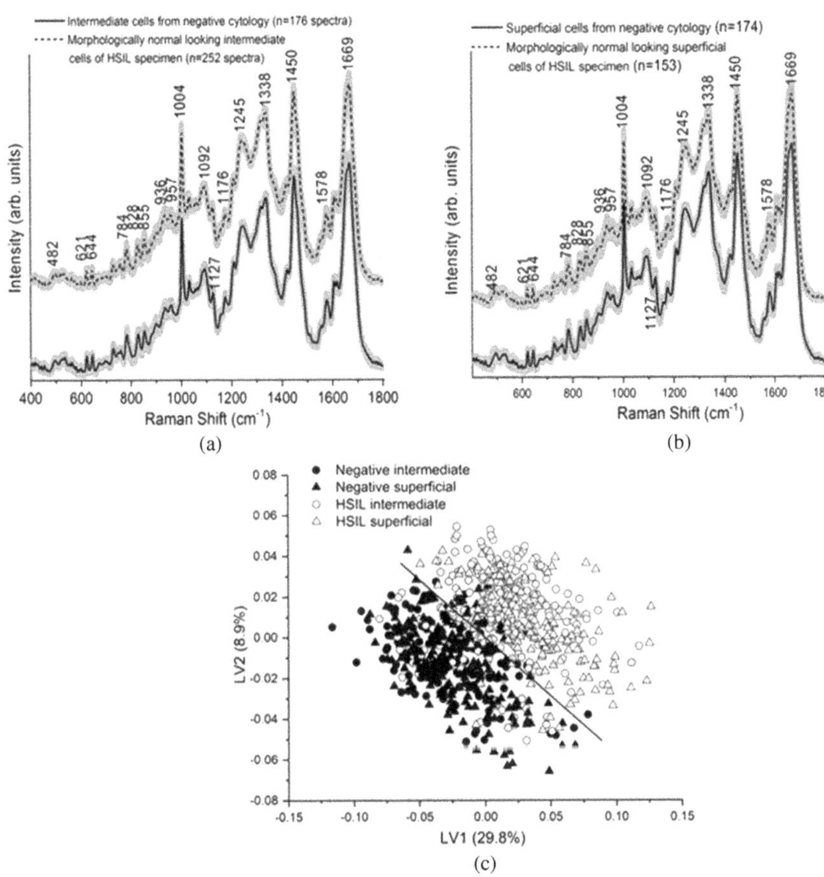

Figure 12.8. (a) Mean Raman spectra from intermediate cells of negative cytology samples (black) and from morphologically normal-appearing intermediate cells of HSIL samples. (b) Mean Raman spectra from superficial cells of negative cytology samples (black) and from morphologically normal-appearing superficial cells of HSIL samples. Shading denotes the standard deviation. (c) LV scores scatter plot of spectra from intermediate (circles) and superficial (triangles) cells from negative (black) and HSIL samples (white). Reproduced from Ref. [95] with permission.

(60–600 integrated copies of HPV16)) can be discriminated from each other using both Raman and FTIR spectroscopy based on spectral features of nucleic acids, proteins and lipids [45] (Figure 12.10).

As well as identifying HPV infection, it is important to distinguish between a transient and a transforming HPV infection to ensure better clinical management of women. Women with a transient infection, in which the HPV DNA has not integrated into the cellular DNA, are unlikely to need treatment,

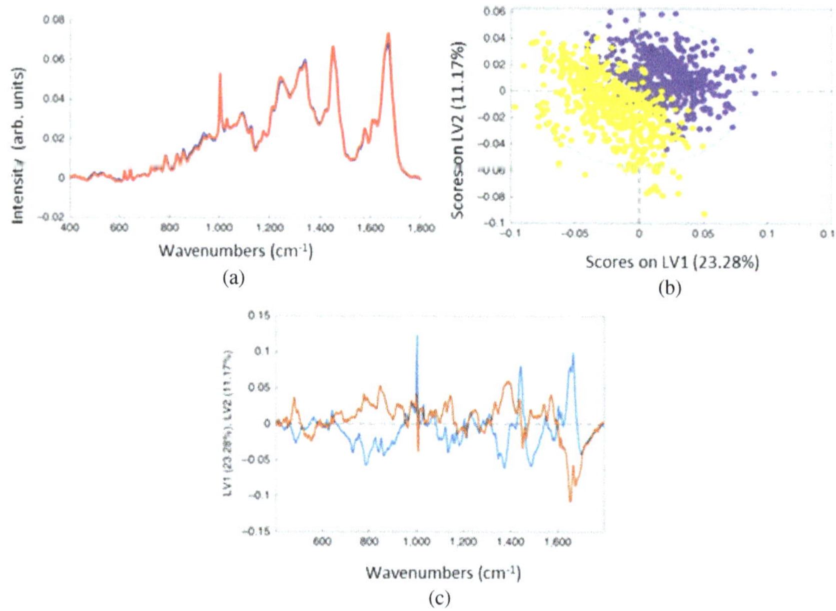

Figure 12.9. (a) Mean Raman spectra recorded from the nuclei of cervical cells with negative cytology (red) and high-grade cytology (blue). (b) PLSDA LV score scatter plot of spectra from cells with negative cytology (yellow) and high-grade cytology (blue). (c) LV1 and LV2 loading. Reproduced from Ref. [97] with permission.

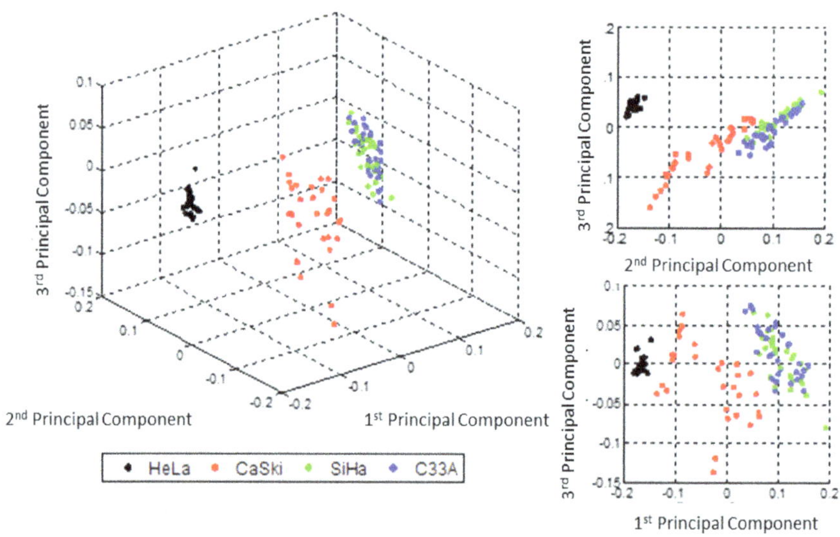

Figure 12.10. PCA scatterplots (3D, left and 2D, right) of Raman spectra from cervical cancer cell lines, C33A (blue), SiHa (green), HeLa (black) and CaSki (red) cells. Reproduced from Ref. [45] with permission.

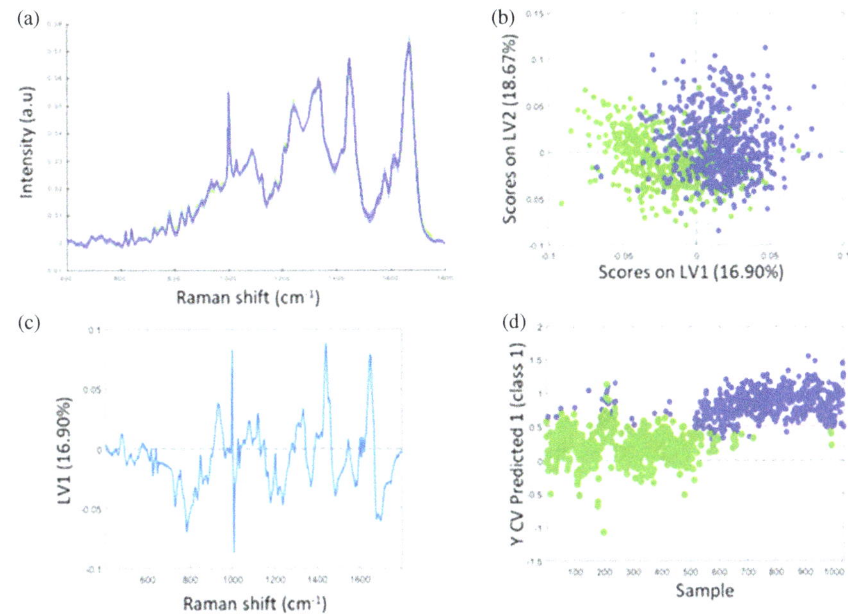

Figure 12.11. (a) Mean spectra of samples with transient HPV infection and transforming HPV infection. Shading indicates the standard deviation. (b) Latent variable (LV) score scatter plot. (c) LV1 loadings. (d) PLSDA plot. Reproduced from Ref. [55] with permission.

while women with a transforming infection, in which the HPV DNA has integrated into the cellular DNA, should be followed up at colposcopy and treated if necessary. Raman spectroscopy can distinguish between transient and transforming HPV infection based on spectral features at 482 (glycogen), 727 (nucleic acids), 782 (nucleic acids), 826 (nucleic acids), 852 (glycogen), 937 (glycogen), 1082 (glycogen), 1123 (glycogen), 1152 (proteins), 1334 (glycogen), 1380 (glycogen), 1238 (amide III), 1450 (proteins/lipids), 1485 (nucleic acids), 1580 (nucleic acids), 1642 (proteins) and 1670 cm^{-1} (amide I) (Figure 12.11) [55].

12.5 Summary and Future Perspectives

From the early observations of the biological cell in the 16th century [6], cytology has hugely impacted on our understanding of lifeforms and their function. Recognizing signatures of cellular dysfunction and the association with disease led to the later emergence of cytopathology [7, 8], which in turn led to population screening programs in the latter half of the 20th century, particularly for cervical cancer [13], a development which has been considered one of the most significant in the battle against cancer [10, 14]. Despite the major impact of the technique, its low sensitivity has been recognized as a source of a high rate of false negative diagnoses, and this has led to the search for more chemically specific techniques.

The technique of spectral cytopathology, and particularly Raman microspectroscopy, is ideally suited to this task, as it can provide a classification of a cell based on its biochemistry, rather than simply its morphology. Since its early development in the 1990s, biomedical applications of vibrational spectroscopy have seen significant recent developments, including the emergence of commercial companies for spectral histology [98, 99], *in vivo* analysis of resection margins [100, 101], spectroscopic endoscopes [102, 103], and blood serum measurement for cancer screening [104, 105]. Spectral cytopathology has been identified as an ideal strategic target for the field, given that screening programs are well established in the "developed world" and so sample throughput is very high [88, 106]. The process of screening cytological slides has become increasingly automated [18], and O'Dwyer *et al.* have demonstrated that the process of Raman-based classification of cell lines prepared as a Thinprep sample can be fully automated, with a high-throughput rate of ten cells per second [107].

Although cells from different anatomical origin may require additional pre-treatment before the Thinprep procedure [50, 51, 74], the sample preparation, measurement and analysis procedures are the same for all samples, and are readily integrated into the clinical workflow [80]. A number of potentially confounding factors have been identified, which are specific to the anatomical site [54, 67], although these have been demonstrated not to obscure the biochemical differences associated with the disease. Adoption of the technique may differ for different clinical pathways.

For cervical cancer, the recent adoption of HPV primary screening means that the test is more of risk than of the presence of disease. A triage test is required to reduce unnecessary referral of HPV-positive women for further investigation and treatment. Cytology is currently utilized for triage after a HPV positive result and research is ongoing into molecular biomarkers of transforming HPV infection.

In the case of oral health screening, spectral cytology may be beneficial as an initial screening of patients with suspicious lesions in their oral cavity. The observation that Raman spectral cytopathology can identify field cancerization suggests that site-specific biopsies may not be required for such screening [69] and the technique may be used for regular screening in follow-up dysplasia clinics. Similarly, in the case of lung cancer screening, spectral cytopathological screening may be invaluable to reduce the requirements for tissue biopsies and, in cases of positive diagnoses, may be employed to identify lung cancer subtypes, and thus guide targeted therapies.

It has been well demonstrated that Raman spectral cytopathology can potentially lead the next stage of impact of cytology on human health and wellbeing, based on automated, objective screening for disease diagnostics, supported by increasingly sophisticated machine learning and artificial intelligence-based algorithms. Importantly, the technique is fundamentally a high-content analytical tool [42] and research is ongoing to further develop its capabilities in analysis of disease origin and progression [45], and development of therapeutic interventions [44].

References

1. Bell, S., O'Dowd, G. and Wright, S. (2020) *Wheater's Pathology: A Text, Atlas and Review of Histopathology.* Elsevier.
2. Koss, L. G. and Melamed, M. R., Eds. (2006) *Koss' Diagnostic Cytology and Its Histologic Bases* 5th ed. Lippincott Williams and Wilkins.
3. Karimi-Zarchi, M., Zanbagh, L., Shafii, A., Shokouh, T.-Z., Teimoori, S. and Yazdian-Anari, P. (2015) Comparison of Pap smear and colposcopy in screening for cervical cancer in patients with secondary immunodeficiency. Electron Physician **7**, 1542–1548.
4. Bobdey, S., Balasubramanium, G., Kumar, A. and Jain, A. (2015) Cancer screening: Should cancer screening be essential component of primary health care in developing countries? Int. J. Prev. Med. **6**, 56.
5. Nath, J., Bhattacharyya, A. and Deka, H. (2015) Comparative study between pap smear and visual inspection with acetic acid (via) in screening of CIN and early cervical cancer. J. Midlife. Health **6**, 53.
6. Micrographia — Robert Hooke.
7. Diamantis, A. and Magiorkinis, E. (2014) Pioneers of exfoliative cytology in the 19th century: The predecessors of George Papanicolaou. Cytopathology **25**, 215–224.
8. Triolo, V. A. (1965) Nineteenth century foundations of cancer research advances in tumor pathology, nomenclature, and theories of oncogenesis. Cancer Res. **25**, 75–106.
9. Elgert, P. A. and Gill, G. W. (2009) George N. Papanicolaou, MD, PhD. Lab. Med. **40**, 245–246.

10. Vilos, G. A. (1998) The history of the Papanicolaou smear and the Odyssey of George and andromache papanicolaou. Obstet. Gynecol. **91**, 479–483.
11. Papanicolaou, G. N. and Traut, H. F. (1941) The diagnostic value of vaginal smears in carcinoma of the uterus. Am. J. Obstet. Gynecol. **42**, 193–206.
12. Papanicolaou, G. N. and Traut, H. F. (1943) Diagnosis of uterine cancer by the vaginal smear. Arch. Intern. Med. **72**, 707.
13. Albrow, R., Kitchener, H., Gupta, N. and Desai, M. (2012) Cervical screening in England: The past, present, and future. Cancer Cytopathol. **120**, 87–96.
14. The History of Cervical Cancer Screening — Labtag Blog.
15. Gill, G. W. (2013) *Cytopreparation: Principles & Practice*. Springer.
16. Papanicolaou, G. N. (1942) A new procedure for staining vaginal smears. Science **95**, 438–439.
17. Rozemeijer, K., Penning, C., Siebers, A. G., Naber, S. K., Matthijsse, S. M., van Ballegooijen, M., van Kemenade, F. J. and de Kok, I. M. C. M. (2016) Comparing SurePath, ThinPrep, and conventional cytology as primary test method: SurePath is associated with increased CIN II+ detection rates. Cancer Causes Control **27**, 15–25.
18. Arbyn, M., Bergeron, C., Klinkhamer, P., Martin-Hirsch, P., Siebers, A. G. and Bulten, J. (2008) Liquid compared with conventional cervical cytology: A systematic review and meta-analysis. Obstet. Gynecol. **111**, 167–177.
19. Naylor, B. (2000) The century for cytopathology. Acta Cytol. **44**, 709–725.
20. Zink, D., Fischer, A. H. and Nickerson, J. A. (2004) Nuclear structure in cancer cells. Nat. Rev. Cancer **4**, 677–687.
21. Pangarkar, M. A. (2022) The Bethesda System for reporting cervical cytology. Cytojournal **19**, 28.
22. Standards for Quality Assurance in Cervical Screening Standards for Quality Assurance in Colposcopy-Interim Document.
23. Nanda, K., McCrory, D. C., Myers, E. R., Bastian, L. A., Hasselblad, V., Hickey, J. D. and Matchar, D. B. (2000) Accuracy of the papanicolaou test in screening for and follow-up of cervical cytologic abnormalities: A systematic review. Ann. Intern. Med. **132**, 810–819.
24. Baker, R. W., O'Sullivan, J. P., Hanley, J. and Coleman, D. V. (1999) The characteristics of false negative cervical smears — Implications for the UK cervical cancer screening programme. J. Clin. Pathol. **52**, 358–362.
25. Castillo, M., Astudillo, A., Clavero, O., Velasco, J., Ibáñez, R. and Desanjosé, S. (2016) Poor cervical cancer screening attendance and false negatives. A call for organized screening. PLoS One **11**, e0161403.
26. Sun, B., Yang, X., Ping, B., He, Y. and Zhang, Z. (2015) Impact of inconclusive endoscopic ultrasound-guided fine-needle aspiration results in the management and outcome of patients with solid pancreatic masses. Dig. Endosc. **27**, 130–136.

27. Yao, X., Gomes, M. M., Tsao, M. S., Allen, C. J., Geddie, W. and Sekhon, H. (2012) Fine-needle aspiration biopsy versus core-needle biopsy in diagnosing lung cancer: A systematic review. Curr. Oncol. **19**, 16–27.
28. Mendoza, P., Lacambra, M., Tan, P.-H. and Tse, G. M. (2011) Fine needle aspiration cytology of the breast: the nonmalignant categories. Patholog. Res. Int. **2011**, 1–8.
29. (2014) Cervical cancer and HPV — Management. NICE Clin. Knowl. Summ.
30. Garland, S. M., Kjaer, S. K., Muñoz, N., Block, S. L., Brown, D. R., Dinubile, M. J., Lindsay, B. R., Kuter, B. J., Perez, G., Dominiak-Felden, G., *et al.* (2016) Impact and effectiveness of the quadrivalent human papillomavirus vaccine: A systematic review of 10 years of real-world experience. Clin. Infect. Dis. **63**, 519–527.
31. Wong, A. A., Fuller, J., Pabbaraju, K., Wong, S. and Zahariadis, G. (2012) Comparison of the hybrid capture 2 and cobas 4800 tests for detection of high-risk human papillomavirus in specimens collected in PreserVcyt medium. J. Clin. Microbiol. **50**, 25–29.
32. Poljak, M., Kocjan, B. J., Oštrbenk, A. and Seme, K. (2016) Commercially available molecular tests for human papillomaviruses (HPV): 2015 update. J. Clin. Virol. **76**, S3–S13.
33. Haedicke, J. and Iftner, T. (2016) A review of the clinical performance of the Aptima HPV assay. J. Clin. Virol. **76**, S40–S48.
34. Tota, J. E., Bentley, J., Blake, J., Coutlée, F., Duggan, M. A., Ferenczy, A., Franco, E. L., Fung-Kee-Fung, M., Gotlieb, W., Mayrand, M. H., *et al.* (2017) Introduction of molecular HPV testing as the primary technology in cervical cancer screening: Acting on evidence to change the current paradigm. Prev. Med. (Baltim). **98**, 5–14.
35. Koliopoulos, G., Nyaga, V. N., Santesso, N., Bryant, A., Martin-Hirsch, P. P. L., Mustafa, R. A., Schünemann, H., Paraskevaidis, E. and Arbyn, M. (2017) Cytology versus HPV testing for cervical cancer screening in the general population. Cochrane Database Syst. Rev. **2017**, CD008587.
36. Shiraz, A., Crawford, R., Egawa, N., Griffin, H. and Doorbar, J. (2020) The early detection of cervical cancer. The current and changing landscape of cervical disease detection. Cytopathology **31**, 258–270.
37. Schubert, J. M., Bird, B., Papamarkakis, K., Miljković, M., Bedrossian, K., Laver, N. and Diem, M. (2010) Spectral cytopathology of cervical samples: Detecting cellular abnormalities in cytologically normal cells. Lab. Invest. **90**, 1068–1077.
38. Bonnier, F., Knief, P., Lim, B., Meade, A. D., Dorney, J., Bhattacharya, K., Lyng, F. M. and Byrne, H. J. (2010) Imaging live cells grown on a three dimensional collagen matrix using Raman microspectroscopy. Analyst **135**, 3169–3177.
39. Farhane, Z., Bonnier, F., Casey, A., Maguire, A., O'Neill, L. and Byrne, H. J. (2015) Cellular discrimination using in vitro Raman micro spectroscopy: the role of the nucleolus. Analyst **140**, 5908–5919.

40. Farhane, Z., Nawaz, H., Bonnier, F. and Byrne, H. J. (2018) In vitro label-free screening of chemotherapeutic drugs using Raman microspectroscopy: Towards a new paradigm of spectralomics. J. Biophotonics **11**, e201700258.
41. Efeoglu, E., Maher, M. A., Casey, A. and Byrne, H. J. (2018) Toxicological assessment of nanomaterials: the role of in vitro Raman microspectroscopic analysis. Anal. Bioanal. Chem. **410**, 1631–1646.
42. Byrne, H. J., Bonnier, F., Casey, A., Maher, M., McIntyre, J., Efeoglu, E. and Farhane, Z. (2018) Advancing Raman microspectroscopy for cellular and subcellular analysis: towards in vitro high-content spectralomic analysis. Appl. Opt. **57**, E11.
43. Meade, A. D., Byrne, H. J. and Lyng, F. M. (2010) Spectroscopic and chemometric approaches to radiobiological analyses. Mutat. Res. **704**, 108–114.
44. Meade, A. D., Howe, O., Unterreiner, V., Sockalingum, G. D., Byrne, H. J. and Lyng, F. M. (2016) Vibrational spectroscopy in sensing radiobiological effects: Analyses of targeted and non-targeted effects in human keratinocytes. Faraday Discuss. **187**, 213–234.
45. Ostrowska, K. M., Malkin, A., Meade, A., O'Leary, J., Martin, C., Spillane, C., Byrne, H. J. and Lyng, F. M. (2010) Investigation of the influence of high-risk human papillomavirus on the biochemical composition of cervical cancer cells using vibrational spectroscopy. Analyst **135**, 3087–3093.
46. WHO. (2020) Cancer Today. Int. Agency Res.
47. Vargis, E., Tang, Y. W., Khabele, D. and Mahadevan-Jansen, A. (2012) Near-infrared Raman microspectroscopy detects high-risk human papillomaviruses1. Transl. Oncol. **5**, 172–179.
48. Rubina, S., Amita, M., Kedar K., D., Bharat, R. and Krishna, C. M. (2013) Raman spectroscopic study on classification of cervical cell specimens. Vib. Spectrosc. **68**, 115–121.
49. Hole, A., Tyagi, G., Sahu, A., Shaikh, R. and Krishna, C. M. (2018) Exploration of Raman exfoliated cytology for oral and cervical cancers. Vib. Spectrosc. **98**, 35–40.
50. Bonnier, F., Traynor, D., Kearney, P., Clarke, C., Knief, P., Martin, C., O'Leary, J. J., Byrne, H. J. and Lyng, F. (2014) Processing ThinPrep cervical cytological samples for Raman spectroscopic analysis. Anal. Methods **6**, 7831–7841.
51. Traynor, D., Duraipandian, S., Martin, C. M., O'Leary, J. J. and Lyng, F. M. (2018) Improved removal of blood contamination from ThinPrep cervical cytology samples for Raman spectroscopic analysis. J. Biomed. Opt. **23**, 1.
52. Ramos, I. R., Meade, A. D., Ibrahim, O., Byrne, H. J., McMenamin, Ma., McKenna, M., Malkin, A. and Lyng, F. M. (2016) Raman spectroscopy for cytopathology of exfoliated cervical cells. Faraday Discuss. **187**, 187–198.
53. Kearney, P., Traynor, D., Bonnier, F., Lyng, F. M., O'Leary, J. J. and Martin, C. M. (2017) Raman spectral signatures of cervical exfoliated cells from liquid-based cytology samples. J. Biomed. Opt. **22**, 1.

54. Traynor, D., Kearney, P., Ramos, I., Martin, C. M., O'Leary, J. J. and Lyng, F. M. (2018) A study of hormonal effects in cervical smear samples using Raman spectroscopy. J. Biophotonics **11**, e201700240.
55. Traynor, D., Martin, C. M., White, C., Reynolds, S., D'arcy, T., O'leary, J. J. and Lyng, F. M. (2021) Raman spectroscopy of liquid-based cervical smear samples as a triage to stratify women who are hpv-positive on screening. Cancers (Basel) **13**, 2008.
56. Traynor, D., Duraipandian, S., Bhatia, R., Cuschieri, K., Tewari, P., Kearney, P., D'arcy, T., O'leary, J. J., Martin, C. M. and Lyng, F. M. (2022) Development and validation of a Raman spectroscopic classification model for cervical intraepithelial neoplasia (CIN). Cancers (Basel). **14**, 1836.
57. Aljakouch, K., Hilal, Z., Daho, I., Schuler, M., Krauß, S. D., Yosef, H. K., Dierks, J., Mosig, A., Gerwert, K. and El-Mashtoly, S. F. (2019) Fast and noninvasive diagnosis of cervical cancer by coherent anti-Stokes Raman scattering. Anal. Chem. **91**, 13900–13906.
58. Sitarz, K., Czamara, K., Bialecka, J., Klimek, M., Zawilinska, B., Szostek, S. and Kaczor, A. (2020) HPV infection significantly accelerates glycogen metabolism in cervical cells with large nuclei: Raman microscopic study with subcellular resolution. Int. J. Mol. Sci. **21**, 2667.
59. Sitarz, K., Czamara, K., Bialecka, J., Klimek, M., Szostek, S. and Kaczor, A. (2021) Dual switch in lipid metabolism in cervical epithelial cells during dysplasia development observed using raman microscopy and molecular methods. Cancers (Basel). **13**, 1997.
60. Karunakaran, V., Saritha, V. N., Joseph, M. M., Nair, J. B., Saranya, G., Raghu, K. G., Sujathan, K., Kumar, K. S. and Maiti, K. K. (2020) Diagnostic spectro-cytology revealing differential recognition of cervical cancer lesions by label-free surface enhanced Raman fingerprints and chemometrics. Nanomedicine **29**, 102276.
61. Karunakaran, V., Saritha, V. N., Ramya, A. N., Murali, V. P., Raghu, K. G., Sujathan, K. and Maiti, K. K. (2021) Elucidating Raman image-guided differential recognition of clinically confirmed grades of cervical exfoliated cells by dual biomarker-appended SERS-Tag. Anal. Chem. **93**, 11140–11150.
62. H. Alsarraf, A., Kujan, O. and Farah, C. S. (2018) The utility of oral brush cytology in the early detection of oral cancer and oral potentially malignant disorders: A systematic review. J. Oral Pathol. Med. **47**, 104–116.
63. Mehrotra, R. (2012) The role of cytology in oral lesions: A review of recent improvements. Diagn. Cytopathol. **40**, 73–83.
64. Sahu, A., Tawde, S., Pai, V., Gera, P., Chaturvedi, P., Nair, S. and Krishna, C. M. (2015) Raman spectroscopy and cytopathology of oral exfoliated cells for oral cancer diagnosis. Anal. Methods **7**, 7548–7559.
65. Sahu, A., Gera, P., Pai, V., Dubey, A., Tyagi, G., Waghmare, M., Pagare, S., Mahimkar, M. and Murali Krishna, C. (2017) Raman exfoliative cytology for oral precancer diagnosis. J. Biomed. Opt. **22**, 1.

66. Behl, I., Calado, G., Ibrahim, O., Malkin, A., Flint, S., Byrne, H. J. and Lyng, F. M. (2017) Development of methodology for Raman microspectroscopic analysis of oral exfoliated cells. Anal. Methods **9**, 937–948.
67. Behl, I., Calado, G., Malkin, A., Flint, S., Galvin, S., Healy, C. M., Pimentel, M. L., Byrne, H. J. and Lyng, F. M. (2020) A pilot study for early detection of oral premalignant diseases using oral cytology and Raman micro-spectroscopy: Assessment of confounding factors. J. Biophotonics **13**, e202000079.
68. Sahu, A., Gera, P., Malik, A., Nair, S., Chaturvedi, P. and Murali Krishna, C. (2019) Raman exfoliative cytology for prognosis prediction in oral cancers: A proof of concept study. J. Biophotonics **12**, e201800334.
69. Behl, I., Calado, G., Vishwakarma, A., Flint, S., Galvin, S., Healy, C. M., Leite Pimentel, M., Malkin, A., Byrne, H. J. and Lyng, F. M. (2020) Raman microspectroscopic study for the detection of oral field cancerisation using brush biopsy samples. J. Biophotonics **13**, e202000131.
70. Behl, I., Calado, G., Vishwakarma, A., Traynor, D., Flint, S., Galvin, S., Healy, C. M., Pimentel, M. L., Malkin, A., Byrne, H. J., *et al.* (2022) Classification of cytological samples from oral potentially malignant lesions through Raman spectroscopy: A pilot study. Spectrochim. Acta — Part A Mol. Biomol. Spectrosc. **266**, 120437.
71. Lewis, D. R., Check, D. P., Caporaso, N. E., Travis, W. D. and Devesa, S. S. (2014) US lung cancer trends by histologic type. Cancer **120**, 2883–2892.
72. Houston, K. A., Henley, S. J., Li, J., White, M. C. and Richards, T. B. (2014) Patterns in lung cancer incidence rates and trends by histologic type in the United States, 2004–2009. Lung Cancer **86**, 22–28.
73. Almeida, F. A. (2012) Bronchoscopy and endobronchial ultrasound for diagnosis and staging of lung cancer. Cleve. Clin. J. Med. **79**, 11–16.
74. O'Dea, D. (2020) Raman microspectroscopy for the discrimination of thyroid and lung cancer subtypes for application in clinical cytopathology. Doctoral Thesis, Technological University Dublin.
75. Murphy, W. M., Soloway, M. S., Jukkola, A. F., Crabtree, W. N. and Ford, K. S. (1984) Urinary cytology and bladder cancer. The cellular features of transitional cell neoplasms. Cancer **53**, 1555–1565.
76. Koss, L. G., Deitch, D., Ramanathan, R. and Sherman, A. B. (1985) Diagnostic value of cytology of voided urine. Acta Cytol. **29**, 810–816.
77. Shapiro, A., Gofrit, O. N., Pizov, G., Cohen, J. K. and Maier, J. (2011) Raman molecular imaging: A novel spectroscopic technique for diagnosis of bladder cancer in urine specimens. Eur. Urol. **59**, 106–112.
78. Yosef, H. K., Krauß, S. D., Lechtonen, T., Jütte, H., Tannapfel, A., Käfferlein, H. U., Brüning, T., Roghmann, F., Noldus, J., Mosig, A., *et al.* (2017) Noninvasive diagnosis of high-grade urothelial carcinoma in urine by Raman spectral imaging. Anal. Chem. **89**, 6893–6899.

79. Hu, D., Xu, X., Zhao, Z., Li, C., Tian, Y., Liu, Q., Shao, B., Chen, S., Zhao, Y., Li, L., *et al.* (2021) Detecting urine metabolites of bladder cancer by surface-enhanced Raman spectroscopy. Spectrochim. Acta A **247**, 119108.
80. Traynor, D., Behl, I., O'Dea, D., Bonnier, F., Nicholson, S., O'Connell, F., Maguire, A., Flint, S., Galvin, S., Healy, C. M., *et al.* (2021) Raman spectral cytopathology for cancer diagnostic applications. Nat. Protoc. **16**, 3716–3735.
81. Byrne, H. J., Knief, P., Keating, M. E. and Bonnier, F. (2016) Spectral pre and post processing for infrared and Raman spectroscopy of biological tissues and cells. Chem. Soc. Rev. **45**, 1865–1878.
82. Liland, K. H., Kohler, A. and Afseth, N. K. (2016) Model-based pre-processing in Raman spectroscopy of biological samples. J. Raman Spectrosc. **47**, 643–650.
83. Storey, E. E. and Helmy, A. S. (2019) Optimized preprocessing and machine learning for quantitative Raman spectroscopy in biology. J. Raman Spectrosc. **50**, 958–968.
84. Bonnier, F., Knief, P., Meade, A. D., Dorney, J., Bhattacharya, K., Lyng, F. M. and Byrne, H. J. (2011) Collagen matrices as an improved model for in vitro study of live cells using Raman microspectroscopy. In *Clinical and Biomedical Spectroscopy and Imaging II* (Ramanujam, N. and Popp, J., Eds.), Vol. 8087 of Proceedings of SPIE-OSA Biomedical Optics (Optica Publishing Group, 2011), paper 80870F.
85. Fullwood, L. M., Griffiths, D., Ashton, K., Dawson, T., Lea, R. W., Davis, C., Bonnier, F., Byrne, H. J. and Baker, M. J. (2013) Effect of substrate choice and tissue type on tissue preparation for spectral histopathology by Raman microspectroscopy. Analyst **139**, 446–454.
86. Kerr, L. T., Byrne, H. J. and Hennelly, B. M. (2015) Optimal choice of sample substrate and laser wavelength for Raman spectroscopic analysis of biological specimen. Anal. Methods **7**, 5041–5052.
87. Gargotti, M., Efeoglu, E., Byrne, H. J. and Casey, A. (2018) Raman spectroscopy detects biochemical changes due to different cell culture environments in live cells in vitro. Anal. Bioanal. Chem. **410**, 7537–7550.
88. Baker, M. J., Byrne, H. J., Chalmers, J., Gardner, P., Goodacre, R., Henderson, A., Kazarian, S. G., Martin, F. L., Moger, J., Stone, N., *et al.* (2018) Clinical applications of infrared and Raman spectroscopy: State of play and future challenges. Analyst **143**, 1735–1757.
89. Behl, I., *et al.* (2019) Raman microspectroscopy for detection of oral potentially malignant disorders using minimally invasive brush biopsy samples. J. Biophotonics **13**, e202000131.
90. Morais, C. L. M., Lima, K. M. G., Singh, M. and Martin, F. L. (2020) Tutorial: multivariate classification for vibrational spectroscopy in biological samples. Nat. Protoc. **15**, 2143–2162.

91. Bonnier, F. and Byrne, H. J. (2012) Understanding the molecular information contained in principal component analysis of vibrational spectra of biological systems. Analyst **137**, 322–332.
92. Lyng, F. M., Faoláin, E. Ó., Conroy, J., Meade, A. D., Knief, P., Duffy, B., Hunter, M. B., Byrne, J. M., Kelehan, P. and Byrne, H. J. (2007) Vibrational spectroscopy for cervical cancer pathology, from biochemical analysis to diagnostic tool. Exp. Mol. Pathol. **82**, 121–129.
93. Dixon, S. J. and Brereton, R. G. (2009) Comparison of performance of five common classifiers represented as boundary methods: Euclidean Distance to Centroids, Linear Discriminant Analysis, Quadratic Discriminant Analysis, Learning Vector Quantization and Support Vector Machines, as dependent on. Chemom. Intell. Lab. Syst. **95**, 1–17.
94. Kyrgiou, M., Arbyn, M., Bergeron, C., Bosch, F. X., Dillner, J., Jit, M., Kim, J., Poljak, M., Nieminen, P., Sasieni, P., *et al.* (2020) Cervical screening: ESGO-EFC position paper of the European Society of Gynaecologic Oncology (ESGO) and the European Federation of Colposcopy (EFC). Br. J. Cancer **123**, 510–517.
95. Duraipandian, S., Traynor, D., Kearney, P., Martin, C., O'Leary, J. J. and Lyng, F. M. (2018) Raman spectroscopic detection of high-grade cervical cytology: Using morphologically normal appearing cells. Sci. Rep. **8**, 15048.
96. Shambayati, B. (2011) *Cytopathology.* Oxford University Press.
97. Traynor, D., Duraipandian, S., Bhatia, R., Cuschieri, K., Martin, C. M., O'Leary, J. J. and Lyng, F. M. (2019) The potential of biobanked liquid based cytology samples for cervical cancer screening using Raman spectroscopy. J. Biophotonics **12**, e201800377.
98. Sarri, B., Appay, R., Heuke, S., Poizat, F., Franchi, F., Boissonneau, S., Caillol, F., Dufour, H., Figarella-Branger, D., Giovaninni, M., *et al.* (2021) Observation of the compatibility of stimulated Raman histology with pathology workflow and genome sequencing. Transl. Biophotonics **3**, e202000020.
99. Instant Tissue Histology with the BondXplorer microscope — Lightcore Technologies.
100. Made in Quebec: Illuminating hidden brain cancer cells | Reveal Surgical.
101. Pinto, M., Zorn, K. C., Tremblay, J.-P., Desroches, J., Dallaire, F., Aubertin, K., Marple, E., Kent, C., Leblond, F., Trudel, D., *et al.* (2019) Integration of a Raman spectroscopy system to a robotic-assisted surgical system for real-time tissue characterization during radical prostatectomy procedures. J. Biomed. Opt. **24**, 1–10.
102. InSplorer Endoscope — Lightcore Technologies.
103. Septier, D., Mytskaniuk, V., Habert, R., LABAT, D., Baudelle, K., Cassez, A., Brevalle, G., Conforti, M., Bouwmans, G., Rigneault, H., *et al.* (2022) Label-free highly multimodal nonlinear endoscope. Opt. Express **30**, 25020–25033.
104. Technology | Dxcover.
105. CanSense — Innovation in cancer diagnostics.

106. Byrne, H. J., Baranska, M., Puppels, G. J., Stone, N., Wood, B., Gough, K. M., Lasch, P., Heraud, P., Sulé-Suso, J. and Sockalingum, G. D. (2015) Spectropathology for the next generation: Quo vadis? Analyst **140**, 2066–2073.
107. O'Dwyer, K., Domijan, K., Dignam, A., Butler, M. and Hennelly, B. M. (2021) Automated Raman micro-spectroscopy of epithelial cell nuclei for high-throughput classification. Cancers (Basel) **13**, 4767.

https://doi.org/10.1142/9789811264610_0013

Chapter 13

Exploring the Hidden Realms: New Frontiers for Raman Spectroscopy in Life Sciences

Jeong Hee Kim,[1] Swati Tanwar,[1] Zhenhui Liu,[1] Ishan Barman[1-3,*]

[1]*Department of Mechanical Engineering, Johns Hopkins University, Baltimore, MD, 21218, USA*
[2]*Department of Oncology, Johns Hopkins University School of Medicine, Baltimore, MD, 21287, USA*
[3]*The Russell H. Morgan Department of Radiology and Radiological Science, Division of Cancer Imaging Research, Johns Hopkins University School of Medicine, Baltimore, MD, 21205, USA*
**Corresponding author: ibarman@jhu.edu*

13.1 Introduction

For the last several decades, Raman spectroscopy has demonstrated its value in the study of life sciences as a powerful analytical technique [1, 2]. Raman spectroscopy can provide molecular information of various biological samples with respect to their composition, concentration, and structure in an objective, quantitative, and non-invasive manner [3, 4]. Some of the main applications of Raman spectroscopy in the life sciences include cell and tissue analysis [5–8], drug discovery and development [9, 10], diagnostics [11–13], bacteria and virus identification [14–16], protein and nucleic acid analysis [17–19] and pharmaceuticals [20–22]. Among those, its use in cancer diagnostics and treatment [23–28] and cell and tissue analysis across various pathological states [29–31] have received considerable contemporary attention.

Also, the advent of highly sensitive variants of Raman spectroscopy has expanded its applications within biomedical research and accelerated its translation from a lab to a clinical setting [32–36]. One of the most prominent techniques is surface-enhanced Raman spectroscopy (SERS), which provides significantly improved molecular sensitivity and specificity compared to what Raman spectroscopy can offer [37–42]. Such amplification in SERS signal is facilitated by surface plasmon phenomena with the use of metallic nano substrates [43–46].

In this chapter, we aim to introduce and discuss two relatively underexplored applications of Raman spectroscopy in the life sciences: [1] decoding the interactions between cancer and microbiota and [2] unraveling the formation of amyloid proteins from molecular to tissue level. Despite their clinical significance and the promise of Raman spectroscopy for these use cases, the investigation using Raman spectroscopy has not been as active as other highly recognized areas. We demonstrate current studies covering these topics in the following two sections, and highlight the potential use of Raman spectroscopy to further stimulate investigations. Additionally, in this chapter, we feature four topics at the forefront of SERS applications ranging from studying basic cellular processes to detection of infectious diseases, cancer imaging and image-guided surgery.

13.2 Decoding the Cancer-Microbiota Interactions

Raman spectroscopy has been extensively used for the study of cancer and human microbiome, with each of them being a huge topic that demands dedicated research efforts. Recently the two fields have started to overlap, as the role of human microbiota in cancer initiation and progression is getting recognized. With our understanding of the interactions between cancer and microbiota still being limited, a comprehensive analysis with various molecular techniques is desired to improve our knowledge base. Raman spectroscopy, owing to its advantages in molecular specificity and being non-perturbative and label-free, could bring new insights into this interdisciplinary area [47], in addition to the techniques already deployed such as next-generation sequencing and fluorescence or magnetic tagging. In this section, we highlight two areas where Raman spectroscopy can be applied for the characterization of cancer microbiota interactions: intratumor microbiota, and the effects of microbial metabolites on cancer cells.

13.2.1 *Intratumor Microbiota*

Bacteria are known to be present in many types of human tumors. Recently, efforts have been made to profile the bacterial composition in different tumor types [48], but it still remains unclear how bacteria affect the growth of cancer cells or vice versa. These bacteria were found to be mostly intracellular, residing inside cancer or immune cells. Therefore, in order to study the interactions between cancer cells and intratumor bacteria, the desired technique should be capable of first distinguishing between the two counterparts, and second extracting genotype or phenotype information from them. Raman spectroscopy is a promising candidate for such applications because its compatibility with optical microscopy allows researchers to achieve high spatial resolution and molecular specificity simultaneously, which can help identify bacteria inside cancer cells, and characterize the molecular compositions of both.

The identification of intracellular bacteria with Raman microspectroscopy has been achieved in different cell types. For example, Große *et al.* conducted Raman imaging on EA.hy926 endothelial cells infected with *Staphylococcus aureus* [49]. 3D Raman spectra were collected in the fingerprint region of 400–1850 cm^{-1}, as well as the high-wavenumber region of 2770–3025 cm^{-1}. An unsupervised unmixing algorithm, N-FINDR, was used to identify bacteria and cellular components, according to the similarity of each spectrum to the individual endmember calculated from the algorithm. Such analysis yields realistic false color images to visualize the intracellular *S. aureus* with high spatial resolution and specificity, which was confirmed with immunostaining and fluorescence microscopy (Figure 13.1). In a similar study, Silge *et al.* conducted 3D Raman mapping on *Mycobacterium gordonae*-infected macrophages [50]. The intracellular *M. gordonae* could be identified based on the Raman peaks at 1155 and 1524 cm^{-1}, which were attributable to carotenoids synthesized by the bacteria. These two studies showcased the versatility of Raman spectroscopy for intracellular bacteria detection. It can either use single peaks unique to the bacteria or, in the absence of such peaks, be followed by multivariate analysis to extract and differentiate the molecular compositions of bacteria and host cells, using the full Raman spectrum.

While the cancer research community has been mostly focusing on the bacteria in the human microbiota, other components such as fungi, viruses, and protozoans might be equally important. Raman spectroscopy, unlike some other techniques specific to bacteria, is versatile and can be used to

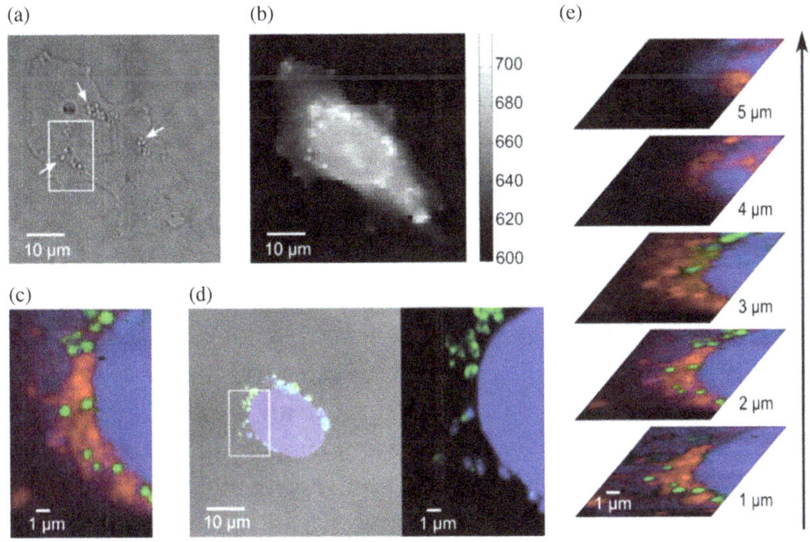

Figure 13.1. Raman-based imaging and identification of intracellular bacteria. (a) Bright field image showing *S. aureus* in an infected EA.hy926 endothelial cell, appearing as spherical particles of ~1 μm in diameter. (b) Raman mapping of the same cell based on the Raman peak intensity at 2938 cm^{-1}, which corresponds to CH stretching vibration. (c) False-color Raman image of the marked section in (a). The relative RGB color shows the intensity of Raman signals assigned to bacteria (green), cellular nucleus (blue), perinuclear region (red), and background (black). (d) Fluorescence image of the same cell stained for *S. aureus* (green) and DNA (blue), confirming the Raman analysis. (e) Raman images taken in Z stacks, showing the 3D distribution of *S. aureus* inside the host cell. Reproduced from Ref. [49] with permission.

elucidate the interactions between cancer cells and other types of microbes. In addition, Raman spectroscopy can achieve more sophisticated analysis on top of intracellular microbe detection. Since the Raman spectrum reflects the molecular composition of the samples, with certain benchmarks, it will inform us about the change in the molecular phenotypes of the cells. This works for both the intracellular microbes and the host cells. Naemat *et al.* used Raman microspectroscopy to characterize the spatial and temporal molecular changes in *T. gondii* tachyzoites and *T. gondii*-infected human retinal cells [51]. Principal component analysis (PCA) was performed to resolve the different molecular components such as proteins, lipids, nucleic acids, and water background. Interestingly, they found a significant increase in the lipid and protein contents in the *T. gondii* tachyzoites as the infection progressed inside the host cells. In another study, Sinjab *et al.* integrated Raman microspectroscopy with holographic optical tweezers to allow for spatial manipulation of *T. gondii* and control their infection on human cerebrovascular endothelial cells [52]. Stable isotope labeling in culture was used to track the exchange of phenylalanine between them. Live cell monitoring of the infection process revealed that as soon as 15 minutes after infection initiation, there had been phenylalanine transfer from the host cells to *T. gondii*.

The aforementioned studies were performed on different host cell types, including endothelial cells, retinal cells, and macrophages, as well as different microbes such as bacteria and parasites, which demonstrated the feasibility of applying Raman spectroscopy on a system of cancer cells and intratumor microbes. Many insights could potentially be gained from such investigations. For example, the change in lipid and protein contents and the material transfer between cancer cells and microbes suggest an important role of intratumor microbes in tumor growth. Increased energy expenditure and rapid metabolism and proliferation are hallmarks of cancer cells, and the accumulation of intracellular lipids can serve as an additional energy reserve to support cancer cell growth. However, these studies indicate that the intracellular microbes acquire energy and materials from cancer cells, a process appearing in favor of the microbes but not the cancer cells. It is still too early to say whether the intratumor microbiota is beneficial or detrimental to tumor growth, but these studies opened the door for further investigations using Raman spectroscopy.

13.2.2 *Effects of Microbial Metabolites on Cancer Cells*

Apart from direct microbial infections, the human microbiota can also impact cancer initiation and growth indirectly, through the synthesis and secretion of metabolites, signaling intermediates, and toxins. For example, three groups of bacterial genotoxins, including the cytolethal distending toxin family, the typhoid toxin, and colibactin have been identified that can induce DNA damage in host cells [53]. DNA damage increases the genomic instability of cells, which leads to a higher chance of cancer development. In addition to bacterial genotoxins, there are various other types of microbial metabolites that could affect cancer cells in ways still unknown to us. Raman spectroscopy, with its capability to probe the ensemble changes in the biomolecular composition of cells, is well suited for such use cases. Raman spectroscopy can be used as a quick first-level characterization tool to find out the major changes in cancer cells caused by microbial metabolites, which can then be followed by more dedicated techniques to pinpoint the exact mechanism of the effect.

As the first attempt to use Raman spectroscopy for such applications, our team studied breast cancer cells exposed to *Bacteroides fragilis* toxin (BFT) [54]. BFT is a toxin secreted by enterotoxigenic *B. fragilis* (ETBF), which are virulent strains of *B. fragilis*, a bacterium commonly found in the human gut microbiota. Previous studies indicated that BFT has a causative effect on colorectal cancer. Interestingly, *B. fragilis* was also found in cancerous breast, and ETBF plays an important role in cell proliferation and tumor metastatic progression.

In this context, our laboratory has used Raman spectroscopy, in combination with machine learning, to investigate the bimolecular responses of breast cancer cells to BFT exposure. Raman spectra were first collected on pellets of cells with or without BFT exposure, and through PCA analysis we found that BFT-treated cells have a higher abundance in Raman features such as tyrosine (831, 1164 cm^{-1}), glucose (911 cm^{-1}) and glycogen (1157 cm^{-1}), and lower abundance in Raman features such as phenylalanine (997, 1581 cm^{-1}), amide I (1640–1680 cm^{-1}), and amide III bands (1241 cm^{-1}) for proteins, ribose (1124 cm^{-1}), and guanine (1312, 1331 cm^{-1}) for nucleic acids (Figure 13.2). Furthermore, we acquired Raman spectra from single cells, and with a machine learning algorithm distinguished between cells with and without BFT exposure with good sensitivity and specificity. Our study demonstrated that Raman spectroscopy is able to recognize biomolecular responses of cancer cells to microbial metabolite exposure. In particular, the assigned Raman bands may suggest that BFT exposure leads to reprogrammed glucose metabolism such as increased glucose uptake. The downstream information from Raman spectroscopy provides directions for further studies to find out the upstream signaling pathway alterations causing the changes.

In addition to the ensemble characterization by spontaneous Raman spectroscopy, other variations of the technique such as stimulated Raman spectroscopy (SRS) and SERS can be used in a more targeted manner to analyze one or a few types of molecules inside cells. One example of this, which has great potential in the context of cancer-microbiota interactions, is the analysis of epithelial-mesenchymal transition (EMT).

EMT is a process where cells with an epithelial phenotype adopt a mesenchymal phenotype that is more motile and invasive. For cancer, this means the cancer cells will have a higher migration and invasion potential, and there is an increased risk of cancer progression and metastasis [55]. Many Gram-negative bacteria are known to secrete metabolites, such as lipopolysaccharide

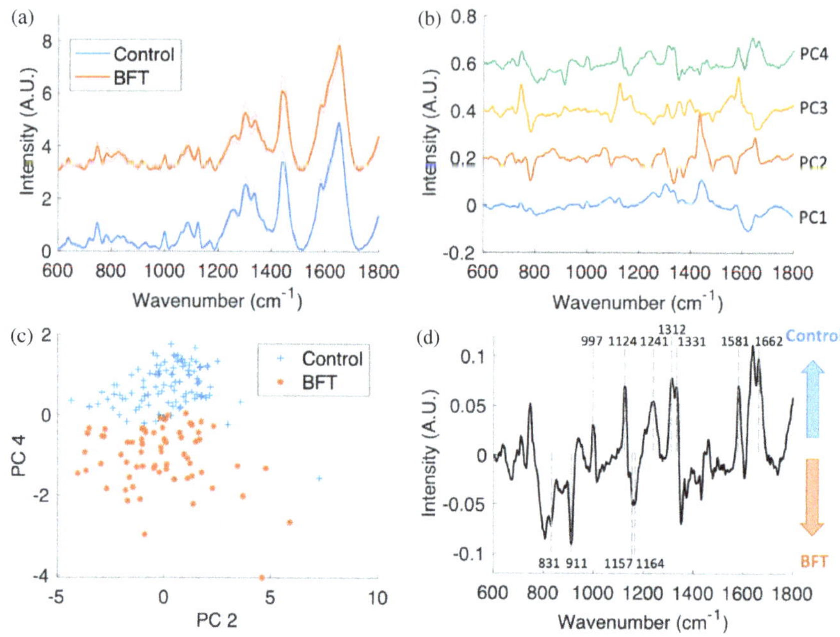

Figure 13.2. Molecular analysis with Raman spectroscopy on MCF7 breast cancer cells exposed to *Bacteroides fragilis* toxin secreted by enterotoxigenic *B. fragilis*. (a) Raman spectra acquired on cells with and without BFT treatment. (b) PCA analysis on the Raman spectra. The first four principal components (PCs) are plotted. (c) Scores of PC2 and PC4, showing that the BFT-treated and control cells are clearly separated in the scores of PC4. (d) Raman band assignment on PC4 with prominent spectral features indicated with the dashed lines. The bands with positive values are more abundant in control cells, and the bands with negative values are more abundant in BFT-treated cells. Reproduced from Ref. [54] with permission.

and acetate, that promote EMT in cancer [56]. Therefore, some microbial metabolites pose a risk of poor prognosis and worse outcomes for cancer patients. Further understanding and detection of the downstream effects, such as EMT, has great significance in the clinical setting.

Raman spectroscopy can reveal the changes in not only the overall cellular composition, but also several specific biomarkers during EMT. In one study, Marro *et al.* analyzed a breast epithelial cell line with Raman spectroscopy and found that EMT is associated with lower keratin, higher tryptophan, and increased fatty acids [57]. In another study, Zhang *et al.* imaged breast cancer cells using SRS, and the intracellular distribution of labeled amino acids, choline, glucose, and palmitate acids suggested that after EMT, the cells have decreased protein synthesis, reduced membrane phospholipid synthesis, and increased fatty acid uptake [58]. Lastly, for clinical translation of diagnosis,

Zhang *et al.* used SERS probes coupled with E-cadherin and N-cadherin antibodies to successfully detect the upregulation of N-cadherin expression and downregulation of E-cadherin expression in the lysate of breast cancer cells after EMT. This assay was further applied to plasma samples from human subjects [59].

To summarize, while the importance of microbiota in cancer is recognized, a lot is still unknown regarding their interactions. With the two use cases described above, we envision the increasing adoption of Raman spectroscopy in the cancer-microbiota research community and expect that it will not only accelerate our progress in understanding this complex system, but also achieve clinical translation in the future.

13.3 The Study of Amyloid Proteins Using Raman Spectroscopy

Proteins, essential macromolecules that constitute the majority of the dry mass of living organisms [60], are one of the most frequently studied biomolecules using Raman spectroscopy and its variants [61–63]. In addition to traditional tools for studying proteins, such as nuclear magnetic resonance spectroscopy and X-ray crystallography, Raman spectroscopy has successfully demonstrated the ability to identify proteins with respect to their structures and conformations. Also, other forms of Raman spectroscopy, such as SERS, tip-enhanced Raman spectroscopy (TERS), and UV resonance Raman spectroscopy have characterized proteins at a single-molecule level [64–66]. For proteins to express biological functionality, they must undergo proper folding, assisted by molecular chaperones, into native, defined three-dimensional structures. Otherwise, misfolded proteins are prone to forming toxic aggregates, including soluble oligomers and fibrillar amyloid deposits, shown in Figure 13.3(a) [67–69]. Amyloid proteins present in tissues and organs across the human body are associated with numerous pathologies, including neurodegenerative diseases and other non-neuropathic organ-specific conditions. Over the years, Raman spectroscopy has been applied to elucidate amyloid proteins and their links to pathology.

In this section, we will concentrate on the study of amyloids using spontaneous Raman spectroscopy. This section will cover 1) the structure of amyloid proteins, 2) their progression into insoluble aggregates, and 3) deposits embedded in tissues, explored by Raman spectroscopy.

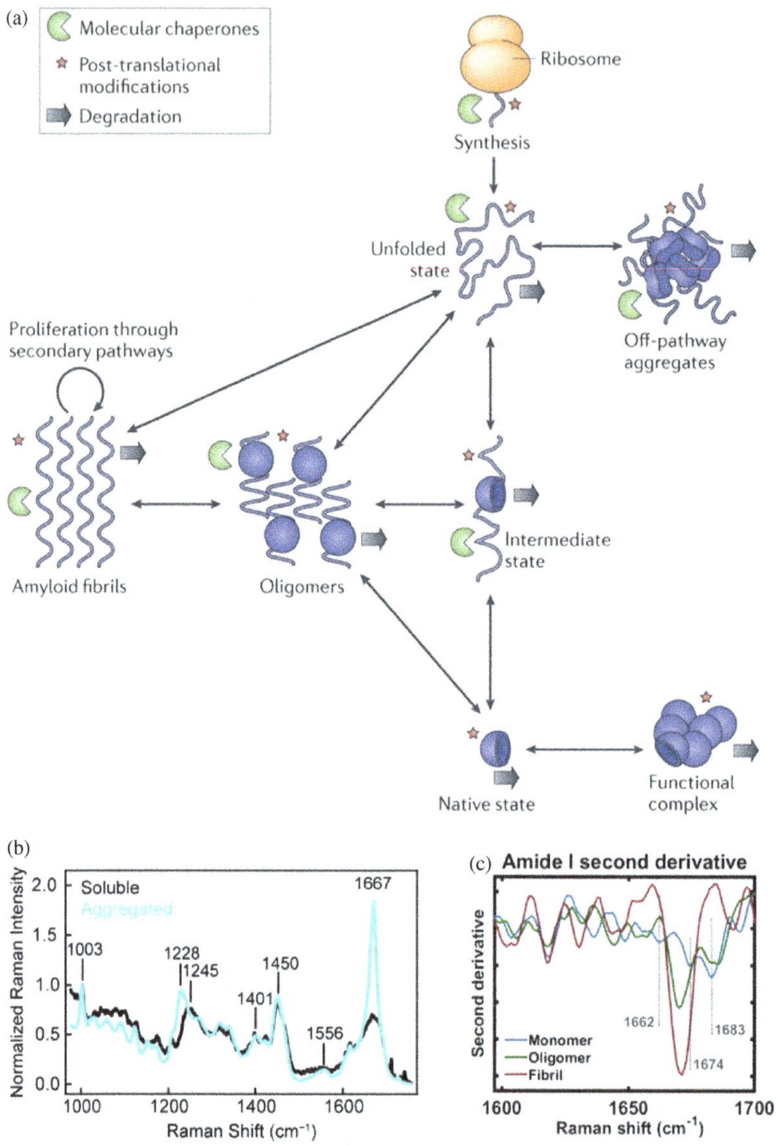

Figure 13.3. (a) Protein chains exhibit various interconvertible conformations at different folding states. Proteins in the amyloid state present a highly ordered form of aggregate with the polypeptide chains adopting a fibrillar structure. Amyloid fibrils are generally formed from unfolded or partially folded protein polypeptide chains. Amyloid fibrils are insoluble, non-crystalline, and rich in β-sheets. (b) Comparison of normalized Raman spectra α-synuclein before (black) and after (cyan) aggregation. Noticeable changes observed at 1667 cm^{-1}. (c) Comparison of Raman second derivative spectra of tau during aggregation from monomer (blue) to oligomer (green) and fibril (red). Noticeable changes observed at amide-I band. Reproduced from (a): Ref. [67]; (b): Ref. [70]; (c): Ref. [71] with permission.

13.3.1 *Amyloid Fibril Structures and Formation*

Raman spectroscopy has been utilized to study the numerous structures and conformations of amyloid fibrils. Structural analysis reveals that different proteins aggregate into filamentous structures in various arrangements, all broadly termed as amyloids. In some cases, peptide strands are stacked in parallel and antiparallel sheets; in others, they form subunit stacks that develop into the fibril. All amyloid fibrils share a cross-β architecture, where β-strands are aligned perpendicular to the axis of the fibril, with hydrogen bonds located between β-strands.

Researchers have applied Raman spectroscopy to investigate the structure of amyloid fibrils, particularly by probing protein secondary structures and their changes. As water does not display a strong spontaneous Raman signature, measurements of amyloid fibrils can be taken in either solution or solid forms with minimal to no sample preparation. Various amyloid proteins have been investigated using Raman spectroscopy. The most prevalently studied ones are α-synuclein (α-syn), amyloid β (Aβ), and tau. α-syn and Aβ are associated with Parkinson's disease and Alzheimer's disease, respectively; tau is broadly associated with neurodegenerative diseases.

Maiti and coworkers studied the environmentally determined conformational plasticity of α-syn [72]. They showed that α-syn, prior to fibril formation, can interchange its secondary structure conformations between α-helix (1653 cm^{-1}) and β-sheet (1667 cm^{-1}), depending on the local environment. Flynn and coworkers have identified α-syn amyloid fibrils in buffer solution [70]. Their work on α-syn fibrils formed in varying conditions, such as pH and ionic strength, demonstrates that Raman spectroscopy can reveal molecular-level conformational changes of amyloid fibrils (Figure 13.3(b)). Also, Imanbekova and coworkers identified Aβ secreted in extracellular vesicles [73]. While probing molecular features of Aβ in such conditions complicates Raman spectra analysis compared to investigation of synthesized fibrils, they could distinguish extracellular vesicles containing Aβ proteins from those that do not, based on characteristic peaks and PCA.

Several studies involved amyloid proteins associated with non-neuropathic diseases. Louros and coworkers examined the structural core of islet amyloid polypeptides (IAPP), a hallmark of type II diabetes. [74]. Second derivate analysis of IAPP and its four mutants with varying peptide residues revealed that they all form into β-sheet structures, regardless of the alternations made in their structural units. Flynn and coworkers extended the study to different types of synthesized amyloid fibrils, including α-syn, Aβ, and apolipoprotein C-III (ApoCIII), which are associated with cardiovascular diseases [75]. Raman spectra of synthesized fibrils showed shared peaks at amide I and III for all types tested. However, second derivative analysis unveiled subtle structural differences, both between the two amyloids linked to neurodegeneration and between them and ApoCIII.

13.3.2 *Amyloid Formation*

To fully understand the mechanisms behind the aggregation process of a given protein, all intermediate conformational states and oligomeric structures incorporating polypeptide chains must be identified. In the aggregation process, different amyloid proteins are influenced by their thermodynamics and kinetics. Also, various environmental or chemical factors, such as pH, temperature, and peptide concentration, play a vital role in aggregation steps. Researchers have elucidated the nature of transitional forms in between various conformational states and the formation of mature amyloid fibrils. Raman spectroscopy has also provided important insights into amyloid formation under various conditions. Ishigaki and coworkers explored the influence of salt conditions and temperature on insulin amyloid formation [76]. They found that changes in secondary β-sheet structure were facilitated by the addition of salt and an increase in heating temperature during aggregation. Also, time-resolved changes in the amide I band matched with the three phases of amyloid fibrillation: nucleation, elongation, and equilibrium. Devitt and coworkers have also monitored conformational changes in the β-sheet structure of three different amyloidogenic proteins: bovine serum albumin, β2-microglobulin, and tau, as they aggregate from monomers into oligomers, and fibrils [71]. Second derivative analysis on the amide I band of all three proteins showed an increase in intensity during aggregation, indicating the formation of β-sheet-rich structures (Figure 13.3(c)).

13.3.3 *Tissue-Embedded Amyloid Fibrils*

Various researchers have used Raman spectroscopy directly on amyloid deposits in tissues to explore its potential for clinical applications. Although the tissue environment adds complexity to amyloid fibril analysis due to other molecules interacting and interfering with the Raman signatures arising from amyloid proteins, Raman spectroscopy demonstrated the possibility for the label-free detection and diagnosis of amyloids within tissues.

Because of the predominant interest in neurodegenerative diseases, brain tissues have received much of the attention in elucidating the connection between amyloid aggregates and these diseases. Fonseca and coworkers have identified Aβ aggregates in mouse brain tissues [77]. They observed the characteristic peak in amide I, which is due to the vibrational frequency of the β-sheet secondary structure, from tissue spectra after conducting unsupervised unmixing analysis of synthesized Aβ fibrils. Corresponding studies were conducted in a rat model with similar results [78]. Hippocampal tissues from rats injected with Aβ_{25-35} also exhibited a Raman peak in amide I attributed to the change in dominant secondary structure after amyloid aggregation, from α-helices to β-sheets. In addition, researchers identified an increase in cholesterol content in the rat Aβ tissues. Another study examined conformational changes of Aβ_{1-42} through longitudinal monitoring of a rat model facilitated by ozone exposure, which induced oxidative stress [79]. Deconvolution analysis of Raman spectra of rat brain tissues in this model demonstrated changes in the amide I band profile: at the beginning of the study, this showed a dominant α-helix peptide profile (1665 cm^{-1}) featuring a β-turn structure. However, over time, this structure continually decreased in abundance, with β-sheets (1672 cm^{-1}) dominating towards the end of monitoring.

Also, several researchers investigated human brain tissues featuring Aβ aggregates from Alzheimer's disease patients. Lochocki and coworkers used formalin-fixed, paraffin-embedded brain tissues after dewaxing [80]. Michael and coworkers identified β-sheet secondary structures and localized them within unstained human brain tissues through hyperspectral Raman data [81]. Coupled with hierarchical cluster analysis, Raman spectra revealed prominent β-sheet structures (1666 cm^{-1}) within both plaque-like and tangle-like morphologies of amyloid aggregates (Figure 13.4(a)). Another recent study revealed the possible role of carotenoids in Aβ aggregates [82].

The application of Raman spectroscopy has also expanded to other parts of the body, including the eyes and cardiovascular tissues. Sevgi and coworkers observed α-syn aggregates within rat brain and colon tissues [83]. This study explored whether α-syn can be detected in peripheral tissues for the diagnosis of Parkinson's disease. Raman spectra of colon tissues showed changes in protein conformation, denoted by α-helix (1317 cm^{-1}) and β-sheet (1248 cm^{-1}) structures in amide III (Figure 13.4(c)). PCA further revealed conformational changes of

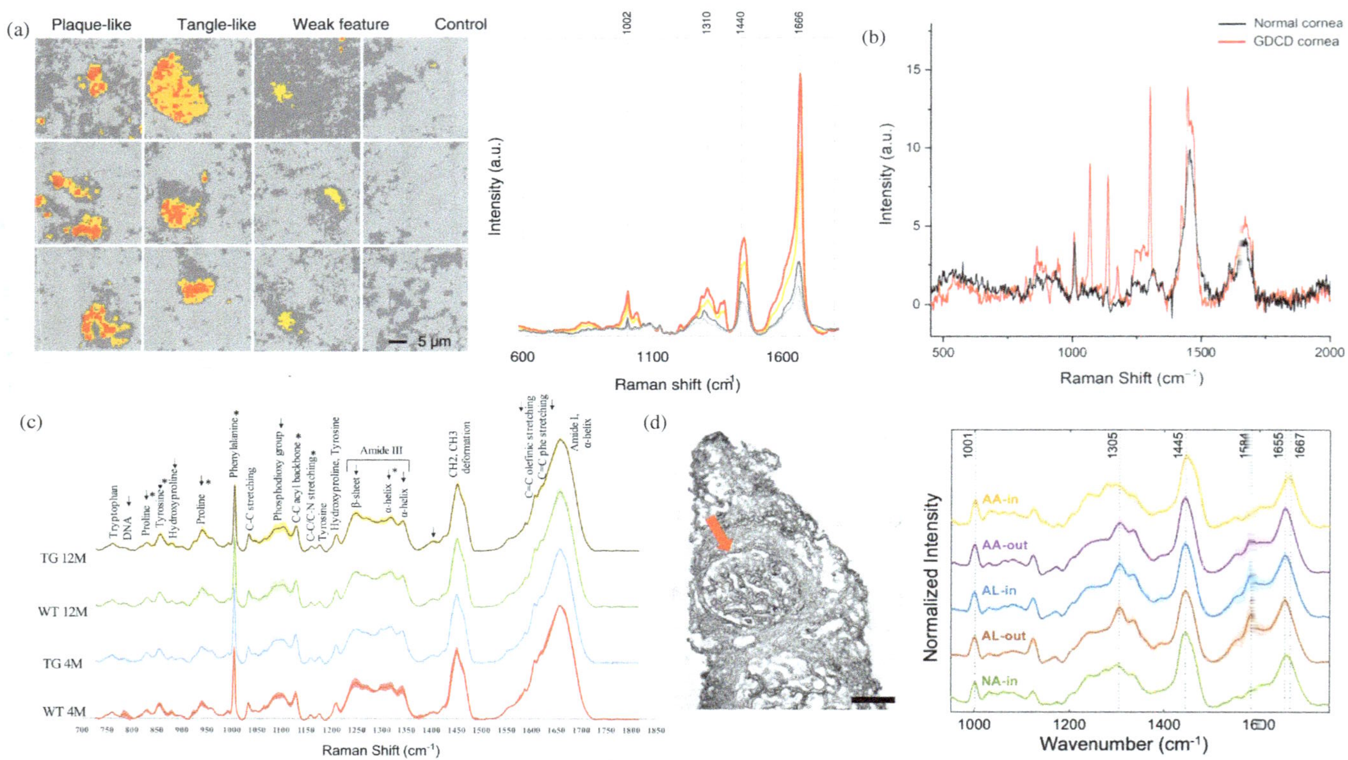

Figure 13.4. Raman spectra of tissues featuring amyloid aggregates. (a) Hierarchical cluster analysis of hyperspectral Raman imaging of human brain tissues featuring Aβ and tau. Red and orange distributions represent the local core and surrounding tissue of amyloids with respective spectra. (b) Raman spectra of normal (black) and GDCD (red) cornea in corneal dystrophy. (c) Raman spectra of colon tissues from Parkinson's disease patients. (d) Raman spectra of human kidney tissues featuring immunoglobin light chain and serum amyloid A proteins. Reproduced from (a): Ref. [81]; (b): Ref. [84]; (c): Ref. [83] with permission.

those in the amide I region as well. Acri and coworkers applied Raman spectroscopy on the human cornea to detect Gelatinous Drop-like Corneal Dystrophy (GDCD) due to amyloid deposits in the stroma (Figure 13.4(b)) [84]. Also, our group has recently characterized immunoglobin light chain and serum amyloid A proteins from human kidney tissues [137] (Figure 13.4(d)). Both amyloid proteins associated with renal conditions demonstrated protein secondary structures in amide I and III. With machine learning analysis, we were able to both distinguish tissues with amyloid fibrils from non-amyloidogenic tissues, and subtypes between the two amyloids.

In summary, Raman spectroscopy has shown its potential applications for the study of amyloidogenesis and clinical diagnosis of label-free tissue biopsies. Its advantages of spectral robustness to water content and non-destructive manner of investigation may allow further probing of the mechanisms underlying amyloid aggregation under various chemical and environmental conditions, which remain poorly understood. Additionally, Raman signal enhancement techniques, such as SERS and TERS, allow the probing of conformational changes in amyloid proteins at single-molecule resolution. Also, while the use of Raman spectroscopy in the study of amyloid fibrils is currently largely confined to those associated with neurodegenerative diseases, it can also be applied to the investigation of other non-neuropathic systemic and hereditary amyloid conditions.

13.4. Surface-Enhanced Raman Scattering for Biomedical Applications

In recent years, there has been a tremendous increase in the application of Raman spectroscopy for the label-free characterization of biological samples [85]. The great appeal of Raman spectroscopy lies in its potential to probe biological samples with exquisite molecular specificity and ultra-high sensitivity without requiring external contrast-enhancing agents [86, 87]. As a result of disease, the molecular makeup of the affected tissues and cells alters, and these changes in the molecular composition are reflected in the Raman spectra. While this has been illustrated by several published reports where differences were observed between Raman spectra of healthy and diseased tissues [88, 89], detection of clinically important biomarkers present in ultra-trace levels using spontaneous Raman measurements remains extremely difficult [90]. This is because: first, their concentration is very low in clinical samples; and second, detection is required in the presence of an abundance of other biomolecules. And, due to the inherently low Raman cross-section of the order of 10^{-29} [91], detection using Raman spectroscopy becomes challenging. This presents a major hurdle to the translation of Raman spectroscopy from optical bench to clinical settings for developing diagnostic tools.

To address this gap, SERS, the plasmonic counterpart of spontaneous Raman spectroscopy, has emerged as a powerful analytical tool for *in vitro* and *in vivo* monitoring of clinically important biomarkers [92–95]. In SERS, the analytes must be placed in the vicinity of noble metal nanostructures, where plasmonic enhancement results in a significant increase in Raman signals, offering unparalleled sensitivity down to the single molecule level [96–98].

13.4.1 *Application of SERS in Biomedicine*

SERS-based sensing techniques can be broadly classified into direct and indirect categories. In direct sensing, analyte molecules are physically adsorbed or bound to a plasmonic substrate, and the resulting spectrum characteristics are the analyte's vibrational modes. In indirect sensing, a reporter molecule—typically a dye or another molecule with a high Raman cross-section rather than the analyte itself—generates the SERS signal. In this section, we seek to present the current literature from the last five years on the use of SERS for human health and biomedicine with a special emphasis on novel design strategies being adopted to advance the field.

13.4.1.1 *SERS for Infectious Disease Detection*

The efficient management of infectious diseases and the readiness for a pandemic such as severe acute respiratory syndrome coronavirus (SARS-CoV-2) depend on the prompt and accurate identification of infectious diseases. Each year, 15 million people die from infectious diseases brought on by parasites, viruses, bacteria, and fungi; more than 95% of these deaths occur in developing nations [99]. The World Health Organization has listed most of the bacterial and mosquito-borne infectious diseases under the neglected tropical disease category that must be controlled by the next decade [100]. Thus, a rapid, inexpensive, sensitive, and widely deployable diagnostic technique is required for managing the current and preventing occurrence of any future pandemic.

To achieve this, very recently we developed a lab-on-chip ultrasensitive field-enhancing metal-insulator antenna (FEMIA) SERS substrate for the rapid and label-free detection of SARS-CoV-2 in a complex body fluid like saliva

(Figure 13.5) [101]. First, the Raman signatures of the purified spike protein and the hemagglutinin protein found on the surface of SARS-CoV-2 were identified, then supervised random forest algorithm classification was used for classification and identification of spectral data in human saliva samples. We observe that high classification accuracy of about 86.8% is achieved in a 1:1 ratio of pooled human saliva spiked with cell lysate. The key feature of the developed technology includes highly accurate results in a short time of fewer than 25 minutes, a possible extension for the detection of other viruses with minimal system modification, and the flexibility of mounting the sensor on surfaces like doorknobs, face masks, and skin for rapid and continuous surveillance. Utilizing a similar approach, a SERS platform for dengue diagnosis was developed [102]. Here, silver nanorod array was used as plasmonic substrate and SERS spectra of pure dengue non-structural protein 1 were recorded and peaks were identified. Next, Raman signatures of spiked serum samples were recorded and by employing PCA, dengue-positive, -negative, and healthy subjects were differentiated. The developed substrate showed potential for early diagnosis of dengue. To further enhance the specificity of SERS-based biosensors, target molecules are captured using antibodies as a biorecognition element. For example, the SERS immunosensor was developed by Chattopadhyay *et al.* [103] for the detection of *Salmonella typhimurium*. The capture probe was prepared by coating gold nanoparticles with Raman reporter and antibodies. Before detection, the pathogen and capture probe solutions were mixed and incubated at 37°C for one hour. The developed sensor showed high specificity towards *S. typhimurium* with a limit of detection of 10 cells/mL in solution and real food matrix samples. So far, many antibody-based SERS biosensors showing significant potential have been reported [104, 105]. However, it is important to note that the specificity of these sensors is highly reliant on the specificity of the antibody and factors like antibody stability, and cost must be considered while designing SERS-based sensors for point-of-care diagnostics. SERS biosensors utilizing aptamers as bioreceptor is a possible alternative to antibodies because they show similar affinity as antibodies, are more stable, and have a minimal cost of synthesis. Several reports have already been published with ongoing efforts to further improve the sensitivity of the SERS-based sensors [106–108].

13.4.1.2 *SERS for Sensing Cellular Functional Molecules*

A subtle irregularity in the concentration, distribution, and interaction of intracellular biomolecules can result in the onset of various diseases [109].

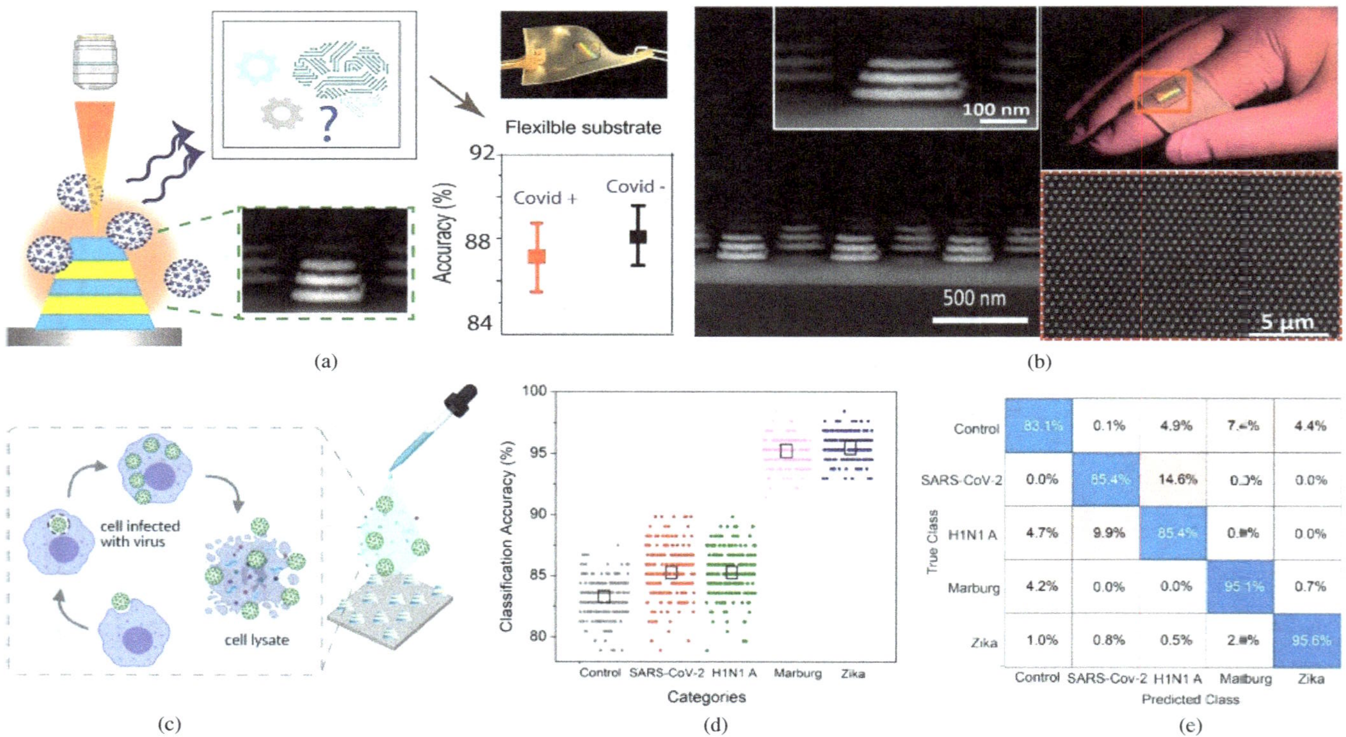

Figure 13.5. (a) Schematic description of the SERS-based detection of SARS-CoV-2 using FEMIA. (b) High- and low-resolution cross-sectional scanning electron microscopy images of FEMIA substrate. (c) Schematic of the sample details and measurement scheme. (d) and (e) Classification accuracy for control, SARS-CoV-2, H1N1 A, Marburg, and Zika samples using multiclass random forest classifier and confusion matrix showing the percentage of a sample getting classified into various classes. Reproduced from Ref. [101] with permission.

Hence, sensitive methods for real-time visualization of cellular processes at the molecular and cellular levels remains in high demand. In recent years, SERS has emerged as a promising and powerful alternative tool for studying cellular and tissue chemistry owing to its ability in long-time live cell monitoring without signal deterioration [93].

In general, these sensors can be classified into two categories; first, where plasmonic nanoparticle core is coated with a Raman reporter that is responsive towards a specific bioorganic molecule or environment. Second, the investigation is performed using Raman signatures of intrinsic biomolecules [110]. The best fit for the former category is SERS-based nanosensors for intracellular pH and redox potential measurement [111–114]. In these cases, the reporter molecules have functional groups sensitive to changes in pH or redox potential [115] and, therefore, can provide information about their immediate environment. For instance, Zhang *et al.* performed 3D profiling of intracellular pH distribution by time-dependent SERS-based monitoring of Au nanoparticles coated with 4-mercaptobenzoic acid from endosomes to lysosomal compartments [111]. For acquiring intrinsic SERS signatures of living cells, two general forms of SERS nanosensors have been developed: label-free colloidal plasmonic nanoparticles and targeting moiety-conjugated plasmonic nanostructures for delivering the nanoparticles to the desired location [116–118]. For example, Zivanovic *et al.* reported that plasmonic nanoparticles enabled direct probing of the molecular aspect of *Leishmania* infection in macrophage cells, a highly beneficial method for gaining detailed insights into host-pathogen interactions that could be further extended to other related diseases [119].

13.4.1.3 *SERS-Based Cancer Imaging*

In the last decade, there has been rapid development in the field of SERS-based precision cancer imaging owing to its non-invasive nature, ultra-high sensitivity, and perennial advantages [95, 120]. A major focus is on the design of active targeting nanoparticles, tailor-engineered for interacting with a specific biomarker within/on tumor cells for enhancing detection specificity [121, 122]. An example is mucin1 targeting SERS nanoprobes for human breast cancer imaging [123]. The nanoprobes were aptamer conjugated and showed enhanced accumulation in tumors due to active targeting. The strategy is claimed to be advantageous over antibody-based targeting where immunogenicity is a major concern.

Numerous studies have been published on the use of SERS for cancer imaging [120, 124]. However, most of the developed nanoprobes have plasmonic cores active in the visible (400–700 nm) and near-infrared I (NIR-1) (700–900 nm) regions, which have restricted the applicability of SERS for *in vivo* biomedical applications in real clinical settings. To address this challenge, recent attention has shifted towards plasmonic nanoparticles that are active in the near-infrared II (NIR-II, 1000–1700 nm) region [125, 126]. The NIR-II region offers advantages such as reduced light scattering and autofluorescence from tissues [127]. Until now, there are few reports about *in vivo* SERS imaging within NIR-II windows. To realize SERS-based imaging technology for actual world problems, further research should focus on SERS imaging driven by higher wavelength lasers.

13.4.1.4 *Intraoperative SERS-Guided Surgery*

Due to the infiltrative nature of tumors, it remains challenging for surgeons to identify tumor margins during surgery. Insufficient surgical resection might result in an early recurrence, and excessive resection can harm nearby functioning tissues. Therefore, a highly sensitive imaging technology capable of endoscopic pathological evaluation before the operative procedure, delineation of lesion margins during surgery, and replacing regular biopsies with objectively assessed target biopsies is highly desirable. Recent reports illustrating the possibility of SERS being used for real-time intraoperative interventions have made this goal easier to achieve [128–130].

In a pioneering study by Kircher and coworkers [131], it was shown that SERS can be used as an image-guiding tool using glioma mouse models. However, it was realized that when using tabletop imaging devices, partially exposed/difficult-to-reach regions of tumors cannot be imaged in real time. Therefore, a handheld Raman scanner was developed and its potential for Raman-guided resection of malignant brain tumors was shown [132]. In another report, Li and coworkers introduced an interesting concept that used acidic tumor microenvironments for the SERS-guided removal of brain tumors (Figure 13.6(a)) [133]. In this example, two Au nanoprobes were created, one with an azide modification and the other with an alkyne modification (Au-AK). The nanoprobes demonstrated monodispersity under neutral conditions and possessed the capability to effectively cross the blood-brain barrier and accumulate within brain tumors. Specifically engineered for pH-induced activation, these nanoprobes initiated the formation of plasmonic nanoassemblies, thereby activating SERS signal. Encouraged by the promising results of the SERS studies, substantial efforts are being carried out to integrate SERS with an endoscope to create fiber-optic Raman endoscopes [134]. With this technology, real-time imaging of malignancy in parts of the body easily accessible to endoscopes such as the colon, esophagus, stomach, cervix, bladder, and oral cavity will become feasible.

Using a combination of biomarker-targeting SERS nanoparticles and a miniaturized mechano-Raman device, Gambhir and coworkers enabled fast circumferential scanning and imaging of human and swine gastrointestinal tracts [134]. In this direction, recently others have reported surface-enhanced resonant Raman scattering (SERRS)-based detection of pre-cancerous GI lesions using an in-house built Raman endoscope (Figure 13.6(c)—(e)) [135]. The animals were first injected with synthesized SERS nanoprobes followed by Raman imaging after they sufficiently accumulated in the pre-malignant precursor lesions. The SERRS-positive lesions were matched with histology and sensitivity, and precision values were found to be 93.1% and 89%, respectively. The developed method holds promise for earlier detection of these tumor types and results in a significant reduction in the rate of morbidity and mortality significantly. Efforts are also being directed towards integrating SERS with other imaging modalities such as photoacoustic and magnetic resonance imaging to combine their complementary capabilities and improve surgical outcomes [133, 136]. The current results underscore the potential of SERS for improved detection and therapeutic intervention of malignancy.

13.4.2 *Perspective*

SERS has demonstrated its potential to be a versatile tool in a myriad of applications to biology and biomedicine. The recent trend is currently moving towards combining SERS with machine learning algorithms due to major improvements in computational methods for complex data analysis. Major objectives in this field of study should be construction of a detailed molecular database for spectrum assignment, development of internal standards for accurate comparison and quantitative analysis, and construction of effective data pre-processing and statistical analysis tools. We anticipate that over the coming decades, the applicability of SERS in the biological and medical sciences will remain active and will address more challenging problems with the goal of improving human healthcare including the discovery of novel drug targets, the elucidation of intricate cellular pathways, and the tracking of the metabolism of small biomolecules.

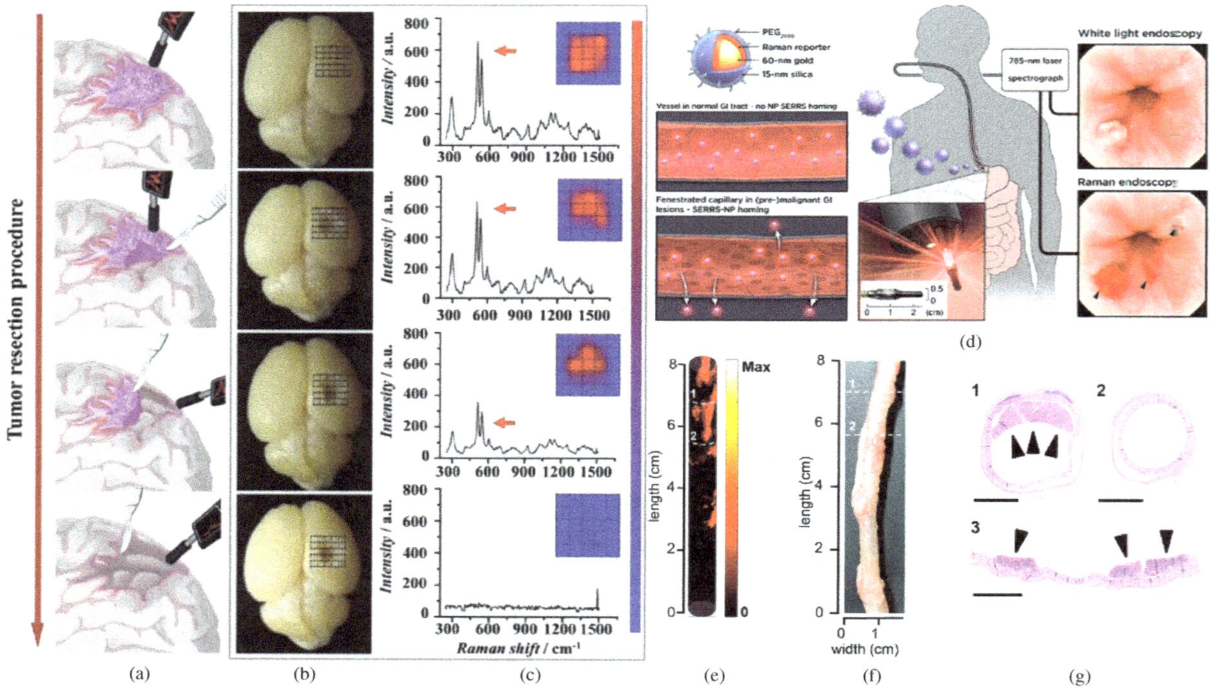

Figure 13.6. (a)–(c) Cartoons illustrating the procedure of Raman spectroscopy-guided glioma resection in U87MG glioma xenografts 24 hours post-intravenous injection of SERS-active nanoparticles, and digital images of the excised mouse brain and Raman spectra acquired on the 5 × 5 grid covering the tumor cutting bed. Reproduced from Ref. [133] with permission. (d) Concept of contrast-enhanced Raman imaging of gastrointestinal lesions. (e) 3D cylindrical projection of the 2D Raman map. (f) *Ex vivo* white-light image of the examined colon. (g) The SERRS signal correlated with the presence of an adenomatous polyp(s) ("1" and "3"), while no lesions were found in the SERRS-negative section ("2"). Reproduced from Ref. [135] with permission.

References

1. Ember, K. J. I., Hoeve, M. A., McAughtrie, S. L., Bergholt, M. S., Dwyer, B. J., Stevens, M. M., *et al.* (2017) Raman spectroscopy and regenerative medicine: a review. NPJ Regen. Med. **2**, 12.
2. Krafft, C. and Popp, J. (2015) The many facets of Raman spectroscopy for biomedical analysis. Anal. Bioanal. Chem. **407**, 699–717.
3. Wróbel, M. S., Kim, J. H., Raj, P., Barman, I. and Smulko, J. (2021) Utilizing pulse dynamics for non-invasive Raman spectroscopy of blood analytes. Biosens. Bioelectron. **180**, 113115.
4. Barman, I., Kong, C.-R., Singh, G. P., Dasari, R. R. and Feld, M. S. (2010) Accurate spectroscopic calibration for noninvasive glucose monitoring by modeling the physiological glucose dynamics. Anal. Chem. **82**, 6104–6114.
5. Suet Man, T., Rafay, A., Noreen, A., Irfan, A., Jingwei, Y., Francis, A. M. M., *et al.* (2020) Single red blood cell analysis reveals elevated hemoglobin in poikilocytes. J. Biomed Opt. **25**, 015004.
6. Sperati, C. J., Zhang, C., Delsante, M., Gupta, R., Bagnasco, S. and Barman, I. (2018) Raman spectroscopy for the diagnosis of intratubular triamterene crystallization. Kidney Int. Rep. **3**, 997–1003.
7. Singh, S. P., Kang, S., Kang, J. W., So, P. T. C., Dasari, R. R., Yaqoob, Z., *et al.* (2017) Label-free characterization of ultra violet-radiation-induced changes in skin fibroblasts with Raman spectroscopy and quantitative phase microscopy. Sci. Rep. **7**, 10829.
8. Yuan, Y., Zhang, J., Qi, X., Li, S., Liu, G., Siddhanta, S., *et al.* (2019) Furin-mediated intracellular self-assembly of olsalazine nanoparticles for enhanced magnetic resonance imaging and tumour therapy. Nat. Mater. **18**, 1376–1383.
9. Wang, W.-T., Zhang, H., Yuan, Y., Guo, Y. and He, S.-X. (2018) Research progress of Raman spectroscopy in drug analysis. AAPS PharmSciTech **19**, 2921–2928.
10. Gala, U. and Chauhan, H. (2015) Principles and applications of Raman spectroscopy in pharmaceutical drug discovery and development. Expert Opin. Drug Discov. **10**, 187–206.
11. Paidi, S. K., Pandey, R. and Barman, I. (2020) Chapter 18 — Emerging Trends in Biomedical Imaging and Disease Diagnosis using Raman Spectroscopy. In *Molecular and Laser Spectroscopy* (Gupta, V. P. and Ozaki, Y., Eds.), pp. 623–652, Elsevier.
12. Barman, I., Dingari, N. C., Singh, G. P., Kumar, R., Lang, S. and Nabi, G. (2012) Selective sampling using confocal Raman spectroscopy provides enhanced specificity for urinary bladder cancer diagnosis. Anal. Bioanal. Chem. **404**, 3091–3099.
13. Pandey, R., Zhang, C., Kang, J. W., Desai, P. M., Dasari, R. R., Barman, I., *et al.* (2018) Differential diagnosis of otitis media with effusion using label-free Raman spectroscopy: A pilot study. J. Biophotonics **11**, e201700259.

14. Pezzotti, G., Ohgitani, E., Fujita, Y., Imamura, H., Shin-Ya, M., Adachi, T., *et al.* (2022) Raman fingerprints of the SARS-CoV-2 delta variant and mechanisms of its instantaneous inactivation by silicon nitride bioceramics. ACS Infect. Dis. **8**, 1563–1581.
15. Ho, C.-S., Jean, N., Hogan, C. A., Blackmon, L., Jeffrey, S. S., Holodniy, M., *et al.* (2019) Rapid identification of pathogenic bacteria using Raman spectroscopy and deep learning. Nat. Commun. **10**, 4927.
16. Pahlow, S., Meisel, S., Cialla-May, D., Weber, K., Rösch, P. and Popp, J. (2015) Isolation and identification of bacteria by means of Raman spectroscopy. Adv. Drug Deliv. Rev. **89**, 105–120.
17. Zhang, C., Springall, J. S., Wang, X. and Barman, I. (2019) Rapid, quantitative determination of aggregation and particle formation for antibody drug conjugate therapeutics with label-free Raman spectroscopy. Anal. Chim. Acta **1081**, 138–145.
18. Barman, I., Dingari, N. C., Kang, J. W., Horowitz, G. L., Dasari, R. R. and Feld, M. S. (2012) Raman spectroscopy-based sensitive and specific detection of glycated hemoglobin. Anal. Chem. **84**, 2474–2482.
19. Pandey, R., Singh, S. P., Zhang, C., Horowitz, G. L., Lue, N., Galindo, L., *et al.* (2018) Label-free spectrochemical probe for determination of hemoglobin glycation in clinical blood samples. J. Biophotonics **11**, e201700397.
20. Esmonde-White, K. A., Cuellar, M., Uerpmann, C., Lenain, B. and Lewis, I. R. (2017) Raman spectroscopy as a process analytical technology for pharmaceutical manufacturing and bioprocessing. Anal. Bioanal. Chem. **409**, 637–649.
21. Nagy, B., Farkas, A., Borbás, E., Vass, P., Nagy, Z. K. and Marosi, G. (2018) Raman spectroscopy for process analytical technologies of pharmaceutical secondary manufacturing. AAPS PharmSciTech **20**, 1–16.
22. Lin, Y. K., Leong, H. Y., Ling, T. C., Lin, D.-Q. and Yao, S.-J. (2021) Raman spectroscopy as process analytical tool in downstream processing of biotechnology. Chin. J. Chem. Eng. **30**, 204–211.
23. Paidi, S. K., Troncoso, J. R., Harper, M. G., Liu, Z., Nguyen, K. G., Ravindranathan, S., *et al.* (2022) Raman spectroscopy reveals phenotype switches in breast cancer metastasis. Theranostics **12**, 5351–5363.
24. Auner, G. W., Koya, S. K., Huang, C., Broadbent, B., Trexler, M., Auner, Z., *et al.* (2018) Applications of Raman spectroscopy in cancer diagnosis. Cancer Metastasis Rev. **37**, 691–717.
25. Barman, I., Dingari, N. C., Saha, A., McGee, S., Galindo, L. H., Liu, W., *et al.* (2013) Application of Raman spectroscopy to identify microcalcifications and underlying breast lesions at stereotactic core needle biopsy. Cancer Res. **73**, 3206–3215.
26. Winnard, P. T., Jr., Zhang, C., Vesuna, F., Kang, J. W., Garry, J., Dasari, R. R., *et al.* (2017) Organ-specific isogenic metastatic breast cancer cell lines exhibit distinct Raman spectral signatures and metabolomes. Oncotarget **8**, 20266–20287.

27. Felipe, L. M., Alexei, M. C. M., Eduardo, P., Sangram, K. S., Ana, M. d. P., Aloísio, M. G., *et al.* (2018) Raman spectroscopy with a 1064-nm wavelength laser as a potential molecular tool for prostate cancer diagnosis: a pilot study. J. Biomed Opt. **23**, 121613.
28. Paidi, S. K., Rodriguez Troncoso, J., Raj, P., Monterroso Diaz, P., Ivers, J. D., Lee, D. E., *et al.* (2021) Raman spectroscopy and machine learning reveals early tumor microenvironmental changes induced by immunotherapy. Cancer Res. **81**, 5745–5755.
29. Mussi, V., Fasolino, I., Paria, D., De Simone, S., Caporali, M., Serrano-Ruiz, M., *et al.* (2022) Label-free morpho-molecular imaging for studying the differential interaction of black phosphorus with tumor cells. Nanomaterials **12**, 1994.
30. Liu, Z., Lee, S. J., Park, S., Konstantopoulos, K., Glunde, K., Chen, Y., *et al.* (2020) Cancer cells display increased migration and deformability in pace with metastatic progression. FASEB J. **34**, 9307–9315.
31. Paidi, S. K., Raj, P., Bordett, R., Zhang, C., Karandikar, S. H., Pandey, R., *et al.* (2021) Raman and quantitative phase imaging allow morpho-molecular recognition of malignancy and stages of B-cell acute lymphoblastic leukemia. Biosens. Bioelectron. **190**, 113403.
32. Nicolson, F., Kircher, M. F., Stone, N. and Matousek, P. (2021) Spatially offset Raman spectroscopy for biomedical applications. Chem. Soc. Rev. **50**, 556–568.
33. Odion, R., Strobbia, P. and Vo-Dinh, T. (2018) Surface-enhanced patially offset Raman spectroscopy (SESORS) for biomedical applications. Proc. SPIE **10484**, 7–14.
34. Pozzi, E. A., Sonntag, M. D., Jiang, N., Klingsporn, J. M., Hersam, M. C. and Van Duyne, R. P. (2013) Tip-enhanced Raman imaging: an emergent tool for probing biology at the nanoscale. ACS Nano **7**, 885–888.
35. Krafft, C., Schie, I. W., Meyer, T., Schmitt, M. and Popp, J. (2016) Developments in spontaneous and coherent Raman scattering microscopic imaging for biomedical applications. Chem. Soc. Rev. **45**, 1819–1849.
36. Zhang, C., Zhang, D. and Cheng, J.-X. (2015) Coherent Raman scattering microscopy in biology and medicine. Annu. Rev. Biomed. Eng. **17**, 415–445.
37. Zheng, P., Raj, P., Wu, L., Szabo, M., Hanson, W. A., Mizutani, T., *et al.* (2022) Leveraging nanomechanical perturbations in Raman spectro-immunoassays to design a versatile serum biomarker detection platform. Small **18**, 2204541.
38. Zhang, C., Paria, D., Semancik, S. and Barman, I. (2019) Composite-scattering plasmonic nanoprobes for label-free, quantitative biomolecular sensing. Small **15**, 1901165.
39. Huang, Z., Siddhanta, S., Zheng, G., Kickler, T. and Barman, I. (2020) Rapid, label-free optical spectroscopy platform for diagnosis of heparin-induced thrombocytopenia. Angew. Chem. Int. Ed. **59**, 5972–5978.
40. Huang, Z., Siddhanta, S., Zhang, C., Kickler, T., Zheng, G. and Barman, I. (2017) Painting and heating: a nonconventional, scalable route to sensitive

biomolecular analysis with plasmon-enhanced spectroscopy. J. Raman Spectrosc. **48**, 1365–1374.

41. Zheng, P., Wu, L., Raj, P., Mizutani, T., Szabo, M., Hanson, W. A., *et al.* (2022) A dual-modal single-antibody plasmonic spectro-immunoassay for detection of small molecules. Small **18**, 2200090.
42. Paria, D., Convertino, A., Mussi, V., Maiolo, L. and Barman, I. (2021) Silver-doated disordered silicon nanowires provide highly sensitive label-free glycated albumin detection through molecular trapping and plasmonic hotspot formation. Adv. Healthc. Mater. **10**, 2001110.
43. Zhang, C., Siddhanta, S., Paria, D., Li, Y., Zheng, C. and Barman, I. (2021) Spectroscopy-assisted label-free molecular analysis of live cell surface with vertically aligned plasmonic nanopillars. Small **17**, 2100161.
44. Paria, D., Zhang, C. and Barman, I. (2019) Towards rational design and optimization of near-field enhancement and spectral tunability of hybrid core-shell plasmonic nanoprobes. Sci. Rep. **9**, 1–9.
45. Li, M., Lin, H., Paidi, S. K., Mesyngier, N., Preheim, S. and Barman, I. (2020) A fluorescence and surface-enhanced Raman spectroscopic dual-modal aptasensor for sensitive detection of cyanotoxins. ACS Sens. **5**, 1419–1426.
46. Liang, L., Zheng, P., Zhang, C. and Barman, I. (2021) A programmable DNA-silicification-based nanocavity for single-molecule plasmonic sensing. Adv. Mater. **33**, 2005133.
47. Liu, Z., Parida, S., Prasad, R., Pandey, R., Sharma, D. and Barman, I. (2022) Vibrational spectroscopy for decoding cancer microbiota interactions: Current evidence and future perspective. Semin. Cancer Biol. **86**, 743–752.
48. Nejman, D., Livyatan, I., Fuks, G., Gavert, N., Zwang, Y., Geller, L. T., *et al.* (2020) The human tumor microbiome is composed of tumor type–specific intracellular bacteria. Science **368**, 973–980.
49. Große, C., Bergner, N., Dellith, J., Heller, R., Bauer, M., Mellmann, A., *et al.* (2015) Label-free imaging and spectroscopic analysis of intracellular bacterial infections. Anal. Chem. **87**, 2137–2142.
50. Silge, A., Abdou, E., Schneider, K., Meisel, S., Bocklitz, T., Lu-Walther, H. W., *et al.* (2015) Shedding light on host niches: label-free in situ detection of Mycobacterium gordonae via carotenoids in macrophages by Raman microspectroscopy. Cell. Microbiol. **17**, 832–842.
51. Naemat, A., Elsheikha, H. M., Al-Sandaqchi, A., Kong, K., Ghita, A. and Notingher, I. (2015) Analysis of interaction between the apicomplexan protozoan Toxoplasma gondii and host cells using label-free Raman spectroscopy. Analyst **140**, 756–764.
52. Sinjab, F., Elsheikha, H. M., Dooley, M. and Notingher, I. (2020) Induction and measurement of the early stage of a host-parasite interaction using a combined optical trapping and Raman microspectroscopy system. J. Biophotonics **13**, e201960065.

53. Martin, O. C. B. and Frisan, T. (2020) Bacterial genotoxin-induced DNA damage and modulation of the host immune microenvironment. Toxins **12**, 63.
54. Liu, Z., Parida, S., Wu, S., Sears, C. L., Sharma, D. and Barman, I. (2022) Label-free vibrational and quantitative phase microscopy reveals remarkable pathogen-induced morphomolecular divergence in tumor-derived cells. ACS Sens. **7**, 1495–1505.
55. Brabletz, T., Kalluri, R., Nieto, M. A. and Weinberg, R. A. (2018) EMT in cancer. Nat. Rev. Cancer **18**, 128–134.
56. Rossi, T., Vergara, D., Fanini, F., Maffia, M., Bravaccini, S. and Pirini, F. (2020) Microbiota-derived metabolites in tumor progression and metastasis. Int. J. Mol. Sci. **21**, 5786.
57. Marro, M., Nieva, C., Sanz-Pamplona, R. and Sierra, A. (2014) Molecular monitoring of epithelial-to-mesenchymal transition in breast cancer cells by means of Raman spectroscopy. Biochim. Biophys. Acta (BBA)-Mol. Cell Res. **1843**, 1785–1795.
58. Zhang, L. and Min, W. (2017) Bioorthogonal chemical imaging of metabolic changes during epithelial–mesenchymal transition of cancer cells by stimulated Raman scattering microscopy. J. Biomed Opt. **22**, 106010.
59. Zhang, Z., Wang, J., Shanmugasundaram, K. B., Yeo, B., Möller, A., Wuethrich, A., *et al.* (2020) Tracking drug-induced epithelial–mesenchymal transition in breast cancer by a microfluidic surface-enhanced Raman spectroscopy immunoassay. Small **16**, 1905614.
60. Milo, R. and Phillips, R. (2015) *Cell Biology by the Numbers.* Routledge.
61. Rygula, A., Majzner, K., Marzec, K. M., Kaczor, A., Pilarczyk, M. and Baranska, M. (2013) Raman spectroscopy of proteins: a review. J. Raman Spectrosc. **44**, 1061–1076.
62. Benevides, J. M., Overman, S. A. and Thomas Jr., G. J. (2003) Raman spectroscopy of proteins. Curr. Protoc. Protein Sci. **33**, 17.18.11–17.18.35.
63. Kuhar, N., Sil, S. and Umapathy, S. (2021) Potential of Raman spectroscopic techniques to study proteins. Spectrochim. Acta A **258**, 119712.
64. Jakubek, R. S., Handen, J., White, S. E., Asher, S. A. and Lednev, I. K. (2018) Ultraviolet resonance Raman spectroscopic markers for protein structure and dynamics. Trends Anal. Chem. **103**, 223–229.
65. Oladepo, S. A., Xiong, K., Hong, Z. and Asher, S. A. (2011) Elucidating peptide and protein structure and dynamics: UV resonance Raman spectroscopy. J. Phys. Chem. Lett. **2**, 334–344.
66. Kurouski, D., Van Duyne, R. P. and Lednev, I. K. (2015) Exploring the structure and formation mechanism of amyloid fibrils by Raman spectroscopy: a review. Analyst **140**, 4967–4980.
67. Knowles, T. P. J., Vendruscolo, M. and Dobson, C. M. (2014), The amyloid state and its association with protein misfolding diseases. Nat. Rev. Mol. Cell Biol. **15**, 384–396.
68. Hartl, F. U. (2017) Protein misfolding diseases. Annu. Rev. Biochem. **86**, 21–26.

69. Eisenberg, D. and Jucker, M. (2012) The amyloid state of proteins in human diseases. Cell **148**, 1188–1203.
70. Flynn, J. D., McGlinchey, R. P., Walker, R. L. and Lee, J. C. (2018) Structural features of α-synuclein amyloid fibrils revealed by Raman spectroscopy. J. Biol. Chem. **293**, 767–776.
71. Devitt, G., Rice, W., Crisford, A., Nandhakumar, I., Mudher, A. and Mahajan, S. (2019) Conformational evolution of molecular signatures during amyloidogenic protein aggregation. ACS Chem. Neurosci. **10**, 4593–4611.
72. Maiti, N. C., Apetri, M. M., Zagorski, M. G., Carey, P. R. and Anderson, V. E. (2004) Raman spectroscopic characterization of secondary structure in natively unfolded proteins: α-synuclein. J. Am. Chem. Soc. **126**, 2399–2408.
73. Imanbekova, M., Suarasan, S., Rojalin, T., Mizenko, R. R., Hilt, S., Mathur, M., *et al.* (2021) Identification of amyloid beta in small extracellular vesicles via Raman spectroscopy. Nanoscale Adv. **3**, 4119–4132.
74. Louros, N. N., Tsiolaki, P. L., Baltoumas, F. A., Chryssikos, G. D., Gionis, V., Hamodrakas, S. J., *et al.* (2017) Tracking the amyloidogenic core of IAPP amyloid fibrils: Insights from micro-Raman spectroscopy. J. Struct. Biol. **199**, 140–152.
75. Flynn, J. D. and Lee, J. C. (2018) Raman fingerprints of amyloid structures. Chem. Commun. (Camb) **54**, 6983–6986.
76. Ishigaki, M., Morimoto, K., Chatani, E. and Ozaki, Y. (2020) Exploration of insulin amyloid polymorphism using Raman spectroscopy and imaging. Biophys. J. **118**, 2997–3007.
77. Fonseca, E. A., Lafetá, L., Cunha, R., Miranda, H., Campos, J., Medeiros, H. G., *et al.* (2019) A fingerprint of amyloid plaques in a bitransgenic animal model of Alzheimer's disease obtained by statistical unmixing analysis of hyperspectral Raman data. Analyst **144**, 7049–7056.
78. Chen, P., Shen, A., Zhao, W., Baek, S.-J., Yuan, H. and Hu, J. (2009) Raman signature from brain hippocampus could aid Alzheimer's disease diagnosis. Appl. Opt. **48**, 4743–4748.
79. Rivas-Arancibia, S., Rodríguez-Martínez, E., Badillo-Ramírez, I., López-González, U. and Saniger, J. M. (2017) Structural changes of amyloid beta in hippocampus of rats exposed to ozone: a Raman spectroscopy study. Front. Mol. Neurosci. **10**, 137.
80. Lochocki, B., Morrema, T. H. J., Ariese, F., Hoozemans, J. J. M. and de Boer, J. F. (2020) The search for a unique Raman signature of amyloid-beta plaques in human brain tissue from Alzheimer's disease patients. Analyst **145**, 1724–1736.
81. Michael, R., Lenferink, A., Vrensen, G., Gelpi, E., Barraquer, R. I. and Otto, C. (2017) Hyperspectral Raman imaging of neuritic plaques and neurofibrillary tangles in brain tissue from Alzheimer's disease patients. Sci. Rep. **7**, 15603.
82. Ettema, L., Lochocki, B., Hoozemans, J. J. M., de Boer, J. F. and Ariese, F. (2022) Label-free Raman and fluorescence imaging of amyloid plaques in human

Alzheimer's disease brain tissue reveal carotenoid accumulations. J. Opt. **24**, 054005.

83. Sevgi, F., Brauchle, E. M., Carvajal Berrio, D. A., Schenke-Layland, K., Casadei, N., Salker, M. S., *et al.* (2021) Imaging of α-synuclein aggregates in a rat model of Parkinson's disease using Raman microspectroscopy. Front. Cell Dev. Biol. **9**, 664365.
84. Acri, G., Micali, A., D'Angelo, R., Puzzolo, D., Aragona, P., Testagrossa, B., *et al.* (2022) Raman spectroscopic study of amyloid deposits in gelatinous drop-like corneal dystrophy. J. Clin. Med. **11**, 1403.
85. Smith, R., Wright, K. L. and Ashton, L. (2016) Raman spectroscopy: an evolving technique for live cell studies. Analyst **141**, 3590–3600.
86. Byrne, H. J., Bonnier, F., McIntyre, J. and Parachalil, D. R. (2020) Quantitative analysis of human blood serum using vibrational spectroscopy. Clin. Spectrosc. **2**, 100004.
87. Paidi, S. K., Pandey, R. and Barman, I. (2006) Medical Applications of Raman Spectroscopy. In *Encyclopedia of Analytical Chemistry*, John Wiley & Sons.
88. Tanwar, S., Paidi, S. K., Prasad, R., Pandey, R. and Barman, I. (2021) Advancing Raman spectroscopy from research to clinic: Translational potential and challenges. Spectrochim. Acta A **260**, 119957.
89. Choo-Smith, L.-P., Edwards, H. G. M., Endtz, H. P., Kros, J. M., Heule, F., Barr, H., *et al.* (2002) Medical applications of Raman spectroscopy: From proof of principle to clinical implementation. Biopolymers **67**, 1–9.
90. Kelley, S. O. (2017) What are clinically relevant levels of cellular and biomolecular analytes?. ACS Sens. **2**, 193–197.
91. Lee, H. K., Lee, Y. H., Koh, C. S. L., Phan-Quang, G. C., Han, X., Lay, C. L., *et al.* (2019) Designing surface-enhanced Raman scattering (SERS) platforms beyond hotspot engineering: emerging opportunities in analyte manipulations and hybrid materials. Chem. Soc. Rev. **48**, 731–756.
92. Kaur, V., Tanwar, S., Kaur, G. and Sen, T. (2021) DNA-origami-based assembly of Au@Ag nanostar dimer nanoantennas for label-free sensing of pyocyanin. ChemPhysChem **22**, 160–167.
93. Tanwar, S., Kim, J. H., Bulte, J. W. M. and Barman, I. (2022) Surface-enhanced Raman scattering: An emerging tool for sensing cellular function. WIREs Nanomed. Nanobiotechnol. **14**, e1802.
94. Cialla, D., Pollok, S., Steinbrücker, C., Weber, K. and Popp, J. (2014) SERS-based detection of biomolecules. Nanophotonics **3**, 383–411.
95. Moore, T. J., Moody, A. S., Payne, T. D., Sarabia, G. M., Daniel, A. R. and Sharma, B. (2018) In vitro and in vivo SERS biosensing for disease diagnosis. Biosensors **8**, 46.
96. Schlücker, S. (2014) Surface-enhanced Raman spectroscopy: concepts and chemical applications. Angew. Chem. Int. Ed. **53**, 4756–4795.

97. Tanwar, S., Haldar, K. K. and Sen, T. (2017) DNA origami directed Au nanostar dimers for single-molecule surface-enhanced Raman scattering. J. Am. Chem. Soc. **139**, 17639–17648.
98. Kneipp, J., Kneipp, H., Rice, W. L. and Kneipp, K. (2005) Optical probes for biological applications based on surface-enhanced Raman scattering from indocyanine green on gold nanoparticles. Anal. Chem. **77**, 2381–2385.
99. Hamm, L., Gee, A. and De Silva Indrasekara, A. S. (2019) Recent advancement in the surface-enhanced Raman spectroscopy-based biosensors for infectious disease diagnosis. Appl. Sci. **9**, 1448.
100. Mabey, D., Peeling, R. W., Ustianowski, A. and Perkins, M. D. (2004) Diagnostics for the developing world. Nat. Rev. Microbiol. **2**, 231–240.
101. Paria, D., Kwok, K. S., Raj, P., Zheng, P., Gracias, D. H. and Barman, I. (2022) Label-free spectroscopic SARS-CoV-2 detection on versatile nanoimprinted substrates. Nano Lett. **22**, 3620–3627.
102. Gahlaut, S. K., Savargaonkar, D., Sharan, C., Yadav, S., Mishra, P. and Singh, J. P. (2020) SERS platform for dengue diagnosis from clinical samples employing a hand held Raman spectrometer. Anal. Chem. **92**, 2527–2534.
103. Chattopadhyay, S., Sabharwal, P. K., Jain, S., Kaur, A. and Singh, H. (2019) Functionalized polymeric magnetic nanoparticle assisted SERS immunosensor for the sensitive detection of S. typhimurium. Anal. Chim. Acta **1067**, 98–106.
104. Bi, L., Wang, X., Cao, X., Liu, L., Bai, C., Zheng, Q., *et al.* (2020) SERS-active Au@Ag core-shell nanorod (Au@AgNR) tags for ultrasensitive bacteria detection and antibiotic-susceptibility testing. Talanta **220**, 121397.
105. Shen, H., Xie, K., Huang, L., Wang, L., Ye, J., Xiao, M., *et al.* (2019) A novel SERS-based lateral flow assay for differential diagnosis of wild-type pseudorabies virus and gE-deleted vaccine. Sens. Actuators B Chem. **282**, 152–157.
106. Duan, N., Shen, M., Qi, S., Wang, W., Wu, S. and Wang, Z. (2020) A SERS aptasensor for simultaneous multiple pathogens detection using gold decorated PDMS substrate. Spectrochim. Acta A **230**, 118103.
107. Zhang, C., Wang, C., Xiao, R., Tang, L., Huang, J., Wu, D., *et al.* (2018) Sensitive and specific detection of clinical bacteria via vancomycin-modified Fe3O4@Au nanoparticles and aptamer-functionalized SERS tags. J. Mater. Chem. B **6**, 3751–3761.
108. Ngo, H. T. and Vo-Dinh, T. (2022) Chapter 4 — SERS Biosensors for Point-of-Care Infectious Disease Diagnostics. In *SERS for Point-of-Care and Clinical Applications* (Fales, A., Ed.), pp. 115–134, Elsevier.
109. Zong, C., Xu, M., Xu, L.-J., Wei, T., Ma, X., Zheng, X.-S., *et al.* (2018) Surface-enhanced Raman spectroscopy for bioanalysis: reliability and challenges. Chem. Rev. **118**, 4946–4980.
110. Kneipp, J. (2017) Interrogating cells, tissues and live animals with new generations of surface-enhanced Raman scattering probes and labels. ACS Nano **11**, 1136–1141.

111. Zhang, Y., Jimenez de Aberasturi, D., Henriksen-Lacey, M., Langer, J. and Liz-Marzán, L. M. (2020) Live-cell surface-enhanced Raman spectroscopy imaging of intracellular pH: from two dimensions to three dimensions. ACS Sens. **5**, 3194–3206.
112. Shen, Y., Liang, L., Zhang, S., Huang, D., Zhang, J., Xu, S., *et al.* (2018) Organelle-targeting surface-enhanced Raman scattering (SERS) nanosensors for subcellular pH sensing. Nanoscale **10**, 1622–1630.
113. Zhang, Z., Bando, K., Mochizuki, K., Taguchi, A., Fujita, K. and Kawata, S. (2019) Quantitative evaluation of surface-enhanced Raman scattering nanoparticles for intracellular pH sensing at a single particle level. Anal. Chem. **91**, 3254–3262.
114. Cui, K., Fan, C., Chen, G., Qiu, Y., Li, M., Lin, M., *et al.* (2018) para-Aminothiophenol radical reaction-functionalized gold nanoprobe for one-to-all detection of five reactive oxygen species in vivo. Anal. Chem. **90**, 12137–12144.
115. Scarpitti, B. T., Morrison, A. M., Buyanova, M. and Schultz, Z. D. (2020) Comparison of 4-mercaptobenzoic acid surface-enhanced Raman spectroscopy-based methods for pH determination in cells. Appl. Spectrosc. **74**, 1423–1432.
116. Kuku, G., Altunbek, M. and Culha, M. (2017) Surface-enhanced Raman scattering for label-free living single cell analysis. Anal. Chem. **89**, 11160–11166.
117. Živanović, V., Seifert, S., Drescher, D., Schrade, P., Werner, S., Guttmann, P., *et al.* (2019) Optical nanosensing of lipid accumulation due to enzyme inhibition in live cells. ACS Nano **13**, 9363–9375.
118. Shin, H. J., Lee, J. H., Kim, Y. D., Shin, I., Sim, T. and Lim, D.-K. (2019) Raman-based in situ monitoring of changes in molecular signatures during mitochondrially mediated apoptosis. ACS Omega **4**, 8188–8195.
119. Živanović, V., Semini, G., Laue, M., Drescher, D., Aebischer, T. and Kneipp, J. (2018) Chemical mapping of Leishmania infection in live cells by SERS microscopy. Anal. Chem. **90**, 8154–8161.
120. Du, Z., Qi, Y., He, J., Zhong, D. and Zhou, M. (2021) Recent advances in applications of nanoparticles in SERS in vivo imaging. WIREs Nanomed. Nanobiotechnol. **13**, e1672.
121. Maeda, H. (2001) The enhanced permeability and retention (EPR) effect in tumor vasculature: the key role of tumor-selective macromolecular drug targeting. Adv. Enzyme Regul. **41**, 189–207.
122. Ruoslahti, E. (2017) Tumor penetrating peptides for improved drug delivery. Adv. Drug Deliv. Rev. **110**, 3–12.
123. Pal, S., Harmsen, S., Oseledchyk, A., Hsu, H.-T. and Kircher, M. F. (2017) MUC1 aptamer targeted SERS nanoprobes. Adv. Funct. Mater. **27**, 1606632.
124. Liu, H., Gao, X., Xu, C. and Liu, D. (2022) SERS tags for biomedical detection and bioimaging. Theranostics **12**, 1870–1903.
125. Lane, L. A., Xue, R. and Nie, S. (2018) Emergence of two near-infrared windows for in vivo and intraoperative SERS. Curr. Opin. Chem. Biol. **45**, 95–103.

126. Song, C., Li, F., Guo, X., Chen, W., Dong, C., Zhang, J., *et al.* (2019) Gold nanostars for cancer cell-targeted SERS-imaging and NIR light-triggered plasmonic photothermal therapy (PPTT) in the first and second biological windows. J. Mater. Chem. B 7, 2001–2008.
127. Shan, B., Li, L., Zhao, Y., Wang, H. and Li, M. (2021) Near-infrared II plasmonic Au@Au–Ag dot-in-cubic nanoframes for in vivo surface-enhanced Raman spectroscopic detection and photoacoustic imaging. Adv. Funct. Mater. **31**, 2103186.
128. Andreou, C., Neuschmelting, V., Tschaharganeh, D.-F., Huang, C.-H., Oseledchyk, A., Iacono, P., *et al.* (2016) Imaging of liver tumors using surface-enhanced Raman scattering nanoparticles. ACS Nano **10**, 5015–5026.
129. Han, L., Duan, W., Li, X., Wang, C., Jin, Z., Zhai, Y., *et al.* (2019) Surface-enhanced resonance Raman scattering-guided brain tumor surgery showing prognostic benefit in rat models. ACS Appl. Mater. Interfaces **11**, 15241–15250.
130. Wang, Y. W., Reder, N. P., Kang, S., Glaser, A. K., Yang, Q., Wall, M. A., *et al.* (2017) Raman-encoded molecular imaging with topically applied SERS nanoparticles for intraoperative guidance of lumpectomy. Cancer Res. **77**, 4506–4516.
131. Kircher, M. F., de la Zerda, A., Jokerst, J. V., Zavaleta, C. L., Kempen, P. J., Mittra, E., *et al.* (2012) A brain tumor molecular imaging strategy using a new triple-modality MRI-photoacoustic-Raman nanoparticle. Nat. Med. **18**, 829–834.
132. Karabeber, H., Huang, R., Iacono, P., Samii, J. M., Pitter, K., Holland, E. C., *et al.* (2014) Guiding brain tumor resection using surface-enhanced Raman scattering nanoparticles and a hand-held Raman scanner. ACS Nano **8**, 9755–9766.
133. Gao, X., Yue, Q., Liu, Z., Ke, M., Zhou, X., Li, S., *et al.* (2017) Guiding brain-tumor surgery via blood–brain-barrier-permeable gold nanoprobes with acid-triggered MRI/SERRS signals. Adv. Mater. **29**, 1603917.
134. Heng, H. P. S., Shu, C., Zheng, W., Lin, K. and Huang, Z. (2021) Advances in real-time fiber-optic Raman spectroscopy for early cancer diagnosis: Pushing the frontier into clinical endoscopic applications. Transl. Biophotonics **3**, e202000018.
135. Harmsen, S., Rogalla, S., Huang, R., Spaliviero, M., Neuschmelting, V., Hayakawa, Y., *et al.* (2019) Detection of premalignant gastrointestinal lesions using surface-enhanced resonance Raman scattering–nanoparticle endoscopy. ACS Nano **13**, 1354–1364.
136. Wen, Y., Truong, V. X. and Li, M. (2021) Real-time intraoperative surface-enhanced Raman spectroscopy-guided thermosurgical eradication of residual microtumors in orthotopic breast cancer. Nano Lett. **21**, 3066–3074.
137. Kim, J. H., Zhang, C., Sperati, C. J., Bagnasco, S. M. and Barman, I. (2023) Non-perturbative identification and subtyping of amyloidosis in human kidney tissue with Raman spectroscopy and machine learning. Biosensors **13**(4), 466.

https://doi.org/10.1142/9789811264610_0014

Chapter 14

Translating Biomedical Raman Spectroscopy into Clinical Endoscopic Diagnosis and Post-Treatment Monitoring in Head and Neck Cancer Patients

Chi Shu, Wei Zheng, Kan Lin, Zhiwei Huang*

Optical Bioimaging Laboratory, Department of Biomedical Engineering, College of Design and Engineering, National University of Singapore, Singapore 117576

**Corresponding author: biehzw@nus.edu.sg*

14.1 Introduction

Head and neck cancer (HNC) is the sixth most common cancer worldwide, affecting over 1.4 million people and resulting in over 510,000 deaths in 2020 [1]. The malignancies of HNC could be found at various locations in the head and neck region (e.g., nasal, nasopharynx, pharynx, oral cavity, etc.) [2–4]. Nasopharyngeal carcinoma (NPC) is a special type of HNC with its unique epidemiology, etiology and clinical behavior [5]. In 2020, there were 133,000 newly diagnosed NPC cases and 80,000 death cases reported globally [1]. Geographically, the distribution of newly diagnosed NPC cases is extremely unbalanced with over 70% of the reported NPC cases located in the regions of East and Southeast Asia [6]. The main cause of NPC is Epstein-Barr virus infection [6]. The other risk factors related to the incurrence of NPC include family history, consumption of preserved food and alcohol, tobacco smoking and oral hygiene [6]. The clinical gold standard for NPC diagnosis relies on the histopathological assessment of formalin-fixed, hematoxylin and eosin (H&E)-stained tissue cryostat slides acquired through tissue biopsy under the white light reflectance (WLR) endoscope guidance [7]. Due to the fact that endoscopic visualizations of early NPC lesions (i.e., structural and morphological details) are mostly indistinguishable from normal or benign tissues, the detection accuracy of NPC based on WLR endoscopy is low [8]. Consequently, a large number of NPC patients are detected at locally advanced stages [6, 7, 9–11].

Since NPC tissue is particularly sensitive to ionizing radiation, radiotherapy is the main treatment modality for non-metastatic NPC patients [6]. A combination of radio- and chemotherapy (e.g., concurrent chemoradiotherapy, adjuvant chemotherapy, induction chemotherapy, etc.) is adopted for locoregional advanced NPC patients [6]. Around 85% of the small NPC tumor and ~55% of late-stage NPC can be controlled by the treatment [6, 7]. Unfortunately, around 10–58% of the NPC tumor could relapse after the treatment due to treatment resistance and tumor recurrence. The prognosis of the recurrent NPC (rNPC) patients is usually poor with ~17.5% progression control rate and ~47.2% 3-year survival rate [12]. Currently, clinical NPC recurrence detection mainly relies on physical assessment, WLR endoscopic screening and radiological imaging (e.g., computed tomography (CT), magnetic resonance imaging (MRI), etc.) [6]. Due to the subtle morphological and structural differences between the recurrent tumor and benign nasopharyngeal mucosa, especially when its morphology is highly variable after the treatment (e.g., edema, tumor necrosis, fibrosis, acute/chronic inflammation, etc.), current clinical modalities are encountering difficulties in rNPC diagnosis with limited accuracies (e.g., reported diagnostic accuracy for CT: 64% and MRI: 78%) [9, 13]. Hence, it is of great clinical value to develop advanced biomolecular-sensitive methods for real-time, accurate detection and diagnosis of NPC and even rNPC in the head and neck clinic.

Biomedical Raman spectroscopy is an optical vibrational spectroscopy technique with the advantage of high specificity to biomolecular fingerprints of tissue and cells without labeling [14, 15]. The utility of biomedical Raman spectroscopy has been widely explored for cancer diagnosis and detection at various organs (e.g., brain [16], larynx [17–19], oral cavity [20–23], esophagus [24], gastric [25], colon [26], etc.). Preliminary *ex vivo* Raman studies of the nasopharynx have shown promising results for detecting NPC from normal tissues with accuracies of 85~95% [27, 28]. The recent development of fiber-optic Raman endoscopy techniques [24, 29–31] further allows the translation of biomedical Raman spectroscopy into real-time, *in vivo* tissue diagnosis and characterization in clinical settings [14, 24, 29, 31–34].

In this chapter, we will concentrate on the development and translation of biomedical Raman spectroscopy technique for tackling the clinical challenges in HNC diagnosis, treatment efficacy follow-up and tumor recurrence detection at endoscopy. Specifically, we will focus on:

(1) Rapid *in vivo* diagnosis of NPC using fiber-optic Raman endoscopy technique.

(2) Post-treatment (PT) NPC patients' follow-up surveying of treatment efficacy and cancer recurrence detection using fiber-optic Raman endoscopy technique.

(3) Development of deep learning-guided fiber-optic Raman spectroscopy for real-time *in vivo* diagnosis of NPC and PT efficacy assessment during endoscopy.

14.2 Materials and Methods

14.2.1 *Fiber-Optic Raman Endoscopy System*

We have developed a fiber-optic Raman endoscopy system for *in vivo* tissue Raman measurements with the ability of simultaneous collection of Raman spectra in both fingerprint (FP) and high-wavenumber (HW) regions [25, 32, 35, 36]. Figure 14.1(a) depicts the schematic of the fiber-optic Raman endoscopy technique, and Figure 14.1(b) shows the photograph of the fiber-optic Raman endoscopy system placed in trolley for *in vivo* tissue Raman measurements in clinical settings. The developed fiber-optic Raman endoscopy system consists of a near-infrared (NIR) Raman excitation diode laser (excitation wavelength (λ_{ex}): 785 nm; maximum output power: 300 mW; B&W TEK Inc.), a high-throughput reflective imaging spectrograph (Acton LS-785, *f*/2, Princeton Instruments Inc.) equipped with a customized gold-coated 830 gr/mm grating, an NIR-optimized charge-coupled device (CCD) camera (PIXIS 400BR-eXcelon, Teledyne Princeton Instruments Inc.), as well as a specially fabricated miniaturized fiber-optic Raman probe [14, 29, 31, 32, 37–40]. The system is capable of capturing Raman spectra in the spectral range of 400–3600 cm^{-1} with a resolution of ~8 cm^{-1}. The uniquely designed and fabricated 1.9 meters long fiber-optic Raman probe with ~ 1.8 mm outer

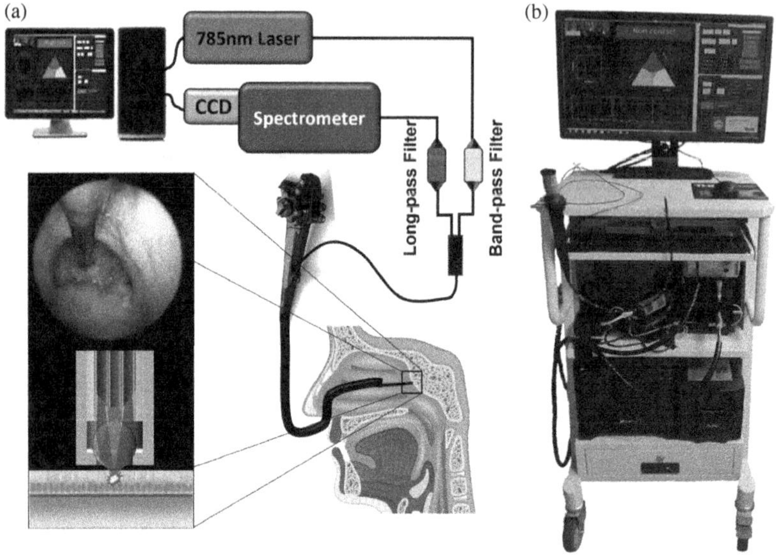

Figure 14.1. (a) Fiber-optic Raman endoscopy system for *in vivo* head and neck tissue Raman measurements. (b) Photograph of a Raman endoscopy system in the clinic. Reproduced from Ref. [14] with permission.

diameter is used for both excitation laser delivery and back-scattered tissue Raman signal collection at endoscopy. The depth-selective capability and the excitation/collection efficiency of the fiber-optic Raman probe have been further improved by coupling a 1 mm diameter sapphire ball-lens on the tip of the probe [40]. This configuration allows the tight focus of excitation light onto the tissue surface as well as the effective Raman signal collection from the epithelial lining [32, 40]. The probing volume of the probe designed is <0.02 mm^3 with a shallower tissue interrogation (<200 μm), eliminating the signal interference and dilution from deeper stromal tissue layer while selectively interrogating the tissue epithelium where the malignancies normally occur and progress [29]. An in-line bandpass filter (LL01-785, Semrock, Inc.) and an in-line edge long-pass filter (LP02-785RU, Semrock, Inc.) are coupled onto the proximal end of the Raman probe to eliminate the laser noise in the excitation optical path and to guarantee that the tissue-scattered Raman signal can be coupled into the Raman spectrometer with excitation laser eliminated in the collection optical path, respectively. The excitation laser power on the tissue surface is controlled to ~12 mW (~1.5 W/cm^2 within the laser spot size of ~ 300 μm) which is permissible under the laser safety guidance of American National Standards Institute [41]. The wavelength calibration in the FP region uses the atomic emission lines of mercury-argon spectral calibration lamps (HG-1 and AR-1, Ocean Optics, Inc., Dunedin, FL), while the HW region is calibrated using signature peaks of 4-acetamidophenol at 2931 cm^{-1} and 3064 cm^{-1} (ASTM E1840 standard) [36]. The relative intensity is calibrated using standard reference material 2241 (U.S. National Institute of Standards and Technology) [42].

To further achieve rapid, online tissue Raman measurement and diagnosis *in vivo* (e.g., the sub-second Raman data collection and real-time data pre-processing and tissue diagnosis), a set of optimization methods have been developed for both software and hardware [39]:

(1) A real-time Raman diagnostic software has been developed for Raman spectra acquisition, processing, and diagnosis with computation time <30 ms (2.2 GHz, Dell CPU) [43].

(2) A uniquely designed round-to-parabolic fiber bundle has been coupled into the entrance slit of the Raman spectrometer to correct the spectrometer-introduced image aberration. This design allows the hardware binning of the entire CCD height (PIXIS 400BR-eXcelon, 1340 × 400, 20 × 20 μm pixels, Teledyne Princeton Instruments Inc.), enhancing the spectral resolution to ~5 cm^{-1} and signal-to-noise ratio of the system by 20-fold ($\sqrt{400}$) [44].

(3) A special miniaturized ball-lens fiber-optic Raman probe has been designed to enhance the surface and subsurface Raman excitation and collection efficiency by ~19-fold at endoscopy [29, 30].

14.2.2 *Clinical Raman Measurement Protocol*

The *in vivo* tissue Raman spectra utilized in this chapter were measured on NPC patients at endoscopy in the Head and Neck Clinic at the National University Hospital, Singapore. The ethical protocol of the clinical study was reviewed and approved by the Institutional Review Board of the National Healthcare Group (NHG), Singapore (NHG DSRB Ref No: 2014/00323). Before the endoscope screening, informed consent forms of clinical Raman measurements were explained to and signed by the patients. During the clinical measurements, the fiber-optic Raman probe was introduced into the instrument channel of the endoscope and contacted to the nasopharyngeal mucosal surface under the guidance of WLR endoscope. The measurement sites were determined by an experienced head and neck surgeon. For each measurement site, ~15 to 20 tissue Raman spectra were acquired with the integration time of ~0.5 s to reduce the influence of patients' breathing and organ motions during the measurement [37]. For NPC patients, suspicious sites measured by Raman spectroscopy were immediately biopsied. The biopsied tissue was then made into formalin-fixed, H&E-stained tissue slides and sent to three pathologists who were blinded to the Raman-based diagnosis results separately. Only the tissue sites with the inter-agreement among pathologists assessed by Cohen's Kappa statistics ($\kappa >$ 0.9) [45] will be included into the Raman database. For the healthy volunteers and PT NPC patients whose nasopharynx were normal under the otolaryngologist's assessment, biopsy was not taken. The PT NPC patients involved in the study was observed for six months after the Raman measurements, and cancer recurrence sign was not discovered during this period.

14.2.3 *Data Pre-Processing and Statistical Analysis*

The *in vivo* Raman spectra are pre-processed in real-time using a customized Raman processing algorithm developed on MATLAB (Mathworks Inc.). The tissue Raman spectra of nasopharyngeal mucosa show a combination of relatively weak tissue Raman signal, intense tissue autofluorescence (AF) background and noise. Due to the existence of a so-called silent region that does not exhibit tissue Raman peaks, only the Raman spectra in the region of 800–1800 cm^{-1} and 2800–3600 cm^{-1} are fed into the pre-processing algorithm. Firstly, the Raman spectra in FP (800–1800 cm^{-1}) and HW (2800–3600 cm^{-1}) regions are smoothed using a Savitzky-Golay filter with window width of 5 and 7 pixels, respectively, to suppress the noise. The AF background of the tissue is then removed using an iterative polynomial fitting algorithm with the fifth and first polynomial fitting order in FP and HW regions, respectively [14, 46, 47].

The statistical analysis in the study is conducted using a two-sided Student's *t*-test [48]. After the spectral pre-processing, the Raman peaks associated with lipids and proteins in both FP and HW regions (i.e., 1078 cm^{-1} and 1665 cm^{-1} in FP, and 2885 cm^{-1} and 2940 cm^{-1} in HW) are selected for the protein-to-lipid ratios estimation. The ratios are calculated using the Raman intensities of the peak together with Eqs. (14.1) and (14.2) [38]:

Raman estimated protein to lipid ratio (FP)

$$= (I_{1665\ cm^{-1}} - I_{1078\ cm^{-1}}) / I_{1078\ cm^{-1}} \tag{14.1}$$

Raman estimated protein to lipid ratio (HW)

$$= (I_{2940\ cm^{-1}} - I_{2885\ cm^{-1}}) / I_{2885\ cm^{-1}} \quad (14.2)$$

Principal components analysis-linear discriminant analysis (PCA-LDA) and partial least squares-linear discriminant analysis (PLS-LDA) models are further implemented for tissue diagnosis model development [37, 38]. Leave-one-subject-out cross-validation (LOOCV) is used together with PCA-LDA for the diagnostic model evaluation with unbiased manner, and the majority voting strategy is utilized for the final classification of each measured tissue site. To evaluate the diagnostic performance of tissue Raman spectroscopy in rNPC detection, PLS-LDA model is used for diagnostic model development. The determination of loading vectors (LVs) numbers in the PLS-LDA model is achieved using two training datasets containing 90% of the randomly sampled tissue Raman spectra together with 10-split Venetian blinds cross-validation. The trained PLS-LDA models are further tested using the testing tissue Raman spectra dataset. Accuracy together with sensitivity and specificity are calculated for the diagnostic models developed. Receiver operating characteristic (ROC) curves together with the areas under the curve (AUCs) are calculated for the model performance evaluation.

14.2.4 *Raman-Specified Convolutional Neural Network Model and Model Evaluation*

Raman-specified convolutional neural network (RS-CNN) models are developed based on PyTorch (Facebook Inc.) for NPC detection from normal and PT tissues, respectively [39]. The structure of the RS-CNN model optimized using the training and validation Raman datasets is shown in Figure 14.2(a). The designed RS-CNN model structure consists of three parts: the feature extraction layers, the feature mapping layers, and the classification layers. The number of input and output feature vectors is marked in Figure 14.2(a) for each convolutional layer. In detail, the feature extraction layers consist of a 1-to-64 and a 64-to-64 convolutional layer, while the feature mapping layers are made up of two 64-to-64 convolutional layers. All the convolutional layers are followed by a batch normalization layer [49] and a rectified linear unit layer [50]. The classification layers include an adaptive averaging pooling layer, a flatten layer and a decision-making output layer [39]. Data augmentation is performed in the model training process by randomly flipping the input Raman spectra (i.e., horizontal flipping: reversing the x-wavenumber

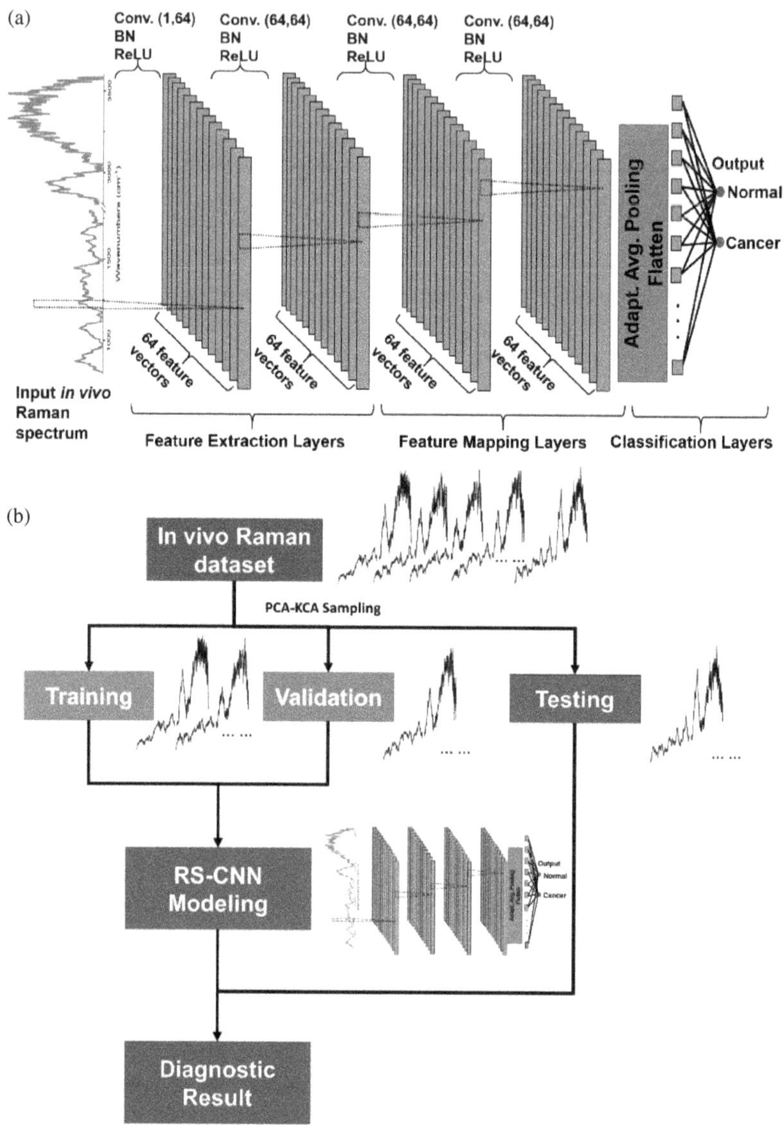

Figure 14.2. (a) Structure of the RS-CNN model designed. The first and second numbers in the parentheses represent, respectively, the input and output numbers of the 1D vectors of the respective convolutional layers; (b) workflow of the dataset preparation using PCA-KCA and the RS-CNN model training, validation, and testing processes. Abbreviations: Conv.: convolution layer, BN: batch normalization, ReLU: rectified linear unit, and Adapt. Avg. Pooling: adaptive averaging pooling layer. Reproduced from Ref. [39] with permission.

display of the Raman spectra; vertical flipping: multiplying a factor of −1 to the Raman spectra) to prevent the overfitting of the training data during the model training process [39]. The hyperparameters of the RS-CNN models are optimized through solving the cross-entropy loss function (Eq. (14.3)) using the stochastic gradient descent method [51, 52]. In Eq. (14.3), f_θ represents the deep learning model prediction using the tissue Raman spectra x_i, θ denotes the model hyperparameters, y_i denotes the clinical gold standard diagnosis of Raman spectra x_i, and N denotes the total number of Raman spectra in the training datasets.

$$\min_{\theta} \sum_{i}^{N} l(f_\theta(x_i), y_i) \tag{14.3}$$

The RS-CNN model training, validating, testing, as well as evaluation process are illustrated in Figure 14.2(b). Firstly, the tissue Raman spectra in each category (i.e., healthy control, NPC, and PT) are uniformly sampled using PCA and k-means clustering analysis (KCA) methods developed to prevent the biased evaluation of the model performance. In detail, the Raman spectral dataset are projected into PCA space, and then the first 10 principal components are picked to separate the dataset into four clusters using KCA. Two datasets are prepared in the study to address the clinical challenges in NPC detection in HNC patients:

(1) In the task of discriminating NPC from healthy volunteers, 10% of the healthy control tissue sites (n = 14) in each KCA cluster are put into the testing set, while another 10% of the control sites (n = 13) are put into the validation set. The rest of the control tissue sites (n = 55) were put into the training set. To balance the performance estimation in both validation and testing process, a similar number of the NPC tissue sites are put into the testing (n = 15) and validation sets (n = 13). The rest of the NPC tissue sites (n = 126) are put into the training set.

(2) In the task of classifying NPC from PT tissues, 10% of the NPC tissue sites (n = 24) in each cluster are put into the testing set, while 10% of the NPC sites in each cluster (n = 23) are put into the validation set. The rest of the NPC tissue sites (n = 121) were put into the training set. Meanwhile, a similar number of the PT tissue sites are put into the testing (n = 25) and validation sets (n = 23), and the rest of the PT tissue sites (n = 210) are put into the training set.

The RS-CNN models are then trained with hyperparameters optimized using the prepared training and validation Raman sets together with Eq. (14.3). PLS-LDA models are also trained using the merged training and validation Raman sets. The number of LVs in the PLS-LDA model training is determined by 10-split Venetian blind cross-validation. To evaluate the model performance and robustness, we also down-sample the Raman database with a factor of 2 and 4, and then feed them into the RS-CNN and PLS-LDA models. The model accuracy together with sensitivity and specificity are calculated for classification results of the testing datasets. The operating points of the RS-CNN models and the ROC curves of the PLS-LDA models are further calculated for the comparison of model performance in testing dataset.

We also calculated the saliency maps for the RS-CNN models trained for a better interpretation of the learning process. The saliency maps are calculated using the 100 randomly sampled testing Raman spectra with correct predictions. The calculation of the saliency map can be expressed as follows [53]:

$$\mathbb{E}_{\delta \sim N(0,\sigma^2)} \partial l(f_\theta(x+\delta), y) / \partial(x+\delta) \tag{14.4}$$

As illustrated in Eq. (14.4), to remove the oscillation of the gradient and to obtain a smooth saliency map, we add the Gaussian noise $\delta \sim N(0, \sigma^2)$ into the input Raman spectra as well as to the expected gradient of the loss between the prediction and the output with respect to the input [54]. The calculated saliency maps are sequentially averaged, and the top 10 wavenumbers with the highest absolute values in the saliency maps are picked out for the analysis of the possible biomolecules related to NPC carcinogenesis.

14.3 Results

14.3.1 *Real-Time In Vivo Diagnosis of NPC Using Fiber-Optic Raman Endoscopy*

We have acquired 15,354 *in vivo*, high-quality FP/HW tissue Raman spectra (healthy control: 1,761; NPC: 4,147; and non-recurring PT (PT): 9,446) from 888 tissue sites (control: 142; NPC: 237; and PT: 509) of 418 patient subjects (control: 85; NPC: 82; and PT: 251) in the past 5-year *in vivo* NPC measurements using fiber-optic Raman endoscopy system [38, 39]. The mean nasopharyngeal Raman spectra of healthy control, non-recurring PT and NPC are depicted in Figure 14.3(a) with ±1 standard deviation (SD) in shades. Representative nasopharyngeal tissue Raman peaks can be observed

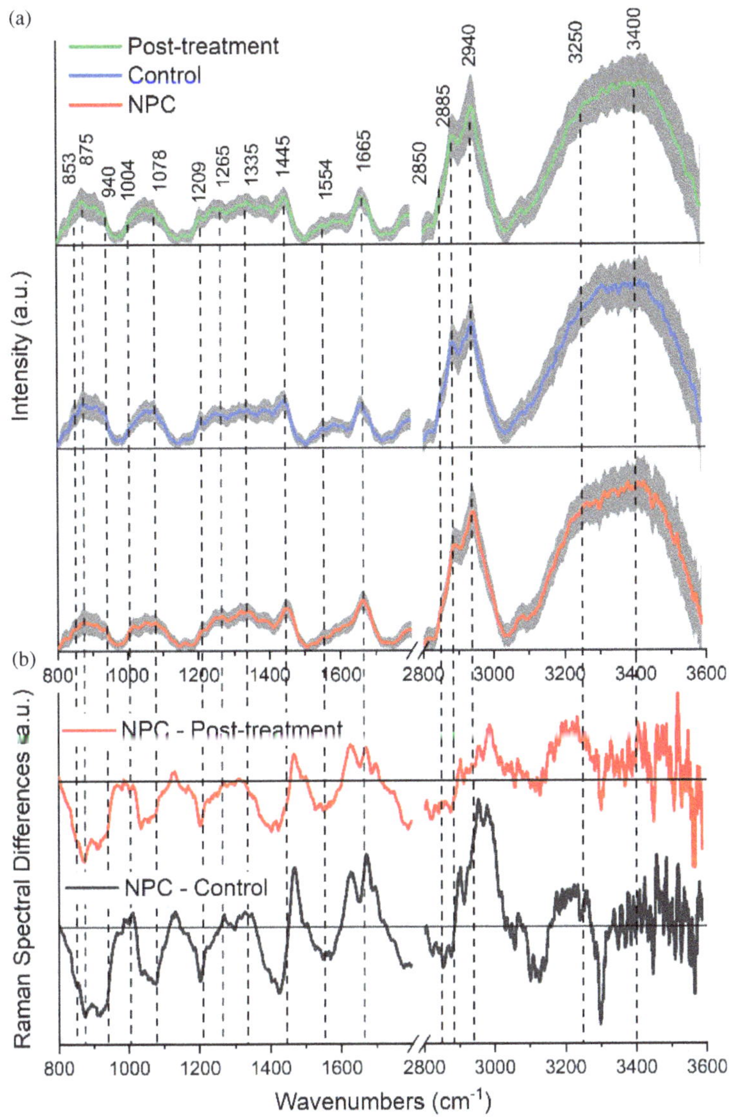

Figure 14.3. (a) Mean FP/HW Raman spectra of NPC, control and PT nasopharyngeal tissues acquired at endoscopy from 888 tissue sites of 418 patient subjects, with ±1 SD (shaded). (b) Raman spectral differences between different tissue types (i.e., between NPC and PT, and between NPC and control). Reproduced from Ref. [39] with permission.

in all three types of nasopharyngeal tissues in both FP (e.g., 853 cm^{-1} (ν(C–C) proteins), 875 cm^{-1} (ν(C–C) stretching of hydroxyproline), 940 cm^{-1} (proline and valine), 1078 cm^{-1} (ν(C–C) of lipids), 1209 cm^{-1} (tryptophan and phenylalanine), 1265 cm^{-1} (amide III, ν(C–N) and δ(N–H) of proteins), 1335 cm^{-1}

(CH_3CH_2 twisting of proteins and nucleic acids), 1445 cm^{-1} ($\delta(CH_2)$ deformation of proteins and lipids), 1554 cm^{-1} ($\nu(C=C)$ of amide III), 1665 cm^{-1} (amide I and $\nu(C=O)$ of lipids)), and HW regions (e.g., 2850 cm^{-1} and 2885 cm^{-1} (symmetric and asymmetric CH_2 stretching of lipids), 2940 cm^{-1} (CH_3 stretching of proteins), and the broad Raman bands of water (OH stretching vibrations peaking at ~3250 and ~3400 cm^{-1})) [14, 37–39, 55, 56]. Tissue Raman spectral differences are further compared between NPC and PT as well as NPC and control in Figure 14.3(b), reflecting the contribution of difference Raman-active biomolecules in the NPC malignancy progression from healthy and PT tissues. For instance, Raman spectral differences can be identified at the peaks of 853, 875, 940, 1078, 1209, 1335, 1445, 1554, and 1665 cm^{-1} in the FP region and the Raman peaks of 2850, 2940, 3250 and 3400 cm^{-1} in the HW region in the comparison between healthy and NPC tissues, showing the potential of using fiber-optic Raman spectroscopy for early NPC detection from healthy subjects at endoscopy [14, 37–39, 55, 56].

The development of Raman model for early NPC diagnosis involves a total of 3,731 high-quality FP/HW Raman spectra (healthy control: 1,765; NPC: 1,966) acquired *in vivo* from 204 tissue sites (healthy control: 95; NPC: 109) of 95 patient subjects (healthy control: 57; NPC: 38) at endoscopy [37]. The Raman spectral differences between healthy control and NPC are firstly investigated using PCA together with Student's *t*-test. The PCs with statistical significance (unpaired two-sided Student's, $p < 0.01$) between healthy control and NPC are selected which explain 64.2% (PC1), 18.9% (PC2) and 7.5% (PC3) of the total variance of the tissue Raman spectra [37]. The selected PCs with diagnostically significant Raman features are then fed into the LDA model together with LOOCV to evaluate early NPC detection capability of tissue Raman spectra. In the cross-validation process, the Raman spectra of one subject are excluded as validation dataset while the rest of the Raman spectra are fed into the model as training dataset. The validation results of the PCA-LDA training processing calculated using LOOCV are shown in the scattered plots in the form of posterior probability (Figure 14.4). Three types of tissue Raman spectra covering different Raman spectral ranges are fed into the model (i.e., integrated FP/HW, FP only and HW only), and the diagnostic results are calculated based on majority voting [37]. The PCA-LDA model using integrated FP/HW tissue Raman spectra reports the diagnostic accuracy of 93.1% with a sensitivity of 93.6% and specificity of 92.6% in discriminating NPC from control tissue sites, which is superior to the diagnostic performance using either FP (accuracy of 89.2%, sensitivity of 89.9% and specificity of

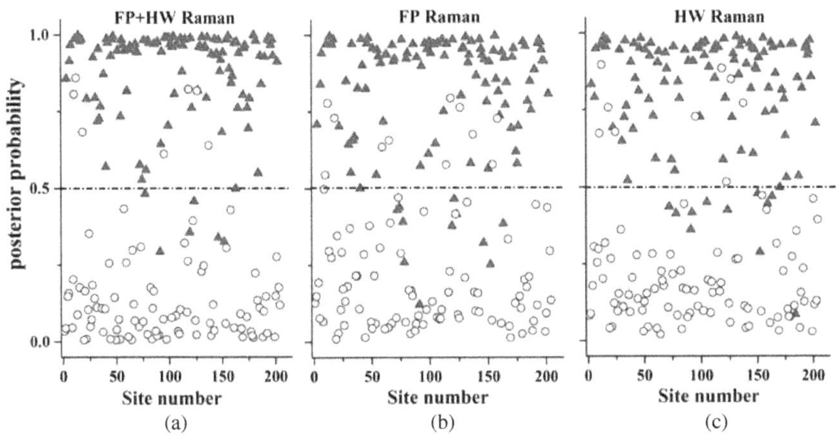

Figure 14.4. The posterior probability plots for detecting NPC tissue sites from healthy control using PCA-LDA model and LOOCV as well as the tissue Raman spectra covering the spectral range of (a) integrated FP/HW, (b) FP and (c) HW. Reproduced from Ref. [37] with permission.

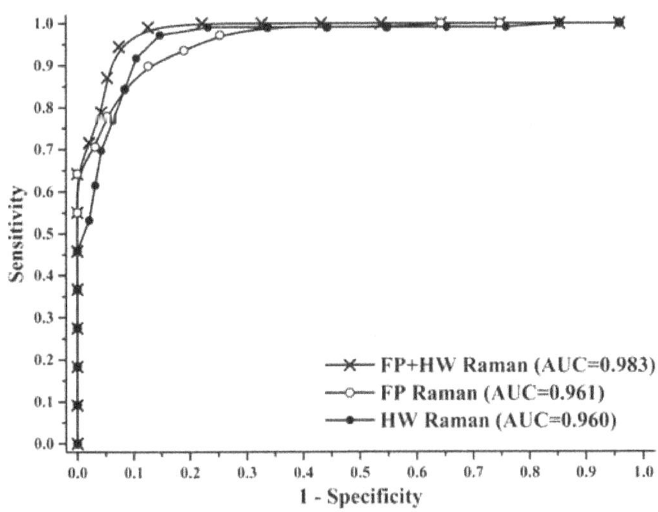

Figure 14.5. ROC curves of the PCA-LDA models for detecting early NPC from normal tissue using the integrated FP/HW Raman, FP, and HW Raman techniques together. The AUCs are 0.983, 0.961 and 0.960, respectively, by using the integrated FP/HW, FP, and HW Raman spectra. Reproduced from Ref. [37] with permission.

88.4%) or HW regions (accuracy of 89.7%, sensitivity of 89.0% and specificity of 90.5%) only [37]. We further calculate the ROC curve for the PCA-LDA model generated (Figure 14.5). The AUC for the PCA-LDA model generated using simultaneous FP/HW tissue Raman spectra is 0.983, while the ROCs of using FP or HW only are 0.961 and 0.960, respectively [37].

14.3.2 *Label-Free Follow-up of NPC Patient Post-Treatment Efficacy and Recurrent NPC Detection Using Fiber-Optic Raman Endoscopy*

In the study of PT NPC patients' follow-up and rNPC detection, 396 patient subjects (primary NPC (pNPC): 82, rNPC: 6, healthy control: 57, non-recurring PT: 251) are involved with a total of 15,052 tissue FP/HW Raman spectra (pNPC: 4,147, rNPC: 275, healthy control: 1,184, PT: 9,446) acquired from 860 tissue sites (pNPC: 237, rNPC: 13, healthy control: 101, PT: 509) at endoscopy [38]. The *in vivo* tissue Raman spectral variations of non-recurring PT NPC patients at different PT duration time points (i.e., number of months from the last day of treatment to the date of Raman measurement) are firstly investigated longitudinally. Figure 14.6(a) shows the mean tissue Raman spectra of healthy control as well as non-recurring PT patients grouped on a monthly basis from 1 month (PT 1-m) to over 6 months (PT ≥ 6-m) with ±1 SD in shades, and Figure 14.6(b) compares the mean tissue Raman spectral differences between the healthy control and PT NPC patients (PT 1-m to PT ≥ 6-m). Statistically significant Raman spectral differences are discovered in the comparison between control and PT 3-m group at Raman peaks of 1665 and 2940 cm^{-1} ($p < 0.001$). The tissue Raman spectral differences at the peaks of 1665 and 2940 cm^{-1} can also be observed between the control and PT 4-m to PT ≥ 6-m groups with similar level as shown in Figure 14.6(b). On the other hand, no statistically significant Raman changes are identified between control and PT 1-m or PT 2-m ($p = 0.8$). The increase of Raman peaks at 1665 and 2940 cm^{-1} in the non-recurring PT tissue from PT 3-m to PT ≥ 6-m compared to healthy control indicates the protein and lipid variations in the PT nasopharynx at the time point of 60 days after the treatment [38].

The in-depth analysis of protein and lipids variation of the PT nasopharyngeal tissue is then achieved by calculating the Raman-estimated protein-to-lipid ratios (Eq. (14.1) and Eq. (14.2)) using the selected representative Raman bands of protein and lipids (i.e., 1078 and 1665 cm^{-1} in FP region and 2885 and 2940 cm^{-1} in HW region). Figure 14.6(c) and (d) show the calculated protein-to-lipid ratios using the Raman bands in FP and HW regions with ±1 SD for healthy control (0-m) and PT (1-m to ≥ 6-m). Obvious increasing trend of protein-to-lipid ratio within the first 3 months after the treatment is shown in both Figure 14.6(c) and (d) for the PT patients. In contrary, the

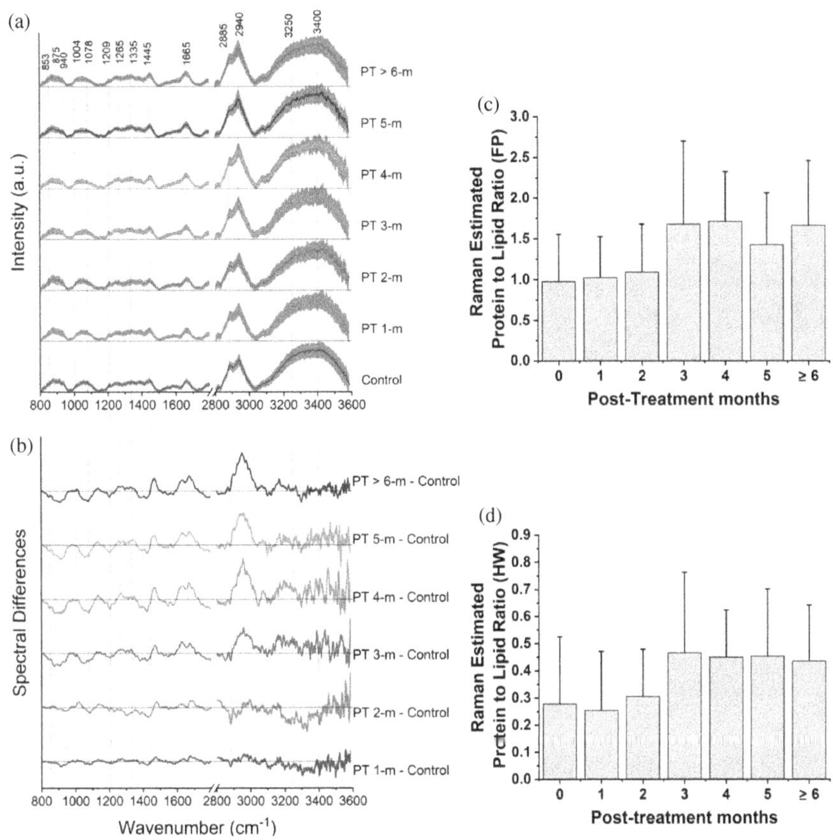

Figure 14.6. (a) Mean tissue Raman spectral of healthy control and PT 1-m to PT ≥ 6-m with ±1 SD in grey shades. (b) Raman spectral differences between control and PT 1-m to PT ≥ 6-m, showing the distinct Raman spectral changes after the treatment. (c) Raman-estimated protein-to-lipid ratio of control (0-m) and PT 1-m to PT ≥ 6-m calculated using the Raman intensity ratio of the band at 1665 and 1078 cm^{-1}. (d) Raman-estimated protein-to-lipid ratio of control (0-m) and PT 1-m to PT ≥ 6-m calculated using the Raman intensity ratio of the band at 2885 and 2940 cm^{-1}. Reproduced from Ref. [38] with permission.

protein-to-lipid ratios of PT 4-m to PT ≥ 6-m groups remain at a similar level as the PT 3-m group, suggesting that the long-term protein content accumulation in the nasopharyngeal tissues starts from around 60 days after the treatment. This increasing trend discovered through tissue Raman spectra is probably related to the PT tissue fibrosis, which normally occurs at around 4 months after the radiotherapy [6, 57].

Based on previous observation, we separate the Raman spectra of PT patients into two groups: PT duration < 3 months (PT < 3-m) and PT duration

≥ 3 months (PT ≥ 3-m). Figure 14.7 shows the comparison between the two groups of PT Raman spectra and NPC spectra. Figure 14.7(a) depicts the mean *in vivo* tissue Raman spectra of PT < 3-m, PT ≥ 3-m, pNPC and rNPC with ±1 SD in shades. Representative Raman peaks of nasopharyngeal tissue can be observed in Figure 14.7(a) for all four categories of tissue Raman spectra.

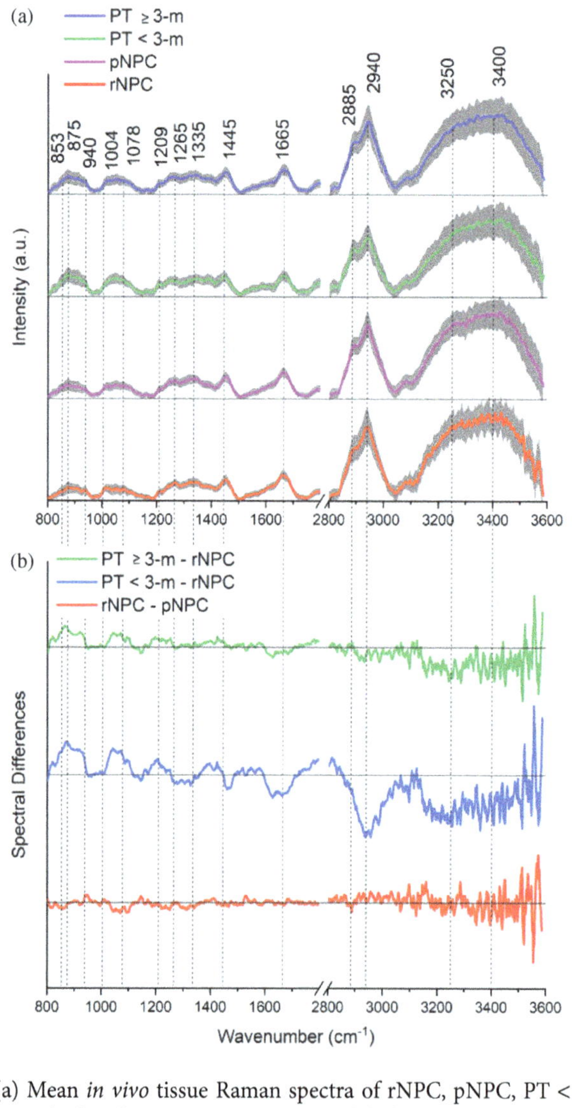

Figure 14.7. (a) Mean *in vivo* tissue Raman spectra of rNPC, pNPC, PT < 3-m and PT ≥ 3-m with ±1 SD in shades. (b) Tissue Raman spectral differences between rNPC, PT ≥ 3-m, PT < 3-m, and pNPC, showing significant Raman spectral differences between NPC and PT. Reproduced from Ref. [38] with permission.

Figure 14.7(b) compares the tissue Raman spectral differences between rNPC, pNPC, PT < 3-m, and PT ≥ 3-m. The Raman spectral differences between rNPC and pNPC are almost negligible as shown in Figure 14.7(b), reflecting that they are almost the same grade of malignancies in the biomolecular scale observed by fiber-optic Raman spectroscopy. On the other hand, significant Raman spectral differences are shown between rNPC and both PT groups. In the comparison of Raman spectra between rNPC and PT < 3-m, both FP and HW regions show obvious Raman spectral differences, showing the distinct biomolecular variation between early PT nasopharyngeal tissues and rNPC. The tissue Raman spectral differences can also be easily identified in the region of 850–1209 cm^{-1} when we compare the tissue Raman spectra of rNPC and PT ≥ 3-m, reflecting the biomolecular differences between rNPC and long-term PT patients [38].

Raman diagnosis models for rNPC detection have been further developed using *in vivo* tissue Raman spectra acquired together with the PLS-LDA method. To identify rNPC from early PT patients (PT < 3-m), a training dataset is prepared with 90% randomly sampled PT < 3-m patients (patient n = 26, tissue site n = 53) and pNPC patients (patient n = 82, tissue site n = 237). In the task of detecting rNPC from long-term PT patients (PT ≥ 3-m), we randomly sample 90% of the PT ≥ 3-m subjects (patient n = 200, tissue site n = 407) and merge it with the pNPC subjects to generate the training dataset. The training datasets are then fed into the PLS-LDA model, the diagnostic capabilities are sequentially evaluated using the testing datasets prepared with rNPC patient subjects (patient n = 6, tissue site n = 13) as well as the remaining 10% of the PT < 3-m (patient n = 3, tissue site n = 6) and PT ≥ 3-m (patient n = 22, tissue site n = 43) patient subjects. Figure 14.8(a) and (b) show the posterior probability scattering plots provided by the NPC detection model using training datasets. The trained PLS-LDA models achieve the accuracy of 99.66% (sensitivity: 99.58%, specificity: 100%) in detecting NPC from the PT < 3-m group, and the accuracy of 99.69% (sensitivity: 99.16%, specificity: 100%) for discriminating NPC from PT ≥ 3-m group [38]. The ROC curves and the AUCs are also calculated to evaluate the training process (Figure 14.8(c)). The AUCs for detecting NPC from PT < 3-m group and PT ≥ 3-m group are 0.997 and 0.996, respectively [38], showing the clinical potential of *in vivo* fiber-optic Raman spectroscopy for NPC detection in PT patient subjects.

The trained models are further tested using the testing datasets prepared using the real rNPC patients and remaining PT patient to examine the rNPC detection ability of the model. The testing results in the form of posterior

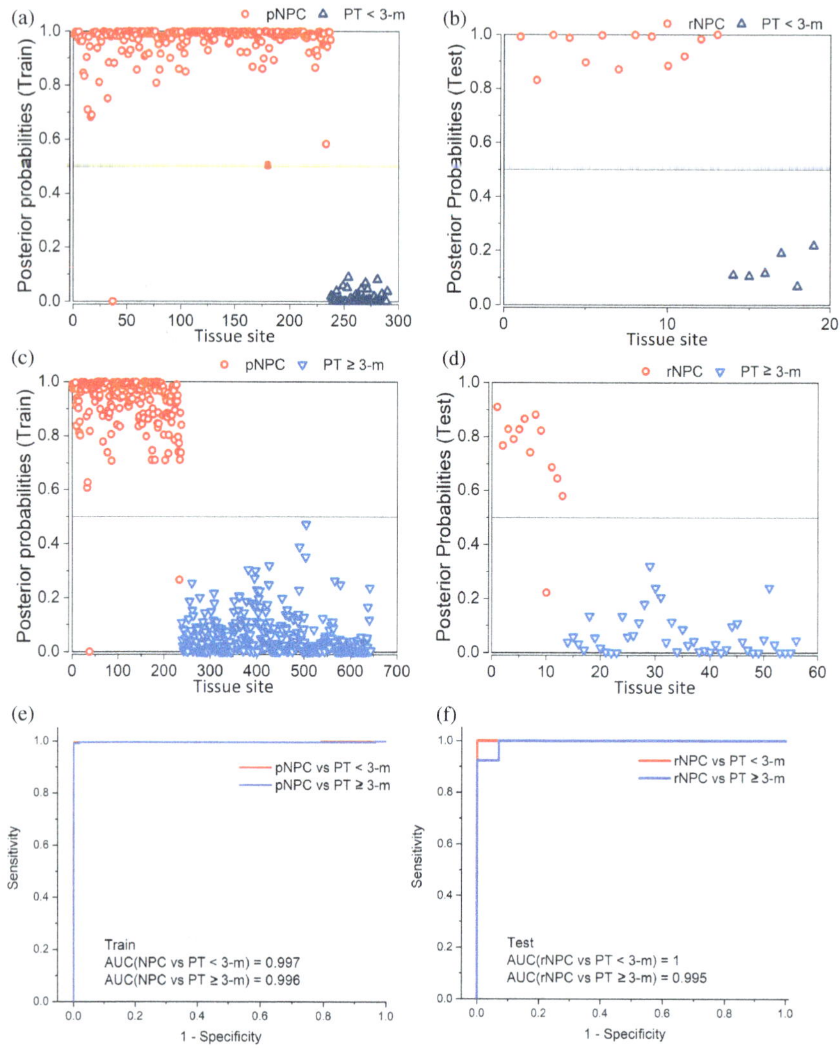

Figure 14.8. The posterior probability scatter plots of training PLS-LDA models for classifying (a) pNPC from PT < 3-m group, and (b) pNPC from PT ≥ 3-m group. (c) ROC curves comparison between the two training PLS-LDA models. The posterior probability scatter plots of testing PLS-LDA models for detecting (d) rNPC in PT < 3-m group, and (e) rNPC in PT ≥ 3-m group. (f) ROC curves comparison between the two testing PLS-LDA models. Reproduced from Ref. [38] with permission.

probability are shown in Figure 14.8(d) and (e) as scattering plots. The trained PLS-LDA models report a testing accuracy of 100% (sensitivity: 100%, specificity: 100%) for detecting rNPC from PT < 3-m group and 98.21% (sensitivity: 92.31%, specificity: 100%) for detecting rNPC from PT ≥ 3-m group. The

ROC curves and AUCs are calculated using the testing results by PLS-LDA (Figure 14.8(f)). The testing models report AUCs of 1 and 0.995 for detecting rNPC in PT < 3-m and PT ≥ 3-m groups, confirming the capability of rNPC detection from PT patients using *in vivo* fiber-optic Raman spectroscopy [38].

14.3.3 *Deep Learning-Guided Fiber-Optic Raman Spectroscopy for NPC Patient Diagnosis and Post-Treatment Efficacy Assessment*

To further enhance the clinical diagnosis capability of fiber-optic Raman spectroscopy for discriminating NPC from healthy and PT subjects, RS-CNN models have been developed. The robustness, generalization and spectral information sensitiveness of the RS-CNN model are comprehensively evaluated and compared with the widely used PLS-LDA model. Three types of tissue Raman spectra are fed into the models during the evaluation (i.e., full FP/HW Raman spectra (Full Spec), the tissue Raman spectra down-sampled by factors of 2 (DS-2) and 4 (DS-4)). The signature Raman peaks as well as the Raman spectral differences are mostly preserved during the down-sampling process, indicating that the down-sampling process with a factor less than 4 will not affect the Raman feature differences among NPC, control and PT [39]. The tissue Raman spectra are then separated into training, validation and testing datasets as described in Section 14.2.4 using the PCA-KCA method developed. The RS-CNN and PLS-LDA models are then trained and optimized using the prepared training and validation datasets. Figure 14.9 compares the diagnostic accuracy between RS-CNN and PLS-LDA models in the tasks of detecting NPC from both healthy control and PT subjects, classifying NPC from healthy

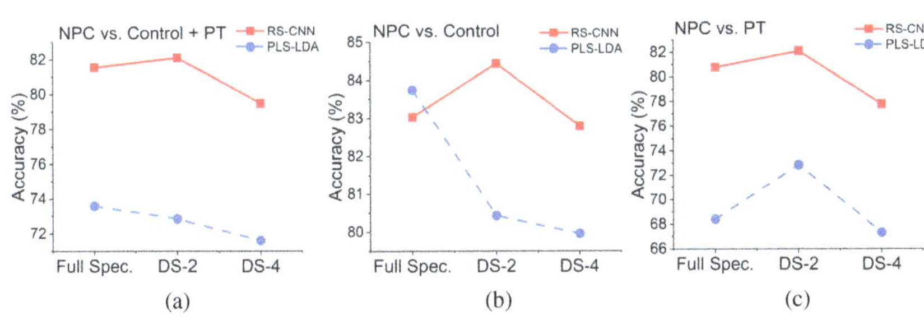

Figure 14.9. Comparison of Raman diagnostic accuracy between RS-CNN and PLS-LDA using full tissue Raman spectra (Full Spec), down-sampled tissue Raman spectra with a factor of 2 (DS-2), and down-sampled tissue Raman spectra with a factor of 4 (DS-4) for detecting NPC from (a) healthy control and PT, (b) healthy control and (c) PT. Reproduced from Ref. [39] with permission.

control subjects, and discriminating NPC from PT subjects using three kinds of tissue Raman spectra (i.e., Full Spec, DS-2 and DS-4). The RS-CNN model reaches its optimal diagnostic performance when using the DS-2 Raman spectra dataset while PLS-LDA is reporting the highest diagnostic accuracy when using the full tissue Raman spectra. Specifically, the RS-CNN model achieves an overall diagnostic accuracy of 82.09% (sensitivity of 92.18%, specificity of 73.99%) using the DS-2 dataset for detecting NPC from healthy control and PT subjects, while the PLS-LDA model is providing the overall accuracy of 73.57% only (sensitivity: 89.74%, specificity: 58.10%) for discriminating NPC from healthy control and PT patient subjects [39]. These results indicate that the RS-CNN model can achieve a better detection capability in the tasks of discriminating NPC from healthy control and PT subjects.

The operating points for RS-CNN models and ROC curves for PLS-LDA models in the tasks of NPC detection from healthy control and PT tissues are also calculated (Figure 14.10). As shown in the figure, the operating points calculated by RS-CNN models are above the ROC curves of PLS-LDA models in most of the tasks, showing the higher diagnostic capability of RS-CNN compared to PLS-LDA models in NPC detection from both healthy control and PT subjects [39]. These results affirm the superior performance of RS-CNN model for improving rapid NPC diagnosis at endoscopy.

Saliency maps are then calculated using the correctly predicted tissue Raman spectra in the DS-2 dataset to gain an in-depth understanding of the biomolecular information identified during the RS-CNN model classification process (Figure 14.11). The most representative Raman bands during the separating of NPC from control and PT sites are identified in the saliency maps as shown in Figure 14.11(a) and (b), reflecting the relative biomolecular

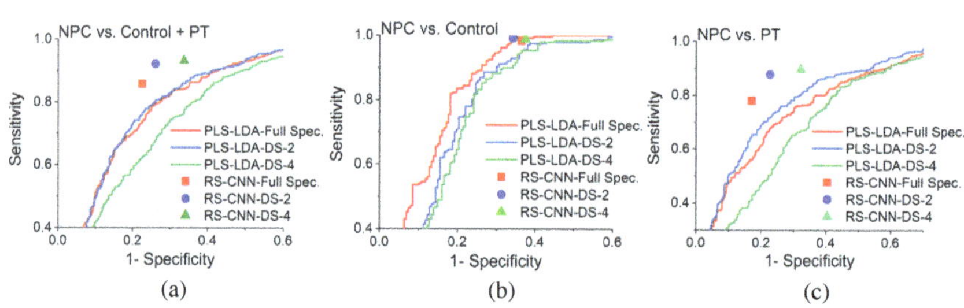

Figure 14.10. Calculated operating points of RS-CNN models and ROC curves of PLS-LDA model using Full Spec, DS-2 and DS-4 tissue Raman dataset for discriminating NPC from (a) both control and PT, (b) control and (c) PT tissues. Reproduced from Ref. [39] with permission.

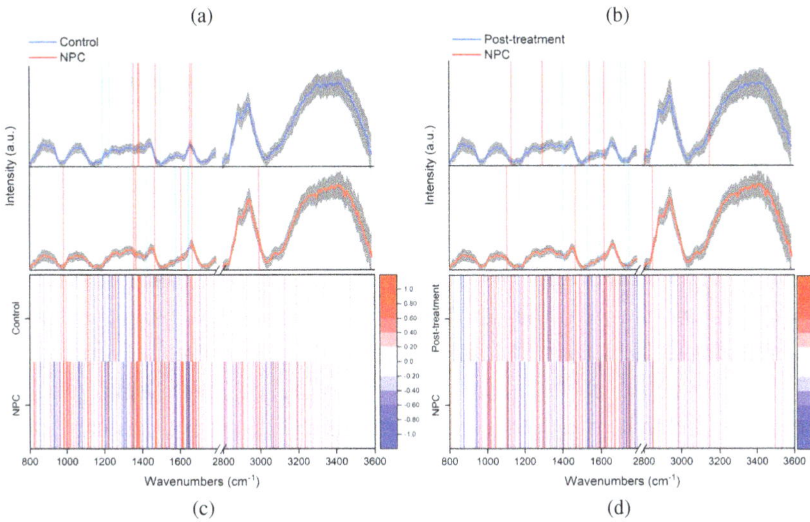

Figure 14.11. Mean tissue Raman spectra (DS-2) with RS-CNN identified signature tissue Raman bands in the tasks of (a) discriminating NPC from healthy control tissues, and (b) separating NPC with PT tissues. The entire saliency maps calculated by RS-CNN model for (c) discriminating NPC from healthy control tissues, and (d) separating NPC from PT tissues. Reproduced from Ref. [39] with permission.

changes in the Raman diagnosis based on RS-CNN models. For instance, the RS-CNN model mainly focuses on the relative intensity increase at the Raman peaks of 1367 cm^{-1} (phospholipids), 1466 cm^{-1} (lipids), 1607 cm^{-1} (tyrosine and phenylalanine), 1668 cm^{-1} (amide I), and 2994 cm^{-1} (cholesterol easter) and the intensity decrease of the Raman peaks at 1646 cm^{-1} and 1651 cm^{-1} (amide I) in the NPC tissues as compared to control tissue sites in discriminating control tissue sites from NPC tissue sites. To discriminate NPC from PT tissues, the RS-CNN model identified the Raman intensity increase at the peaks of 1104 cm^{-1} (phenylalanine), 1466 cm^{-1} (lipids), 1618 cm^{-1} (proteins and tryptophan), and 2848 cm^{-1} (lipids and fatty acids) and the intensity decrease of Raman peaks at 1403 cm^{-1} (collagen) and 1596 cm^{-1} (amide I) in the NPC tissue Raman spectra as compared to the PT tissue sites [37–39, 58]. The entire calculated saliency maps for the two tasks are also depicted in Figure 14.11, indicating the RS-CNN working process in nasopharyngeal tissue diagnosis.

14.4 Discussions

Development of a rapid but accurate NPC detection method is of high clinical value for the accurate diagnosis of NPC and PT patients' treatment efficacy management. Different from traditional histopathology assessment of NPC which mainly relies on cellular morphology, biochemical and biomolecular variations (e.g., proteins, lipids, DNA and water) of the nasopharyngeal tissues associated with NPC carcinogenesis are identified in the high-quality FP/HW Raman spectra acquired *in vivo* at endoscopy. The significant tissue Raman spectral differences are uncovered in both FP (e.g., 800–955, 1000–1120, 1180–1230, 1235–1265, 1400–1470, 1500–1580 and 1590–1683 cm^{-1}) and HW regions (e.g., 2850, 2885, and 2940 cm^{-1}) (Figure 14.3), revealing the diagnostically significant biomolecular information changes in NPC progression [37]. For instance, the reduction of Raman peaks at 853 cm^{-1} (ν(C–C) proteins) and 875 cm^{-1} (ν(C–C) stretching of hydroxyproline) can be observed in NPC tissue compared to healthy control, showing the collagen reduction in NPC tissues [37]. The nasopharyngeal mucosa thickenings of the NPC patients are reflected in the reduction of Raman peaks at 853 and 1078 cm^{-1}, where the thickened mucosa will attenuate the excitation laser while reducing the Raman emission from nasopharyngeal sub-layers [37, 59]. The DNA content increase in the NPC transformation is also reflected in the tissue Raman spectra (e.g., higher intensity of Raman peak at 1335 cm^{-1} (CH_3CH_2 twisting of proteins and nucleic acids)) [37, 60, 61]. The over-expression of various protein-related biomolecules in NPC tissues can also be observed through the increased protein-related Raman peaks of NPC tissue (e.g., 1265 cm^{-1} (amide III, ν(C–N) and δ(N–H) of proteins), 1335 cm^{-1} (CH_3CH_2 twisting of proteins and nucleic acids), 1445 cm^{-1} ($\delta(CH_2)$ deformation of proteins and lipids), etc.) [37, 62, 63]. On the other hand, the Raman spectral differences between healthy control and NPC in HW region can provide further insight into the CH_2 and CH_3 information, as well as the interactions of intra- and inter-cellular water *in situ* [37]. For example, the Raman spectral differences at the peaks of 2850 cm^{-1} and 2885 cm^{-1} (symmetric and asymmetric CH_2 stretching of lipids) as well as 2940 cm^{-1} (CH_3 stretching of proteins) are related to the proliferation activity of epithelial cells during NPC development [37, 62, 63]. The water region increasing at the peaks ~3250 cm^{-1} in the NPC tissue shows the hydrogen-bonded network rearrangement in the nasopharyngeal epithelium [37].

Relying on the distinct Raman spectral differences between NPC and healthy control, PCA-LDA model has been developed with LOOCV for early NPC diagnosis at endoscopy. Compared with using FP and HW regions only in the diagnosis model which incorrectly predict 22 (normal: 11 and NPC: 11) and 21 (normal: 9 and NPC: 12) sites of the total 204 tissue sites measured, only 14 tissue sites are mistakenly classified by using simultaneous FP/HW Raman spectra for NPC diagnosis. The diagnostic results are further investigated by tracing back on the misclassified tissue sites. The misdiagnosed tissue sites by using FP region only have a relatively more intense AF background while the Raman signal in FP region is weaker. By adding the Raman spectra in the HW region where the AF background is comparably diminutive, the overall signal-to-noise ratio of the Raman spectral can be improved in the diagnosis model development [37]. The encouraging results of early NPC detection using FP/HW Raman spectroscopy suggests that fiber-optic Raman spectroscopy has great potential to be a rapid but accurate tool for *in vivo* NPC diagnosis at endoscopy.

Distinct Raman spectral differences can also be identified among the PT NPC patients at different PT time points compared to the healthy control (Figure 14.6). These spectral differences are mainly related with the biomolecular changes of the nasopharyngeal epithelium after the treatment, such as proteins, lipids, and nucleic acids, suggesting the underlying biomolecular and morphological changes caused by the toxicity accumulation at the nasopharynx after the radio/chemotherapy treatment as well as the concurrent tissue fibrosis process [37, 38, 56, 57, 62]. We have further semi-quantitatively analyzed this biomolecular change using the protein-to-lipid Raman ratio of the PT patients using the representative Raman bands in FP and HW regions as well as Eqs. (14.1) and (14.2). A significant increasing trend of protein-to-lipid ratios can be found from PT 1-m to PT 3-m groups, while the level of protein-to-lipid ratios remains unchanged from PT 3-m to PT $\geq$ 6-m (Figure 14.6(c)–(d)), reflecting the stability of the accumulated protein contents in the PT nasopharyngeal epithelium after the treatment. The increasing trend of the protein-to-lipid ratio discovered in the tissue Raman spectra agrees with the tissue fibrosis progression, which normally happens from ~4 months after the treatment. During the fibrosis process, the extracellular collagen matrix is regenerated to repair the tissue damaged by the radio/chemotherapy-induced toxicity [6, 38, 57]. Hence, this discovery shows that the biomolecular sensitiveness of the fiber-optic Raman spectroscopy enables the longitudinal label-free, rapid follow-up of the biochemical changes in the PT NPC patients at endoscopy.

To provide an objective and unbiased evaluation of the rNPC diagnosis capability using fiber-optic Raman spectroscopy, the training and testing dataset are strictly separated. The PLS-LDA mode for NPC recurrence detection from early and long-term PT patients are trained and tested separately. Attributed to the significant biomolecular and morphological differences between NPC and early PT nasopharynx reflected in the tissue Raman spectra (Figure 14.7), only one tissue site is misdiagnosed in the training dataset and all the tissue sites in the testing dataset are correctly classified for discriminating rNPC from PT < 3-m group (Figure 14.8(a), (d)). This result confirms the ability of fiber-optic Raman spectroscopy in capturing the key biomolecular differences between rNPC and early PT nasopharynx tissue. Although both rNPC and PT fibrosis show protein overexpression and mucosal thickening [37, 57], which may diminish the Raman spectral differences, significant Raman spectral dissimilarity can still be observed in the region of 850–1209 cm^{-1} due to a plethora of biomolecular differences between rNPC and PT ≥ 3-m (Figure 14.7). Consequently, only two NPC tissue sites and one rNPC tissue site are misclassified in the task of discriminating NPC from PT ≥ 3-m groups (Figure 14.8(b), (e)), confirming that biomolecular features of rNPC can be accurately identified by fiber-optic Raman spectroscopy from tissue PT fibrosis. Furthermore, the AUCs of the ROC curves calculated for all models are larger than 0.995, affirming the clinical diagnostic capability of fiber-optic Raman spectroscopy for label-free PT NPC patient follow-up and tumor recurrence detection.

We further evaluated the utility of RS-CNN model for rapid NPC detection and PT patient assessment. The Raman spectra diagnosis accuracy is calculated on a single spectrum basis with an integration time of >1 s per spectrum to evaluate the real-time diagnosis capability of fiber-optic Raman spectroscopy. Compared to the PLS-LDA model whose overall diagnostic accuracy drops from 73.57% to 71.58% in discriminating NPC from control and PT tissue sites using Full Spec, DS-2 and DS-4 datasets, the RS-CNN model shows an overall accuracy of >79% (Figure 14.9(a)), reflecting a superior spectral information sensitiveness and higher fitting capability with less parameters required for RS-CNN models for NPC detection. In detail, both PLS-LDA and RS-CNN models show a diagnostic accuracy of >82% for discriminating NPC from healthy control sites due to the distinct Raman spectral differences between control and NPC (Figure 14.9). However, the Raman spectra of PT NPC patients are changing with respect to their PT duration due to the progression of the PT fibrosis induced by radio/chemotherapy toxicity [6, 38, 57]. This Raman spectral variation will largely prevent the linear classification models from making an accurate judgement in the Raman spectral-based NPC diagnosis [55]. Owing to a better fitting capability of convolutional neural networks, the RS-CNN model shows a superior prediction capability, accurately diagnosing 672 out of 832 tissue Raman spectra for detecting NPC from PT patients, while only 569 out of 832 spectra are classified correctly by PLS-LDA. These results indicate that RS-CNN can more effectively unveil subtle but diagnostically relevant Raman spectral features in NPC diagnosis, as compared to traditional multivariate linear models (e.g., PLS-LDA).

The performance of the RS-CNN model can be further optimized by reducing the redundant information and noise in the input dataset through the down-sampling process [64, 65]. In this study, the RS-CNN model reaches its optical performance with the DS-2 dataset, where 1,041 out of 1,256 tissue Raman spectra are correctly predicted in all testing datasets, while only 924 out of 1,256 spectra are classified correctly by PLS-LDA model with Full Spec datasets, affirming the enhanced NPC detection ability of the RS-CNN model. Meanwhile, the operating points provided by RS-CNN models are remarkably higher compared to the ROC curves provided by PLS-LDA models, showing that RS-CNN-based Raman diagnosis models can provide a more accurate and robust diagnostic result for differentiating NPC from both healthy and PT subjects.

Further understanding of the Raman spectral features identified by the RS-CNN model in the diagnosis process is achieved by drawing the saliency maps using the correctly predicted Raman spectra in DS-2 testing datasets. The most sensitive Raman bands are selected in the maps (e.g., 1104, 1367, 1402, 1466, 1596, 1607, 1646, 1651, 1668, 2848, 2994 cm^{-1}, etc.), showing the new insights of NPC-related biomolecular information which is useful in RS-CNN tissue diagnosis. Specifically, the relative Raman intensity changes related to proteins or amino acids in the NPC Raman spectra are recognized by the RS-CNN model in the diagnosis (e.g., the increase of 1607 cm^{-1} (tyrosine and phenylalanine) and 1668 cm^{-1} (amide I) and the decrease of 1646 cm^{-1} (amide I) and 1651 cm^{-1} (amide I) compared to control tissues, and the increase of 1104 cm^{-1} (phenylalanine) and 1618 cm^{-1} (proteins and tryptophan) and the decrease of 1402 cm^{-1} (collagens) and 1596 cm^{-1} (amide I) compared to PT tissues), reflecting the extracellular matrix remodeling and protein translation in the NPC tissues [37, 38, 58, 66]. On the other hand, there are also lipid-related Raman peak variations in NPC tissue Raman spectra which draw RS-CNN models' attention in the decision-making process (e.g., the increase of 1367 cm^{-1} (phospholipids), 1466 cm^{-1} (lipids), and 2994 cm^{-1} (cholesterol ester) compared to control tissues, and the increase of 1466 cm^{-1} (lipids) and 2848 cm^{-1} (lipids and fatty acids) compared to PT tissues), indicating the possible accumulation of the lipid or fatty acid biochemicals in the NPC tissues due to the elevated metabolism process [37, 38, 58, 67]. Overall, the diagnostically significant Raman features identified by the RS-CNN model in the diagnosis process further proves the biomolecular sensitiveness of *in vivo* fiber-optic Raman spectroscopy for accurate and rapid NPC diagnosis at the biomolecular level.

14.5 Conclusions

In conclusion, we have presented the development and clinical utility of fiber-optic Raman spectroscopy for HNC diagnosis and PT patient management. We have developed a fiber-optic Raman spectroscopy system associated with diagnostic algorithms for the rapid, label-free collection of tissue Raman spectra at endoscopy. The effectiveness and robustness of the fiber-optic Raman spectroscopy in HNC diagnosis have been demonstrated through solving the clinical challenges of real-time NPC detection and PT NPC patient follow-ups. A novel RS-CNN model has been further developed with high diagnostic accuracy, affirming the clinical effectiveness of fiber-optic Raman spectroscopy for enhancing NPC diagnosis and rapid PT follow-up in NPC patients. Further clinical trials involving a larger scale of HNC patients at multiple clinical centers can be launched in the near future to truly assess the clinical merits of fiber-optic Raman spectroscopy in the head and neck clinic. We anticipate that with the advantages of high diagnostic accuracy, real-time detection, minimal invasiveness, as well as cost effectiveness and ease of operation, fiber-optic Raman spectroscopy has great promise to serve as a powerful clinical diagnostic tool for mass screening and surveyance of HNC patients, ultimately improving HNC management and patients' quality of life.

Acknowledgements

This work was supported in part by the Academic Research Fund Tier 2 (A-8000117-01-00) and Tier 1 (R397-000-334-114, R397-000-371-114, and R397-000-378-114) from the Ministry of Education, Merlion Fund (R397-000-356-133), and the National Medical Research Council (A-0009502-01-00 and A-8001143-00-00), Singapore.

References

1. Sung, H., Ferlay, J., Siegel, R. L., Laversanne, M., Soerjomataram, I., Jemal, A., *et al.* (2021) Global cancer statistics 2020: GLOBOCAN estimates of incidence and mortality worldwide for 36 cancers in 185 countries. CA. Cancer J. Clin. **71** (3), 209–249.

2. Frazell, E. L. and Martin, H. (1962) Cancer of the head and neck. CA. Cancer J. Clin. **12** (1), 27–30.
3. Cohen, E. E. W., LaMonte, S. J., Erb, N. L., Beckman, K. L., Sadeghi, N., Hutcheson, K. A., *et al.* (2016) American Cancer Society head and neck cancer survivorship care guideline. CA. Cancer J. Clin. **66** (3), 203–239.
4. Jawa, Y., Yadav, P., Gupta, S., Mathan, S. V., Pandey, J., Saxena, A. K., *et al.* (2021) Current insights and advancements in head and neck cancer: emerging biomarkers and therapeutics with cues from single cell and 3D model omics profiling. Front. Oncol. **11**, 676948.
5. Argiris, A. and Eng, C. (2003) Epidemiology, staging, and screening of head and neck cancer. Cancer Treat. Res. **114**, 15–60.
6. Chen, Y.-P., Chan, A. T. C., Le, Q.-T., Blanchard, P., Sun, Y. and Ma, J. (2019) Nasopharyngeal carcinoma. Lancet **394** (10192), 64–80.
7. Chua, M. L. K., Wee, J. T. S., Hui, E. P. and Chan, A. T. C. (2016) Nasopharyngeal carcinoma. Lancet **387** (10022), 1012–1024.
8. Chen, Y., Zhao, W., Lin, L., Xiao, X., Zhou, X., Ming, H., *et al.* (2015) Nasopharyngeal Epstein-Barr virus load: an efficient supplementary method for population-based nasopharyngeal carcinoma screening. PLoS One **10** (7), e0132669.
9. Ng, S.-H., Liu, H.-M., Ko, S.-F., Hao, S.-P. and Chong, V. F. H. (2002) Posttreatment imaging of the nasopharynx. Eur. J. Radiol. **44** (2), 82–95.
10. Tabuchi, K., Nakayama, M., Nishimura, B., Hayashi, K. and Hara, A. (2011) Early detection of nasopharyngeal carcinoma. Int. J. Otolaryngol. **2011**, 638058.
11. Mohandas, A., Marcus, C., Kang, H., Truong, M.-T. and Subramaniam, R. M. (2014) FDG PET/CT in the management of nasopharyngeal carcinoma. Am. J. Roentgenol. **203** (2), W146–W157.
12. Zhan, Y. and Fan, S. (2020) Multiple mechanisms involving in radioresistance of nasopharyngeal carcinoma. J. Cancer. **11** (14), 4193–4204.
13. Chong, V. F. and Fan, Y. F. (1997) Detection of recurrent nasopharyngeal carcinoma: MR imaging versus CT. Radiology **202** (2), 463–470.
14. Heng, H. P. S., Shu, C., Zheng, W., Lin, K. and Huang, Z. (2021) Advances in real-time fiber-optic Raman spectroscopy for early cancer diagnosis: Pushing the frontier into clinical endoscopic applications. Transl. Biophotonics **3** (1), e202000018.
15. Raman, C. V. and Krishnan, K. S. (1928) A new type of secondary radiation. Nature **121** (3048), 501–502.
16. Desroches, J., Jermyn, M., Pinto, M., Picot, F., Tremblay, M.-A., Obaid, S., *et al.* (2018) A new method using Raman spectroscopy for in vivo targeted brain cancer tissue biopsy. Sci. Rep. **8** (1), 1792.
17. Lin, K., Zheng, W., Lim, C. M. and Huang, Z. (2016) Real-time in vivo diagnosis of laryngeal carcinoma with rapid fiber-optic Raman spectroscopy. Biomed. Opt. Express **7** (9), 3705.

18. Teh, S. K., Zheng, W., Lau, D. P. C. and Huang, Z. (2009) Spectroscopic diagnosis of laryngeal carcinoma using near-infrared Raman spectroscopy and random recursive partitioning ensemble techniques. Analyst **134** (6), 1232.
19. Lin, K., Lau, D. P. C. and Huang, Z. (2012) Optical diagnosis of laryngeal cancer using high wavenumber Raman spectroscopy. Biosens. Bioelectron. **35** (1), 213–217.
20. Singh, S. P., Deshmukh, A., Chaturvedi, P. and Krishna, C. M. (2012) In vivo Raman spectroscopic identification of premalignant lesions in oral buccal mucosa. J. Biomed. Opt. **17** (10), 105002.
21. Yan, H., Yu, M., Xia, J., Zhu, L., Zhang, T. and Zhu, Z. (2019) Tongue squamous cell carcinoma discrimination with Raman spectroscopy and convolutional neural networks. Vib. Spectrosc. **103**, 102938.
22. Yu, M., Yan, H., Xia, J., Zhu, L., Zhang, T., Zhu, Z., *et al.* (2019) Deep convolutional neural networks for tongue squamous cell carcinoma classification using Raman spectroscopy. Photodiagnosis Photodyn. Ther. **26**, 430–435.
23. Singh, S. P., Sahu, A., Deshmukh, A., Chaturvedi, P. and Krishna, C. M. (2013) In vivo Raman spectroscopy of oral buccal mucosa: a study on malignancy associated changes (MAC)/cancer field effects (CFE). Analyst **138** (14), 4175.
24. Bergholt, M. S., Zheng, W., Ho, K. Y., Teh, M., Yeoh, K. G., Yan So, J. B., *et al.* (2014) Fiber-optic confocal Raman spectroscopy for real-time in vivo diagnosis of dysplasia in barrett's esophagus. Gastroenterology **146** (1), 27–32.
25. Wang, J., Lin, K., Zheng, W., Ho, K. Y., Teh, M., Yeoh, K. G., *et al.* (2016) Fiber-optic Raman spectroscopy for in vivo diagnosis of gastric dysplasia. Faraday Discuss. **187**, 377–392.
26. Bergholt, M. S., Zheng, W., Lin, K., Wang, J., Xu, H., Ren, J., *et al.* (2015) Characterizing variability of in vivo Raman spectroscopic properties of different anatomical sites of normal colorectal tissue towards cancer diagnosis at colonoscopy. Anal. Chem. **87** (2), 960–966.
27. Lau, D. P., Huang, Z., Lui, H., Man, C. S., Berean, K., Morrison, M. D., *et al.* (2003) Raman spectroscopy for optical diagnosis in normal and cancerous tissue of the nasopharynx—preliminary findings. Lasers Surg. Med. **32** (3), 210–214.
28. Li, S., Chen, Q.-Y., Zhang, Y.-J., Liu, Z., Xiong, H., Guo, Z., *et al.* (2012) Detection of nasopharyngeal cancer using confocal Raman spectroscopy and genetic algorithm technique. J. Biomed. Opt. **17** (12), 125003.
29. Wang, J., Bergholt, M. S., Zheng, W. and Huang, Z. (2013) Development of a beveled fiber-optic confocal Raman probe for enhancing in vivo epithelial tissue Raman measurements at endoscopy. Opt. Lett. **38** (13), 2321–2323.
30. Wang, J., Lin, K., Zheng, W., Ho, K. Y., Teh, M., Yeoh, K. G., *et al.* (2015) Comparative study of the endoscope-based bevelled and volume fiber-optic Raman probes for optical diagnosis of gastric dysplasia in vivo at endoscopy. Anal. Bioanal. Chem. **407** (27), 8303–8310.

31. Duraipandian, S., Zheng, W., Ng, J., Low, J. J. H., Ilancheran, A. and Huang, Z. (2012) Simultaneous fingerprint and high-wavenumber confocal Raman spectroscopy enhances early detection of cervical precancer in vivo. Anal. Chem. **84** (14), 5913–5919.
32. Bergholt, M. S., Lin, K., Wang, J., Zheng, W., Xu, H., Huang, Q., *et al.* (2016) Simultaneous fingerprint and high-wavenumber fiber-optic Raman spectroscopy enhances real-time in vivo diagnosis of adenomatous polyps during colonoscopy. J. Biophotonics **9** (4), 333–342.
33. Heng, H. P. S., Shu, C., Zheng, W. and Huang, Z. (2022) Development of coaxial DCF-GRIN fiber-optic Raman probe for enhancing in vivo epithelial tissue Raman measurements. Opt. Lett. **47** (22), 5989–5992.
34. Shu, C., Zheng, W., Wang, Z., Yu, C. and Huang, Z. (2021) Development and characterization of a disposable submillimeter fiber optic Raman needle probe for enhancing real-time in vivo deep tissue and biofluids Raman measurements. Opt. Lett. **46** (20), 5197–5200.
35. Lin, K., Wang, J., Zheng, W., Ho, K. Y., Teh, M., Yeoh, K. G., *et al.* (2016) Rapid fiber-optic Raman spectroscopy for real-time in vivo detection of gastric intestinal metaplasia during clinical gastroscopy. Cancer Prev. Res. **9** (6), 476–483.
36. Wang, J., Lin, K., Zheng, W., Yu Ho, K., Teh, M., Guan Yeoh, K., *et al.* (2015) Simultaneous fingerprint and high-wavenumber fiber-optic Raman spectroscopy improves in vivo diagnosis of esophageal squamous cell carcinoma at endoscopy. Sci. Rep. **5** (1), 12957.
37. Lin, K., Zheng, W., Lim, C. M. and Huang, Z. (2017) Real-time in vivo diagnosis of nasopharyngeal carcinoma using rapid fiber-optic Raman spectroscopy. Theranostics **7** (14), 3517–3526.
38. Shu, C., Zheng, W., Lin, K., Lim, C. and Huang, Z. (2021) Label-free follow-up surveying of post-treatment efficacy and recurrence in nasopharyngeal carcinoma patients with fiberoptic Raman endoscopy. Anal. Chem. **93** (4), 2053–2061.
39. Shu, C., Yan, H., Zheng, W., Lin, K., James, A., Selvarajan, S., *et al.* (2021) Deep learning-guided fiberoptic Raman spectroscopy enables real-time in vivo diagnosis and assessment of nasopharyngeal carcinoma and post-treatment efficacy during endoscopy. Anal. Chem. **93** (31), 10898–10906.
40. Mo, J., Zheng, W. and Huang, Z. (2010) Fiber-optic Raman probe couples ball lens for depth-selected Raman measurements of epithelial tissue. Biomed. Opt. Express. **1** (1), 17–30.
41. American National Standards Institute and The Laser Institute of America, Eds. (2007) American National Standard for safe use of lasers: approved March 16, 2007. The Laser Institute of America, Orlando, FLa.
42. Choquette, S., Etz, E. S., Hurst, W., Blackburn, D. H. and Leigh, S. D. (2007) Relative intensity correction of Raman spectrometers: NIST SRMs 2241 through 2243 for 785 nm, 532 nm and 488 nm/514.5 nm excitation. Appl. Spectrosc. **61**, 117–129.

43. Duraipandian, S., Zheng, W., Ng, J., Low, J. J. H., Ilancheran, A. and Huang, Z. (2013) Near-infrared-excited confocal Raman spectroscopy advances in vivo detection of cervical precancer. J. Biomed. Opt. **18** (6), 67007.
44. Huang, Z., Zeng, H., Hamzavi, I., McLean, D. I. and Lui, H. (2001) Rapid near-infrared Raman spectroscopy system for real-time in vivo skin measurements. Opt. Lett. **26** (22), 1782–1784.
45. Carletta, J. (n.d.) Squibs and discussions: assessing agreement on classification tasks: the kappa statistic. Comput. Linguist. **22** (2), 6.
46. Lieber, C. A. and Mahadevan-Jansen, A. (2003) Automated method for subtraction of fluorescence from biological Raman spectra. Appl. Spectrosc. **57** (11), 1363–1367.
47. Zhao, J., Lui, H., McLean, D. I. and Zeng, H. (2007) Automated autofluorescence background subtraction algorithm for biomedical Raman spectroscopy. Appl. Spectrosc. **61** (11), 1225–1232.
48. Haynes, W. (2013) Student's t-Test BT-Encyclopedia of Systems Biology. In *Encyclopedia of Systems Biology* (Dubitzky, W., Wolkenhauer, O., Cho, K.-H. and Yokota, H., Eds.), pp. 2023–2025, Springer.
49. Ioffe, S. and Szegedy, C. (2015) Batch normalization: accelerating deep network training by reducing. J. Mol. Struct. **1134**, 63–66.
50. He, K., Zhang, X., Ren, S. and Sun, J. (2016) Deep residual learning for image recognition. Proc. IEEE Comput. Soc. Conf. Comput. Vis. Pattern Recognit., 770–778.
51. Le, Q. V, Ngiam, J., Coates, A., Lahiri, A., Prochnow, B. and Ng, A. Y. (2011) On optimization methods for deep learning. In: Proc. 28th Int. Conf. Mach. Learn., Omnipress, Madison, WI, USA, 265–272.
52. LeCun, Y., Bottou, L., Bengio, Y. and Haffner, P. (1998) Gradient-based learning applied to document recognition. Proc. IEEE. **86** (11), 2278–2323.
53. Selvaraju, R.R., Cogswell, M., Das, A., Vedantam, R., Parikh, D. and Batra, D. (2016) Grad-CAM: Visual explanations from deep networks via gradient-based localization. Int. J. Comput. Vis. **128** (2), 336–359.
54. Smilkov, D., Thorat, N., Kim, B., Viégas, F. and Wattenberg, M. (2017) SmoothGrad: removing noise by adding noise [Preprint]. arXiv:1706.03825.
55. Lim, C. M., Gangodu, N. R., Loh, T., Zheng, W., Wang, J., Lin, K., *et al.* (2017) Real time near-infrared Raman spectroscopy for the diagnosis of nasopharyngeal cancer. Oncotarget **8** (30), 49443–49450.
56. Žuvela, P., Lin, K., Shu, C., Zheng, W., Lim, C. M. and Huang, Z. (2019) Fiber-optic Raman spectroscopy with nature-inspired genetic algorithms enhances real-time in vivo detection and diagnosis of nasopharyngeal carcinoma. Anal. Chem. **91** (13), 8101–8108.
57. Straub, J. M., New, J., Hamilton, C. D., Lominska, C., Shnayder, Y. and Thomas, S. M. (2015) Radiation-induced fibrosis: mechanisms and implications for therapy. J. Cancer Res. Clin. Oncol. **141** (11), 1985–1994.

58. Movasaghi, Z., Rehman, S. and Rehman, I. (2007) Raman spectroscopy of biological tissues. Appl. Spectrosc. Rev. **42**, 493–541.
59. Sakr, W. A., Gale, N., Gnepp, D. R. and Crissman, J. D. (2009) Chapter 1 — Squamous Intraepithelial Neoplasia of the Upper Aerodigestive Tract. In *Diagnostic Surgical Pathology of the Head and Neck* 2nd ed. (Gnepp, D. R., Ed.), pp. 1–44, Saunders.
60. Dai, W., Zheng, H., Cheung, A. K. L. and Lung, M. L. (2016) Genetic and epigenetic landscape of nasopharyngeal carcinoma. Chinese Clin. Oncol. **5** (2), 16.
61. Tong, J. H. M., Tsang, R. K. Y., Lo, K.-W., Woo, J. K. S., Kwong, J., Chan, M. W. Y., *et al.* (2002) Quantitative Epstein-Barr virus DNA analysis and detection of gene promoter hypermethylation in nasopharyngeal (NP) brushing samples from patients with NP carcinoma. Clin. Cancer Res. **8** (8), 2612–2619.
62. Chou, J., Lin, Y.-C., Kim, J., You, L., Xu, Z., He, B., *et al.* (2008) Nasopharyngeal carcinoma--review of the molecular mechanisms of tumorigenesis. Head Neck. **30** (7), 946–963.
63. Ouyang, J., Wu, M., Huang, C., Cao, L. and Li, G. (2013) Overexpression of oxidored-nitro domain containing protein 1 inhibits human nasopharyngeal carcinoma and cervical cancer cell proliferation and induces apoptosis: Involvement of mitochondrial apoptotic pathways. Oncol. Rep. **29** (1), 79–86.
64. Wang, C.-W. and You, W.-H. (2013) Boosting-SVM: Effective learning with reduced data dimension. Appl. Intell. **39**, 465–474.
65. Xu, A. and Raginsky, M. (2017) Information-theoretic analysis of generalization capability of learning algorithms. Proceedings of the 31st International Conference on Neural Information Processing Systems, pp. 2521–2530.
66. Xu, S., Xu, H., Wang, W., Li, S., Li, H., Li, T., *et al.* (2019) The role of collagen in cancer: from bench to bedside. J. Transl. Med. **17** (1), 309.
67. Currie, E., Schulze, A., Zechner, R., Walther, T. C. and Farese Jr., R. V. (2013) Cellular fatty acid metabolism and cancer. Cell Metab. **18** (2), 153–161.

https://doi.org/10.1142/9789811264610_0015

Chapter 15

Raman Probe and Live Tissue Analysis for Monitoring Biological Activity

Akinori Taketani,[1] Hidetoshi Sato[2,*]

[1]*Research Center for Pre-Disease Science, University of Toyama*
2630, Sugitani, Toyama, Toyama, 930-0194 Japan
[2]*School of Biological and Environmental Sciences, Kwansei Gakuin University*
1, Gakuen Uegahara, Sanda, Hyogo, 669-1330 Japan
**Corresponding author: hidesato@kwansei.ac.jp*

15.1 Introduction

Raman spectroscopy is one of the few label-free techniques that are able to obtain molecular information in both live tissues and cells. It is useful to apply the knowledge obtained from cells to tissues. Many Raman studies of live cells have been published in which commercially available Raman microscopes have often been used for the measurements [1–7]. An inversed Raman microscope is preferable but an upright one is also applicable for short-time monitoring of the live cells. For Raman measurement of live mammal cells, a CO_2 incubator may be required to keep the cells under cultivation conditions. As the CO_2 incubator is commercially available for microscopy, it is not difficult to prepare a Raman microscope system for live cell analysis. In contrast, it is rather difficult to make Raman measurements for live tissues, because there are many variations for tissue locations. One of the difficulties is how to bring an optical head near the tissue to be measured. A small handheld Raman instrument with an optical head is commercially available. This type of instrument is useful when the sample has strong Raman signal and weak autofluorescence, but it is not efficient enough for most tissue analysis. The excitation light of

785 nm is often used for tissue analysis to avoid autofluorescence of the tissue sample. Dark current of a charge-coupled detector (CCD) is generated by self-absorption of the light generated by blackbody emission that is stronger in the near-infrared region than in the visible region at room temperature. Therefore, the CCD must be cooled down to suppress the dark current noise for measurement with 785 nm excitation. The container size and electrical consumption of the near-infrared (NIR) optimized CCD unit are usually too large for a handheld Raman instrument. If the tissue was inside of the inner organ of a body, it would be impossible to bring the whole instrument, even if it was the handheld one, into the body. It means that a remote optical head is required, and the head must be guided under visual observation. For this purpose, several types of Raman probes made with optical fibers have been developed and introduced [8–20]. The Raman probes are designed for all over the surface area which is not able to be put under an objective lens of the microscope and/or for use with an endoscope. The former is relatively thick and can be purchased from vendors of Raman instruments recently. However, the latter is not commercially available as far as we know. The users must design and develop their own Raman probes to fit their purposes. In this chapter, optical designs, materials and properties of miniaturized Raman probes are introduced, and then their applications to medical and health sciences are discussed.

15.2 Optical Design and Property of Miniaturized Raman Probes

15.2.1 *Property of Bundled Optical Fibers*

An optical fiber made of glass materials is useful to deliver light. The optical fiber usually consists of two kinds of glass materials to deliver light and a protective sheath made of resin, plastic or metal. As the glass optical fiber has core and clad parts with higher and lower refraction indexes, respectively, the light inserted in the fiber is confined by total reflection at the border of the core and clad. The clad material may be a plastic in some cases. The maximum angle of the acceptable ray of light to the optical fiber depends on the angle of total reflection according to Snell's law and refraction indices of its fiber materials. Although the optical fiber is a great device for transmission of light, some problems should be addressed to use for Raman probes, especially that due to noise lights arising from various origins in the optical fiber. Suppression of such optical noises is important especially for medical and health applications, as the Raman spectra of tissues and biomaterials are often remarkably weak.

Ma *et al.* reported about Raman background spectra of fused silica fibers which were due to the glass material of the fiber itself [21]. Although the Raman scattered light of quartz is not strong, the accumulated Raman scattered light in the fiber easily overwhelms the Raman signal of the sample, because the total excitation volume of quartz (core material) is quite large and the generated Raman scattered light is enclosed in the fiber and transmitted with the laser light. Moreover, high numerical aperture (NA) fibers often emit stronger background due to the varied ions which are doped to the core and/or clad materials, such as Ge. The ions are doped to control the refraction indices of the materials. It is necessary to pay careful attention to use a gradient index lens as well as graded index fiber for use in the miniaturized Raman probe because of the strong background due to the doped glasses. The Raman noise of the doped fibers were compared in the literature by Komachi *et al.* [15] (Figure 15.1). The noise light generated in the Ge-doped optical fiber (a) is stronger than those in fused silica fibers (b and c).

The total reflection is in one direction. When the side wall of the optical fiber is irradiated from the outside, part of the light can reach the core, scattered and trapped in the fiber. Therefore, the optical fiber part of the Raman probe must be covered with a light shield. When the fiber is bent sharply, a ray which irradiates at the core-clad border more than the angle of total reflection

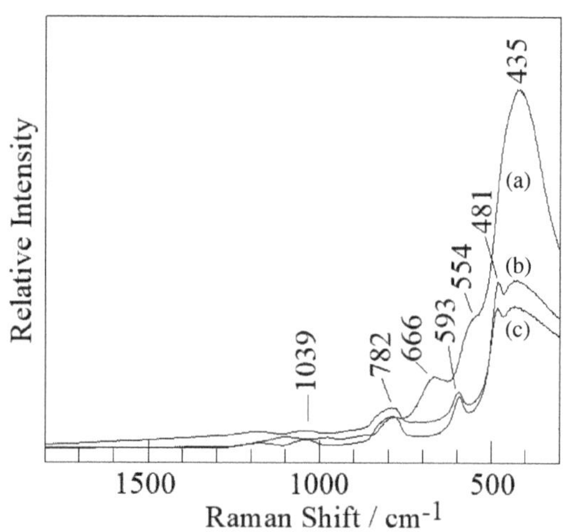

Figure 15.1. Raman spectra of the FRB of (a) GeO_2-doped fused silica, (b) pure fused silica, and (c) low-OH fused silica optical fibers measured for 720 nm excitation. Reproduced from Ref. [15] with permission.

can be released from the core. Moreover, the released laser light irradiates the sheath material, such as polyimide, and generates strong fluorescence due to the sheath material. A part of the leaked laser light and resulting fluorescence can be trapped in other fibers in the bundle. This optical cross-talk is sometimes an origin of noise light and should be avoided. The leaked and noise light often trapped in the clad can be transmitted partly in the fiber and can sometimes become a noise source. The probe head must be designed to suppress all the possible optical noises.

15.2.2 *Coupling of Optical Fibers to a Spectrometer*

High NA optical fibers are commercially available and their use seems to be favorable for higher efficiency in collecting scattered light from the sample. However, it may not be a good choice. When designing a miniaturized Raman probe, it is necessary to consider optical properties of other devices, too, in the entire Raman system. NA of a quartz fiber is usually about 0.20–0.22, of which the acceptable angle of the fiber is about 12°. As discussed above, optical filters must be placed in the distal optical head of the miniaturized Raman probe to suppress the noise generated in the optical fibers, a band-pass (BP) filter for the laser light delivery fiber and a long-pass (LP) filter for the scattered light collection fibers. If the optical head was enough large to equip an efficient lens coupling, incoming beam to the filters would be collimated correctly. However, the miniaturized Raman probe, with typically 2 mm or less diameter, does not have enough room for such collimating lens. The BP and LP filters, which are usually dielectric multilayer filters, are attached on the optical fibers without a collimation lens. Their sharp spectral cutting edge and high shield property are trade-offs against their acceptable angle. The acceptable angle of a high-performance filter is usually less than 10°, which is smaller than that of a normal quartz fiber. Hence, use of high NA optical fiber will result in the increment of optical noise due to the light leaked from the filters.

The aperture of the normal quartz fiber, NA 0.21, corresponds to 2.32 of F number. The typical F number of a usual dispersion polychromator with 300 mm focal length is about 4.0. It means that the NA of the normal quartz fiber is already too large to couple with a normal spectrometer. Figure 15.2(a) depicts an optical design of a typical coupling stage of an optical fiber and a spectrometer. Now, we consider to couple an optical fiber, NA 0.21, 100 μm diameter to a spectrometer, F 4.0. When the ratio of the focal lengths of lens A to lens B is 1.72 (= 2.32/4.0), the acceptable angles of the optical fiber and

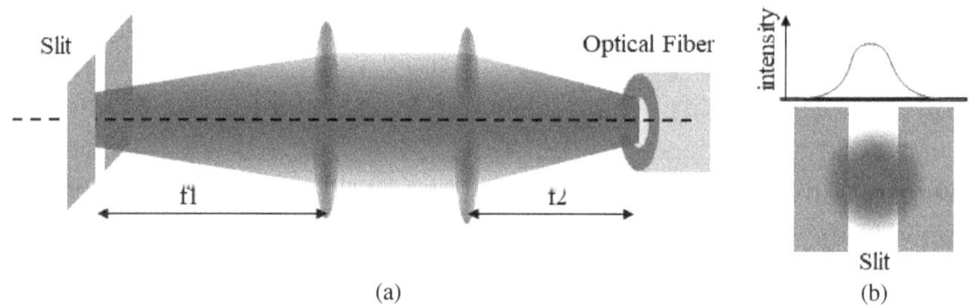

Figure 15.2. (a) An optical design of coupling stage connecting optical fiber and Raman spectrometer and (b) a transferred image of the optical fiber on a slit of the spectrometer.

the spectrometer are matched. The image of the core of the fiber is transferred onto the slit of the spectrometer, which is 172 μm in diameter. It means that the slit width of the spectrometer must be larger than 172 μm to accept all light. Although the slit width of a polychromator depends on the number of grooves of the grating and pixel size of the CCD, it is usually around 100 μm. The ray emitted from the fiber core does not fully pass through the slit (Figure 15.2(b)). This is another reason that the high NA fiber may not be suitable for a Raman probe in theory. Use of thick optical fiber for collection is not recommended for the same reason, although a large cross-sectional area of the core seems to give better efficiency for collection of scattered light. However, the optical loss of this deviation is, in fact, rather smaller than that estimated merely from the image transfer of the core. As the optical density of the delivered light by a multimode optical fiber has a hat top distribution, the photon density in the peripheral area is much lower than in the center. Nevertheless, attention should be paid to any optical loss because any optical fiber has its specific optical property. Instead, multiple collection fibers, which are usually placed surrounding the excitation fiber at the distal end, are aligned in the vertical direction along the longitudinal direction of the slit to improve the coupling efficiency [8, 15].

15.2.3 *Miniaturized Raman Probes*

A miniaturized Raman probe made of bundled optical fibers was developed by Shim *et al.* in 1999 [10]. The diameter of the probe was about 2.0 mm which is narrow enough to insert into a forceps channel of gastric and colon endoscopes. The probe head was designed to shift the focusing axis of the collection fibers toward the excitation fiber to improve the collection efficiency.

Behind the optical head, BP and LP filters are placed at the distal end of optical fibers. The excitation light delivered in an optical fiber excites the optical fiber itself and generates strong background noise due to the glass material, which overwhelms the weak Raman signal of the tissue samples. The glass material usually has Raman bands near 450, 800 and 1100 cm^{-1} due to Si–O bonding. Shim *et al.* applied their Raman probe for use with gastrointestinal endoscope, and Bushman *et al.* for observation of artery wall [11, 12]. Motz *et al.* developed their own Raman probe in 2004 with a ball lens of which the total diameter was about 2 mm [14].

Our research group developed a fiber-optic micro Raman probe in 2005 (MRP; Figure 15.3) of which the total diameter was only about 600 μm [15]. Since our MRP was much narrower than the previously developed Raman probes, we faced problems attributing to the small size of the probe during the development. One of the problems was heat degradation of the filter attached on the laser delivery fiber due to the strong laser illumination. When the filter was glued on the fiber, the optical loss due to the glue layer generated heat and burnt the materials. To solve the problem, a short metal pipe was induced to hold the filter and the fiber by their side and to keep a small interspace in between. The pipe also improved the heat conduction around the BP filter. Moreover, the metal pipe worked to avoid cross-talks of the laser delivery fiber to the light collection fibers. We developed an improved MRP with lenses at its distal end of which total diameter was 750 μm [19]. The central fiber for excitation light was with a flat, thin BP filter and the surrounding fibers for collection light was with a thick LP filter of which the glass substrate side was polished to be a convex lens. When the focal length of the lens was 0.58 mm, its working distance (WD) was 0.3 mm. The sensitivity of MRP with 0.58 mm focal length lens was seven times better than MRP without lens. The WD of the probe could be tuned up to about 1.0 mm by selecting the convex lens.

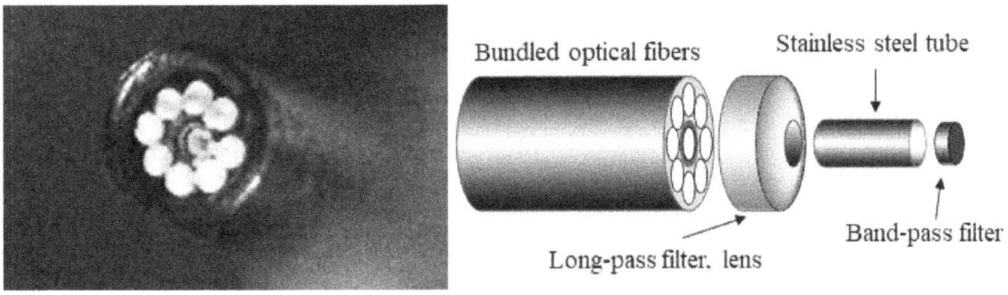

Figure 15.3. A photo of MRP head and its structure.

15.2.4 *Hollow Optical Fiber Raman Probes*

The hollow optical fiber (HOF) is made of an empty quartz tube of which the inside wall is coated with a very smooth silver mirror. HOF was originally developed for the purpose of infrared light delivery [22]. Although the silver mirror has relatively high reflection efficiency among metal mirrors, the transmission efficiency of HOF is lower than that of a usual glass optical fiber. The transmission efficiency is decreased further when HOF is bent, because its NA is about 0.07, much smaller than that of a glass fiber. Since the light is delivered by reflection at the silver surface in the empty core, HOF is free from noise due to the core material. It gives a great advantage despite the drawback of the low transmission efficiency, especially for optical design of a miniaturized Raman probe. There is no filter required at the distal end of the probe, resulting in that one fiber is able to be used bi-directionally for excitation and Raman scattered lights. As the optical axes of delivery and collection rays are identical, the optical design of the probe head can be very simple.

We developed a ball lens top hollow optical fiber Raman probe (BHRP; Figure 15.4) in 2009 [20]. BHRP does not equip the BP or LP filter at its distal head. Instead, it has a ball lens to focus and collect the excitation and Raman scattered lights. The HOF used for BHRP had 320 and 435 μm of core and total diameter, respectively. The WD of BHRP depends on the diameter and the material of the ball lens installed at the distal end. Since only the rather collimated incident light is accepted for transmission because of the low NA, BHRP has an optical property of pseudo-confocal effect. The WD and focal

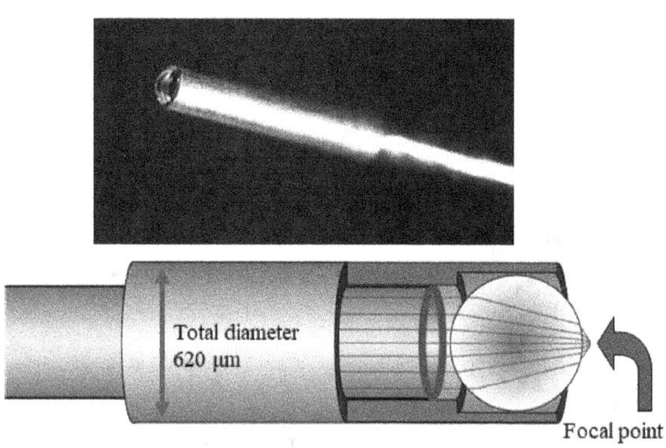

Figure 15.4. A photo of BHRP head and its structure. Adapted from Ref. [20] with permission.

depth of BHRP with a sapphire ball lens of 500 μm diameter is about 58 and 92 μm [23]. In contrast, the WD of BHRP with a quartz ball lens of 500 μm is estimated to be about 230 μm. It is possible to extend WD more with a larger ball lens, but it is with drawback of reduction in the collection efficiency for the scattered light. As endothelial tissues usually have layer structure, the Raman probe with variable WD is useful to analyze the specific subsurface layer in the tissues. The NA 0.07 of HOF corresponds to 4.0° of the acceptable angle and to 7.13 of F number. It is recommended to use a single-mode laser and a coupling lens with relatively long focal length, 150–200 mm to put the laser light into the HOF. If the spectrometer with F 4.0 is correctly coupled with the HOF, the hollow core image transferred onto the slit shrinks down to about 180 μm diameter. The designs of the probes and coupling stage were discussed in detail in a previous book edited by Matousek and Morris [24].

15.3 Application Studies of the Miniaturized Raman Probe

15.3.1 *Study on Development of Colorectal Cancer*

Cancer is not a single disease. Normal tissues are similar to each other but cancer tissues have large variation depending on patients. Many oncogenes have been found, and there are several stages in cancer development. Although cancer tissues have some common properties, such as collagen increment and having a necrosis part, they are not specific only to cancers. Cancer development starts from chronic inflammation, advances to tumors, and then a part turns into malignant tumors. The malignant tumor is usually referred to as cancer. A benign tumor stays on the basal membrane that is made of collagen. When a tumor cell gains the function to dissolve collagen, the cell penetrates the basal membrane and spreads all over the body such that metastasis takes place. Although the process of advancing cancer has been studied mostly through comprehensive medical observations for human patients, experiments on animal models give valuable information on molecular metabolism and reaction to drugs. Moreover, since each patient has different genes, cause, history and type of cancer, it is not possible to make reproducible observations for human patients. The advance of tumor attributes involves slow accumulation of genetic and/or epigenetic mutations. It suggests that the character and molecular composition of the tumor tissue changes along with its advance. As many reports have demonstrated, Raman spectroscopy is one of the most powerful tools to discriminate cancer tissue from normal tissues [25, 26]. In order to carry out Raman analysis of cancer, it should take into account the advancing stages of tumors. It is also important to evaluate the viability of the analytical techniques as well as the instruments for actual clinical use in a body, because live tissues always have blood current and activity which induce difficulties that are not modeled well in *ex vivo* application studies. For example, a resected tissue is usually rinsed with normal saline before Raman measurement, whereas a live tissue in a body is filled with blood. Hemoglobin in blood gives pre-resonance-enhanced Raman bands even with near-infrared excitation light, which can overwhelm weak bands due to minor materials in a tissue [27–29].

We have developed a miniaturized endoscope for mouse and rat to use with MRP and BHRP [18]. It has 2.5 mm total diameter which includes a channel of 1.2 mm inner diameter and a bending mechanism at the head. The endoscope is narrow enough to insert into the stomach of rat and colon of mouse. The endoscope is equipped with a bundled image fiber, 0.5 mm diameter, consisting of 10,000 elemental fibers instead of a CCD camera on the distal end. It was designed for autofluorescence imaging, as the fluorescent light was induced into a filter spectrometer to obtain hyperspectral images. Moreover, the usage of imaging fibers was necessary to avoid heating due to electric current driving the CCD chip because the head of the endoscope was too small to disperse heat efficiently. The miniaturized Raman endoscope (mRE) system was applied to a rodent cancer model [30, 31]. As mice are developed within several months and are syngenetic, they are useful to study advancing cancer with high reproducibility and to demonstrate the potential of Raman spectroscopy in cancer analysis. We employed an azoxymethane-dextran sodium sulfate (AOM-DSS) colon cancer mouse model because the tumor advances rapidly into adenocarcinoma with high probability within only one month. The endoscopic images and Raman spectra of the tumor tissues were recorded in live animals under anesthesia without any invasive procedure [30]. The Raman spectra of advancing tumors were successfully obtained in the live AOM-DSS mouse models under the endoscopic visual guide. It should be noted that Raman data with photo image was repeatedly recorded on a live intact tissue of each specific advancing tumor.

The AOM-DSS administrations were made by intraperitoneal injection to 8-week-old healthy mice. The laser wavelength and power were 785 nm and typically 60 mW, and the exposure time was 60 s. There was no trace of laser illumination observed after the Raman measurement, even at 2 and 4 weeks later, showing that the laser light of 60 mW with 785 nm wavelength was safe to the mucosal and epithelial tissues in colon. The endoscopic observation and

Raman measurements were carried out on each specific tumor for 3 times with 2-week intervals. The distance from anus and the angle of the rotation were recorded for the locations of tumors found under the endoscopic observation [30] (Figure 15.5(A)). The experiments were made under inherent anesthesia. (The mask of anesthesia was removed to take photo in Figure 15.5(A)). Since the mouse models having relatively large and fewer tumors were selected for the study, it was not difficult to discern each lesion. Raman spectra were measured at about 8 different spots in each tumor lesion. Figure 15.5(B) depicts images of a single tumor lesion in a mouse recorded 3 times. It is difficult to estimate if the tumor is benign or malignant from the visual observation. The distal head of BHRP is seen at right up in Figure 15.5B(a). BHRP employed for the mouse colon measurement was equipped with a 500 μm diameter

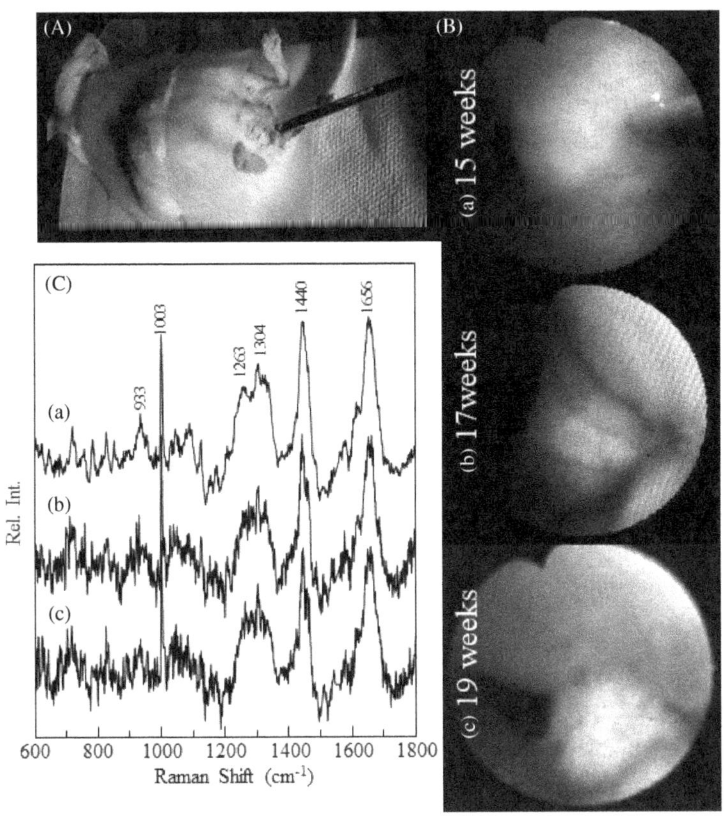

Figure 15.5. (A) An experimental setup for mRE observation, (B) endoscopic images of advancing tumors and (C) their Raman spectra observed in a live mouse model at (a) 15, (b) 17 and (c) 19 weeks old. Adapted from Ref. [30] with permission.

sapphire ball lens, of which WD and focal depth were about 50 and 100 μm, respectively. As the thickness of the mucosal layer of mouse colon was about 100 μm thick and the tumor in the AOM-DSS model arose from the epithelial cell, this BHRP was ideal for the observation. Figure 15.5(C) shows Raman spectra of the live tumor tissues measured with the mRE system. The spectra were slightly noisy but had enough high quality to analyze their molecular changes along with the advancing tumor. Bands at 1656, 1440, 1263, and 1003 cm^{-1} are assigned to amide I, CH bending, amide III and phenylalanine ring modes of protein, respectively. No or very weak band was observed near 1735 cm^{-1} due to C = O stretching mode of ester in fat. Moreover, bands attributed to hemoglobin did not appear. Since the colon has a muscle layer beneath the mucosa layer that is rich in fat and blood vessels, the spectra indicate that the present BHRP had its WD and focal depth perfectly matched to the thickness of the mucosa layer and successfully picked up the spectra of the tumor lesion only. The spectra were analyzed with partial least square regression (PLSR) method to emphasize the difference among the data obtained at 15, 17, and 19 weeks old. The score and loading plots for factors 1 and 2 are shown in Figure 15.6 [30]. The score and loading plots of 3 mice (A and C) and single mouse (B and D) reflect molecular compositional changes due to the tumor advancing. The major spectral change due to the tumor advance is explained with factor 1, as the data dispersion transfers from low to high value along with the advancing of tumor. In the score plot for 3 mice (A), the datasets have wider distributions in the factor 1 axis. The datasets also transfer slightly from low to high value in the factor 2 axis along with the advancing of tumor. In contrast, the datasets in the score plot for the single mouse (B) distribute mostly in the factor 1 axis. The results suggested that the progression rates of the tumors varied among the models, but all of them went in a similar direction and progression rate. In the loading plot of single mouse (D), weak negative bands are observed near 850 and 940 cm^{-1} that are assignable to collagen. It suggests reduction of collagen density in the advancing tumor.

In the AOM-DSS mouse model, it was rumored among the researchers that a tumor would disappear. It happened very rarely but was observed in our study. Raman spectra and endoscopic images were successfully recorded in one of the cases of the shrinking tumor. Figure 15.7 exhibits images (A) and Raman spectra (B) of the shrinking tumor lesion [30]. The head of BHRP and cavity of the colon are marked with asterisks in Figure 15.7(A). A tumor lesion slightly protruded on the colon wall in the image (a), divided into smaller lesions in the image (b), and disappeared in the image (c). Difference spectra (d) and (e) show the difference of (b) and (c) from (a). The Raman

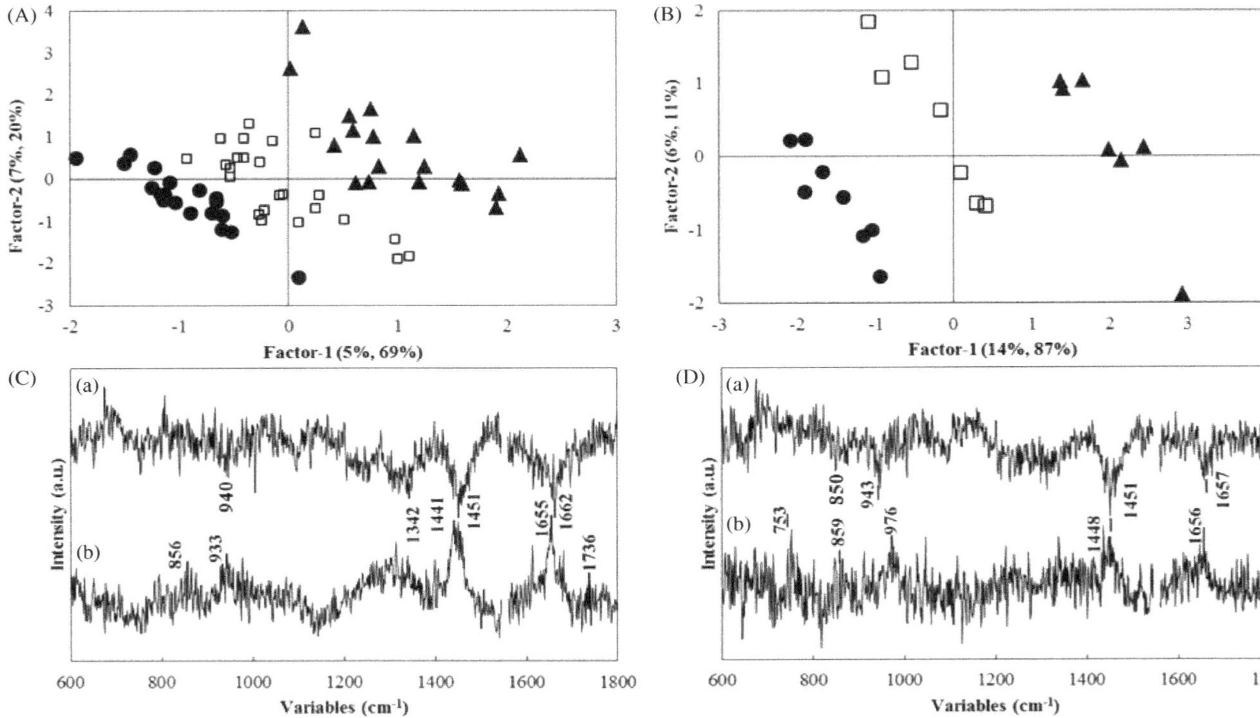

Figure 15.6. (A, B) Score and (C, D) loading plots for factors (a) 1 and (b) 2 of PLSR models obtained for the spectra measured in three tumor mouse models and in a single tumor mouse model, respectively. Marks of ●, □ and ▲ represent the spectral data measured at 15, 17 and 19 weeks of age, respectively. The Raman spectra were measured at several tumor lesions in the mouse; for the three tumor mouse models, the total number of spectra are 19, 24 and 19 for 15, 17 and 19 weeks, respectively; for the single tumor mouse model, the total number of spectra are 8, 7 and 7 for 15, 17 and 19 weeks, respectively. Reproduced from Ref. [30] with permission.

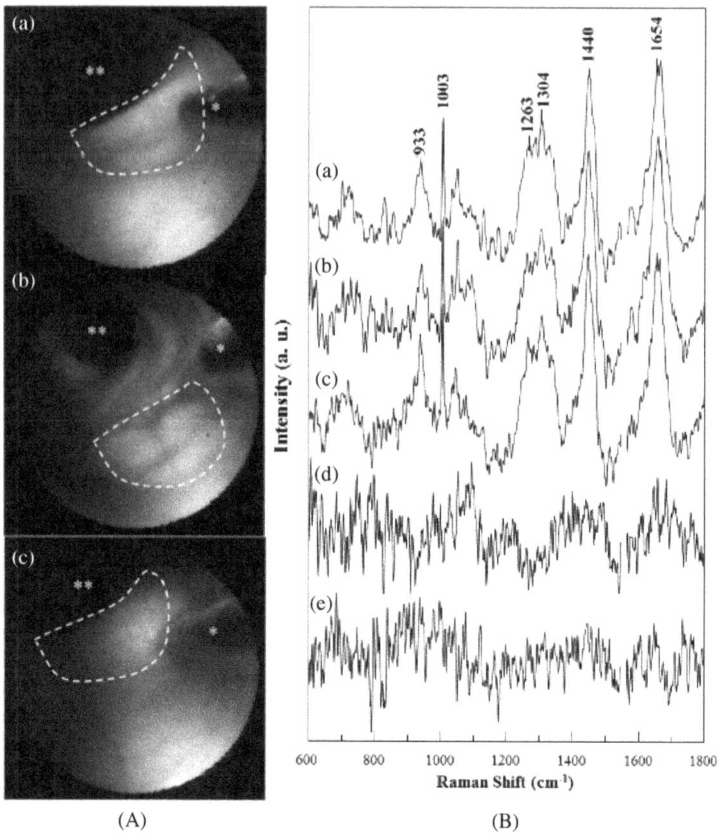

Figure 15.7. (A) The pictures of a shrinking tumor taken at mouse ages of (a) 15, (b) 17, and (c) 19 weeks; (B) the Raman spectra of tumors measured at mouse ages of (a) 15, (b) 17, and (c) 19 weeks, and (d) the subtraction spectra of 17 weeks minus 15 weeks and (e) 19 weeks minus 15 weeks. Reproduced from Ref. [30] with permission.

spectra of the lesion (15.7B(a), (b) and (c)) are similar to each other and show no clear difference. A linear discrimination analysis model was built with the usual advancing tumor lesions and surrounding normal tissues (including tissues with inflammation) and was applied for the analysis of the shrinking tumor. The result suggested that the Raman spectra of the shrinking tumor were all classified as tumorous. It implied that the tumor did not disappear but changed its appearance to be a diffuse infiltration type of cancer. This result of Raman analysis agreed with the commonly recognized knowledge that an advanced cancer does not cure itself. Since the case that we succeeded in the measurement of Raman spectra was only one, it was difficult to confirm the result. However, this study demonstrated that the Raman analysis could help visual endoscope observations.

15.3.2 *Monitoring Effect of Anticancer Drug*

Anticancer drugs are a mainstay in treating any cancer. Although there are many kinds of anticancer drugs, they sometimes cause severe side effects. To reduce the side effects, it would be ideal if we could select the most effective one from various drugs for each case. It is, however, not easy to do that because the sensitivity of each patient, as well as the type of each cancer, are always different. Moreover, a higher dose is better to suppress cancer cells but lower dose is better to minimize its side effect. If it was possible to monitor the effect of an anticancer drug in a short enough time before the side effect appears, doctors could select the suitable drug and dose to each patient during the chemotherapy. The mRE system was applied to the live AOM-DSS mouse model to validate the potential of Raman analysis for monitoring the effect of anticancer drugs [31].

The AOM-DSS mouse model was treated with three types of anticancer drugs: 5-fluorouracil (5-FU), cisplatin (CDDP) and docetaxel. Since the lifetime of a mouse is relatively short, and it is not allowed to keep mouse models for a prolonged period of time because of ethical reasons, the effects of the anticancer drugs were estimated in two weeks of treatments. There was no morphological alteration, such as shrinking of the tumor lesion, found during the two weeks by endoscopic visual observation. The Raman spectra of the same cancer lesions were compared before (a) and after (b) 5-FU treatments in Figure 15.8(A) [31]. Their difference is the spectrum (c). The spectra were categorized into two groups in a PCA score plot for PCs 2 and 3 in Figure 15.8(B). The loading plots of PCs shown in Figure 15.8(C) did not reflect the reduction of collagen, which had been observed in the spectra of the advancing tumor measured in two-week intervals. The result demonstrated that it was technically possible to detect molecular compositional changes in live tumor tissues via Raman analysis without any invasion. However, it was not enough to distinguish the effect of anticancer drug treatment, because the advance of tumor in the AOM-DSS model was so quick that the molecular changes could be attributed to the advance of tumor. The molecular changes due to the anticancer drug treatments were compared among the mouse models with the same ages. Figure 15.9 exhibits score plots of PCA models built for non-tumor and tumor tissues without and with 5-FU (a), CDDP (b) and docetaxel (c) treatments [31]. The non-tumor tissues were those surrounding the tumor, which included chronic inflammation parts. The datasets with and without drug treatments were well categorized in the score plots, indicating that the anticancer drugs gave effects to normal tissues as well as cancer lesions.

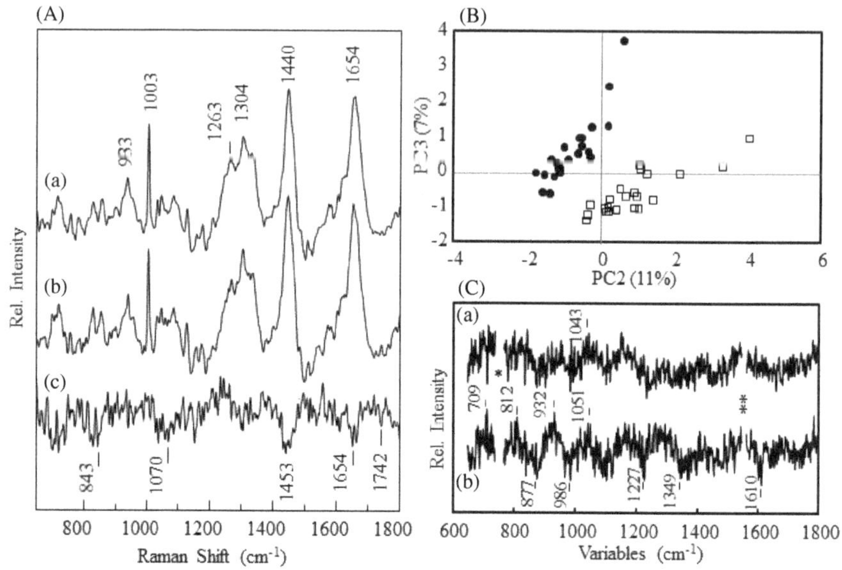

Figure 15.8. (A) Raman spectra of tumors measured (a) before and (b) after anticancer drug treatment, and (c) their difference spectra. (B) A score plot for PC2 and 3 of the PCA model built for the datasets of tumor tissue before (●) and after 5-FU treatment (□). (C) Loading plots of (a) PC2 and (b) PC3. Adapted from Ref. [31] with permission.

The results suggested that Raman analysis was able to detect infiltration of anticancer drugs to the tissues. However, the potential to evaluate the efficacy of the drugs was not revealed. The present study demonstrated the technical possibility of Raman endoscopic analysis in real time and *in situ* analysis of anticancer drug efficacy. It would be necessary to conduct further research to determine the therapeutic effect induced by anticancer drugs with human patients.

15.4 Summary

Raman probes are highly useful for Raman measurement of live tissues *in situ*. To use the probes efficiently, users must understand the optical property of the probes correctly. The Raman probes must be designed to match the sample shape and structure. As BHRP has a simple structure and potential to adjust its WD, it is one of the most feasible miniaturized probes for live tissue analysis, despite the drawback of low transmission efficiency. Raman endoscopy has strong potential to detect the molecular compositional changes in tumor tissues in a totally non-invasive and real-time manner. The multivariate

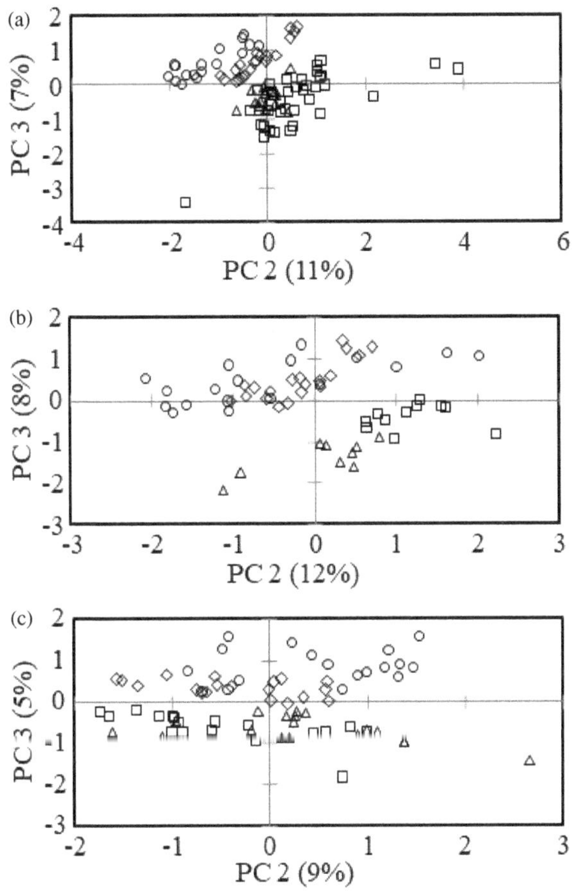

Figure 15.9. Score plots of PCA models built with datasets of non-tumor and tumor tissues with and without drug treatments. Datasets of tumor lesions and non-tumor tissue of a control mouse are marked with ◊ and ○; those of tumor lesions and non-tumor tissue with drug treatment are marked with □ and △, respectively. Anticancer drugs are (a) 5-FU, (b) CDDP and (c) docetaxel. Adapted from Ref. [31] with permission.

analytical techniques are very strong in extracting useful information from data with large noise and fluctuation such as Raman spectra of live tissues. As it was shown in the application studies described above, Raman endoscopy has technically high viability for application in cancer diagnosis. In the same time, however, the studies indicate to us a pressing question — how can we build sophisticated discrimination models for cancer diagnosis?

Raman analysis shows that the molecular composition of a cancer always changes with its development. Since it is possible to control the objective samples in a scientific study, a discrimination analysis can be applied to a specific cancer type. If the molecular change of a cancer is not linear (and it is probably not), a usual multivariate analytical model is difficult to cover all stages of advancing tumors. It would be necessary to build a nonlinear discrimination model to cover the different stages of tumors, even for a specific type of cancer. Although new types of analytical techniques such as artificial intelligence give foresight to develop a comprehensive model of cancer diagnosis, it is necessary to know the mechanisms and regularity of the changes to deal with unknown cases. As Raman data is often treated in multivariate analytical techniques, it has high affinity to mathematical treatments, such as big data analysis. In the last two decades, big data analysis on DNA sequences opened a new era for various biological research fields. Biomedical Raman data could be analyzed based on genetic information of the biological samples. Imaging technology could also be used efficiently for analysis of Raman data. For example, mass spectrometry imaging of whichever total system is commercially available has a high potential to couple with biomedical Raman imaging technique for detailed molecular analysis. Biology has been the last science which has not yet adopted mathematics, but it is changing now and mathematical and informational techniques are developing quickly in biology and life sciences. Raman spectroscopy is a strong technique to translate biological information into "values", which can be analyzed with mathematical treatments. Moreover, it is one of the few techniques able to analyze molecular composition in live tissues and cells. It is necessary to expand the application of Raman spectroscopy more in the health and biomedical sciences.

References

1. Puppels, G. J., de Mul, F. F. M., Otto, C., Greve, J., Robert-Nicoud, M., Arndt-Jovin D. J. and Jovin, T. M. (1990) Studying single living cells and chromosomes by confocal Raman microspectroscopy. Nature **347**, 301–303.
2. Smith, R., Wright, K. L. and Ashton L. (2016) Raman spectroscopy: an evolving technique for live cell studies. Analyst **141**, 3590–3600.
3. Ishigaki, M., Hitomi, H., Ozaki, Y. and Nishiyama A. (2022) Exposing intracellular molecular changes during the differentiation of human-induced pluripotent stem cells into erythropoietin-producing cells using Raman spectroscopy and imaging. Sci. Rep. **12**, 20454.
4. Paramitha, P. N., Zakaria, R., Maryani, A., Kusaka, Y., Andriana, B. B., Hashimoto, K. Nakazawa, H., Kato, S. and Sato H. (2021) Raman study on lipid droplets in hepatic cells co-cultured with fatty acids. Int. J. Mol. Sci. **22**, 7378–7391.

5. Hashimoto, K., Andriana, B. B., Matsuyoshi H. and Sato, H. (2018) Discrimination analysis of excitatory and inhibitory neurons using Raman spectroscopy Analyst **143**, 2889–2894.
6. Moor, K., Terada, Y., Taketani, A. Matsuyoshi, H., Ohtani, K. and Sato, H. (2018) Early detection of virus infection in live human cells using Raman spectroscopy. J. Biomed. Opt. **23**, 097001-1-7.
7. Oshima, Y., Shinzawa, H., Takenaka, T., Furihata, C. and Sato, H. (2010) Discrimination analysis of human lung cancer cells associated with histological type and malignancy using Raman spectroscopy. J. Biomed. Opt. **15**, 017009-1-8.
8. Shim, M. G. and Wilson, B. C. (1997) Development of an in vivo Raman spectroscopic system for diagnostic applications. J. Raman Spectrosc. **28**, 131–142.
9. Mahadevan-Jansen, A., Mitchell, M. F., Ramanujam N., Malpica, A., Thomsen, S., Utzinger U. and Richards-Kortum, R. (1998) Development of a fiber optic probe to measure NIR Raman spectra of cervical tissue in vivo. Photochem. Photobiol. **68**, 427–431.
10. Shim, M. G., Wilson, B. C., Marple, E. and Wach, M. (1999) Study of fiber-optic probes for in vivo medical Raman spectroscopy. Appl. Spectrosc. **53**, 619–627.
11. Shim, M. G., Song, L.-M. W. K., Marcon, N. E. and Wilson B. C. (2000) In vivo near-infrared Raman spectroscopy: demonstration of feasibility during clinical gastrointestinal endoscopy. Photochem. Photobiol. **72**, 146–150.
12. Buschman, H. P., Marple, E. T., Wach, M. L., Bennett, B., Bakker Schut, T. C. Bruining, H. A., Bruschke, A. V., van der Laarse, A. and Puppels, G. J. (2000) In vivo determination of the molecular composition of artery wall by intravascular Raman spectroscopy. Anal. Chem. **72**, 3771–3775.
13. Molckovsky, A., Song, L.-M. W. K., Shim, M. G., Marcon, N. E. and Wilson, B. C. (2003) Diagnostic potential of near-infrared Raman spectroscopy in the colon: Differentiating adenomatous from hyperplastic polyps. Gastrointest. Endosc. **57**, 396–402.
14. Motz, J. T., Hunter, M., Galindo, L. H. Gardecki, J. A., Kramer, J. R., Dasari, R. R. and Feld, M. S. (2004) Optical fiber probe for biomedical Raman spectroscopy. Appl. Opt. **43**, 542–554.
15. Komachi, Y., Sato, H., Aizawa, K. and Tashiro, H. (2005) Micro-optical fiber probe for use in an intravascular Raman endoscope. Appl. Opt. **44**, 4722–4732.
16. Motz, J. T., Gandhi, S. J., Scepanovic, O. R., Haka, A. S., Kramer, J. R., Dasari, R. R. and Feld, M. S. (2005) Real-time Raman system for in vivo disease diagnosis. J. Biomed. Opt. **10**, 031113-1.
17. Komachi, Y., Sato, H. and Tashiro, H. (2006) Intravascular Raman spectroscopic catheter for molecular diagnosis of atherosclerotic coronary disease. Appl. Opt. **45**, 7938–7943.
18. Hattori, Y., Komachi, Y., Asakura, T., Shimosegawa, T., Kanai, G., Tashiro, H. and Sato, H. (2007) In vivo Raman study of the living rat esophagus and stomach using a micro-Raman probe under an endoscope. Appl. Spectrosc. **61**, 579–584.

19. Komachi, Y., Katagiri, T., Sato, H. and Tashiro, H. (2009) Improvement and analysis of a micro Raman probe. Appl. Opt. **48**, 1683–1696.
20. Katagiri, T., Yamamoto, Y. S., Ozaki, Y., Matsuura, Y. and Sato, H. (2009) High axial resolution Raman probe made of a single hollow optical fiber. Appl. Spectrosc. **63**, 103–107.
21. Ma, J. and Li, Y.-S. (1996) Optical-fiber Raman probe with low background interference by spatial optimization. Appl. Opt. **35**, 2527–2533.
22. Komachi, Y., Sato, H., Matsuura, Y., Miyagi, M. and Tashiro, H. (2005) Raman probe using a single hollow waveguide. Opt. Lett. **30**, 2942–2944.
23. Yamamoto, Y. S., Shinzawa, H., Matsuura, Y., Ozaki, Y. and Sato, H. (2011) Noninvasive subsurface analysis using multiple miniaturized Raman probes, part I: basic study of thin-layered transparent models of biomedical tissues. Appl. Spectrosc. **65**, 844–848.
24. Matousek, P. and Morris, M. D., Eds. (2010) *Emerging Raman Applications and Techniques in Biomedical and Pharmaceutical Fields.* Springer.
25. Kallaway, C., Almond, L. M., Barr, H., Wood, J., Hutchings, J., Kendall, C. and Stone, N. (2013) Advances in the clinical application of Raman spectroscopy for cancer diagnostics. Photodiagnosis Photodyn. Ther. **10**, 207–221.
26. Ishigaki, M., Maeda, Y., Taketani, A., Andriana, B. B., Ishihara, R., Wongravee, K., Ozaki, Y. and Sato, H. (2016) Diagnosis of early-stage esophageal cancer by Raman spectroscopy and chemometric techniques. Analyst **141**, 1027–1033.
27. Sato, H., Chiba, H., Tashiro, H. and Ozaki, Y. (2001) Excitation wavelength-dependent changes in Raman spectra of whole blood and hemoglobin: comparison of the spectra with 514.5-, 720-, and 1064-nm excitation. J. Biomed. Opt. **6**, 366–370.
28. Sato, H., Wada, S., Ozaki, Y. and Tashiro, H. (2004) Qualitative analysis of trace Raman bands of non-resonant species in near-infrared excited pre-resonance Raman spectra of hemoglobin by partial least square regression-Raman excitation profile method. Vib. Spectrosc. **34**, 149–156.
29. Zakaria, R., Andriana, B. B., Watanabe, T., Maryani, A., Parmitha, P. N., Kuntana, Y. P., Kusaka, Y., Noothalapati, H., Iwasaki, K., Oshima, N., Hashimoto, K., Matsuyoshi, H., Ishihara, S. Yamamoto, T. and Sato, H. (2023) Development of in-situ Raman diagnosis technique of eosinophil esophagitis. Spectrochim. Acta A **285**, 121804.
30. Taketani, A., Hariyani, R., Ishigaki, M., Andriana, B. B. and Sato, H. (2013) Raman endoscopy for the in situ investigation of advancing colorectal tumors in live model mice. Analyst **138**, 4183–4190.
31. Taketani, A., Andriana, B. B., Matsuyoshi, H. and Sato, H. (2017) Raman endoscopy for monitoring the anticancer drug treatment of colorectal tumors in live mice. Analyst **142**, 3680–3688.

https://doi.org/10.1142/9789811264610_0016

Chapter 16

Clinical Aspects of Raman Spectroscopy in Surgical Applications

Katherine Ember,[1,2] Jean-Philippe Dulude,[1,4,5] Trang Tran,[1,2] Mai-Kim Gervais,[4,5] Sarkis Meterissian,[6] Roy Dudley,[7] Kevin Petrecca,[8] Frédéric Leblond[1-3,*]

[1]*Department of Engineering Physics, Polytechnique Montréal, Montreal, Canada*
[2]*Centre de recherche du Centre hospitalier de l'Université de Montréal, Montreal, Canada*
[3]*Institut du cancer de Montréal, Montreal, Canada*
[4]*Division of Surgical Oncology, Department of Surgery, Maisonneuve-Rosemont Hospital, Université de Montréal, Montreal, Quebec, Canada*
[5]*Department of Surgery, Université de Montréal, Montreal, Quebec, Canada*
[6]*Department of Surgery, McGill University Health Center (MUHC), Montreal, Quebec, Canada*
[7]*Department of Pediatric Surgery, McGill University Health Center (MUHC), Montreal, Quebec, Canada*
[8]*Montreal Neurological Institute-Hospital, McGill University, Montreal, Canada*
**Corresponding author: frederic.leblond@polymtl.ca*

16.1 Introduction

Surgery involves an incision into the body and is defined as a technical intervention of dissecting tissue, repairing organs, treating infection and disease or resecting tumors. It has been part of medical practice for thousands of years. Neolithic skulls have been found with trepanned holes and there is evidence of amputations taking place in ancient Greece [1]. Since then, the risks of mortality, pain and scarring due to surgery have diminished due to advances in medical science such as general anesthetic, the sterile technique [2] and laparoscopic "keyhole" surgeries [3].

Surgery entered the third millennium with high promises for the future of healthcare. Impressive advances were made in robotic surgery, with several techniques already translated to the clinic using commercial robotic platforms. These include the Da Vinci system from Intuitive Surgical [4], the ROSA knee system from ZIMMER BIOMET [5] and the upcoming Ottava surgical robot from Johnson & Johnson. Applications using robotic surgeries include radical prostatectomy [6], arthroplasty [5] and hysterectomy [7]. Concurrently, the rapid pace at which artificial intelligence (AI) advances is remarkable, to the point where ethical concerns are raised about its use in all layers of society, particularly with regard to task automation, job replacement and reliability [8]. Pertaining to medicine, there are debates as to whether AI models could eventually substitute clinical specialties such as radiology and pathology [9] where it has made impressive strides, partly due to efforts by tech giants like Google. An area where AI perhaps offers the most enticing prospect is in omics-based medicine, where models will be trained to rapidly decipher genomic and metabolomic molecular profiles [10]. This will help provide high-precision personalized diagnostics information, ensuring that tailored treatment options are offered to patients. These methods are rich in information content and, when combined with an ever-expanding artillery of cancer treatments such as immunotherapy, will provide actionable information towards truly personalized medicine [11].

Despite these advances in molecular diagnostics and prognostics, surgery will likely remain a quintessential component of patient care in medicine for centuries to come. The prospect of synergistic advances combining AI and robotics with new and emerging intraoperative molecular diagnostic technologies is highly enticing, and perhaps represents the future of surgery.

16.1.1 *Electromagnetic Radiation in Surgery*

When referring to a surgical tool, the term *intraoperative* must be defined further as it is sometimes used loosely. In the literature, it often refers to any tool that has the potential to be used as a surgical aid within timeframes compatible with surgical decision making. Such tools could take the form of instruments, such as *ex vivo* imaging microscopes, designed to rapidly interrogate tissue specimens that were biopsied by the surgeon, for confirmation of histopathological status [12, 13]. These techniques are often positioned as candidates to replace current frozen section pathology, which can take up to an hour typically and provides limited pathology detection accuracy due to the damage incurred to tissue. Another class of techniques relate to *in situ* tissue characterization methods, here also to provide information similar to histopathology, albeit at a faster pace, ideally in real time and as many times as is required by the surgeon.

There are multiple emerging technologies that can be made compatible with intraoperative use and for which there has been a lot of innovative scientific activity in the last decades. These include advanced methods that can be developed to interrogate tissue live *in situ* during surgical procedures using electromagnetic (EM) radiation. Several such techniques using either near-infrared (near-IR) or visible light have already made it to clinical use (or are close), either for diagnostics or as a support to decision making during surgery. These include: optical coherence tomography in ophthalmology [14], 5-aminolevulinic acid-induced protoporphyrin IX (ALA-PpIX) fluorescence imaging during glioblastoma neurosurgery [15], spatial frequency domain imaging for diabetes ulcer detection [16], and the albumin marker indocyanine green (ICG) for real-time imaging detection of blood vessels [17]. Other methods are currently used in clinical practice using radiation from other regions of the EM spectrum. These include intraoperative versions of standard medical imaging techniques (e.g., magnetic resonance imaging (MRI), tomodensimetry, and nuclear imaging).

Near-IR and optical techniques can reveal biomolecular contrast that is often unavailable using standard imaging tools, e.g., ultrasound and MRI. This information enhances the ability of the surgeons to achieve safer and more precise high-quality surgical procedures, hence this area of research is expanding rapidly. The intended use of these techniques is often as adjoints to currently adopted surgical methods, rather than as replacement. For example, these methods can be integrated into current surgical robotic platforms as done with the Intuitive Surgical Firefly system, where a near-IR fluorescence ICG imaging subunit was integrated into a Da Vinci surgical robot [18]. For the blood marker ICG, optical methods are mostly used to provide more precise information relating to the locations of vessels, capillaries, veins, and arteries [17]. This extra information reinforces the confidence of surgeons in their interventions. Other applications have led to the development of fluorescent agents with affinity to proteins expressed in nerves [19]. This affords yet another way to minimize the damage to normal tissue, as can be critical for example in orthopedics and prostate surgery. The requirement to minimize the amount of normal tissue being resected is especially true in neurosurgery for which normal brain must be spared to minimally impact the cognitive and motor functions of a patient. Whilst fluorescence is a well-established optical technique in biomedicine, it requires exogenous fluorophores (contrast agents) to be administered. Development and safety assessment of such fluorophores can take decades. ICG, methylene blue, fluorescein and 5-ALA are the only four fluorescence contrast agents approved by the US Food and Drug Administration for medical use [20].

Surgical oncology applications, such as tumor resection, pose their own colossal challenges. The current suite of available standard imaging modalities — including MRI, X-ray techniques and nuclear imaging — are generally not sensitive enough to detect the dysplastic processes which are precursors to the onset of carcinogenesis. They are also limited in their ability to image subtler oncogenic processes at tumor margins. Since these methods are usually utilized preoperatively (before surgery), another limitation is the lack of precise spatial alignment between the radiological images and the 3D coordinates within the operating theatre. This can further limit the ability of those techniques to precisely locate the tumor location and its contrast-enhancing boundaries. For surgical applications requiring a particularly high degree of spatial accuracy, as is the case for neurosurgery, this is addressed using navigation systems. These systems can track surgical tools live in the operating room, and they provide 3D maps associated with their location superimposed onto preoperative radiological images. Furthermore, sophisticated algorithms and software have been developed to compensate for tissue deformation occurring during surgery (e.g., brain shift from craniotomy) compared to images acquired preoperatively.

16.1.2 *Added Value of Vibrational Spectroscopy*

Vibrational spectroscopy is a class of techniques that includes IR spectroscopy and Raman spectroscopy (RS). Both techniques rely on the interrogation of biological material with near-IR light. IR spectroscopy, often implemented as Fourier Transform IR (FTIR) spectroscopy, and RS have the potential to further improve outcomes by informing surgeons about the molecular status of tissues in real time intraoperatively [21–24]. This could help address a wide range of surgical challenges including: avoiding blood vessels, ensuring complete tumor resection [24], guiding biopsies [25], assessing viability of donor organs [26] and monitoring patient recovery. Many of these surgical problems are currently addressed by imaging techniques such as computed tomography scans and MRI which are highly expensive and lack molecular specificity, or ultrasound which can lack sensitivity.

RS leads to complex spectra that are often composed of more than one thousand spectral bins. The number of individual intensity bins, or actual Raman bands, that are required for a given tissue detection task can vary greatly, depending on the intrinsic biomolecular contrast between the different tissue types that need to be discriminated. For example, discriminating fatty tissue from protein-rich tissue is usually a very simple task that can require only one spectral band, e.g., the phenylalanine peak at around 1003 mm^{-1}, that is not present in purely adipose tissue. Similarly, discriminating between bone and any other tissue type in orthopedic applications can be trivial because of the presence of the distinguishing mineral peak at 955 cm^{-1} [27]. However, applications of medical interest are most of the time associated with more complex tasks, such as discriminating cancer from normal tissue, which can be further complicated by the high levels of heterogeneity associated with these two classes [28]. As a result, for tumor detection applications, complex statistical techniques are required, relying on the optical contrast associated with a larger number of spectral features.

16.1.3 *Machine Learning and Clinical Spectroscopy*

Clinical applications of RS typically rely on advanced statistical approaches, commonly in the form of supervised machine learning techniques. Several groups have considered other predictive modeling approaches relying on deep learning techniques or neural networks, but these are usually more appropriate when considering big data applications, where thousands of learning instances are available. This has not yet been the case for surgical applications of RS where most published studies rely on datasets acquired from 10–50 patients, and rarely in the hundreds of patients. This is likely the case because of difficulties in patient recruitment, plus the tedious and costly nature of the supervised learning process requiring, for training purposes, that each acquired spectral fingerprint be labeled with histopathology information. For example, in cancer detection applications, model training typically requires that a pathologist analyzes each area where a spectrum is acquired to provide an assessment on whether cancer cells are present. The complexity of that task can vary dramatically depending on the application, as will be seen in Section 16.2.

For a given application, the predictive modeling paradigm requires a dataset to be acquired for which a subset is used to train and validate a model. A hold-out subset that has been pre-selected to ensure no biases remain is then used to quantify the performance of the model when applied to independent spectral data not used during the training phase. Quantitatively assessing the generalizability of the model to new data is essential for the clinical deployment of those models along with the instruments that were used to collect them. Another crucially important aspect associated with model development is to ensure patient enrollment in surgical RS techniques is made to avoid biases, to ensure the models are applicable for the whole population. As an example, the structure of the brain and its specific biomolecular composition is known to change with age [29, 30], and differences can be observed between females and males [31]. Training a model to detect a specific lesion type must then not only be made from age- and sex-matched active and control groups, but the study design must also ensure patients are enrolled for all age groups, both sexes as well as accounting for other demographic characteristics that lead to initially unsuspected spectral fingerprint changes [32, 33]. Another example is the detection of skin lesions, where skin pigmentation must be explicitly included as part of the machine learning models to ensure model applicability to people with all skin colors [34].

The machine learning model training, validation, and testing processes result in multiple models. Each is associated with a different parametric value between 0 and 1, and that effectively corresponds to different points on a receiver-operating-characteristic curve (Figure 16.1). The value of the parameter ultimately chosen for intraoperative use will depend on the clinical requirements in terms of tolerated risk associated with false negatives and false positives. In other words, surgeons will need to decide whether detection performance should be tuned more towards higher sensitivity (lower number of false positive predictions) or higher specificity (lower number of false negative predictions). In surgical oncology, the goal is to maximize the volume of resected tumor tissue to make the patient cancer-free. The specific models used (higher sensitivity, higher specificity, or a more balanced model) for surgical applications will usually depend on the organ site and the chances of cancer recurrence. Minimizing the impact to normal tissue may be a requirement in neurosurgery, where a high-specificity model may be required. Specificity will then be favored over sensitivity because minimizing the number of false positives will allow cancer tissue to be ruled-in at the borders of a resection, thus sparing the erroneous resection of normal brain in keeping with the first principle of clinical medicine: First, do not harm. On the other hand, in applications such as breast-conserving surgery, liposarcoma or skin cancer

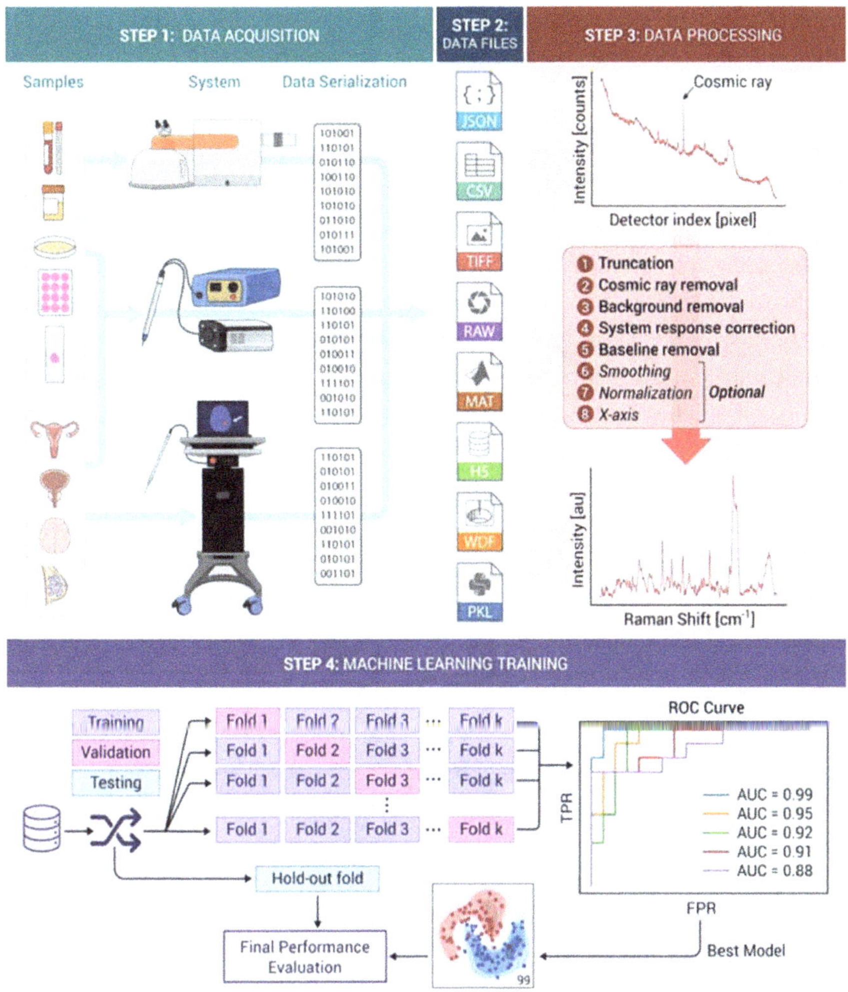

Figure 16.1. Depiction of all steps involved in acquiring spectroscopic data using Raman spectroscopy devices and the development of predictive machine learning models. STEP 1: Spectra are acquired in different contexts (different organs (*in situ*, *ex vivo* or fixed) or body fluids) with different instruments, including commercial Raman microscopes, handheld surgical guidance probes or optical biopsy needles. STEP 2: Data (Raman spectra and metadata, including patient information) are stored in files with formats that can be processed using readily available tools (e.g., Python, Matlab). STEP 3 illustrates all pre-processing algorithms include in the ORPL open-sourced data processing package. STEP 4 illustrates the process involved in training, validation and testing of machine learning models with performance assessment based on receiver-operating-characteristic (ROC) analysis. Reproduced from Ref. [52] with permission.

surgery, resecting normal tissue may not be as critical and, as a result, the utilization of a high-specificity model may be appropriate.

A critical step prior to machine learning model development is spectral data pre-processing to ensure models are trained based only on the inelastic scattering contributions to the signal (Figure 16.1). Related to this, perhaps the most challenging aspect of intraoperative RS is to achieve high spectral quality Raman detection in the face of those large background sources that are not specific to the tissue itself. Some of these sources can be managed externally, as is the case of ambient light or even the white-light source from a surgical microscope or surgical googles that are required to maneuver the spectroscopy instrument to the location where a measurement needs to be made. Such sources of background can be dealt with either by temporarily shutting off all potentially contaminating light sources (e.g., through external triggers sent from those sources to the Raman system) or by introducing optical components in the operating room, ensuring their impact is mitigated. For example, to allow Raman measurements to be achieved without completely shutting off a surgical microscope, custom filters cutting off IR light (e.g., xenon lamps have near-IR light peaks) could be positioned on the microscope front lens [35].

Other background sources, however, are inherent to the tissue itself and come in the form of a fluorescence background associated with biomolecules emitting fluorescence light upon tissue excitation with the laser. Those molecules include structural proteins such as collagen and elastin [36], specific amino acids such as tryptophan, as well as factors associated with metabolic cellular processes, including NADH, FAD, as well as porphyrins [37]. This background contribution is more elevated when ultraviolet and visible excitation wavelengths are used, which explains why most Raman tissue optics applications are using near-IR laser, oftentimes either 785 nm or higher wavelengths. Another source of background signal can be associated with intrinsic luminescence from components of the instruments, such as optical fibers, lenses, and even epoxies which can be highly fluorescent. The impact of those sources on the overall detected signal can be attenuated through careful optical design and selection of optical components with known low fluorescence and inelastic scattering response [38].

In principle, the endogenous tissue fluorescence within the background signal could itself be used as a potential optical biomarker, along with Raman spectroscopic features. However, several factors can prevent effective use of this. Most instruments are tailored towards RS detection and are not equipped to collect signals that can be used to normalize signals to account for variability in the tissue-instrument coupling and tissue variability associated with other intrinsic tissue optical properties. These optical properties include the absorption from tissue chromophores (e.g., oxygenated, deoxygenated hemoglobin) [39] and elastic scattering from microscopic scatterers, including cell membranes and the various organelles. Therefore, absolute fluorescence values cannot be used as a reliable biomarker with most Raman systems. However, signal normalization methods based on multispectral or hyperspectral reflectance measurements could be developed to implement a correction factor allowing the underlying fluorescence spectrum to be used as yet another set of variables towards the development of classification models [40, 41].

From our experience collecting datasets in multiple organ sites towards the development of surgical oncology applications, we have seen that the signal-to-background ratios (SBRs) measured in *ex vivo* and *in situ* biological tissues vary approximately from 100 up to more than 1,000. The Raman SBR background challenge in tissues affects the choice of sensors used when designing tissue RS instruments. For example, high-sensitivity sensors developed for low-light applications would not necessarily be required, but cooled low-noise sensors with a large dynamical range should be preconized to ensure the often-subtle inelastic scattering can be detected.

16.1.4 *Microscopic vs. Macroscopic Systems for Surgery*

The operating room poses many unique challenges to optical diagnostic devices. Most RS studies of biological systems use RS coupled with microscopy, giving high-resolution, spatially resolved measurements from tissue sections and cells [42–44]. However, such microscopes can be impractical for the operating room. They are expensive, not portable, time consuming, and only a small field of view (FOV) can be probed. For example, if a two-second acquisition time is used, a 1 mm × 1 mm Raman map of brain tissue with 10 μm resolution takes 5.5 hours. Another key problem is that sample preparation is complex, requiring samples to be processed in formaldehyde and paraffin or prepared as frozen sections, sliced onto microscope slides, and then analyzed by pathologists or specialized technicians. For surgery, we can make a trade-off between spatial resolution and speed of measurement. To achieve this, single-point, endoscopic, and widefield RS systems with lower spatial resolution but larger FOVs can be employed [24, 45, 46]. Such devices must also be rapid, portable, and sterilizable for use in the operating room. They should be integrated into the surgical workflow with minimal disruption and hence should be easy to use, with a graphical user interface and hardware that is suitable for rapid data acquisition by the operating surgeon. Furthermore, the diagnosis should be reliable, rapid, and unambiguous.

Single-point devices interrogating tissue *in situ* at sub-millimetric scales are the most common when it comes to intraoperative RS applications. In particular, handheld probes (e.g., the probes developed by the company EMVision) are commonplace in the development of open-surgery applications. However, different fiber optics designs were developed for tissue interrogation from within commercial biopsy needles or integrated with clinical endoscopic systems. Over the years, several companies developed intraoperative inelastic scattering measurement systems. Those include Endofotonics for colorectal cancer screening [47], Reveal Surgical for neurosurgical guidance [24], and RiverD for mouth and throat cancer surgical guidance [48].

16.1.5 *Signal to Noise and Spectral Processing*

The lasers used for intraoperative systems are usually at 785 nm, with output powers usually <200 mW at the tissue surface. Typically, multiple measurements are made at the same spot that are subsequently averaged to increase overall signal-to-noise ratio (SNR). The number of repeat measurements per point (known as accumulations) can vary as well as the exposure time per spectrum. However, these parameters are usually set to ensure that the skin maximum permissible exposure (MPE), independent of whether skin or another organ site is interrogated, is respected [49]. In fact, a barrier to clinical translation and adoption for tissue interrogation techniques is that the underlying interactions between radiation and tissue should be non-damaging. This means that exposure of the tissue to radiation will not induce any biological processes resulting in cell death, permanent modifications to the conformation of proteins or damage to nucleic acids. For example, tissue exposure to ultraviolet light is known to cause DNA/RNA damage [50], triggering apoptotic processes as well as mutations, potentially leading to dysplasia that has the risk of maturing into neoplasia. For future clinical applications, specific photo-diagnostic MPE values should be determined for all organ sites, which are likely going to be significantly larger than the skin MPE set by the American National Standards Institute for laboratory laser safety.

Measurements always include a dark noise background measurement made with the laser switched off. The tissue fingerprint measurement should always be done with interrogation parameters such as laser power and integration time set to optimize the fraction of the sensor dynamical range that is used, whilst avoiding saturation [51]. Nowadays, the best academic systems allow the collection of high-quality single-point spectra in less than five seconds, and even in less than one second in some organ sites.

Prior to using the spectroscopic data towards the development of predictive models, several pre-processing steps must be implemented to isolate the inelastic scattering signature from background contributions. These include the following steps: 1) averaging of the accumulations to increase SNR, 2) averaging and subtraction of background spectra acquired with the laser turned off between measurements to mitigate the impact or background sources that could not be eliminated, 3) normalization of the spectrum with a National Institute of Standards and Technology Raman standard (SRM 2214), or another material with known fluorescence profile, to correct for the instrument response, 4) x-axis (wavenumber shift) calibration based on a Raman spectrum acquired on a material for which all Raman peak locations (wavenumber positions in cm^{-1}) are known (e.g., polycarbonate, acetaminophen), 5) removal of background signals using specialized algorithms, and 6) normalization of the resulting spectrum, e.g., using standard normal variate (SNV) normalization. This last step is important to ensure that measured Raman bands are not fed to machine learning pipelines as absolute values, but rather use numerical values relative to other band intensities. For example, a given band on a SNV-normalized spectrum effectively represents the Raman intensity of a given molecular vibrational bond with respect to the average associated with all other measured intensities [52].

Further to these spectral pre-processing steps, some groups developed numerical techniques that can used to evaluate, in real-time during spectral data acquisition, the spectral quality of the measurements. For example, our group developed a quantitative quality factor metric that can be computed from each resulting spectrum. It provided a statistical assessment of the likelihood the SNV-normalized signals are associated with tissue Raman peaks or stochastic noise [52]. Spectra with a quality factor metric inferior to a given threshold could be excluded as they do not always clearly show all the ubiquitous Raman peaks encountered in biological tissue (e.g., amide bands for protein-rich tissue). This metric can be evaluated during the data acquisition process for iterative interrogation parameter adjustments leading to specific targeted values pre-determined to be required for a given application.

16.2 Advances in Clinical Raman Spectroscopy: Current and Future Applications

This chapter is divided into organ types, with each section detailing the clinical workflow of surgery, the challenges that RS can address and the current Raman systems that have been developed for each organ type. There may be potential biases in this chapter towards work that the authors have been involved with or are familiar with. In particular, we have an expertise in RS for surgical oncology and we acknowledge that surgical RS is a rapidly growing field worldwide. We encourage readers to keep updated with surgical RS groups worldwide and those aligned with different surgical disciplines.

The ultimate challenge for RS devices is whether results can be reproduced using different RS units, different surgical teams, and different hospital workflows. In many approaches, this challenge has not yet been met, or has not been made public by companies involved in RS device development. In particular, non-biological sources of Raman background may not be consistent between RS devices and clinical settings. To address this, Picot *et al.* have demonstrated progress made using machine learning models trained with one system on independent data acquired with other systems [53].

16.2.1 *Neurosurgery*

Neurosurgery is any surgical procedure that is carried out to alleviate disorders of the central nervous system including the brain, spinal cord, and peripheral nervous system. Neurosurgery can be used to treat Parkinson's disease, epilepsy, and brain cancer. Most Raman-based advances in neurosurgery are those that involve surgical guidance within the brain, as described below.

Accurate guidance is paramount in the case of brain cancer, as disruption of functional tissue can have profound implications on patient quality of life. Both biopsies and tumor removal may cause problems in vision, movement, sensory processing, and language. Neurosurgeries can aim to cure the patient by total tumor removal (meningioma, possibly low-grade gliomas), or extend patient lifespan and improve quality of life in the case of cancers such as glioblastomas — cancers of the glial cells — which have a poor five-year survival rate (6% in patients aged 55–64) [54]. Tumor margin detection can be assisted by using 5-ALA-induced porphyrin fluorescence which is specific to tumor tissue [15, 55–60]. However, in cases of infiltrated tumors, 5-ALA fluorescence detection is limited and mostly restricted to glioblastoma surgery.

Meningiomas (cancers of the membranes surrounding the brain) are slower growing with a 64% 5-year survival rate, but 24–32% of meningiomas recur and they are the second most common cancer affecting the brain after metastases. Therefore, accurate tumor removal (resection) here is vital. ALA fluorescence is currently only at the experimental stage in guiding meningioma surgery. Quantitative fluorescence could help in some cases, particularly to detect fluorescence that is not visible by eye [61, 62]. However, the studies suggest that this technique fails in 20% of meningioma cases. In 10–26% of malignant cancer cases, cancers metastasize to the brain and 60% of metastases recur within one year after surgical resection, which is likely due to invasion of cancer cells into adjacent brain [63]. There is an unmet need for a device which can detect brain tumor tissue intraoperatively with high sensitivity and specificity across grades and types of brain tumor. In addition, an optical device could potentially detect malignant tumor areas that are missed by MRI.

16.2.1.1 *Neurosurgical Oncology*

In 2015, Jermyn *et al.* developed and tested a brain tumor detection RS probe for use during surgery [24, 64]. The probe is sterilizable and similar in size to a pen or other surgical tool. Moreover, the design of the probe facilitated clinical use: it is handheld, ergonomic, durable, and has a flexible fiber. The spectrometer itself is portable and can be wheeled into the operating room on a cart with a footprint around the size of a microwave oven. The research prototype demonstrated glioma detection with 90% accuracy in 17 patients (161 spectral fingerprint measurements). However, this device was used with a researcher on hand rather than the surgical team alone. It also did not meet the criteria of detecting tumors across grades. Finally, there was no evidence that this device could be applied to different clinics: this was carried out with a single device, by one surgical team at one clinic.

Since this publication, the lab has made strides in dealing with ambient lights, such as surgical microscope lamps [65, 66], and found that multimodal detection coupling endogenous fluorescence spectroscopy with RS enhances brain cancer detection accuracy [67]. The team has also made advances in data processing prior to machine learning to extract information on specific molecular bands implicated in brain cancer [68, 69]. Furthermore, it seems RS can detect cancer in regions that are non-enhancing on MRI [70]. However, more work needs to be done to apply this to larger datasets.

To address these shortcomings, a multi-centric study was established using the device commercialized as the Reveal Surgical Sentry system. In 2023, this was proven to be able to detect tumor tissue amongst non-tumor tissue in patients with glioblastomas, meningiomas and metastases [71]. This was demonstrated in a multi-centric study between the Mount Sinai Hospital (MSH) and the Montreal Neurological Institute and Hospital (MNI-H) with two Sentry units and two different surgical teams. 985 Raman spectra were included in the study, from 67 patients (49 at MNI-H and 18 at MSH). Colocalized biopsies for gold standard histopathology were also taken and assessed for classification of tumor (>90% tumor burden) and non-tumor (0% tumor cells) tissue. The Sentry device achieved accuracies of 91% for glioblastoma, 97% for brain metastases, and 96% for meningiomas. Using a classification model which was not specific to tumor type, the device discriminated brain versus tumor with 87% sensitivity and 93% specificity.

Several key modifications also facilitated clinical translation and commercialization; for example, hardware and signal-processing advances that ensured good reproducibility between instruments. Modifications to instrument design also allowed optimization of Raman SNR during measurements and identification of poor-quality data in real time. Furthermore, the control software has a graphical user interface that is suitable for use by a surgical team alone.

16.2.1.2 *Brain Biopsy Guidance*

Biopsies are one of the main forms of brain cancer diagnosis and there are non-negligible risks associated with each biopsy procedure. Risks of complication are 6–12% whilst mortality risks are 0.7–3.3% [72–74]. Furthermore, some studies suggest diagnostic accuracy of biopsies is approximately 75% compared to the resection, suggesting a quarter of biopsies could lead to either unnecessary treatment or repeat surgeries [75–77]. Our lab has produced a Raman-guided probe for brain biopsies (Figure 16.1) [25, 78]. As with the brain resection guidance probe, this is similar to current microsurgical tools (900 μm diameter), is integrated into a biopsy needle and can gain Raman spectra in both the fingerprint and high wavenumber regions (Figure 16.2).

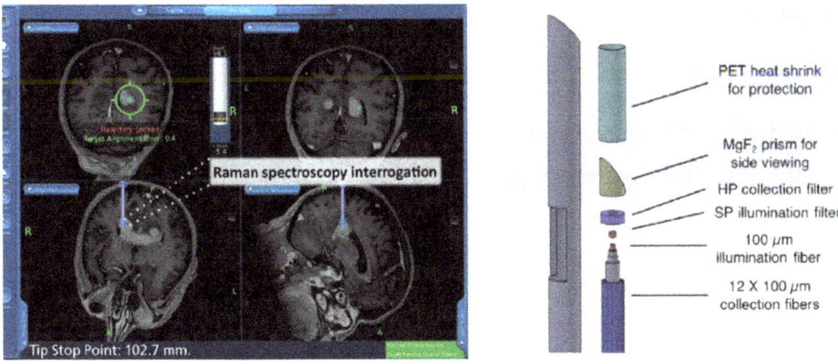

(a) (b)

Figure 16.2. (a) Images from the neuronavigation system. The needle trajectory is identified in the green circle on the top-left scan. On the bottom-left coronal image, the approximate location of the tip of the needle is provided. The corresponding Raman acquisition is depicted for visualization purposes. (b) Exploded view of the Raman microprobe components alongside the internal cannula of the commercial brain biopsy needle. PET, polyethylene terephthalate; MgF_2, magnesium fluoride; HP, high-pass; SP, short-pass. Reproduced from Ref. [78] with permission.

An earlier iteration of the device had been able to measure Raman spectra from the high wavenumber region only, whilst the optical fibers were on the outside of the needle cannula, making sterilization and reuse difficult [25]. This second iteration also made it easier for spatial co-registration between the optical measurement and the biopsy sample. Such considerations are vital when creating Raman tools for surgery. The resulting device can collect Raman spectra with integration times compatible with the surgical workflow (approximately 5 s per acquisition).

16.2.1.3 *Epilepsy*

Patients with epilepsy can have tens to hundreds of seizures per day, and a poor response to medication can make seizure control extremely difficult [79]. The only effective first line of treatment for such cases is brain surgery to remove the area responsible for seizures. Surgery has become the first-line standard of care for focal epilepsy. This form of epilepsy is where the *epileptogenic zone* (EZ, area where seizures originate) in patients is well localized and safe to remove, with no overlap with the eloquent cortex essential for movement, language, vision, and memory. Focal cortical dysplasia (FCD) is the most common cause of focal epilepsy in the pediatric and young adult populations, representing almost 75% of all cases of cortical development malformations [80]. The biggest challenge is to remove all the pathological lesions completely; however, those regions sometimes cannot be distinguished on MRI. Therefore, the modern multimodal neuroimaging and neurophysiological evaluation involves multiple technologies: electroencephalogram (EEG), MRI, positron emission tomography, single-photon emission computed tomography, EEG-functional MRI, magnetoencephalography, as well as intracranial recording. Surgical success depends on the ability to resect the EZ completely while minimizing damage to perilesional normal tissue [81]. This remains extremely challenging for FCD, because these pathologies are very difficult to detect even with the most advanced neuroimaging and electrophysiology techniques. Even when the epicenter of FCD is localized reasonably well after an exhaustive multimodal presurgical evaluation, the borders, where the abnormal tissue stops and where normal brain begins, remain ill-defined.

Although RS is still taking its first steps into the field of epilepsy, the rise of the technique has started to catch the eyes of neurosurgeons treating the disorder. In 2017, Anand *et al.* evaluated the diagnostic capability of a multimodal spectroscopic approach for classifying normal brain tissue and epileptogenic FCD in children. They coupled RS with fluorescence and found that they could detect FCD from normal tissues with 100% sensitivity and 90% specificity [82]. In the same year, Sacharz *et al.* measured Raman spectra on epileptic brain slices in artificial cerebrospinal fluid and showed different organization in proteins, lipid and fatty acid composition of investigated brain areas in rats [83]. Indeed, RS would allow surgeons to save time and improve the rapidity of the whole procedure. It is essentially pivotal to have an intraoperative method to perform the histopathological part indirectly, such that real-time surgical guidance would be attained.

Tran *et al.* recently investigated the ability of RS to discriminate between FCD and normal tissue in *ex vivo* specimens from pediatric epilepsy surgeries. Using Raman micro-spectroscopy on *ex vivo* surgical samples from 30 patients (70 specimens, 1,420 RS measurements) they found that the RS signature of dysmorphic neurons and balloon cells have molecular features distinct from normal brain cells (sensitivity/specificity: 100%/95%), and that FCD types IIa and IIb have distinct Raman-predicted molecular content. With this promising data in hand, they are currently assessing the performance of a new single-point RS probe and training machine learning models for real-time *in vivo* FCD type II detection during resective surgery. The use of novel indirect measures to identify epileptogenic histopathology has the potential to revolutionize intraoperative epilepsy surgery. However, it remains to be seen if extensive research and time will confirm their effectiveness.

16.2.2 *Breast Cancer Surgery*

Breast cancer is projected to have the second highest incidence rate and the fourth highest mortality in Canada in 2022 [84]. Standard of care of localized invasive breast cancer includes breast-conserving surgery (BCS) followed by radiotherapy [85]. Positive resection margins following BCS often require re-excision — a second surgery to remove the breast tissue surrounding the previously resected specimen. This is costly, causes the patient added stress and adds time until they are fully recovered. There has been debate surrounding the definition of positive margins in invasive breast cancer. After the tumor and surrounding tissue have been removed, the removed tissue is coated in ink and examined by histopathology. If ink is found directly on tumor tissue, this suggests that there may still be tumor tissue remaining in the surgical cavity. The Society of Surgical Oncology and American Society of Radiation Oncologists guidelines define negative tumor margins as 'no ink on tumor'. This protocol has lowered the re-excision rate by 35%, and yet 14% of patients must still return for the re-excision process [86]. Cavity shaving has been used to reduce the rate of positive resection margins during BCS [87], but the systematic increase in volume of resected breast tissue entails potentially significant loss of cosmesis [88]. The ability of RS to detect tumors *in situ* makes it an attractive adjunct tool to help identify positive margins during BCS, in order to optimize the volume of resected tissue while maintaining satisfying cosmetic results.

There has been a high level of research activity regarding the use of RS in the diagnosis and treatment of breast cancer in the last 25 years. This was pioneered by Haka *et al.*, who demonstrated the potential for RS to discriminate infiltrating carcinoma from healthy breast tissue, in both *ex vivo* [89] and *in vivo* [90] settings. Subsequent studies have yielded similarly positive results, and a recent meta-analysis evaluating RS's accuracy in diagnosing patients with breast cancer by Wang *et al.* resulted in a pooled sensitivity and specificity of 97% and 96%, respectively [91]. This meta-analysis was based on 16 studies conducted between 2008 and 2021, including those on serum and biopsies.

Although these works were less about detecting tumor tissue intraoperatively, they form a foundation towards using the technique to accurately detect positive resection margins immediately following BCS. Here, the goal would be reducing the number of re-excision surgeries performed. Multiple other RS applications are being pursued, such as analysis of benign and malignant microcalcifications found on mammography [92, 93], and characterizing the molecular composition of breast cancer tissue [94]. The latter helps in better understanding the neoplastic transformation process, and has been used to determine the molecular subtype of breast cancer samples [95]. However, over 50% of new breast cancer patients in the United States underwent BCS between 2005 and 2016 [96], so reducing the rate of positive resection margins holds the greatest potential for significant economic and efficiency impacts from a healthcare system point of view.

David *et al.* have been using single-point RS to detect the biomolecular alterations associated with breast cancer (Figure 16.3). In particular, they show clear discrimination between pure fat tissue, other normal breast structures, and invasive ductal or lobular carcinoma [97].

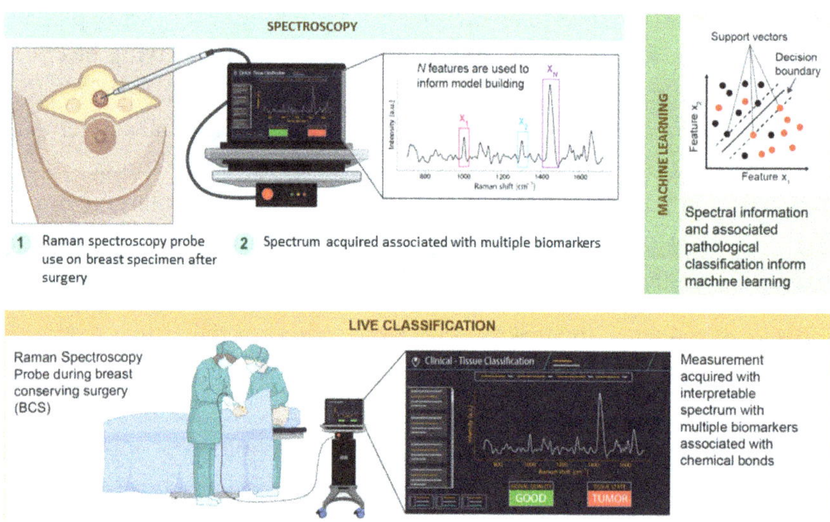

Figure 16.3. Schematic representation of the Raman spectroscopy handheld probe workflow developed for surgical guidance during breast-conserving surgery. *Ex vivo* spectroscopic measurements were made on breast surgery specimen to train machine learning models. The machine learning techniques selected the biomolecular spectral features with the most contrast between cancer and normal breasts, and those features were used to train and test the cancer detection predictive models. The intent is to use those models for live *in situ* cancer detection during breast-conserving surgery. Reproduced from Ref. [97] with permission.

In contrast to the single-point system developed for brain cancer detection, a widefield system with a larger FOV would be ideal for BCS. In brain cancer surgery, it is more important to avoid healthy functional tissue to avert side effects. In BCS, it is preferable to excise all tumor tissue and minimize re-excision likelihood, so a larger surface area should be investigated and repeated use of a single-point system is impractical. Furthermore, the surgical setup of BCS allows widefield systems to be a more practical approach than the smaller surgical cavity available in neurosurgery. The Leblond group have been working on such a system [46, 98] and in recent years, Daoust *et al.* [99] have developed the first widefield RS system for clinical use. This is a device that can be wheeled into the operating room on a cart. A bundle of optical fibers is used to transmit light between the laser/spectrometer and the tissue under investigation. The system is able to collect Raman spectra from a 1×1 cm^2 FOV using a line-scanning approach, and images with information about biomolecular distributions can be built from these. The proof of concept discriminated between porcine adipose and muscle tissue and, in the future, tumor and non-tumor tissues could be rapidly imaged on a large scale.

16.2.3 *Prostate Biopsy Guidance*

Prostate cancer is the second biggest cause of death from cancer for men in the United States — accounting for 11% of male deaths [100]. Transrectal ultrasound (TRUS) biopsy procedures are the standard of care for prostate cancer patients. However, this approach of taking prostate biopsies can have a false negative rate of over 30%, leaving many cancers undiagnosed [101, 102]. MRI can be used to add sensitivity by using preoperative MRI images and combining them with TRUS guidance [103]. However, there are issues with spatial registration of the MRI images and the TRUS guidance, and EM tracking is used to solve this.

Our lab has developed a RS navigation system for targeting biopsy acquisition in conjunction with MRI, TRUS and EM tracking [23, 104, 105] (Figure 16.4). The molecular specificity of RS could be used to accurately assess the guidance of prostate biopsies, reducing bleeding and infection, whilst ensuring the tumor is properly assessed. EM tracking and RS were integrated into the same device, with 671 nm laser excitation for the high wavenumber region and 785 nm illumination for the fingerprint region. The EM-tracked RS system was used to perform MRI-TRUS biopsies on 18 patients, giving 49 *in situ* spectra. These spectra were used to train a support vector machine

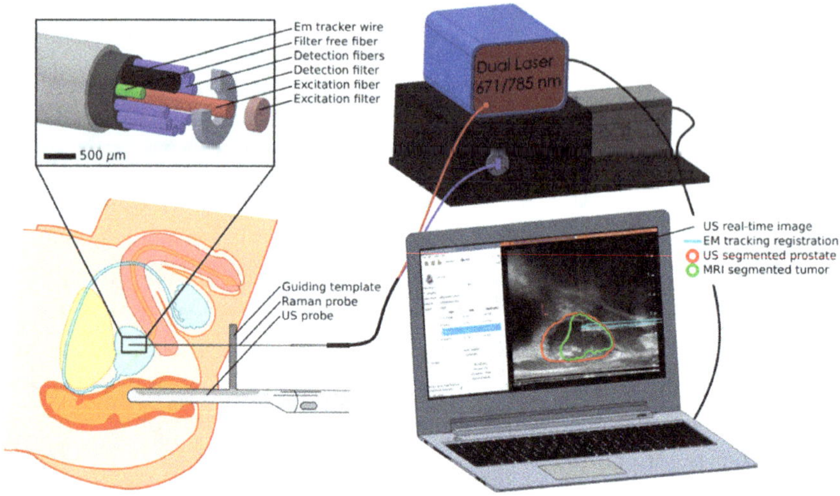

Figure 16.4. Schematic representation of the Raman probe obtaining measurements of the prostate through the guiding template, with a magnified view of the probe's tip. The probe is connected to the laser source and the spectrometer, which are controlled by a computer, and the optical system is combined with a TRUS system to perform the prostate biopsy procedure through the surgical guiding template. The computer displays the fused TRUS-MRI guiding image and the raw optical spectra after spectral acquisition for each site. Reproduced from Ref. [104] with permission.

classification model differentiating between prostate cancer and normal prostate tissue [104]. The trained cancer detection models yielded an accuracy of 79%, a sensitivity of 86%, and a specificity of 72% compared to gold standard histopathology. The key aspects of this device are the fusion of EM and RS, as well as the dual laser allowing both the fingerprint and high wavenumber regions to be probed. In the future, larger datasets could be used to a) help further train the model and b) test the model on an independent dataset. The RS system could also help guide therapeutic strategies, e.g., brachytherapy seed placement.

16.2.4 *Retroperitoneal Soft Tissue Sarcoma*

Retroperitoneal soft tissue sarcoma (RSTS) is a rare form of cancer arising from mesenchymal cells, with an incidence rate of 2.8/100,000 population in the United States in 2018 [106]. RSTS presents a particular challenge to surgical and medical oncologists, as the natural history and biological features of these cancers differ from most of the usual cancer types. Liposarcoma represents the most common subtype of RSTS, and has a 5-year recurrence rate of 23–43% depending on differentiation and grade [107, 108]. Most subtypes tend to recur locally, with a relatively low metastatic potential. Neoadjuvant and adjuvant therapy have limited impact on patient outcomes. Radiotherapy has not shown local recurrence rates nor overall survival improvement in RSTS, although a sub-group analysis showed reduced local recurrence rates in well-differentiated liposarcomas (WDLPS) [109]. Adjuvant chemotherapy has no proven benefit, and neoadjuvant chemotherapy can be used for certain chemosensitive subtypes with limited benefits [110].

Because of the limited efficacy of the aforementioned treatment modalities, complete surgical resection remains the cornerstone in the treatment of RSTS. More specifically, resection margin status significantly correlates with recurrence rate and patient survival [111]. In this particular surgical context, adjunct tools for intraoperative tissue analysis can be particularly useful to surgical oncologists. RS has the potential to help finetune surgical decision making during extensive multi-organ resection surgeries. It is clear that such complex surgical interventions should never be iterative based on intraoperative discoveries, but should rather be carefully planned considering radiological characteristics and tumor biology. Yet, RS offers the possibility to obtain fast, accurate, and non-destructive tissue analysis during RSTS resection surgery. This additional information can help provide a more accurate assessment of the extent of locoregional disease spread to optimize the completeness of resection.

The literature remains relatively scarce in research involving the use of RS with sarcomas. Recent work has shown RS's ability to differentiate between some subtypes of soft tissue sarcomas and surrounding healthy tissues [112, 113]. Notably, Nguyen *et al.* have demonstrated that RS could be used to correctly differentiate healthy fat and muscle tissue from multiple subtypes of RSTS when excluding WDLPS, with a sensitivity of 89.5% and specificity of 96.4% [114]. WDLPS is the second most frequent RSTS subtype after dedifferentiated liposarcoma, accounting for 26.1% of primary RSTS [107]. It also presents a particular surgical challenge, as it is very similar to normal retroperitoneal adipose tissue, both macroscopically and to the surgeon's touch [110]. Demonstrating RS's ability to differentiate WDLPS from retroperitoneal adipose tissue would strongly contribute in making RS a valuable tool during RSTS resection. Our research group is currently recruiting patients for a project that aims to do so, as well as exploring the chemometric modifications caused by neoplastic transformation in soft tissue sarcomas.

16.2.5 *Melanoma*

Malignant melanoma (MM) represents one histologic subtype of skin cancer arising from melanocytes. It is projected to be the cancer type with the seventh highest incidence rate, and was the fifth most prevalent cancer type in 2022 in Canada, with 9,000 new diagnoses [84]. Its prognosis and treatment course are heavily dependent on its histopathological features on initial biopsy, most importantly its Breslow depth (thickness). Different biopsy techniques can be used, with excisional biopsy providing the most accurate histopathologic evaluation.

The use of RS to diagnose MM has been the subject of a significant body of work in recent literature with interesting results, yet no progress has been made towards being incorporated in contemporary management guidelines. The answer as to why that is probably lies in the low specificities achieved in most of these studies, despite sensitivities generally above 90%. For example, Lui *et al.* demonstrated that RS could differentiate MM from non-melanoma pigmented lesions with a sensitivity up to 99%, but with specificity of only 68% [115]. In 2020, Zhang *et al.* proposed a novel approach using RS as a second opinion following visual examination to better inform dermatologists on the probability of a pigmented lesion being MM and requiring biopsy. The aim was to demonstrate that using RS in a screening setting has the potential to significantly reduce the number of unnecessary biopsies performed on non-melanoma pigmented lesions. The results obtained showed that RS could reduce the number needed to treat from 8.6 to 4.1, with a sensitivity of 100% and specificity of 58.5% [116].

RS could be used as a solution to a problem particular to the management of MM. Indeed, pigmented skin lesions are very common, and the great majority of these are benign. Reducing the number of negative biopsies could reduce the burden on healthcare systems from melanoma. With the same goal in mind, RS could potentially have a significant impact in reducing the number of wide local excision (WLE) surgeries performed for low-risk, thin melanomas that have already been completely excised during excisional biopsy.

Once the pathological diagnosis of melanoma is made, the treatment remains a WLE (5 mm to 2 cm margin) of the skin surrounding the melanoma. A recent study by Wee *et al.* [117] showed that 59.5% of MM had a Breslow depth <1mm, with 23.4% being *in situ*. Combined with recent results indicating that residual melanoma following negative-margin excisional biopsy is present in less than 5% of cases [118, 119], an argument could be made that WLE could be altogether avoided if additional information could be obtained at the time of biopsy regarding the probability of residual disease. RS could be used for such a purpose.

Indeed, with its demonstrated high sensitivity in detecting the presence of melanoma *in vivo*, quick acquisition time and non-destructivity, RS could be used to assess the presence of residual MM in the excisional biopsy wound. A negative result would consolidate a negative margin histopathology evaluation and increase the probability of no residual disease at the primary site. Such an application would be well suited for widefield RS, which could accommodate in its FOV a significant proportion of excisional biopsy wounds. The potential to significantly lower the number of surgical interventions has significant financial and organizational appeal, especially in a post-pandemic context of widespread increasing surgical wait-list time.

16.3 Conclusion

Raman spectroscopy has many possible roles to play in surgery. It brings molecular contrast without exogenous agents or ionizing radiation, and it has the capacity to be integrated into systems compatible with the operating room. When designing RS systems for surgery, hardware and software must be tailored to the specific clinical application. Although many may see this as a hurdle to overcome, we would argue that this is testament to the versatility of RS and the ability to be a user-friendly device throughout the surgical disciplines.

References

1. Ellis, H. and Abdalla, S. (2018) *A History of Surgery* 3rd ed., CRC Press.
2. Pitt, D. and Aubin, J.-M. (2012) Joseph Lister: father of modern surgery. Can. J. Surg. **55**, E8–9.
3. Mamidanna, R., Burns, E. M., Bottle, A., Aylin, P., Stonell, C., Hanna, G. B. and Faiz, O. (2012) Reduced risk of medical morbidity and mortality in patients selected for laparoscopic colorectal resection in England: A population-based study. Arch. Surg. **147**, 219–227.
4. Broeders, I. A. M. J. and Ruurda, J. (2001) Robotics revolutionizing surgery: the Intuitive Surgical "Da Vinci" system. Ind. Rob. **28**, 387–392.
5. Batailler, C., Hannouche, D., Benazzo, F. and Parratte, S. (2021) Concepts and techniques of a new robotically assisted technique for total knee arthroplasty: the ROSA knee system. Arch. Orthop. Trauma Surg. **141**, 2049–2058.

6. Tewari, A., Kaul, S. and Menon, M. (2005) Robotic radical prostatectomy: A minimally invasive therapy for prostate cancer. Curr. Urol. Rep. **6**, 45–48.
7. Sarlos, D., Kots, L., Stevanovic, N. and Schaer, G. (2010) Robotic hysterectomy versus conventional laparoscopic hysterectomy: Outcome and cost analyses of a matched case–control study. Eur. J. Obstet. Gynecol. Reprod. Biol. **150**, 92–96.
8. (2015) Robotics: Ethics of artificial intelligence. Nature **521**, 415–418.
9. Liew, C. (2018) The future of radiology augmented with Artificial Intelligence: A strategy for success. Eur. J. Radiol. **102**, 152–156.
10. Quazi, S. (2022) Artificial intelligence and machine learning in precision and genomic medicine. Med. Oncol. **39**, 120.
11. Offit, K. (2011) Personalized medicine: new genomics, old lessons. Hum. Genet. **130**, 3–14.
12. Hollon, T. C., Pandian, B., Adapa, A. R., Urias, E., Save, A. V., Khalsa, S. S. S., Eichberg, D. G., D'Amico, R. S., Farooq, Z. U., Lewis, S., *et al.* (2020) Near real-time intraoperative brain tumor diagnosis using stimulated Raman histology and deep neural networks. Nat. Med. **26**, 52–58.
13. Ma, L. and Fei, B. (2021) Comprehensive review of surgical microscopes: technology development and medical applications. J. Biomed. Opt. **26**.
14. Fujimoto, J. G., Drexler, W., Schuman, J. S. and Hitzenberger, C. K. (2009) Optical Coherence Tomography (OCT) in ophthalmology: introduction. Opt. Express **17**, 3978–3979.
15. Stummer, W., Stocker, S., Wagner, S., Stepp, H., Fritsch, C., Goetz, C., Goetz, A. E., Kiefmann, R. and Reulen, H. J. (1998) Intraoperative detection of malignant gliomas by 5-aminolevulinic acid-induced porphyrin fluorescence. Neurosurgery **42**, 518–525; discussion 525–526.
16. Weinkauf, C., Mazhar, A., Vaishnav, K., Hamadani, A. A., Cuccia, D. J. and Armstrong, D. G. (2019) Near-instant noninvasive optical imaging of tissue perfusion for vascular assessment. J. Vasc. Surg. **69**, 555–562.
17. Namikawa, T., Sato, T. and Hanazaki, K. (2015) Recent advances in near-infrared fluorescence-guided imaging surgery using indocyanine green. Surg. Today **45**, 1467–1474.
18. Meershoek, P., KleinJan, G. H., van Willigen, D. M., Bauwens, K. P., Spa, S. J., van Beurden, F., van Gennep, E. J., Mottrie, A. M., van der Poel, H. G., Buckle, T., *et al.* (2021) Multi-wavelength fluorescence imaging with a da Vinci Firefly — a technical look behind the scenes. J. Rob. Surg. **15**, 751–760.
19. Gibbs-Strauss, S. L., Nasr, K. A., Fish, K. M., Khullar, O., Ashitate, Y., Siclovan, T. M., Johnson, B. F., Barnhardt, N. E., Tan Hehir, C. A. and Frangioni, J. V. (2011) Nerve-highlighting fluorescent contrast agents for image-guided surgery. Mol. Imaging **10**, 91–101.
20. Bateman, L. M., Hebert, K. A., Nunziata, J. A., Streeter, S. S., Barth, C. W., Wang, L. G., Gibbs, S. L. and Henderson, E. R. (2023) Preclinical evaluation of

molecularly targeted fluorescent probes in perfused amputated human limbs. J. Biomed. Opt. **28**, 082802.

21. Santos, I. P., Barroso, E. M., Bakker Schut, T. C., Caspers, P. J., van Lanschot, C. G. F., Choi, D.-H., van der Kamp, M. F., Smits, R. W. H., van Doorn, R., Verdijk, R. M., *et al.* (2017) Raman spectroscopy for cancer detection and cancer surgery guidance: translation to the clinics. Analyst **142**, 3025–3047.
22. Gatin, E., Nagy, P., Paun, I., Dubok, O., Bucur, V. and Windisch, P. (2019) Raman spectroscopy: application in periodontal and oral regenerative surgery for bone evaluation. IRBM **40**, 279–285.
23. Shams, R., Picot, F., Grajales, D., Sheehy, G., Dallaire, F., Birlea, M., Saad, F., Trudel, D., Menard, C., Leblond, F., *et al.* (2020) Pre-clinical evaluation of an image-guided in-situ Raman spectroscopy navigation system for targeted prostate cancer interventions. Int. J. Comput. Assist. Radiol. Surg. **15**, 867–876.
24. Jermyn, M., Mok, K., Mercier, J., Desroches, J., Pichette, J., Saint-Arnaud, K., Bernstein, L., Guiot, M. C., Petrecca, K. and Leblond, F. (2015) Intraoperative brain cancer detection with Raman spectroscopy in humans. Sci. Transl. Med. 7, 1–10.
25. Desroches, J., Jermyn, M., Pinto, M., Picot, F., Tremblay, M.-A., Obaid, S., Marple, E., Urmey, K., Trudel, D., Soulez, G., *et al.* (2018) A new method using Raman spectroscopy for in vivo targeted brain cancer tissue biopsy. Sci. Rep. **8**, 1792.
26. Ember, K. J. I., Hunt, F., Jamieson, L. E., Hallett, J. M., Esser, H., Kendall, T. J., Clutton, R. E., Gregson, R., Faulds, K., Forbes, S. J., *et al.* (2021) Noninvasive detection of ischemic vascular damage in a pig model of liver donation after circulatory death. Hepatology **0**, 1–16.
27. Mandair, G. S. and Morris, M. D. (2015) Contributions of Raman spectroscopy to the understanding of bone strength. Bonekey Rep. **4**, 620.
28. Fisher, R., Pusztai, L. and Swanton, C. (2013) Cancer heterogeneity: implications for targeted therapeutics. Br. J. Cancer **108**, 479–485.
29. Bourre, J. M. (2009) 12 — Brain Lipids and Ageing. In *Food for the Ageing Population* (Raats, M., de Groot, L., and van Staveren, W., Eds.), pp. 219–251, Woodhead Publishing.
30. Seidler, R. D., Bernard, J. A., Burutolu, T. B., Fling, B. W., Gordon, M. T., Gwin, J. T., Kwak, Y. and Lipps, D. B. (2010) Motor control and aging: Links to age-related brain structural, functional, and biochemical effects. Neurosci. Biobehav. Rev. **34**, 721–733.
31. Witte, A. V., Savli, M., Holik, A., Kasper, S. and Lanzenberger, R. (2010) Regional sex differences in grey matter volume are associated with sex hormones in the young adult human brain. NeuroImage **49**, 1205–1212.
32. de Graaf, M. A., Jager, K. J., Zoccali, C. and Dekker, F. W. (2011) Matching, an appealing method to avoid confounding? Nephron Clin. Pract. **118**, c315–c318.
33. Jager, K. J., Zoccali, C., MacLeod, A. and Dekker, F. W. (2008) Confounding: What it is and how to deal with it. Kidney Int. **73**, 256–260.

34. Couch, L., Roskosky, M., Freedman, B. A. and Shuler, M. S. (2015) Effect of skin pigmentation on near infrared spectroscopy. Am. J. Anal. Chem. **6**, 911–916.
35. Zhao, J., Short, M. A., Braun, T. A., Lui, H., McLean, D. I. and Zeng, H. (2014) Clinical Raman measurements under special ambient lighting illumination. J. Biomed. Opt. **19**, 111609.
36. Giovannacci, I., Magnoni, C., Vescovi, P., Painelli, A., Tarentini, E. and Meleti, M. (2019) Which are the main fluorophores in skin and oral mucosa? A review with emphasis on clinical applications of tissue autofluorescence. Arch. Oral Biol. **105**, 89–98.
37. Kolenc, O. I. and Quinn, K. P. (2019) Evaluating cell metabolism through autofluorescence imaging of NAD(P)H and FAD. Antioxid. Redox Signal. **30**, 875–889.
38. Beier, B. D. and Berger, A. J. (2009) Method for automated background subtraction from Raman spectra containing known contaminants. Analyst **134**, 1198–1202.
39. Zijlstra, W. G. and Buursma, A. (1997) Spectrophotometry of hemoglobin: absorption spectra of bovine oxyhemoglobin, deoxyhemoglobin, carboxyhemoglobin, and methemoglobin. Comp. Biochem. Physiol. B **118**, 743–749.
40. Valdés, P. A., Leblond, F., Kim, A., Wilson, B. C., Paulsen, K. D. and Roberts, D. W. (2012) A spectrally constrained dual-band normalization technique for protoporphyrin IX quantification in fluorescence-guided surgery. Opt. Lett. **37**, 1817–1819.
41. Kim, A., Roy, M., Dadani, F. and Wilson, B. C. (2010) A fiberoptic reflectance probe with multiple source-collector separations to increase the dynamic range of derived tissue optical absorption and scattering coefficients. Opt. Express **18**, 5580–5594.
42. Matthäus, C., Bird, B., Miljković, M., Chernenko, T., Romeo, M. and Diem, M. (2008) Chapter 10 Infrared and Raman Microscopy in Cell Biology. In *Methods in Cell Biology*, pp. 275–308, Academic Press.
43. Lee, K. S., Landry, Z., Pereira, F. C., Wagner, M., Berry, D., Huang, W. E., Taylor, G. T., Kneipp, J., Popp, J., Zhang, M., *et al.* (2021) Raman microspectroscopy for microbiology. Nat. Rev. Methods Primers **1**, 80.
44. Swain, R. J. and Stevens, M. M. (2007) Raman microspectroscopy for non-invasive biochemical analysis of single cells. Biochem. Soc. Trans. **35**, 544–549.
45. Lombardini, A., Mytskaniuk, V., Sivankutty, S., Andresen, E. R., Chen, X., Wenger, J., Fabert, M., Joly, N., Louradour, F., Kudlinski, A., *et al.* (2018) High-resolution multimodal flexible coherent Raman endoscope. Light Sci. Appl. **7**, 10.
46. St-Arnaud, K., Aubertin, K., Strupler, M., Jermyn, M., Petrecca, K., Trudel, D. and Leblond, F. (2016) Wide-field spontaneous Raman spectroscopy imaging system for biological tissue interrogation. Opt. Lett. **41**, 4692–4695.

47. Duraipandian, S., Sylvest Bergholt, M., Zheng, W., Yu Ho, K., Teh, M., Guan Yeoh, K., Bok Yan So, J., Shabbir, A. and Huang, Z. (2012) Real-time Raman spectroscopy for in vivo, online gastric cancer diagnosis during clinical endoscopic examination. J. Biomed. Opt. **17**, 081418.
48. Cals, F. L. J., Bakker Schut, T. C., Hardillo, J. A., Baatenburg De Jong, R. J., Koljenović, S. and Puppels, G. J. (2015) Investigation of the potential of Raman spectroscopy for oral cancer detection in surgical margins. Lab. Invest. **95**, 1186–1196.
49. Sliney, D. H. (1989) Radiation safety. The maximum permissible exposure levels: our knowledge of the hazards. Opt. Laser Technol. **21**, 235–240.
50. Rastogi, R. P., Richa, Kumar, A., Tyagi, M. B. and Sinha, R. P. (2010) Molecular mechanisms of ultraviolet radiation-induced DNA damage and repair. J. Nucleic Acids **2010**, 592980.
51. Dallaire, F., Picot, F., Tremblay, J.-P., Sheehy, G., Lemoine, É., Agarwal, R., Kadoury, S., Trudel, D., Lesage, F., Petrecca, K., *et al.* (2020) Quantitative spectral quality assessment technique validated using intraoperative in vivo Raman spectroscopy measurements. J. Biomed. Opt. **25**, 1–8.
52. Sheehy, G., Picot, F., Dallaire, F., Ember, K. J. I., Nguyen, T. and Leblond, F. (2023) Open-sourced Raman spectroscopy data processing package implementing a novel baseline removal algorithm validated from multiple datasets acquired in human tissue and biofluids. J. Biomed. Opt. **28**, 025002.
53. Picot, F., Daoust, F., Sheehy, G., Dallaire, F., Chaikho, L., Bégin, T., Kadoury, S. and Leblond, F. (2021) Data consistency and classification model transferability across biomedical Raman spectroscopy systems. Trans. Biophotonics **3**, e202000019.
54. Ostrom, Q. T., Cioffi, G., Gittleman, H., Patil, N., Waite, K., Kruchko, C. and Barnholtz-Sloan, J. S. (2019) CBTRUS statistical report: primary brain and other central nervous system tumors diagnosed in the United States in 2012–2016. Neuro. Oncol. **21**, v1–v100.
55. Hadjipanayis, C. G., Widhalm, G. and Stummer, W. (2015) What is the surgical benefit of utilizing 5-aminolevulinic acid for fluorescence-guided surgery of malignant gliomas? Neurosurgery **77**, 663–673.
56. Stummer, W., Pichlmeier, U., Meinel, T., Wiestler, O. D., Zanella, F. and Reulen, H.-J. (2006) Fluorescence-guided surgery with 5-aminolevulinic acid for resection of malignant glioma: a randomised controlled multicentre phase III trial. Lancet Oncol. **7**, 392–401.
57. Roberts, D. W., Valdés, P. A., Harris, B. T., Fontaine, K. M., Hartov, A., Fan, X., Ji, S., Lollis, S. S., Pogue, B. W., Leblond, F., *et al.* (2011) Coregistered fluorescence-enhanced tumor resection of malignant glioma: relationships between δ-aminolevulinic acid-induced protoporphyrin IX fluorescence, magnetic resonance imaging enhancement, and neuropathological parameters. Clinical article. J. Neurosurg. **114**, 595–603.

58. Valdés, P. A., Leblond, F., Kim, A., Harris, B. T., Wilson, B. C., Fan, X., Tosteson, T. D., Hartov, A., Ji, S., Erkmen, K., *et al.* (2011) Quantitative fluorescence in intracranial tumor: implications for ALA-induced PpIX as an intraoperative biomarker. J. Neurosurg. **115**, 11–17.
59. Valdés, P. A., Jacobs, V., Harris, B. T., Wilson, B. C., Leblond, F., Paulsen, K. D. and Roberts, D. W. (2015) Quantitative fluorescence using 5-aminolevulinic acid-induced protoporphyrin IX biomarker as a surgical adjunct in low-grade glioma surgery. J. Neurosurg. **123**, 771–780.
60. Valdés, P. A., Kim, A., Leblond, F., Conde, O. M., Harris, B. T., Paulsen, K. D., Wilson, B. C. and Roberts, D. W. (2011) Combined fluorescence and reflectance spectroscopy for in vivo quantification of cancer biomarkers in low- and high-grade glioma surgery. J. Biomed. Opt. **16**, 116007.
61. Bekelis, K., Valdés, P. A., Erkmen, K., Leblond, F., Kim, A., Wilson, B. C., Harris, B. T., Paulsen, K. D. and Roberts, D. W. (2011) Quantitative and qualitative 5-aminolevulinic acid-induced protoporphyrin IX fluorescence in skull base meningiomas. Neurosurg. Focus **30**, E8.
62. Valdes, P. A., Bekelis, K., Harris, B. T., Wilson, B. C., Leblond, F., Kim, A., Simmons, N. E., Erkmen, K., Paulsen, K. D. and Roberts, D. W. (2014) 5-Aminolevulinic acid-induced protoporphyrin IX fluorescence in meningioma: qualitative and quantitative measurements in vivo. Neurosurgery **10 Suppl 1**, 74–82; discussion 82–83.
63. Dankner, M., Caron, M., Al-Saadi, T., Yu, W., Ouellet, V., Ezzeddine, R., Maritan, S. M., Annis, M. G., Le, P. U., Nadaf, J., *et al.* (2021) Invasive growth associated with cold-inducible RNA-binding protein expression drives recurrence of surgically resected brain metastases. Neuro-Oncol. **23**, 1470–1480.
64. Desroches, J., Jermyn, M., Mok, K., Lemieux-Leduc, C., Mercier, J., St-Arnaud, K., Urmey, K., Guiot, M.-C., Marple, E., Petrecca, K., *et al.* (2015) Characterization of a Raman spectroscopy probe system for intraoperative brain tissue classification. Biomed. Opt. Express **6**, 2380.
65. Jermyn, M., Desroches, J., Mercier, J., Tremblay, M.-A., St-Arnaud, K., Guiot, M.-C., Petrecca, K. and Leblond, F. (2016) Neural networks improve brain cancer detection with Raman spectroscopy in the presence of operating room light artifacts. J. Biomed. Opt. **21**, 94002.
66. Desroches, J., Laurence, A., Jermyn, M., Pinto, M., Tremblay, M.-A., Petrecca, K. and Leblond, F. (2017) Raman spectroscopy in microsurgery: impact of operating microscope illumination sources on data quality and tissue classification. Analyst **142**, 1185–1191.
67. Jermyn, M., Mercier, J., Aubertin, K., Desroches, J., Urmey, K., Karamchandiani, J., Marple, E., Guiot, M. C., Leblond, F. and Petrecca, K. (2017) Highly accurate detection of cancer *in situ* with intraoperative, label-free, multimodal optical spectroscopy. Cancer Res. **77**, 3942–3950.

68. Lemoine, É., Dallaire, F., Yadav, R., Agarwal, R., Kadoury, S., Trudel, D., Guiot, M.-C., Petrecca, K. and Leblond, F. (2019) Feature engineering applied to intraoperative in vivo Raman spectroscopy sheds light on molecular processes in brain cancer: a retrospective study of 65 patients. Analyst **144**, 6517–6532.
69. Plante, A., Dallaire, F., Grosset, A.-A., Nguyen, T., Birlea, M., Wong, J., Daoust, F., Roy, N., Kougioumoutzakis, A., Azzi, F., *et al.* (2021) Dimensional reduction based on peak fitting of Raman micro spectroscopy data improves detection of prostate cancer in tissue specimens. J. Biomed. Opt. **26**, 116501.
70. Jermyn, M., Desroches, J., Mercier, J., St-Arnaud, K., Guiot, M.-C., Leblond, F. and Petrecca, K. (2016) Raman spectroscopy detects distant invasive brain cancer cells centimeters beyond MRI capability in humans. Biomed. Opt. Express **7**, 5129.
71. Ember, K., Dallaire, F., Agarwal, R., Selb, J., Plante, A., Umphlette, M., Tsankova, N., Rizea, C., Harb, A., Guiot, M.-C., *et al.* (2023) *In situ* brain tumor detection using the Raman spectroscopy sentry system — results of a multicenter study. 21 July 2023, PREPRINT (Version 1) available at Research Square: https://doi.org/10.21203/rs.3.rs-3161348/v1.
72. Hall, W. A. (1998) The safety and efficacy of stereotactic biopsy for intracranial lesions. Cancer **82**, 1749–1755.
73. Chen, C.-C., Hsu, P.-W., Erich Wu, T.-W., Lee, S.-T., Chang, C.-N., Wei, K., Chuang, C.-C., Wu, C.-T., Wu, C.-T., Lui, T.-N., *et al.* (2009) Stereotactic brain biopsy: Single center retrospective analysis of complications. Clin. Neurol. Neurosurg. **111**, 835—839.
74. Malone, H., Yang, J., Hershman, D. L., Wright, J. D., Bruce, J. N. and Neugut, A. I. (2015) Complications following stereotactic needle biopsy of intracranial tumors. World Neurosurg. **84**, 1084–1089.
75. Khatab, S., Spliet, W. and Woerdeman, P. A. (2014) Frameless image-guided stereotactic brain biopsies: emphasis on diagnostic yield. Acta Neurochir. **156**, 1441–1450.
76. Jain, D., Sharma, M. C., Sarkar, C., Deb, P., Gupta, D. and Mahapatra, A. K. (2006) Correlation of diagnostic yield of stereotactic brain biopsy with number of biopsy bits and site of the lesion. Brain Tumor Pathol. **23**, 71–75.
77. Reithmeier, T., Lopez, W. O., Doostkam, S., Machein, M. R., Pinsker, M. O., Trippel, M. and Nikkhah, G. (2013) Intraindividual comparison of histopathological diagnosis obtained by stereotactic serial biopsy to open surgical resection specimen in patients with intracranial tumours. Clin. Neurol. Neurosurg. **115**, 1955–1960.
78. Desroches, J., Lemoine, É., Pinto, M., Marple, E., Urmey, K., Diaz, R., Guiot, M.-C., Wilson, B. C., Petrecca, K. and Leblond, F. (2019) Development and first in-human use of a Raman spectroscopy guidance system integrated with a brain biopsy needle. J. Biophotonics **12**, e201800396.
79. Sun, Y., Wang, X., Che, N., Qin, H., Liu, S., Wu, X., Wei, M., Cheng, H. and Yin, J. (2017) Clinical characteristics and epilepsy outcomes following surgery

caused by focal cortical dysplasia (type IIa) in 110 adult epileptic patients. Exp. Ther. Med. **13**, 2225–2234.
80. Adler, S., Wagstyl, K., Gunny, R., Ronan, L., Carmichael, D., Cross, J. H., Fletcher, P. C. and Baldeweg, T. (2017) Novel surface features for automated detection of focal cortical dysplasias in paediatric epilepsy. Neuroimage Clin. **14**, 18–27.
81. Krsek, P., Maton, B., Jayakar, P., Dean, P., Korman, B., Rey, G., Dunoyer, C., Pacheco-Jacome, E., Morrison, G., Ragheb, J., *et al.* (2009) Incomplete resection of focal cortical dysplasia is the main predictor of poor postsurgical outcome. Neurology **72**, 217–223.
82. Anand, S., Cicchi, R., Giordano, F., Conti, V., Buccoliero, A. M., Guerrini, R. and Pavone, F. S. (2017) Multimodal fiber-probe spectroscopy allows detecting epileptogenic focal cortical dysplasia in children. J. Biophotonics **10**, 896–904.
83. Sacharz, J., Wesełucha-Birczyńska, A., Zięba-Palus, J., Lewandowski, M. H., Kowalski, R., Palus, K., Chrobok, Ł., Moskal, P., Birczyńska, M. and Sozańska, A. (2018) Epileptic rat brain tissue analyzed by 2D correlation Raman spectroscopy. Spectrochim. Acta A **188**, 581–588.
84. Brenner, D. R., Poirier, A., Woods, R. R., Ellison, L. F., Billette, J.-M., Demers, A. A., Zhang, S. X., Yao, C., Finley, C., Fitzgerald, N., *et al.* (2022) Projected estimates of cancer in Canada in 2022. Can. Med. Assoc. J. **194**, E601.
85. National Comprehensive Cancer Network. (2022) NCCN Clinical Practice Guidelines in Oncology — Breast Cancer (Version 4.2022).
86. Havel, L., Naik, H., Ramirez, L., Morrow, M. and Landercasper, J. (2019) Impact of the SSO-ASTRO margin guideline on rates of re-excision after lumpectomy for breast cancer: a meta-analysis. Ann. Surg. Oncol. **26**, 1238–1244.
87. Chagpar, A. B., Killelea, B. K., Tsangaris, T. N., Butler, M., Stavris, K., Li, F., Yao, X., Bossuyt, V., Harigopal, M., Lannin, D. R., *et al.* (2015) A randomized, controlled trial of cavity shave margins in breast cancer. New Engl. J. Med. **373**, 503–510.
88. Cody, H. S. and Van Zee, K. J. (2015) Reexcision — the other breast cancer epidemic. New Engl. J. Med. **373**, 568–569.
89. Haka, A. S., Shafer-Peltier, K. E., Fitzmaurice, M., Crowe, J., Dasari, R. R. and Feld, M. S. (2005) Diagnosing breast cancer by using Raman spectroscopy. Proc. Natl. Acad. Sci. **102**, 12371–12376.
90. Haka, A. S., Volynskaya, Z., Gardecki, J. A., Nazemi, J., Lyons, J., Hicks, D., Fitzmaurice, M., Dasari, R. R., Crowe, J. P. and Feld, M. S. (2006) In vivo margin assessment during partial mastectomy breast surgery using raman spectroscopy. Cancer Res. **66**, 3317–22.
91. Wang, M.-H., Liu, X., Wang, Q. and Zhang, H.-W. (2022) Diagnosis accuracy of Raman spectroscopy in the diagnosis of breast cancer: a meta-analysis. Anal. Bioanal. Chem. **414**, 7911–7922.
92. Vanna, R., Morasso, C., Marcinnò, B., Piccotti, F., Torti, E., Altamura, D., Albasini, S., Agozzino, M., Villani, L., Sorrentino, L., *et al.* (2020) Raman

spectroscopy reveals that biochemical composition of breast microcalcifications correlates with histopathologic features. Cancer Res. **80**, 1762–1772.

93. Yang, Y., Yang, Y., Liu, Z., Guo, L., Li, S., Sun, X., Shao, Z. and Ji, M. (2021) Microcalcification-based tumor malignancy evaluation in fresh breast biopsies with hyperspectral stimulated Raman scattering. Anal. Chem. **93**, 6223–6231.
94. Lazaro-Pacheco, D., Shaaban, A. M., Titiloye, N. A., Rehman, S. and Rehman, I. U. (2021) Elucidating the chemical and structural composition of breast cancer using Raman micro-spectroscopy. Excli. J. **20**, 1118–1132.
95. Melitto, A. S., Arias, V. E. A., Shida, J. Y., Gebrim, L. H. and Silveira Jr, L. (2022) Diagnosing molecular subtypes of breast cancer by means of Raman spectroscopy. Lasers Surg. Med. **54**, 1143–1156.
96. Jonczyk, M. M., Jean, J., Graham, R. and Chatterjee, A. (2019) Surgical trends in breast cancer: a rise in novel operative treatment options over a 12 year analysis. Breast Cancer Res. Treat. **173**, 267–274.
97. David, S., Tran, T., Dallaire, F., Sheehy, G., Azzi, F., Trudel, D., Tremblay, F., Omeroglu, A., Leblond, F. and Meterissian, S. (2023) *In situ* Raman spectroscopy and machine learning unveil biomolecular alterations in breast cancer. J. Biomed. Opt. **28**(3), 036009.
98. Daoust, F., Nguyen, T., Orsini, P., Bismuth, J., de Denus-Baillargeon, M.-M., Veilleux, I., Wetter, A., Mckoy, P., Dicaire, I., Massabki, M., *et al.* (2021) Handheld macroscopic Raman spectroscopy imaging instrument for machine-learning-based molecular tissue margins characterization. J. Biomed. Opt. **26**, 022911.
99. Daoust, F., Tavera, H., Dallaire, F., Orsini, P., Savard, K., Bismuth, J., Mckoy, P., Veilleux, I., Petrecca, K. and Leblond, F. (2023) A clinical Raman spectroscopy imaging system and safety requirements for *in situ* intraoperative tissue characterization. Analyst **148**, 1991–2001.
100. Siegel, R. L., Miller, K. D., Fuchs, H. E. and Jemal, A. (2021) Cancer statistics, 2021. CA Cancer J. Clin. **71**, 7–33.
101. Bjurlin, M. A., Wysock, J. S. and Taneja, S. S. (2014) Optimization of prostate biopsy: review of technique and complications. Urol. Clin. North. Am. **41**, 299–313.
102. Shah, R. B. and Zhou, M. (2012) Prostate Needle Biopsy Sampling Techniques: Impact on Pathological Diagnosis. In *Prostate Biopsy Interpretation: An Illustrated Guide* (Shah, R. B. and Zhou, M., Eds.), pp. 11–14, Springer.
103. Roethke, M., Anastasiadis, A. G., Lichy, M., Werner, M., Wagner, P., Kruck, S., Claussen, C. D., Stenzl, A., Schlemmer, H. P. and Schilling, D. (2012) MRI-guided prostate biopsy detects clinically significant cancer: analysis of a cohort of 100 patients after previous negative TRUS biopsy. World J. Urol. **30**, 213–218.
104. Picot, F., *et al.* (2022) Image-guided Raman spectroscopy navigation system to improve transperineal prostate cancer detection. Part 1: Raman spectroscopy fiber-optics system and *in situ* tissue characterization. J. Biomed. Opt. **27**, 095003.

105. Grajales, D., Picot, F., Shams, R., Barkati, M., Delouya, G., Béliveau-Nadeau, D., Nicolas, B., Leblond, F., Menard, C. and Kadoury, S. (2021) In vivo confirmation of prostate tumor burden during HDR brachytherapy with a combined Raman spectroscopy and MRI radiomics approach. Int. J. Radiat. Oncol. Biol. Phys. **111**, e279.
106. Porter, G. A., Baxter, N. N. and Pisters, P. W. (2006) Retroperitoneal sarcoma: a population-based analysis of epidemiology, surgery, and radiotherapy. Cancer **106**, 1610–6.
107. Gronchi, A., Strauss, D. C., Miceli, R., Bonvalot, S., Swallow, C. J., Hohenberger, P., Van Coevorden, F., Rutkowski, P., Callegaro, D., Hayes, A. J., *et al.* (2016) Variability in patterns of recurrence after resection of primary retroperitoneal sarcoma (RPS): A report on 1007 patients from the multi-institutional collaborative RPS working group. Ann. Surg. **263**, 1002–1009.
108. Callegaro, D., Fasih, S., Catton, C., Dickson, B. C., Ferguson, P. C., Gupta, A. A. and Gladdy, R. A. (2020) Retroperitoneal and Extremity Soft Tissue Sarcomas. In *Surgical Oncology Manual* 3rd ed., pp. 483–504, Springer.
109. Bonvalot, S., Gronchi, A., Le Péchoux, C., Swallow, C. J., Strauss, D., Meeus, P., van Coevorden, F., Stoldt, S., Stoeckle, E., Rutkowski, P., *et al.* (2020) Preoperative radiotherapy plus surgery versus surgery alone for patients with primary retroperitoneal sarcoma (EORTC-62092: STRASS): a multicentre, open-label, randomised, phase 3 trial. Lancet Oncol. **21**, 1366–1377.
110. Swallow, C. J., Strauss, D. C., Bonvalot, S., Rutkowski, P., Desai, A., Gladdy, R. A., Gonzalez, R., Gyorki, D. E., Fairweather, M., van Houdt, W. J., *et al.* (2021) Management of primary retroperitoneal sarcoma (RPS) in the adult: an updated consensus approach from the transatlantic australasian RPS working group. Ann. Surg. Oncol. **28**, 7873–7888.
111. Dingley, B., Fiore, M. and Gronchi, A. (2019) Personalizing surgical margins in retroperitoneal sarcomas: an update. Expert Rev. Anticancer Ther. **19**, 613–631.
112. Noor Mohamed, M. S., Almond, M., Kendall, C., Dudgeon, A., Mansfield, J., Stone, N. and Barr, H. (2022) 417 Vibrational spectroscopy: a rapid tool for soft tissue sarcoma assessment. Brit. J. Surg. **109 Supp 1**, znac039.283.
113. Li, L., Mustahsan, V. M., He, G., Tavernier, F. B., Singh, G., Boyce, B. F., Khan, F. and Kao, I. (2021) Classification of soft tissue sarcoma specimens with Raman spectroscopy as smart sensing technology. Cyborg Bionic Syst. **2021**, 9816913.
114. Nguyen, J. Q., Gowani, Z. S., O'Connor, M., Pence, I. J., Nguyen, T. Q., Holt, G. E., Schwartz, H. S., Halpern, J. L. and Mahadevan-Jansen, A. (2016) Intraoperative Raman spectroscopy of soft tissue sarcomas. Lasers Surg. Med. **48**, 774–781.
115. Lui, H., Zhao, J., McLean, D. and Zeng, H. (2012) Real-time Raman spectroscopy for in vivo skin cancer diagnosis. Cancer Res. **72**, 2491.
116. Zhang, Y., Moy, A. J., Feng, X., Nguyen, H. T. M., Sebastian, K. R., Reichenberg, J. S., Wilke, C. O., Markey, M. K. and Tunnell, J. W. (2020) Assessment of Raman

spectroscopy for reducing unnecessary biopsies for melanoma screening. Molecules **25**, 2852.

117. Wee, E., Wolfe, R., McLean, C., Kelly, J. W. and Pan, Y. (2020) The anatomic distribution of cutaneous melanoma: A detailed study of 5141 lesions. Australas. J. Dermatol. **61**, 125–133.
118. Jackett, L. A., Satgunaseelan, L., Roper, E., Lo, S. N., Thompson, J. F. and Scolyer, R. A. (2022) Residual melanoma in wide local excision specimens after "complete" excision of primary cutaneous *in situ* and invasive melanomas. Pathology **54**, 71–78.
119. Bolshinsky, V., Lin, M. J., Serpell, J., Leung, M., Wolfe, R., McLean, C. and Kelly, J. W. (2016) Frequency of residual melanoma in wide local excision (WLE) specimens after complete excisional biopsy. J. Am. Acad. Dermatol. **74**, 102–107.

https://doi.org/10.1142/9789811264610_0017

Chapter 17

Exploring Cancer with Raman Spectroscopy: Principles, Progress, and Challenges

Christoph Krafft,[1] Jürgen Popp[1,2,*]

[1]Leibniz-Institute of Photonic Technology, Member of the Leibniz Research Alliance – Leibniz Health Technologies, Member of the Leibniz Center for Photonics in Infectious Research (LPI), Albert-Einstein-Str. 9, 07745 Jena, Germany
[2]Friedrich Schiller University Jena, Institute of Physical Chemistry and Abbe Center of Photonics, Member of the Leibniz Center for Photonics in Infectious Research (LPI), Helmholtzweg 4, Jena, Germany
**Corresponding author: juergen.popp@ipht-jena.de*

17.1 Introduction

According to the World Health Organization, cancer is a large group of diseases that can start in almost every organ or tissue of the body when abnormal cells grow uncontrollably, go beyond their usual boundaries to invade adjoining parts of the body and/or spread to other organs. The latter process is called metastasis and is a major cause of death from cancer. Neoplasm and malignant tumor are other common names of cancer. After cardiovascular diseases, cancer is the second leading cause of death globally, accounting for an estimated 9.6 million deaths, or one in six deaths, in 2018. The global cancer statistics including non-melanoma skin cancer lists almost 20 million new cases in 2020, the latest year available. According to Table 17.1, the five most common cancers are breast, lung, colorectal, skin and prostate cancer contributing to 48.3% of the total number of new cases diagnosed. Cancers of 13 other organs make up a further 36%. The abundance of other cancers is below 1% and they are not considered here.

As the cancer burden continues to grow, prevention, diagnosis and treatment belong to the most significant public health challenges of the 21st century. Many health systems in low- and middle-income countries are least prepared to manage this burden, and large numbers of cancer patients do not have access to timely quality diagnosis and treatment. In countries where health systems are strong, survival rates of many types of cancer are improving thanks to accessible early detection, quality treatment and survivorship care.

Raman spectroscopic-based techniques have been applied to all cancers in Table 17.1. The numbers of original papers were obtained by a PubMed survey (3 Feb. 2023) excluding reviews, coherent Raman scattering (coherent anti-Stokes Raman scattering, stimulated Raman scattering) and surface-enhanced Raman scattering. The latter techniques require dedicated instrumentation and preparation protocols. The advantage of spontaneous Raman spectroscopy is

Table 17.1. Global cancer statistics for the most common cancers in the world in 2020, the latest year available (source: World Cancer Research Fund International). All other cancers are below 1%.

Cancer	New cases	% of all cancers	No. of Raman papers
All cancers	19,292,789		
1. Breast	2,261,419	11.7	345
2. Lung	2,206,419	11.4	140
3. Colorectal	1,931,590	10.0	95
4. Skin	1,522,708	7.9	123
5. Prostate	1,414,259	7.3	109
6. Stomach	1,089,103	5.6	46
7. Liver	905,677	4.7	61
8. Cervix uteri	604,127	3.1	70
9. Thyroid	586,202	3.0	19
10. Bladder	573,278	3.0	35
11. Non-Hodgkin lymphoma	544,352	2.8	18
12. Pancreas	495,773	2.6	18
13. Leukemia	474,519	2.5	77
14. Corpus uteri/ endometrial	417,367	2.2	5
15. Lip, oral cavity	377,713	2.0	94
16. Larynx, nasopharynx	317,969	1.7	9+24
17. Ovary	313,959	1.6	23
18. Brain, central nervous system	308,102	1.6	93
Sum	16,344,536	84.7	1,404

its versatility, minimal or even no sample preparation, and relatively simple instruments. The number of Raman papers roughly follow the number of new cancer cases which served as a criterion for their abundance. Most Raman studies were published in the context of lung and breast cancers followed by skin, prostate, colorectal, oral cancer and brain tumors. The latter two were unexpected because the number of new cases were relatively low. Possible explanations are the good accessibility of the oral cavity for fiber-optic probe Raman systems and the high demand in neurosurgery to delineate tumor borders as accurately as possible (see Chapter 16) that drive the development of advanced intraoperative techniques.

In view of the global challenges to detect, diagnose and monitor treatment of cancer diseases as written above, Raman-based methods offer many opportunities to respond to unmet clinical needs in terms of speed, sensitivity, specificity, usability and costs. Among other optical and spectral technologies, the opportunities of Raman spectroscopy in intraoperative histopathology have recently been described [1]. Generally, intraoperative application of Raman-based techniques includes the *ex vivo* assessment of tissue biopsies or cryosections and the *in vivo* collection of spectra with real-time analysis. Raman spectroscopy can characterize either directly liquid biopsies or after extraction of blood cells, tumor cells or other cells of interest. Here, fundamental experimental details are briefly introduced for cancer cells and tissues in the experimental section. Then, principles, progress, and challenges to explore cancer with Raman spectroscopy will be summarized. Of course, all 1,404 Raman papers mentioned in Table 17.1 cannot be covered here. Instead, a selection of papers from bladder cancer, brain tumors, breast cancer, lung cancer and gastrointestinal cancers are described here.

17.2 Experimental Considerations

17.2.1 *Fundamentals of Raman Spectroscopic Instruments*

Components of state-of-the-art instruments for spontaneous Raman spectroscopy are (1) lasers for monochromatic excitation, (2) a narrow band filter in the excitation path to clean up the light from plasma lines of gas lasers, amplified spontaneous emission radiation of diode laser or spectral contributions of glass fibers, (3) illumination optics to guide the excitation light to the sample, (4) collection optics with an dichroic mirror for the scattered light from the sample, (5) a filter unit in the collection path to separate the inelastic scattered Raman signals from the elastic scattering light, (6) a spectrometer with a dispersive element such as grating or prism, and (7) a multichannel detector such as linear or two-dimensional charge-coupled device (CCD) array. Acquisition of Raman images requires moving the sample relative to the laser using a motorized stage or scanning the laser relative to the sample using movable mirrors. General challenges of Raman spectroscopy in the context of cell and tissue studies are relatively weak signal intensities, phototoxicity at certain excitation wavelengths, photodegradation due to excessive laser intensity and elevated background due to overlap with fluorescence emission. Relatively long exposure times of more than one second per spectrum limits throughput, in particular to collect images. Components should be carefully selected to avoid signal losses. Details of each component were described for biomedical applications of Raman spectroscopy [2].

17.2.2 *Raman Microspectroscopy*

Microscopes are coupled to Raman instruments to study small samples such as single cells or thin samples such as tissue sections. High numerical aperture objective lenses maximize photon density for excitation and photon collection for detection. A pinhole in the collection path offers high confocality, reducing out-of-focus scattered light. The fiber core of a collection fiber also acts as a pinhole of the microscope if it is coupled to the spectrometer via fiber optics. A shielded chamber around the microscope enables one to operate the instrument at ambient light and fulfil the laser safety class 1. Many research grade microscopes can be adapted for Raman spectroscopic use and are commercially available from various manufacturers with options such as epi and dia illumination, digital cameras for visual inspection, upright or inverted geometry, autofocus, polarization, automated single cell detection and full range of objective lenses. This includes lenses with optimized transmission in the ultraviolet or near-infrared range, water or oil immersion lenses with and without cover glass correction. Finally, Raman microscopes can be combined with other modalities to collect fluorescence emission, fluorescence lifetime or multiphoton images. A schematic of a typical Raman microscope that is coupled to an excitation laser and spectrograph via fibers is shown in Figure 17.1.

17.2.3 *Fiber-Optic Probe Raman Spectroscopy*

Instead of microscopes, Raman instruments can also be coupled to fiber-optic probes. Such fiber-optic approaches attract considerable attention in

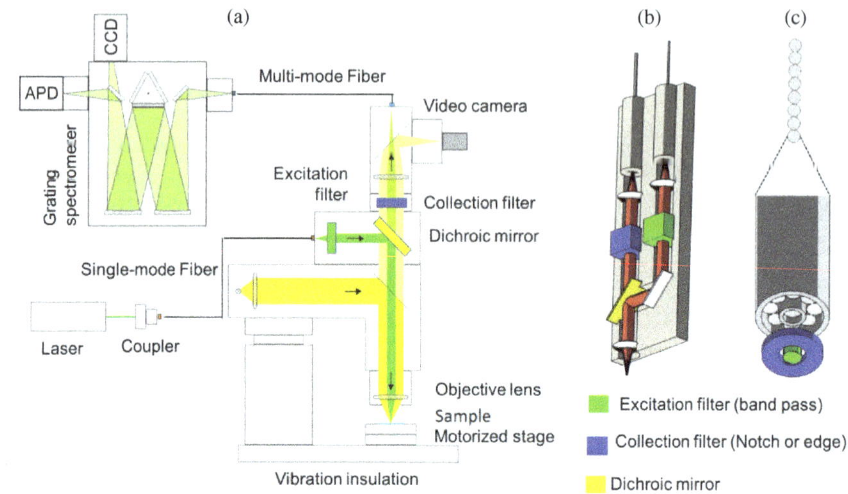

Figure 17.1. (a) Schematic of fiber-coupled Raman microscope. (b) Fiber-optic probes with one collection fiber and a focus lens or (c) with a ring of collection fibers can be coupled to excitation laser and spectrometer with detector as an alternative configuration.

the medical community because they enable us to exploit the fingerprint capability of Raman spectroscopy for *in vivo* applications. The optical layout of fiber-optic Raman probes incorporates all components of a microscope, albeit in miniaturized forms, namely narrow band-pass filter for laser clean-up, and focusing lens and collection filter to suppress the elastic scattered light. Whereas usually one fiber is used to guide the excitation light, two fundamental layouts couple the collected light either via a beam splitter into one fiber (Figure 17.1(b)) or without beam splitter into a ring of fibers that are arranged around the excitation fiber and lined up along the entrance slit of the spectrometer (Figure 17.1(c)). A probe for biomedical applications also has to fulfil the sterilization procedure needs, and size and flexibility constraints for insertion into the working channel of an endoscope. The current development has been reviewed in the *in vivo* context [3].

17.2.4 *Processing of Raman Spectroscopic Data*

As mentioned in Section 17.2.1, weak Raman signals may overlap with background due to fluorescence emission. Further confounding signals arise from buffer, substrate and cosmic spikes from high-energy particles hitting the CCD detector. Scope of processing workflows are to separate unwanted confounding factors from the Raman signals before subjecting the spectra to spectral libraries or classification models. An overview of chemometric analysis in Raman spectroscopy has recently been published [4]. Simple processing algorithms are compiled in toolboxes that are available for programming languages such as MATLAB (The Mathworks), R and Python, or integrated in standalone software programs. The algorithms include correction of cosmic spikes, subtraction of background, normalization of intensities and smoothing the spectrum for better signal-to-noise ratios. Advanced processing algorithms require a set of spectra from several samples or from an image. Then, the variations within the data set can be visualized by principal components analysis which calculates eigenvectors and eigenvalues, hyperspectral unmixing which calculates the most dissimilar components and their abundances, or cluster analysis which segments the spectra according to their similarity, and the results are displayed as mean cluster spectra, cluster membership maps and a dendrogram in case of hierarchical clustering. Recently, artificial intelligence- and deep learning-based methods were developed for processing of Raman data that can further progress this field. As the variations between different cell and tissue types, e.g., the differentiation of cancer versus non-cancer, are often small, instrument stability and instrument-to-instrument variability should be monitored by calibration routines. This includes (i) the stability of the excitation laser, because the position of Raman bands is registered relative to the wavelength of the excitation laser, (ii) calibration of the wavenumber axis of the spectrometer using a material or light source with well-known bands, and (iii) calibration of the intensity axis by a light source with a known emission profile.

17.2.5 *Sample Preparation*

Among the main advantages of Raman-based methods are that tissue and cell samples can be studied without preparation or adding labels for *in vivo* applications and *ex vivo* near the patient and immediately after collection. However, situations might require transporting the sample to a distant location or storing the sample for later studies. To prevent degradation of biological material, freezing and fixation protocols have been developed [5]. Before deep freezing with liquid nitrogen or other cooling agents below −80°C, tissue samples are often embedded in optimal cutting temperature (OCT) medium to prevent freezing artefacts and support tissue during cryosectioning. Raman bands of OCT medium are broad and can be separated from tissue bands during data processing as shown in Section 17.3. The histopathological routine of formalin fixation and paraffin embedding followed by tissue sectioning in a microtome includes washing procedures in organic solvents before paraffin embedding and after sectioning. This routine significantly alters the tissue composition by removing virtually all lipids. Appropriate substrates for thin tissue sections should have weak Raman bands in the fingerprint range between 450 and 1800 cm^{-1}. Raman bands of SiO_2 may occur from glass slides at all excitation wavelengths and other intense bands are evident between 1200 and 1400 cm^{-1} upon near-infrared excitation near 785 nm. Window materials such as CaF_2, BaF_2 and sapphire are better suited because they only show single bands in the low wavenumber range, but are much more expensive. CaF_2 should be used with care because the IR-grade quality has an extraordinarily high background and the even more expensive UV-grade quality (even VUV-grade is specified) should be used in Raman spectroscopy instead. Less expensive alternatives are metal slides (steel, aluminum, etc.) or metal-coated slides (Ag, Au, etc.) which might also offer higher scattering intensities in some situations due to light reflection.

Live cell Raman studies require control of the environment such as buffer medium and for cell cultures even temperature and atmosphere in dedicated chambers. The chamber should be covered with a transparent window of appropriate material (seen previous paragraph) and appropriate thickness for high numerical aperture cover glass-corrected lenses. Because organelles in live cells such as lipid droplets show sub-second dynamics which cannot be resolved by Raman imaging, cells are chemically fixed using 4% formalin solutions. Fixed cells can be conveniently stored in a refrigerator for days. Whereas cancer cell lines can be cultivated directly on substrates for Raman spectroscopic studies, leukemia-derived cell lines are grown in suspension and transferred onto substrates. Drying of cell suspension generates a film with an outer ring of accumulated cells and buffer crystals in the inner portion with only few cells. Cell suspension can also be smeared onto substrates which is a common procedure for blood cells to avoid so-called sessile drop formation with a "coffee ring" and achieve a more even distribution. More details including cell trapping and injecting cells into microfluidic chips combined with Raman spectroscopy will be presented in the following application sections.

17.3 Bladder Cancer

According to the newly diagnosed cancers in Table 17.1, bladder cancer is the sixth most incident neoplasm. Bladder cancer ranges from unaggressive and usually non-invasive cancers that recur and commit patients to long-term invasive surveillance, to aggressive and invasive cancers. Non-muscle-invasive cancers are treated with endoscopic resection and adjuvant intravesical therapy. Patients with high-risk non-muscle-invasive cancers that do not respond to adjuvant therapy with the standard-of-care immunotherapy constitute a challenging population to manage, and many alternative therapies are being studied [6]. For patients with muscle-invasive disease, more aggressive therapy with radical cystectomy and urinary diversion or trimodal therapy with maximal endoscopic resection, radiosensitizing chemotherapy, and radiation is warranted to curb the risk of metastasis and disease-specific mortality [7]. Photodynamic therapy is one of the few treatment options for patients with recurrent non-muscle-invasive bladder cancer.

Enhanced cystoscopy includes technology used to improve the detection of cancers and can reduce the risk of recurrence. In photodynamic diagnosis (PDD), fluorescence contrast is measured with a video system allowing quantitative assessment of the 5-aminolevulinic acid (ALA)-induced fluorescence in cancer tissues. General condition of the bladder can be assessed, and the main foci of the cancer can be determined and intraoperatively resected. The procedure is called transurethral resection. Raman spectroscopic-based techniques have also been suggested for this application. In contrast to fluorescence, Raman spectroscopy provides label-free and non-destructive contrast in tissue sections, *ex vivo* tissue biopsies and *in vivo* during cystoscopy. Furthermore, cells that are shed from the bladder wall can be collected from urine as a liquid biopsy and analyzed by Raman microscopy. Therefore, bladder cancer constitutes an ideal case scenario to demonstrate the capability of Raman-based techniques.

17.3.1 *Bladder Tissue Sections*

An early Raman spectroscopic study on bladder tissue explored the applicability to frozen sections [8]. Two-dimensional maps of 500 to 700 spectra spanned the urothelium, lamina propria and muscle layers that were subdivided by cluster analysis. Raman spectra of lamina propria were dominated by signal contributions of collagen and the smooth muscle layer showed strong signal contributions of actin. The urothelium had a relatively strong lipid signal contribution. In a subsequent paper, the group applied Raman spectroscopic mapping to discriminate between non-cancer and cancer bladder tissue in cryosections from 15 patients and to determine the differences therein [9].

A linear discriminant analysis model was developed and correctly classified 84 out of 90 cluster-averaged spectra with 94% sensitivity and 92% specificity. Non-cancer spectra showed higher collagen content while cancer spectra were characterized by higher lipid, nucleic acid, protein, and glycogen content. A recent publication combined label-free quantitative phase imaging and localized Raman spectroscopy to analyze sliced bladder tissue biopsies [10]. The quantitative phase profile was used to find the best locations for performing Raman measurements. Sparse multinomial logistic regression on the Raman spectra demonstrated that the prior segmentation of the urothelium done by quantitative phase imaging improves the Raman spectra classification accuracy from 85.7% to 94.7%.

17.3.2 *In Vitro Bladder Tissue Assessment*

In another approach towards *in vitro* cancer assessment, human bladder resectates were studied by Raman spectroscopic imaging. For a retrospective study, control and cancer specimens were prepared from resected bladder of ten patients. Raman microspectroscopic images were collected from whole tissue samples in a closed chamber at 785 nm laser excitation using a 20× objective lens and 250 μm step size. Without further pre-processing, Raman images were decomposed by the hyperspectral unmixing algorithm vertex component analysis into endmember spectra and their abundancies. The endmember spectra in Figure 17.2 of the abundance plots are assigned to background, water, OCT medium, necrosis and cancer. The background spectrum is characterized by a maximum near 1340 cm^{-1} from the glass of optical elements in the light path. The sharp band near 1600 cm^{-1} is due to an uncompensated cosmic spike. The water spectrum shows the typical OH deformation vibration near 1630 cm^{-1}. A water immersion lens was used with a water droplet between the window of the sample chamber and objective lens which reduced reflection losses, but contributed to the water signal. The specimen was immersed in OCT medium before storage in the tissue bank, and its broad bands could successfully be separated from the tissue bands. In agreement with the Raman data from tissue sections in Section 17.3.1, cancer spectra show high protein and nucleic acid content. Main protein bands are assigned to aromatic amino acids phenylalanine (621, 1003, 1031, 1209, 1606, 1620 cm^{-1}), tyrosine (643, 827, 855, 1175 cm^{-1}) and tryptophan (756, 1548 cm^{-1}), aliphatic amino acids (1127, 1319, 1340, 1450 cm^{-1}) and the peptide backbone (937, 1249, 1267, 1659 cm^{-1}). Main nucleic acid bands are found at 782, 1082 and 1584 cm^{-1}. Whereas nucleic acids bands were not found in non-cancer bladder, increased nucleic acid content

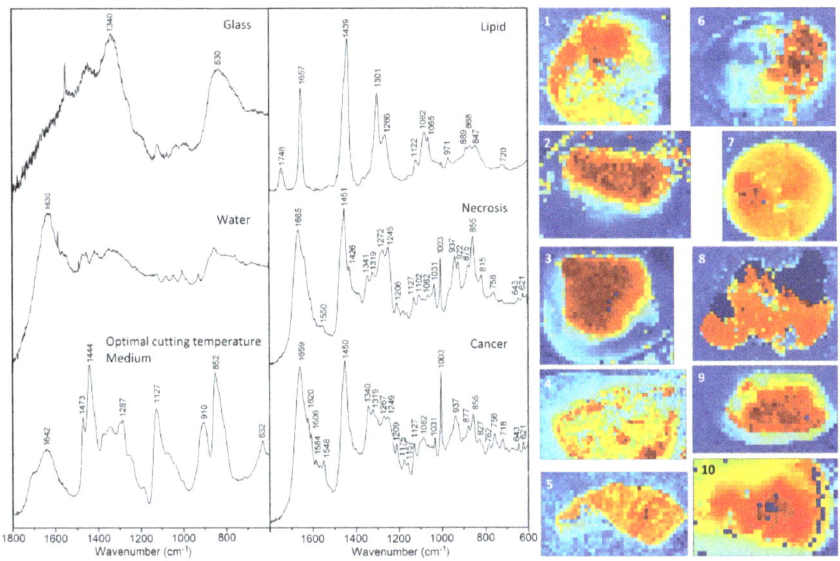

Figure 17.2. Endmember spectra and abundance plots of Raman images from bladder tissue. The spectra from six components were obtained from unsupervised vertex component analysis of specimen 1 without pre-processing. Color-coded plots highlight cancer tissues in red in specimens 1 to 10.

due to DNA is associated with high density and proliferation rate of cancer cells which belong to the hallmarks of cancer. A marker band of the choline group at 718 cm^{-1} is typical for the phospholipid phosphatidylcholine (PC). Altered PC synthesis has been described in cancer and how these changes contributed to malignant growth. These bands can be considered as Raman spectroscopic markers of cancer which will be confirmed by Raman studies of other cancers. The abundance plot of the cancer endmember surrounds necrotic tissue whose endmember spectrum is characterized by elevated bands of fibrous collagenous proteins at 815, 855, 875, 922, 937, 1245, 1272, 1426 and 1665 cm^{-1} relative to cancer protein bands. These bands are typical for triple-helical secondary structures formed by proline-hydroxyproline-glycine-rich primary sequences. As lipid-rich inclusions were found both in cancer and control-specimens, endmember spectra of lipids with main bands assigned to non-saturated fatty acid chains (1065, 1126, 1266, 1301, 1439 and 1657 cm^{-1}) and phospholipids (720, 847, 868, 889, 971, 1082, 1748 cm^{-1}) cannot be considered as cancer marker. An analogous analysis was performed for all specimens. All tumor endmember spectra were similar and were grouped together in the dendrogram of a hierarchical cluster analysis. The color-coded abundance plots highlight the cancer regions in red (Figure 17.2, right). More details have been reported in a recent publication [11].

17.3.3 *Fiber-optic Bladder Tissue Assessment*

A fiber-optic Raman system was used in an early *in vitro* study to collect 220 spectra from 29 snap frozen bladder samples [12]. An algorithm was able to differentiate benign (normal and cystitis) from malignant samples (transitional cell carcinoma) with an overall accuracy of 84%. Because the Raman probe was suitable for use during endoscopic procedures, this work paved the way for *in vivo* studies. A first *in vivo* Raman spectroscopic study used a high-volume probe with deep penetration to investigate the potential of determining the invasiveness of bladder cancer [13]. High-quality spectra were obtained from suspicious and non-suspicious bladder locations during the procedure of transurethral resection with collection times of 1–5 s. Multivariate analysis distinguished bladder cancer from normal bladder locations with a sensitivity of 85% and a specificity of 79%. As the high-volume probe did not reach the expected values of specificity, a confocal Raman probe with a depth of field of approximately 280 μm was proposed to boost the specificity of the diagnostic algorithm based on its suppression of the out-of-focus non-analyte-specific signals emanating from the neighboring normal tissue [14]. Raman spectra were acquired *ex vivo* from normal and cancerous bladder tissues. A diagnostic algorithm yielded comparable sensitivity but significantly higher specificity in relation to high-volume Raman spectral data. A follow-up study compared Raman measurements of a superficial and a non-superficial probe for bladder cancer diagnosis in 104 patients [15]. The area under the receiver operating characteristics curve was 0.95 and 0.80 for the superficial and the non-superficial probe, respectively, which confirmed the better diagnostic ability of the superficial probe.

A low-resolution fiber-optic Raman sensing system was applied to overcome the drawback of intrinsic weak signals [16]. The system collected 262 spectra taken from 32 bladder specimens and evaluated the diagnostic potential of Raman spectroscopy to identify *ex vivo* normal, bladder, low-grade and high-grade bladder tumors. The sensitivities and specificities for normal bladder tissues, low-grade bladder tumors and high-grade bladder tumors were 88.5% and 95.1%, 90.3% and 98%, and 97.5% and 96.4%, respectively. A recent clinical *ex vivo* study on 48 bladder biopsies from 21 patients characterized the tumor grading using a compact fiber probe-based imaging Raman system

[17]. In contrast to the Raman data of bladder tissue in Figure 17.2, Raman spectra exhibited very high tissue autofluorescence in this study that required numerous pre-processing steps including background correction. Partial least squares regression such as dimension reduction technique was combined with linear discriminant analysis to differentiate non-tumor tissue, low-grade and high-grade tumors. Model 1 separated tumor from non-tumor biopsies with a sensitivity of 92% and a specificity of 93%. The values are well within the range reported above. Model 2 achieved an adequate tumor grading in term of predictive performance with a sensitivity of 85% and specificity of 83%. Reduced sensitivities and specificities were also affected by biopsy heterogeneities as the extracted tissue samples not only have the tissue of interest, but also contain other tissues as shown in Figure 17.2.

A multimodal fiber-optic spectroscopy analysis combined fluorescence, Raman spectroscopy and diffuse reflectance for bladder cancer detection, grading and staging [18]. 169 specimens were collected and analyzed from 114 patients of which 129 had bladder cancer with low-grade (34) and high-grade (95). Principal component analysis-linear discriminant analysis classified the *ex vivo* multimodal spectroscopy data between healthy versus bladder cancer with 90% accuracy and high-grade versus low-grade with 83% accuracy which is similar to the study in the previous paragraph.

17.3.4 *Bladder Cancer Cells and Urine Analysis*

Early investigations into the use of Raman optical tweezers to study urological cells were reported with the aim to determine the presence of malignant cells in urine. As a model, live [19] or fixed [20] prostate and bladder cells were trapped with the 514.5 nm Raman excitation laser and analyzed. Principal components analysis afforded discrimination of these cells. Another Raman approach studied epithelial cells in voided urine for diagnosing urothelial carcinoma [21]. Urine samples were obtained from 116 patients without urothelial cancer, 92 patients with low-grade tumors, and 132 patients with high-grade tumors. Raman spectra were obtained from an average of five cells per slide. The height of the Raman band at 1584 cm^{-1} which is assigned to a resonance-enhanced band of cytochromes at 532 nm excitation [22] correlated with the tumor grade. The signal obtained from epithelial cells correctly diagnosed bladder cancer with sensitivity of 92% and even 100% of the high-grade tumors.

Non-invasive urine cytology is usually used in the clinic as an adjunct to cystoscopy. To improve sensitivity of urine cytology, coherent anti-Stokes Raman scattering (CARS) imaging and Raman spectroscopy were combined [23]. In the first step, CARS imaging preselected urothelial cells where high-grade urothelial cancer cells are characterized by a large nucleus-to-cytoplasm ratio. In the second step, Raman spectral imaging was performed. A supervised classifier differentiated normal and cancerous urothelial cells with 100% accuracy. Raman marker bands showed a decrease in the level of glycogen and an increase in the levels of fatty acids in the cancer cells as compared to controls (see Figure 17.3).

A Raman spectroscopy-based chemometric urine analysis called Rametrix was developed as a direct liquid screening method to detect complex molecular signatures in urine associated with bladder cancer and other genitourinary tract pathologies [24]. In study 1, the Rametrix screen was tested using urine specimens from 56 patients from a urologic clinic of which 17 were bladder

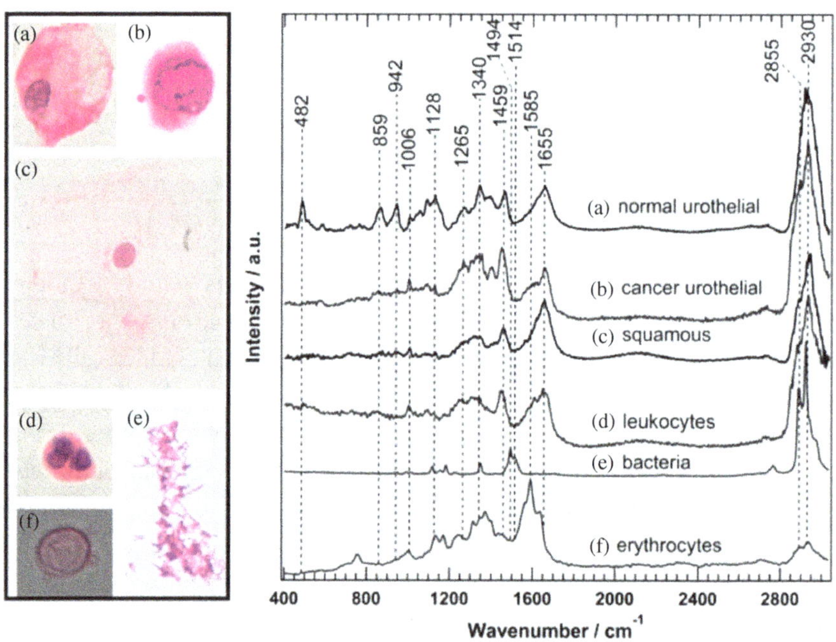

Figure 17.3. Raman spectra and HE-stained images of different cells in urine such as (a) normal and (b) cancerous urothelial cells, (c) a squamous cell, (d) a leukocyte, (e) bacteria, and (f) an erythrocyte. This urine sample was not filtered in order to measure Raman spectra of different cell types in urine. Reproduced from Ref. [23] with permission.

cancer positive. Bladder cancer was detected with 80.4% accuracy, 82.4% sensitivity, 79.5% specificity, 63.6% positive predictive value, and 91.2% negative predictive value. The authors wrote that larger studies are needed to improve classification models and demonstrate clinical relevance.

17.4 Brain Tumors

Brain tumors that originate from brain cells such as glial cells or nearby locations including nerves, the pituitary and pineal glands, and the meninges covering the brain surface are called primary brain tumors. Cancer can spread to the brain from other parts of the body, which are called secondary brain tumors or metastatic brain tumors. Some brain tumors are not cancerous and thus are called non-cancerous brain tumors or benign brain tumors. Whereas benign brain tumors tend to be slow growing, malignant brain tumors tend to be fast growing. Brain tumors range in size from very small to very large. Even small brain tumors can cause symptoms if they start growing in active parts of the brain. Other brain tumors may grow very large before they are found, if they occur in less active parts of the brain. Brain tumor treatment options depend on the type, stage, grade as well as size and location and include surgery, chemotherapy and radiation therapy. Prognosis also depends on the type of cancer. While benign brain tumors have good prognosis, *glioblastoma multiforme* is the most aggressive and most common form of a malignant brain tumor and has a median survival rate of 12 to 17 months. As brain tumors are the most frequent solid tumor in children and adolescents, the average lifetime economic cost is the greatest of any type of cancer.

Brain tumors are diagnosed by computed tomography or MRI after administration of contrast agents. An intact blood-brain barrier sometimes prevents the uptake of contrast agents in benign tumor parts. Stereotactic surgery is a procedure to obtain biopsies from brain tumor for histopathological inspection. Using preoperative MRI information and a stereotactic frame around the skull, a route is defined to insert a rigid stereotactic needle through a hole in the skull and to resect brain tissue. Neuronavigation during brain surgery is an intraoperative guiding tool to project preoperative information such as MRI images into the field of view for three-dimensional orientation and in real time. However, the accuracy is limited due to the so-called brain shift which occurs after a tumor portion is resected and the soft brain tissue moves afterwards. Intraoperative MRI has been introduced in some clinics which requires interruption of surgery and transfer of the patient to a nearby MRI scanner. Similar as in PDD of bladder cancer, the precursor 5-ALA is administered to brain tumor patients and is metabolized in tumor cells to protoporphyrin dyes that emit red fluorescence upon blue excitation [25]. Again, an intact blood-brain barrier may prevent the uptake of 5-ALA in benign tumor parts. Therefore, label-free optical tools such as Raman-based methods are attractive intraoperative tools to maximize tumor resection and to minimize brain function deficits by accurate tumor border delineation. Furthermore, side-viewing fiber-optic probes may be applied during stereotactic surgery to improve collecting biopsies.

17.4.1 *In Vitro Brain Tissue Assessment*

An early *in vitro* study assessed the diagnostic potential of Raman spectroscopic mapping by evaluating its ability to distinguish between normal brain tissue and the human intracranial tumors, gliomas and meningiomas [26]. Variations within seven Raman maps were analyzed by cluster analysis. The dependence of tissue composition on the tissue type in cluster-averaged Raman spectra was shown by linear combinations of reference spectra. Normal brain tissue was found to contain higher levels of lipids, intracranial tumors have more hemoglobin and lower lipid-to-protein ratios, and meningiomas contain more collagen with maximum collagen content in normal meninges. These results were confirmed by subsequent Raman publications of tissue sections.

17.4.2 *Brain Tissue Sections*

Tissue cryosections of the primary intracranial tumors, gliomas, meningiomas and schwannomas were prepared on calcium fluoride windows and studied by Raman and infrared spectroscopic mapping [27]. The autofocus option was activated in order to optimize the laser focus before Raman spectra acquisition of extended maps with 100 μm step size and a high magnification objective lens from uneven surfaces. Cluster-averaged Raman spectra identified spectral contributions of proteins including collagen and hemoglobin, lipids including cholesterol, cholesterolester and PC, hydroxyapatite and tricalciumphosphate as markers for calcification, and nucleic acids. Progress in Raman spectroscopic imaging of brain tumor tissue sections was achieved by lower step size of 2 μm and hyperspectral unmixing by vertex component analysis (VCA) [28]. VCA abundance plots coincided well with histopathologic findings. Cell nuclei were resolved in endmember plots that enabled one to correlate the increase of cell density with tumor grade (see Figure 17.4(a)). Furthermore, the intensity of nucleic acid Raman bands in endmember spectra correlated with the intensity of the hematoxylin staining and with the cell malignancy. Microcrystals were resolved that were formed during the drying process and showed a pure cholesterol Raman spectrum.

In a follow-up study, Raman images were collected at 2 μm step size from non-dried brain tumor sections of astrocytoma, ependymoma and glioblastoma multiforme that were prepared and immersed in aqueous buffer to avoid crystallization of lipids and denaturation of proteins and nucleic acids upon dehydration [29]. Hyperspectral unmixing algorithms VCA and N-FINDR calculated seven endmembers that were assigned to cholesterol, cholesterolester,

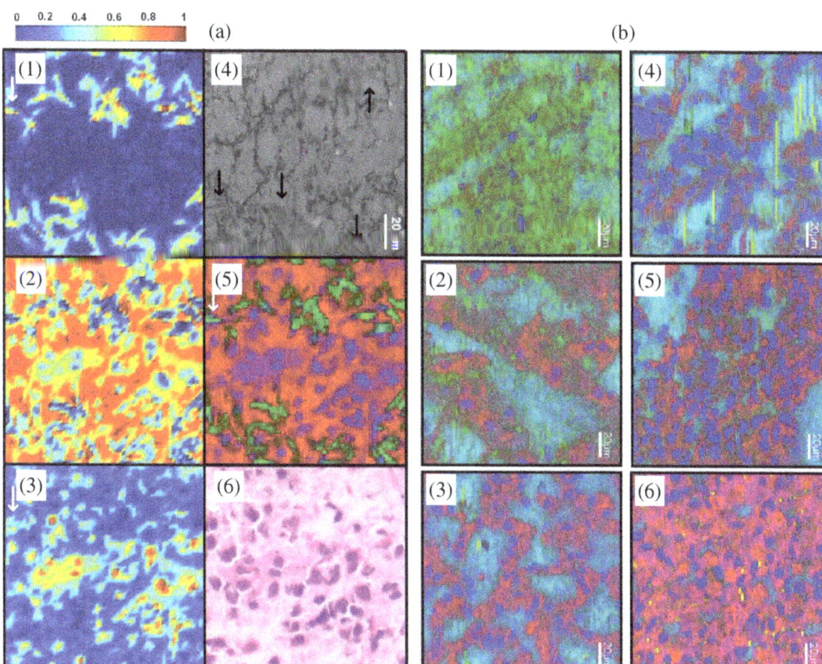

Figure 17.4. (a) Hyperspectral unmixing of Raman images and photomicrographs of dried brain tumor tissue section: components of cholesterol microcrystals (1), proteins (2) and nucleic acids of cell nuclei (3), unstained tissue section with microcrystals (4), composite image of microcrystals (green), proteins (red), nucleic acids (blue) (5), and H&E-stained tissue section (6). (b) Hyperspectral unmixing of Raman images of non-dried brain tissue sections: fitted abundances of phospholipids (green), proteins (red), nucleic acids (blue), cholesterolester (magenta), carotene (yellow) and buffer (cyan) as composite images of glioma brain tumors of grade II (1), grade II-III (2), grade III-IV (3, 4), grade IV (5) and grade IV with sub-necrotic regions (6).

nucleic acids, carotene, proteins, lipids and buffer. The N-FINDR endmember spectra are shown in Figure 17.5 together with the Raman spectra of the reference materials. Typical bands are labeled.

In the next study, 39 Raman images were collected from six glioma brain tumor cryosections in aqueous buffer and processed by VCA [30]. An image segmentation procedure determined morphological parameters in abundance plots like number of cell nuclei and nucleic acid-to-cytoplasm ratios that correlated well with the malignancy ranging from tumor grade II to IV. Representative endmember spectra of proteins, nucleic acids, cholesterol and lipids were obtained from spectral unmixing of the pooled data set and

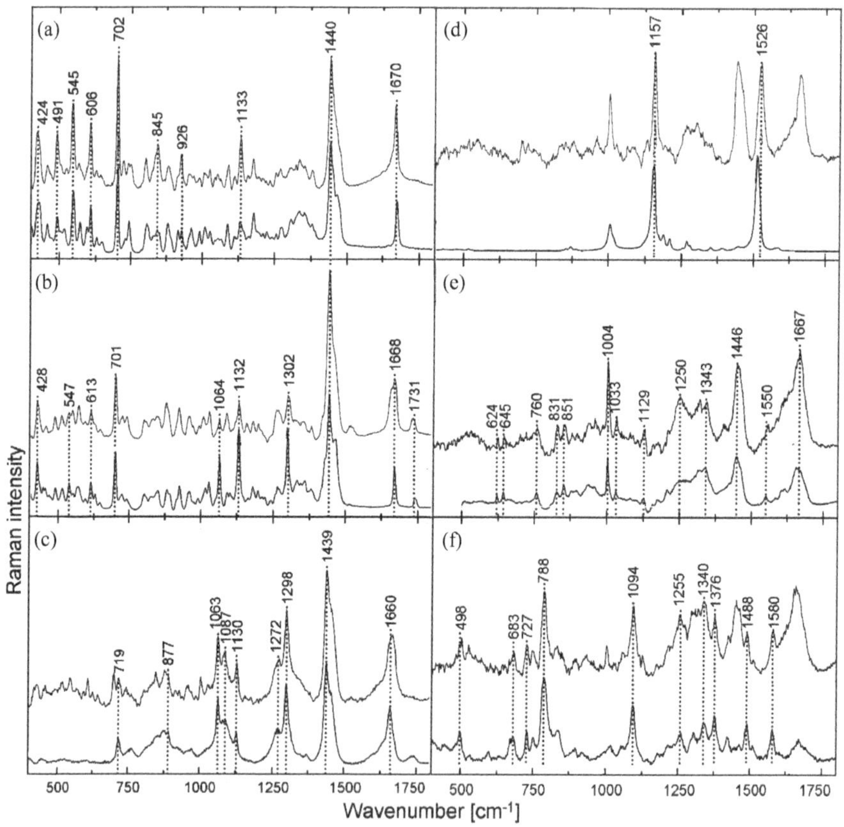

Figure 17.5. Endmember spectra of Raman images from non-dried brain tissue sections (top) and Raman spectra of reference material (bottom of each box): (a) cholesterol, (b) cholesterolester, (c) lipid, (d) brain tissue with carotene, (e) protein and (f) DNA. Only the key bands of each chemical entity were labeled. The Raman spectra of brain tissue and tumor constitute weighted superposition of these components.

chemical parameters were determined by a non-negativity-constrained linear least square fitting of the Raman spectra. The Raman images were reconstructed from the fitting results and included in Figure 17.4(b). The image contrast of cell nuclei was improved in non-dried tissue sections due to more intense nucleic acids bands in hydrated cells compared to dehydrated cells. The color-coded composite images display changes in lipids and cholesterolester that do not crystallize here, density of cell nuclei, and the presence of carotenes. Both lipid-to-protein ratios and nucleic acid-to-protein ratios correlated well with the tumor malignancy. It was concluded that the morphological and chemical information offer new ways to develop Raman-based classification approaches that can complement diagnosis of brain tumors.

The Raman spectroscopic signature can be used as a molecular fingerprint of pathological tissues. In the context of brain metastases of bladder cancer, lung cancer, breast cancer, colon cancer, prostate cancer and renal cell cancer, Raman spectra of cryosections were used to determine the primary tumor [31]. Raman images at 10 μm step size were collected from 22 cryosections. A hierarchical classification model based on support vector machine discriminated Raman spectra of cancer in step 1 that were subjected to classification step 2 to determine the primary tumor. The majority of cancer spectra were correctly assigned to each primary tumor. Fourier transform infrared images were collected from the same specimens and another classification model was trained which confirmed the fingerprint capability of vibrational spectroscopy and complemented the Raman study [32].

17.4.3 *Fiber-Optic Brain Tissue Assessment*

A methodology for Raman mapping of metastases in mouse brains used a fiber-optic probe that was depicted in Figure 17.1(b) [33]. Brain metastases of malignant melanomas were induced by injecting tumor cells into the carotid artery of mice. The procedure mimicked hematogenous tumor spread in one brain hemisphere while the other hemisphere remained tumor-free. The spectral contributions of melanin in tumor cells were resonance enhanced in Raman spectra upon 785 nm excitation which enabled their sensitive detection in Raman maps. Tumor locations were confirmed by consecutive hematoxylin- and eosin-stained tissue sections. This approach was applied in a proof-of-concept experiment to detect intracerebral tumors *in vivo* by surface mapping [34]. Before data acquisition, the mouse was anesthetized, and the cortex was exposed by creating a bony window covered by a calcium fluoride substrate. Raman maps enabled localization of cortical and subcortical tumor cell aggregates at and even below the surface. Most Raman spectra of brain tissue were virtually background-free and main bands were assigned to proteins, lipids, blood and water. Spectra of brain metastases and skull bone showed elevated background and spectral contributions of melanin and hydroxyapatite, respectively.

A laboratory in Montreal (Canada) has published a series of papers since 2015 that confirms the early results and applied novel fiber-optic Raman probes that were developed in collaboration with a company working in this field since the 1990s. In the first paper of this series, Raman spectroscopy was adapted for the operating room that used a handheld, contact, fiber-optic probe [35]. The authors tested the probe intraoperatively in 17 patients with gliomas of different tumor grades and compared the results with 161 biopsy samples. Although a Raman-based detection of both invasive and dense cancer cells achieved an accuracy of 92%, the paper was controversially debated in the scientific community because the underlying spectral signatures deviated from previous data (e.g., in Figure 17.3) due to confounding factors.

Ambient light artefacts can confound Raman spectroscopy measurements performed in clinical settings such as during open surgery. The impact of ambient light sources in the operating room was assessed and recommendations were made for optimal Raman acquisition parameters [36]. Artefacts generated by light have also been overcome by artificial neural networks using non-parametric and adaptive models [37]. As turning off light sources during intraoperative Raman spectral acquisition can be impractical, a filter system was introduced, allowing *in vivo* Raman measurements with light source of a neurosurgical microscope to be turned on without interfering with the standard procedures [38]. The filter system consisted of an adapter, with short-pass filters with a cut-off at 675 nm and one long-pass filter with cut-off at 400 nm. This design avoided interference of the microscope illumination with the Raman spectral range from ca. 785 to 900 nm.

The concept of simple fiber-optic probes for high wavenumber Raman spectroscopy was suggested for tissue characterization in 2005 [39]. This idea was that fused silica show no Raman signals in the high wavenumber region 2400–3800 cm^{-1} which enables the use of a single unfiltered fiber to guide laser light to the tissue and to collect scattered light in this region. Based on high wavenumber Raman spectroscopy, another intraoperative cancer detection system was designed and developed [40]. This device was engineered into a commercially available biopsy system and validated in a swine brain biopsy model. The first in-human use of such Raman spectroscopic guidance system integrated with a brain biopsy needle was reported [41]. The 900 μm diameter probe could detect Raman signal in both the fingerprint and high wavenumber spectral regions.

Similar to the concept of fitting experimental Raman spectra using information from reference spectra [30], feature engineering was used to develop a representation for spectral data tailored for brain tissue diagnosis that improves interpretability of the Raman signal while retaining enough information to accurately predict tissue content [42]. The method consisted of fitting of Raman bands that consistently appeared in the literature. The approach was applied to a dataset of 547 *in situ* Raman spectra from 65 patients undergoing glioma resection and enabled identification of glioma-associated oncogenic processes: increased nucleic acids content, overexpression of collagen and shift in the primary metabolic engine.

17.5 Other Cancers

After the comprehensive presentation of Raman-based techniques in the context of bladder cancer and brain tumors, selected Raman publications are summarized for breast, lung and gastrointestinal cancer.

17.5.1 *Breast Cancer*

In line with breast cancer as the most common cancer among women worldwide, the number of Raman papers is highest. Breast cancer develops from breast tissue, most commonly in cells from the lining of milk ducts called ductal carcinoma and the lobules that supply these ducts with milk called lobular carcinoma. More than 18 other subtypes of breast cancer are also known. Once the diagnosis is confirmed by taking a biopsy, further tests are done to determine if the cancer has spread beyond the breast. In patients who have been diagnosed with cancer, a number of treatments may be used, including surgery, radiation therapy, chemotherapy, hormonal therapy and targeted therapy. Outcomes for breast cancer vary depending on the cancer type, the extent of disease and the person's age. The five-year survival rates in developed countries are between 80 and 90%.

An early, highly cited paper described the Raman spectroscopic diagnosis of human breast cancer [43]. In this study, 130 Raman spectra from 58 patients were acquired from *ex vivo* samples of normal breast tissue, fibrocystic change, fibroadenoma and infiltrating carcinoma. Data were fit by a linear combination model in which nine basis spectra of cell cytoplasm, cell nucleus, collagen, fat, beta-carotene, cholesterol-like, calcium hydroxyapatite and calcium oxalate dihydrate represent the morphologic and chemical features of breast tissue. The fit coefficients for fat and collagen were the key parameters in the resulting diagnostic algorithm, which classified samples according to their specific pathological diagnoses, attaining 94% sensitivity and 96% specificity for distinguishing cancerous tissues from normal and benign tissues. Most of the components were also found in brain tissue and tumors (see Figure 17.5), and calcification due to dedifferentiation of tumor cells were reported in [27].

Raman spectroscopy was used to discriminate between benign lesions such as fibrocystic, fibroadenoma and intraductal papilloma, and cancers such as invasive ductal carcinoma and lobular carcinoma [44]. Different from other Raman studies, Raman maps were recorded from unstained sections of formalin-fixed paraffin preserved tissue. Significant spectral differences were observed between the benign and cancer cases and the benign cases could be differentiated from the cancer cases with good sensitivity and specificity.

The trend to use deep learning and artificial intelligence for analysis of Raman data is also observed for breast cancer. Deep learning was combined with fluorescence imaging and breast cancer diagnosis [45]. First, pseudo-color enhancement algorithm and a convolutional neural network were applied to fluorescence image processing. Second, two different back propagation neural networks were applied to the Raman spectra that mainly comprised collagen and lipid. Finally, the discriminant results of fluorescence images and Raman spectra were arranged into a characteristic variable matrix to predict the breast tissue samples with partial least squares algorithm which correctly predicted all samples. A one-dimensional convolutional neural network algorithm was developed and trained for classification of Raman spectra from breast samples of 20 patients [46]. This model yielded a classification performance of 92% accuracy, 98% sensitivity and 86% specificity. Combining Raman spectroscopy with k-means clustering and stochastic nonlinear neural networks provided quantitative probabilistic brain cancer assessment [47]. The autonomous classification system characterized a dataset of 203 spectra from eight patients. The results showed an increase in nucleic acid signal intensity in the fingerprint

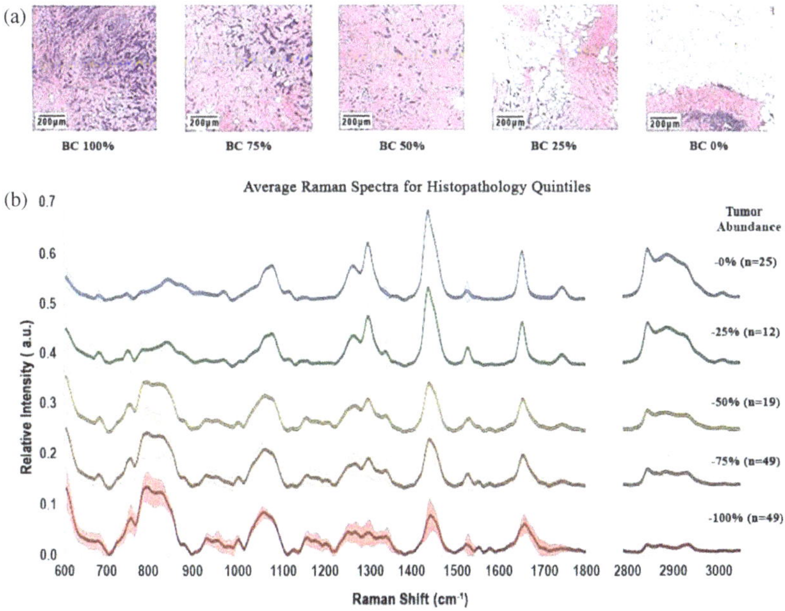

Figure 17.6. Breast cancer histopathology and corresponding laser Raman spectra (n = 154, five patients). Quintile estimates were made by the clinical pathologist (DS) for 1 mm^2 areas surrounding the projected location of the Raman laser probe. (a) Shows the H&E stains for examples of the five tissue categories. Mean low-resolution spectrum for each of the five categories (n0 = 25; n25 = 12; n50 = 19; n75 = 49; n100 = 49) appear in (b). If a region is assigned to the 100% quintile it means that tumor cells are apparent in all portions of the image. If a region is assigned to the 0% quintile it means that there were no clusters of tumor cells apparent throughout the image. Quintile assignment was accomplished for 154 images and spectra acquired from five patients. Average spectra are displayed along with 1-sigma error bars. Scale bars are 200 μm. Reproduced from Ref. [47] with permission.

range and a global loss of high wavenumber signal as warning signs of tumor. Details are given in Figure 17.6.

17.5.2 *Lung Cancer*

Lung cancer is a malignant cancer that begins in the lung and is classified based on the cells it originates from. Around 15% are small cell lung cancers, while the remaining 85% (the non-small cell lung cancers) are adenocarcinomas, squamous cell carcinomas, and large cell carcinomas. Early lung cancer often has no noticeable symptoms. If lung cancer is detected at a late stage, the prognosis will be poor. Lung cancer may be seen on chest radiographs and computed tomography (CT) scans. The diagnosis is confirmed by biopsy, which is usually performed by bronchoscopy or CT guidance. Even with treatment by surgery, radiation therapy and chemotherapy, lung cancer is often deadly, with less than 20% of patients surviving five years from lung cancer diagnosis.

A highly cited Raman paper in the context of lung cancer was an explorative study of 12 normal bronchial tissue specimens, 10 squamous cell carcinoma, and 6 adenocarcinoma [48]. Raman spectra of tumor tissue showed higher signals of nucleic acids, tryptophan and phenylalanine and lower signals of phospholipids, proline and valine compared to normal tissue. The ratio of Raman intensities at 1445 and 1655 cm^{-1} provided good differentiation between normal and malignant bronchial tissue. A more recent Raman study found altered levels of saturated and unsaturated lipids, protein-to-lipid ratios, nucleic acid-to-lipid ratios and protein-to-nucleic acids ratios [49]. Based on these alterations, classification methods including k-nearest neighbors and support vector machines were successfully applied to cytopathologically diagnose lung cancer with an accuracy approaching 99%.

17.5.3 *Gastrointestinal Cancer*

Gastrointestinal cancer refers to the collective term of malignant conditions in the gastrointestinal tract and accessory organs of digestion including esophagus, stomach, biliary system, pancreas, small intestine, large intestine, rectum and anus. The diagnosis often requires endoscopy, followed by biopsy of suspicious tissue.

A laboratory in Singapore published a series of Raman papers to study gastrointestinal cancer and other cancers (see Chapter 14). A fully automated online Raman spectral diagnostics framework was developed which integrated a multimodal image-guided Raman technique for real-time *in vivo* cancer detection at endoscopy [50]. Free-running optical diagnosis and processing time of >0.5 s were achieved which was crucial to realize real-time tissue diagnostics during clinical endoscopic examination. A partial least squares discriminant analysis based on the randomly resampled training database of 2,465 normal and 282 cancer spectra of 309 patients provided a diagnostic accuracy of 85.6%. The algorithm was further applied prospectively on 10 gastric patients at gastroscopy, achieving the predictive accuracy of 80.0%. Earlier papers implemented narrow band imaging to guide Raman endoscopy [51], combined near-infrared autofluorescence and Raman spectroscopy [52], and fitted gastric Raman spectra using a linear combination of eight basis reference from the biochemicals actin, albumin, collagen, DNA, histones, pepsinogen, phospholipids and triolein [53]. The fit coefficients from albumin, nucleic acid, phospholipids and histones were found to be the most significant features for construction of a diagnostic model for gastric cancer recognition. A new beveled fiber-optic probe design provides approximately twofold improvements in tissue Raman to autofluorescence intensity ratios as compared to the use of volume Raman probes [54]. The diagnostic accuracy of 93% for differentiating gastric dysplasia from normal gastric tissue was superior with the beveled probe than with the standard volume probe. However, the autofluorescence background was still high which required baseline corrections. In recent work of this group, a deep learning-guided fiber-optic Raman diagnostic platform was developed to assess its ability of real-time *in vivo* diagnosis of nasopharyngeal carcinoma (NPC) [55]. Progress was also evident from the larger data set. A total of 15,354 fingerprint/high wavenumber Raman spectra were acquired (control: 1,761; NPC: 4,147; and post-treatment (PT): 9,446) from 888 tissue sites of 418 subjects (healthy control: 85; NPC: 82; and PT: 251) during endoscopic examination.

17.6 Conclusion and Outlook

The main principles of Raman-based techniques were described in the context of cancer. The techniques include Raman spectroscopic microscopy, fiber-optic probe Raman spectroscopy, Raman imaging, and Raman spectroscopy combined with other modalities such as fluorescence, light scattering or multiphoton microscopy. A relatively new approach is the combination of infrared and Raman spectroscopy which has been realized as an option in an optical photothermal infrared instrument. Both spectra are complementary to some extent and can be simultaneously registered with such an instrument. Other progress in Raman instrumentation was only marginal within the last years. Main progress was observed in the data analysis by introducing artificial intelligence and deep learning-based approaches besides machine learning concepts. As a promising example, deep convolutional neural networks utilize spectral and spatial information that are expected to improve accuracy and robustness of classification. Big data are needed to train deep learning models which can be achieved by high-throughput Raman instruments, more independent samples, and more clinical partners in multicenter studies. So far, proof-of-concept

Raman studies have been published with relatively low number of independent samples. Recently, initiatives have been initiated to certify Raman instruments for clinical applications which is key to obtain ethical permission for *in vivo* use. It can be expected that more clinical Raman instruments generate more data from more cancer patients which give more robust classification results. This will fully exploit the well-recognized potential of Raman spectroscopy in cancer research and detection in the future.

References

1. Krafft, C. and Popp, J. (2023) Opportunities of optical and spectral technologies in intraoperative histopathology. Optica **10**, 214–231.
2. Krafft, C., Schie, I., Meyer, T., Schmitt, M. and Popp, J. (2016) Developments in spontaneous and coherent Raman scattering microscopic imaging for biomedical applications. Chem. Soc. Rev. **45**, 1819–1849.
3. Cordero, E., Latka, I., Matthäus, C., Schie, I. and Popp, J. (2018) In vivo Raman spectroscopy: from basics to applications. J. Biomed. Opt. **23**, 071210.
4. Guo, S., Popp, J. and Bocklitz, T. (2021) Chemometric analysis in Raman spectroscopy from experimental design to machine learning–based modeling. Nat. Protoc. **16**, 5426–5459.
5. Butler, H. J., Ashton, L., Bird, B., Cinque, G., Curtis, K., Dorney, J., Esmonde-White, K., Fullwood, N. J., Gardner, B., Martin-Hirsch, P. L., Walsh, M. J., McAinsh, M. R., Stone, N. and Martin, F. L. (2016) Using Raman spectroscopy to characterize biological materials. Nat. Protoc. **11**, 664–687.
6. Lenis, A. T., Lec, P. M. and Chamie, K. (2020) Bladder cancer: a review. JAMA **324**, 1980–1991.
7. Patel, V. G., Oh, W. K. and Galsky, M. D. (2020) Treatment of muscle-invasive and advanced bladder cancer in 2020. CA Cancer J. Clin. **70**, 404–423.
8. De Jong, B. W. D., Schut, T. C. B., Wolffenbuttel, K. P., Nijman, J. M., Kok, D. J. and Puppels, G. J. (2002) Identification of bladder wall layers by Raman spectroscopy. J. Urol. **168**, 1771–1778.
9. De Jong, B. W., Schut, T. C., Maquelin, K., van der Kwast, T., Bangma, C. H., Kok, D. J. and Puppels, G. J. (2006) Discrimination between nontumor bladder tissue and tumor by Raman spectroscopy. Anal. Chem. **78**, 7761–7769.
10. Taieb, A., Berkovic, G., Haifler, M., Cheshnovsky, O. and Shaked, N. T. (2022) Classification of tissue biopsies by Raman spectroscopy guided by quantitative phase imaging and its application to bladder cancer. J. Biophotonics **15**, e202200009.
11. Krafft, C., Popp, J., Bronsert, P. and Miernik, A. (2023) Raman spectroscopic imaging of human bladder resectates towards intraoperative cancer assessment. Cancers **15**, 2162.

12. Crow, P., Molckovsky, A., Stone, N., Uff, J., Wilson, B. and WongKeeSong, L. M. (2005) Assessment of fiberoptic near-infrared raman spectroscopy for diagnosis of bladder and prostate cancer. Urology **65**, 1126–1130.
13. Draga, R. O. P., Grimbergen, M. C. M., Vijverberg, P. L. M., Swol, C. F. P. v., Jonges, T. G. N., Kummer, J. A. and Ruud Bosch, J. L. H. (2010) In vivo bladder cancer diagnosis by high-volume Raman spectroscopy. Anal. Chem. **82**, 5993–5999.
14. Barman, I., Dingari, N. C., Singh, G. P., Kumar, R., Lang, S. and Nabi, G. (2012) Selective sampling using confocal Raman spectroscopy provides enhanced specificity for urinary bladder cancer diagnosis. Anal. Bioanal. Chem. **404**, 3091–3099.
15. Stomp-Agenant, M., van Dijk, T., R. Onur, A., Grimbergen, M., van Melick, H., Jonges, T., Bosch, R. and van Swol, C. (2022) In vivo Raman spectroscopy for bladder cancer detection using a superficial Raman probe compared to a nonsuperficial Raman probe. J. Biophotonics **15**, e202100354.
16. Chen, H., Li, X., Broderick, N., Liu, Y., Zhou, Y., Han, J. and Xu, W. (2018) Identification and characterization of bladder cancer by low-resolution fiber-optic Raman spectroscopy. J. Biophotonics **11**, e201800016.
17. Cordero, E., Rüger, J., Marti, D., Mondol, A. S., Hasselager, T., Mogensen, K., Hermann, G. G., Popp, J. and Schie, I. W. (2020) Bladder tissue characterization using probe-based Raman spectroscopy: Evaluation of tissue heterogeneity and influence on the model prediction. J. Biophotonics **13**, e201960025.
18. Morselli, S., Baria, E., Cicchi, R., Liaci, A., Sebastianelli, A., Nesi, G., Serni, S., Pavone, F. S. and Gacci, M. (2021) The feasibility of multimodal fiber optic spectroscopy analysis in bladder cancer detection, grading and staging. Urologia J. **88**, 306–314.
19. Harvey, T. J., Faria, E., Henderson, A., Gazi, E., Ward, A. D., Clarke, N. W., Brown, M., Snook, R. and Gardner, P. (2008) Spectral discrimination of live prostate and bladder cancer cell lines using Raman optical tweezers. J. Biomed. Opt. **13**, 064004.
20. Harvey, T. J., Hughes, C., Ward, A. D., Faria, E. C., Henderson, A., Clarke, N. W., Brown, M. D., Snook, R. D. and Gardner, P. (2009) Classification of fixed urological cells using Raman tweezers. J. Biophotonics **2**, 47–69.
21. Shapiro, A., Gofrit, O. N., Pizov, G., Cohen, J. K. and Maier, J. (2011) Raman molecular imaging: a novel spectroscopic technique for diagnosis of bladder cancer in urine specimens. Eur. Urol. **59**, 106–112.
22. Pätzold, R., Keuntje, M., Theophile, K., Müller, J., Mielcarek, E., Ngezahayo, A. and Anders-von Ahlften, A. (2008) In situ mapping of nitrifiers and anammox bacteria in microbial aggregates by means of confocal resonance Raman microscopy. J. Microbiol. Methods **72**, 241–248.
23. Yosef, H. K., Krauß, S. D., Lechtonen, T., Jütte, H., Tannapfel, A., Käfferlein, H. U., Brüning, T., Roghmann, F., Noldus, J. and Mosig, A. (2017) Noninvasive diagnosis of high-grade urothelial carcinoma in urine by Raman spectral imaging. Anal. Chem. **89**, 6893–6899.

24. Huttanus, H. M., Vu, T., Guruli, G., Tracey, A., Carswell, W., Said, N., Du, P., Parkinson, B. G., Orlando, G., Robertson, J. L. and Senger, R. S. (2020) Raman chemometric urinalysis (Rametrix) as a screen for bladder cancer. PLOS ONE **15**, e0237070.
25. Marbacher, S., Klinger, E., Schwyzer, L., Fischer, I., Nevzati, E., Diepers, M., Roelcke, U., Fathi, A.-R., Coluccia, D. and Fandino, J. (2014) Use of fluorescence to guide resection or biopsy of primary brain tumors and brain metastases. Neurosurg. Focus **36**, E10.
26. Krafft, C., Sobottka, S. B., Schackert, G. and Salzer, R. (2005) Near infrared Raman spectroscopic mapping of native brain tissue and intracranial tumors. Analyst **130**, 1070–1077.
27. Krafft, C., Sobottka, S. B., Schackert, G. and Salzer, R. (2006) Raman and infrared spectroscopic mapping of human primary intracranial tumors: a comparative study. J. Raman Spectrosc. **37**, 367–375.
28. Krafft, C., Belay, B., Bergner, N., Romeike, B. F., Reichart, R., Kalff, R. and Popp, J. (2012) Advances in optical biopsy--correlation of malignancy and cell density of primary brain tumors using Raman microspectroscopic imaging. Analyst **137**, 5533–5537.
29. Bergner, N., Krafft, C., Geiger, K. D., Kirsch, M., Schackert, G. and Popp, J. (2012) Unsupervised unmixing of Raman microspectroscopic images for morphological analysis of non-dried brain tumor specimens. Anal. Bioanal. Chem. **403**, 719–725.
30. Bergner, N., Medyukhina, A., Geiger, K. D., Kirsch, M., Schackert, G., Krafft, C. and Popp, J. (2013) Hyperspectral unmixing of Raman micro-images for assessment of morphological and chemical parameters in non-dried brain tumor specimens. Anal. Bioanal. Chem. **405**, 8719–8728.
31. Bergner, N., Bocklitz, T., Romeike, B. F. M., Reichart, R., Kalff, R., Krafft, C. and Popp, J. (2012) Identification of primary tumors of brain metastases by Raman imaging and support vector machines. Chemometr. Intell. Lab. Syst. **117**, 224–232.
32. Bergner, N., Romeike, B. F. M., Reichart, R., Kalff, R., Krafft, C. and Popp, J. U. (2013) Tumor margin identification and prediction of the primary tumor from brain metastases using FTIR imaging and support vector machines. Analyst **138**, 3983–3990.
33. Krafft, C., Kirsch, M., Beleites, C., Schackert, G. and Salzer, R. (2007) Methodology for fiber-optic Raman mapping and FT-IR imaging of metastases in mouse brains. Anal. Bioanal. Chem. **389**, 1133–1142.
34. Kirsch, M., Schackert, G., Salzer, R. and Krafft, C. (2010) Raman spectroscopic imaging for in vivo detection of cerebral brain metastases. Anal. Bioanal. Chem. **398**, 1707–1713.
35. Jermyn, M., Mok, K., Mercier, J., Desroches, J., Pichette, J., Saint-Arnaud, K., Bernstein, L., Guiot, M.-C., Petrecca, K. and Leblond, F. (2015) Intraoperative brain cancer detection with Raman spectroscopy in humans. Sci. Trans. Med. **7**, 274ra219-274ra219.

36. Desroches, J., Jermyn, M., Mok, K., Lemieux-Leduc, C., Mercier, J., St-Arnaud, K., Urmey, K., Guiot, M.-C., Marple, E., Petrecca, K. and Leblond, F. (2015) Characterization of a Raman spectroscopy probe system for intraoperative brain tissue classification. Biomed. Opt. Express **6**, 2380–2397.
37. Jermyn, M., Desroches, J., Mercier, J., Tremblay, M.-A., St-Arnaud, K., Guiot, M.-C., Petrecca, K. and Leblond, F. (2016) Neural networks improve brain cancer detection with Raman spectroscopy in the presence of operating room light artifacts. J. Biomed. Opt. **21**, 094002.
38. Desroches, J., Laurence, A., Jermyn, M., Pinto, M., Tremblay, M.-A., Petrecca, K. and Leblond, F. (2017) Raman spectroscopy in microsurgery: impact of operating microscope illumination sources on data quality and tissue classification. Analyst **142**, 1185–1191.
39. Koljenovic, S., Bakker Schut, T., Wolthuis, R., de Jong, B., Santos, L., Caspers, P., Kros, J. and Puppels, G. (2005) Tissue characterization using high wave number Raman spectroscopy. J. Biomed. Opt. **10**, 031116.
40. Desroches, J., Jermyn, M., Pinto, M., Picot, F., Tremblay, M.-A., Obaid, S., Marple, E., Urmey, K., Trudel, D., Soulez, G., Guiot, M.-C., Wilson, B. C., Petrecca, K. and Leblond, F. (2018) A new method using Raman spectroscopy for in vivo targeted brain cancer tissue biopsy. Sci. Rep. **8**, 1792.
41. Desroches, J., Lemoine, É., Pinto, M., Marple, E., Urmey, K., Diaz, R., Guiot, M.-C., Wilson, B. C., Petrecca, K. and Leblond, F. (2019) Development and first in-human use of a Raman spectroscopy guidance system integrated with a brain biopsy needle. J. Biophotonics **12**, e201800396.
42. Lemoine, É., Dallaire, F., Yadav, R., Agarwal, R., Kadoury, S., Trudel, D., Guiot, M.-C., Petrecca, K. and Leblond, F. (2019) Feature engineering applied to intraoperative in vivo Raman spectroscopy sheds light on molecular processes in brain cancer: a retrospective study of 65 patients. Analyst **144**, 6517–6532.
43. Haka, A. S., Shafer-Peltier, K. E., Fitzmaurice, M., Crowe, J., Dasari, R. R. and Feld, M. S. (2005) Diagnosing breast cancer by using Raman spectroscopy. Proc. Natl. Acad. Sci. **102**, 12371–12376.
44. Lyng, F. M., Traynor, D., Nguyen, T. N. Q., Meade, A. D., Rakib, F., Al-Saady, R., Goormaghtigh, E., Al-Saad, K. and Ali, M. H. (2019) Discrimination of breast cancer from benign tumours using Raman spectroscopy. PLOS ONE **14**, e0212376.
45. Shang, L.-W., Ma, D.-Y., Fu, J.-J., Lu, Y.-F., Zhao, Y., Xu, X.-Y. and Yin, J.-H. (2020) Fluorescence imaging and Raman spectroscopy applied for the accurate diagnosis of breast cancer with deep learning algorithms. Biomed. Opt. Express **11**, 3673–3683.
46. Ma, D., Shang, L., Tang, J., Bao, Y., Fu, J. and Yin, J. (2021) Classifying breast cancer tissue by Raman spectroscopy with one-dimensional convolutional neural network. Spectrochim. Acta A **256**, 119732.

47. Kothari, R., Jones, V., Mena, D., Bermúdez Reyes, V., Shon, Y., Smith, J. P., Schmolze, D., Cha, P. D., Lai, L. and Fong, Y. (2021) Raman spectroscopy and artificial intelligence to predict the Bayesian probability of breast cancer. Sci. Rep. **11**, 1 17.
48. Huang, Z., McWilliams, A., Lui, H., McLean, D. I., Lam, S. and Zeng, H. (2003) Near-infrared Raman spectroscopy for optical diagnosis of lung cancer. Int. J. Cancer **107**, 1047–1052.
49. Zheng, Q., Li, J., Yang, L., Zheng, B., Wang, J., Lv, N., Luo, J., Martin, F. L., Liu, D. and He, J. (2020) Raman spectroscopy as a potential diagnostic tool to analyse biochemical alterations in lung cancer. Analyst **145**, 385–392.
50. Duraipandian, S., Sylvest Bergholt, M., Zheng, W., Yu Ho, K., Teh, M., Guan Yeoh, K., Bok Yan So, J., Shabbir, A. and Huang, Z. (2012) Real-time Raman spectroscopy for in vivo, online gastric cancer diagnosis during clinical endoscopic examination. J. Biomed. Opt. **17**, 081418.
51. Huang, Z., Bergholt, M. S., Zheng, W., Lin, K., Ho, K.-Y., The, M. and Yeoh, K.-G. (2010) In vivo early diagnosis of gastric dysplasia using narrow-band image-guided Raman endoscopy. J. Biomed. Opt. **15**, 037017.
52. Bergholt, M. S., Zheng, W., Lin, K., Ho, K. Y., Teh, M., Yeoh, K. G., So, J. B. and Huang, Z. (2011) Combining near-infrared-excited autofluorescence and Raman spectroscopy improves in vivo diagnosis of gastric cancer. Biosens. Bioelectron. **26**, 4104–4110.
53. Huang, Z., Teh, S. K., Zheng, W., Lin, K., Ho, K. Y., Teh, M. and Yeoh, K. G. (2010) In vivo detection of epithelial neoplasia in the stomach using image-guided Raman endoscopy. Biosens. Bioelectron. **26**, 383–389.
54. Wang, J., Lin, K., Zheng, W., Ho, K. Y., Teh, M., Yeoh, K. G. and Huang, Z. (2015) Comparative study of the endoscope-based bevelled and volume fiber-optic Raman probes for optical diagnosis of gastric dysplasia in vivo at endoscopy. Anal. Bioanal. Chem. **407**, 8303–8310.
55. Shu, C., Yan, H., Zheng, W., Lin, K., James, A., Selvarajan, S., Lim, C. M. and Huang, Z. (2021) Deep learning-guided fiberoptic Raman spectroscopy enables real-time in vivo diagnosis and assessment of nasopharyngeal carcinoma and post-treatment efficacy during endoscopy. Anal. Chem. **93**, 10898–10906.

https://doi.org/10.1142/9789811264610_bmatter

Index

www.ingramcontent.com/pod-product-compliance
Lightning Source LLC
LaVergne TN
LVHW021055220926
848484LV00021B/829
* 9 7 8 9 8 1 1 2 6 4 6 0 3 *